KINASE INHIBITOR DRUGS

Wiley Series in Drug Discovery and Development
Binghe Wang, Series Editor

KINASE INHIBITOR DRUGS

Edited by

RONGSHI LI
JEFFREY A. STAFFORD

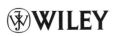

A JOHN WILEY & SONS, INC., PUBLICATION

Published by John Wiley & Sons, Inc., Hoboken, New Jersey
Published simultaneously in Canada

For general information on our other products and services or for technical support, please contact our Customer Care Department within the United States at (800) 762-2974, outside the United States at (317) 572-3993 or fax (317) 572-4002.

Wiley also publishes its books in a variety of electronic formats. Some content that appears in print may not be available in electronic formats. For more information about Wiley products, visit our web site at www.wiley.com.

Library of Congress Cataloging-in-Publication Data:

Li, Rongshi, Ph. D.
    Kinase inhibitor drugs / Rongshi Li, Jeffrey A. Stafford.
        p. ; cm.
    Includes index.
    ISBN 978-0-470-27829-1 (cloth)
    1. Protein kinases–Inhibitors–Therapeutic use. 2. Antineoplastic agents. I. Stafford, Jeffrey A. II. Title.
    [DNLM: 1. Neoplasms–drug therapy. 2. Protein Kinase Inhibitors–therapeutic use. 3. Antineoplastic Agents–therapeutic use. 4. Drug Discovery. 5. Protein Kinase Inhibitors–pharmacology. 6. Protein Kinases–metabolism. QZ 267 L6927k 2009]
    RM666.E548L5 2009
    615'.798–dc22

                                                                                    2009015172

Printed in the United States of America

10 9 8 7 6 5 4 3 2 1

CONTENTS

PREFACE

The field of protein kinase drug discovery has advanced dramatically since the discovery of protein kinase activity in 1954 (G. Burnett, and E. P. Kennedy, *J Biol Chem*. **1954**, 211(2), 969–980). In a landmark paper published in 2002 in the journal *Science*, it was revealed that 518 protein kinases are encoded in the human genome (G. Manning, D. B. Whyte, R. Martinez, et al., *Science*. **2002**, 298, 1912–1934), and the "kinome" was catalogued according to sequence similarity in the catalytic domain and other protein structural comparisons. The protein kinases all share the same catalytic mechanism—the transfer of the terminal phosphate from an ATP molecule, an enzymatic reaction that we now understand controls many crucial cellular processes. With growth and proliferation pathways being regulated by protein kinase activity, the pharmacological inhibition of kinases has been an attractive option for many years. Nonetheless, owing to the high degree of overlapping homology and function, it is fair to acknowledge that, in the 1990s, the challenge to identify selective protein kinase inhibitors (PKIs) was met with a healthy dose of skepticism among industrial and academic drug discovery groups alike. The inhibition of protein kinases using small molecules took a step forward in 1994 when Parke-Davis scientists showed that 4-anilinoquinazolines in general and PD153035 specifically are potent inhibitors of epidermal growth factor receptor (EGFR) kinase, having concomitant cell-based effects on EGFR autophosphorylation (D. W. Fry, A. J. Kraker, A. McMichael, et al., *Science*. **1994**, 265, 1093–1095). The identification of the quinazoline scaffold opened the door for later discoveries leading to the launches of the important PKI drugs, gefitinib (Iressa™), erlotinib (Tarceva™), and lapatinib (Tykerb™).

The impressive clinical success of the Bcr-Abl kinase inhibitor, imatinib (Gleevec™), in the treatment of chronic myelogenous leukemia (CML) validated the use of small molecules in the fledgling field of molecular targeted therapy (R. Capdeville, E. Buchdunger, J. Zimmermann, et al., *Nat Rev Drug Discov*. **2002**, 1(7), 493–502). With 2006 worldwide sales surpassing $2.5 billion,

Gleevec has been rightfully hailed as a "poster child" for targeted cancer therapy and "cancer magic bullet" by drug discovery researchers in the protein kinase field. Its success provides compelling and unequivocal evidence that kinase inhibitors can be highly efficacious, especially in diseases caused by mutations of a protein kinase. The daunting task of discovering selective, ATP-competitive inhibitors has now been achieved in numerous cases, including those profiled in this volume. Since the approval of Gleevec in 2001, seven more PKIs have reached marketing approval (Figure 1), and it is estimated that there are presently well over 100 PKIs in clinical development. The worldwide market for kinase inhibitor drugs is expected to exceed US$10 billion by 2011, and efforts to discover new inhibitors continue vigorously in both industry and academic laboratories.

Not surprisingly, the first marketed PKIs were witnessed in oncology, where kinase gene mutations or disregulated kinase activity is often associated with hyperproliferation of cells, a hallmark phenotype of cancer. To date, there have been dozens of protein kinases implicated in human cancer, with undoubtedly more to be identified. Beyond the direct causal role of the Bcr-Abl kinase in CML, a noteworthy example is B-Raf kinase, a member of the Ras-Raf-Mek-Erk growth pathway. Somatic mutations in the B-Raf *gene* are observed in 66% of malignant melanomas and at lower frequency in a range of other human cancers (H. Davies, G. R. Bignell, C. Cox, et al., *Nature.* **2002**, 417, 949–954). Similarly, mutations in the phosphatidylinositol-3 kinase (PI3K) are associated with gastric and colon cancers (S. Velho, C. Oliveira, A. Ferreira, et al., *Eur J Cancer.* **2005**, 41(11), 1649–1654). Overexpression of the oncogene, human epidermal growth factor 2 (Her2, also known as erbB2), has been widely characterized in human breast carcinomas and its overexpression correlates with more aggressive disease (S. Menard, S. M. Pupa, M. Campiglio, et al., *Oncogene.* **2003**, 22(42), 6570–6578). These are only three examples among the dozens of protein kinases that have been implicated in human cancer to date, with undoubtedly more to be identified. In addition to oncology, kinase inhibitors are being investigated in other disease areas such as inflammation, diabetes, neuroscience, and virology.

Kinase Inhibitor Drugs represents our effort to compile, within a single volume, important discovery case studies of marketed kinase drugs and several of the more advanced kinase inhibitors. These case studies are authored by leading investigators and experts in the field of protein kinase research and provide a first-hand account of kinase inhibitor discovery. The reader is exposed to current thinking on kinase structure, biochemistry, and signaling. State-of-the-art technologies and tools such as structure-based and fragment-based drug discovery are also addressed in this book. The discoveries of the marketed inhibitors, sunitinib (Sutent™, Chapter 1) and lapatinib (Tykerb™, see Fig 1 Chapter 2), highlight a lineup of clinical-phase growth factor inhibitors, including several VEGFR2 kinase and multitargeted, antiangiogenic agents from investigators at Abbott, Amgen, BMS, GSK, and Pfizer. There are several chapters on inhibitors of the cell cycle kinases, Aurora and PLK, contributed

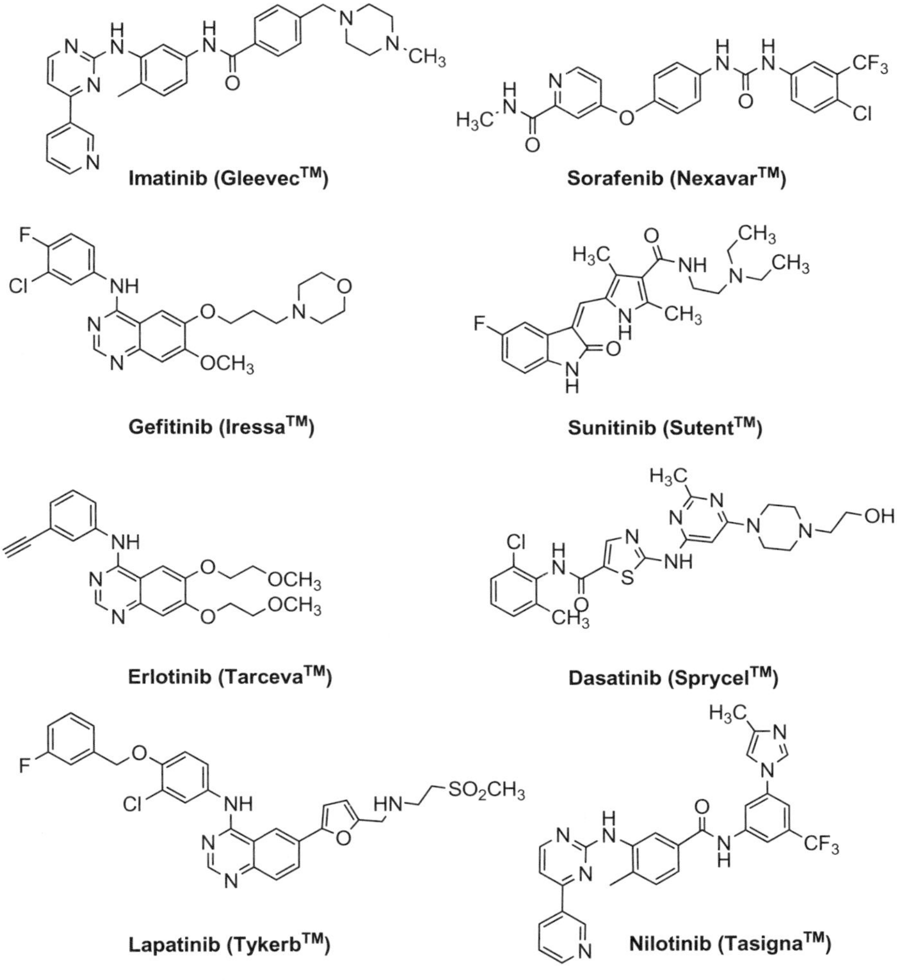

Figure 1. Kinase inhibitor drugs to reach market approval by the US Food and Drug Administration (2001–2008).

by investigators from AstraZeneca, GSK, Millenium, Nerviano, and Vertex. Additional case study chapters from Pfizer and Array Biopharma, respectively, are dedicated to the discovery of allosteric inhibitors of MEK kinase. Allosteric kinase inhibition engenders a kinase selectivity profile that is unequaled by inhibitors that occupy that ATP binding pocket. The field of pharmacogenomics and its application to kinase inhibitor clinical development is highlighted in the context of the marketed Src/Abl kinase inhibitor, dasatinib (Sprycel™). And finally, there are chapters dedicated to topics that are vital to efficient and intelligent kinase drug discovery, such as computational chemistry, fragment-based discovery, and methods in structural biology. We are grateful to all of the authors for their dedication to this project, which we believe is unique even within the richly informed and documented field of protein kinase research. Our intent is that the present volume serves the reader as an informative text or supplementary reading on successful small-molecule drug discovery, specifically as it pertains to PKIs. The descriptions on contemporary applications of medicinal chemistry, including lead optimization and in vivo profiling, should find great interest among medicinal chemists and pharmacologists alike. Of course, it is fair to acknowledge that an undertaking of the present, limited scope will exclude informative case studies, including, notably, the Gleevec discovery story, case studies from the p38 MAPK inhibitor class, for example, SB203580 (A. M. Badger, J. N. Bradbeer, B. Votta, et al., *J Pharm Exp Ther.* **1996**, 279(3), 1453–1461) and BIRB796 (C. Pargellis, L. Tong, L. Churchill, et al., *Nat Structural Biol.* **2002**, 9(4), 268–272), and the search for second-generation inhibitors to kinases that have undergone active site mutation to become drug resistant (M. E. Gorre, M. Mohammed, K. Ellwood, et al., *Science.* **2001**, 293, 876–880; S. Kobayashi, T. Boggon, T. Dayaram, et al., *N Engl J Med.* **2005**, 352(8), 786–792).

We would like to recognize and thank the individuals whose efforts were essential to the successful completion of this volume. First, we acknowledge the following drug discovery researchers, each of whom provided thoughtful and critical reviews of portions of the manuscript: Shane Atwell (SGX Pharmaceuticals), Chris Buhr (Exelixis), David Campbell (Phenomix), Edcon Chang (Takeda San Diego), Sam Chu (Takeda San Diego), Erick Co (Takeda San Diego), Ron deJong (Takeda San Diego), Qing Dong (Takeda San Diego), David Drewry (GlaxoSmithKline), Pamela Farrell (Takeda San Diego), Stephen Gwaltney (Takeda San Diego), Gavin Hirst (MPEX Pharmaceuticals), Jason Kahana (Takeda San Diego), David Lawson (Takeda San Diego), James Leahy (Exelixis), Michael Peel (Scynexis), Kirk Stevens (Gilead Sciences), and Amy Tsuhako (Exelixis). Administrative assistance was kindly and generously provided by Ms. Tara Brown and Ms. Jacqueline Fernandez, both of Takeda San Diego. We also extend our sincere thanks to Ms. Angie Vassar, who was responsible for organizing and formatting the individual chapters for submission, while also providing valuable advice to enrich the technical style and content of the volume. We wish to thank the Wiley staff, in particular Jonathan Rose, Lauren Hilger, and Kellsee Chu, for their support and advice during the preparation of this volume. We also extend our gratitude to Stephanie Sakson at SNP Best-set Typesetters, who offered patience and guidance to us in the final stages.

Color figures that supplement this book can be found at: ftp://ftp.wiley.com/public/sci_tech_med/kinase_drugs

RONGSHI LI, Ph.D.
Tampa, Florida
JEFFREY A. STAFFORD, Ph.D.
San Diego, California
August 2009

CONTRIBUTORS

Daniel H. Albert, Abbott Laboratories, Abbott Park, IL 60064

Rajeev S. Bhide, Research and Development, Bristol-Myers Squibb Company, Princeton, NJ 08543

James F. Blake, Drug Discovery, Array BioPharma, Boulder, CO 80301

Alexander J. Bridges, Oncovera Therapeutics, Inc., Ann Arbor, MI 48103

James G. Christensen, Pfizer Global Research and Development, La Jolla, CA 92121

Christopher F. Claiborne, Department of Oncology Chemistry, Millennium Pharmaceuticals, Inc., Cambridge, MA 02139

Edwin A. Clark, Oncology Clinical Biomarkers, Discovery Medicine & Clinical Pharmacology, Bristol-Myers Squibb Company, Princeton, NJ 08540

G. Stuart Cockerill, Arrow Therapeutics, London SE1 1DB, United Kingdom

Kyle A. Emmitte, GlaxoSmithKline R&D, Research Triangle Park, NC 27709

Daniel A. Erlanson, Sunesis Pharmaceuticals, Inc., South San Francisco, CA 94080

Daniele Fancelli, Congenia S.r.l. (Genextra Group), Via Adamello 16, I-20139 Milan, Italy

Joseph Fargnoli, Research and Development, Bristol-Myers Squibb Company, Princeton, NJ 08543

Victoria A. Feher, Department of Computational Sciences, Takeda San Diego, Inc., San Diego, CA 92121

Kevin M. Foote, Chemistry, AstraZeneca Pharmaceuticals, Macclesfield, Cheshire SK10 4TG, United Kingdom

Julian M. C. Golec, Vertex Pharmaceuticals (Europe) Ltd, Oxfordshire OX14 4RY, United Kingdom

Philip A. Harris, GlaxoSmithKline R&D, Collegeville, PA 19426

David J. Hosfield, Department of Structural Biology, Takeda San Diego, Inc., San Diego, CA 92121

Fei Huang, Oncology Clinical Biomarkers, Discovery Medicine & Clinical Pharmacology, Bristol-Myers Squibb Company, Princeton, NJ 08540

Robert S. Kania, Pfizer Global Research and Development, San Diego, CA 92121

Kevin W. Kuntz, GlaxoSmithKline R&D, Research Triangle Park, NC 27709

Karen Lackey, Molecular Discovery Research, GlaxoSmithKline, Research Triangle Park, NC 27709

J. David Lawson, Department of Computational Sciences, Takeda San Diego, Inc., San Diego, CA 92121

Mark G. Manfredi, Department of Cancer Pharmacology, Millennium Pharmaceuticals, Inc., Cambridge, MA 02139

Gerald McMahon, Poniard Pharmaceuticals, Inc., South San Francisco, CA 94080

Michael Michaelides, Abbott Laboratories, Abbott Park, IL 60064

Clifford D. Mol, Department of Structural Biology, Takeda San Diego, Inc., San Diego, CA 92121

Jürgen Moll, Nerviano Medical Sciences S.r.l., Viale Pasteur 10, I-20014 Nerviano (Mi), Italy

Andrew A. Mortlock, Oncology, AstraZeneca Pharmaceuticals, Macclesfield, Cheshire SK10 4TG, United Kingdom

Kengo Okada, Department of Structural Biology, Takeda San Diego, Inc., San Diego, CA 92121

Vinod F. Patel, Chemistry Research and Discovery, Amgen, Inc., Cambridge, MA 02139

Judith S. Sebolt-Leopold, Oncovera Therapeutics, Inc., Ann Arbor, MI 48103

Jeffrey A. Stafford, Takeda San Diego, Inc., San Diego, CA 92121

Connie L. Sun, Poniard Pharmaceuticals, Inc., South San Francisco, CA 94080

Andrew S. Tasker, Chemistry Research and Discovery, Amgen, Inc., Thousand Oaks, CA 91320

James M. Veal, Structural Chemistry and Informatics, Serenex, Inc., Durham, NC 27701

Eli Wallace, Drug Discovery, Array BioPharma, Boulder, CO 80301

PART I

GROWTH FACTOR INHIBITORS: VEGFR2, ERBB2, AND OTHER KINASES

1

DISCOVERY AND DEVELOPMENT OF SUNITINIB (SU11248): A MULTITARGET TYROSINE KINASE INHIBITOR OF TUMOR GROWTH, SURVIVAL, AND ANGIOGENESIS

CONNIE L. SUN, JAMES G. CHRISTENSEN, AND GERALD McMAHON

1.1. SUNITINIB

Sunitinib (SU11248, Sutent™; Pfizer, Inc.) is an oral, multitargeted tyrosine kinase inhibitor of vascular endothelial growth factor receptors (VEGFRs 1, 2, and 3), platelet-derived growth factor receptors (PDGFRs α and β), stem-cell factor receptor (KIT), FMS-like tyrosine kinase 3 (FLT3), colony-stimulating factor 1 receptor (CSF1R), and glial cell line-derived neurotrophic factor receptor (REarranged during Transfection; RET) and currently approved multinationally for the treatment of advanced renal cell carcinoma (RCC) and for gastrointestinal stromal tumors (GISTs) after disease progression or intolerance to imatinib mesylate (IM) therapy. Sunitinib (SU11248) emerged from a drug discovery program within the biotechnology company (SUGEN, South San Francisco). An original aim of the SU11248 program was to understand cellular signaling mechanisms and design novel agents that would modulate signaling mechanisms for the treatment of human disease. Sunitinib resulted from many years of iterative chemistry and pharmacologic testing. Herein, we summarize the historical discovery and rationale, clinical pharmacology, nonclinical and translational medicine studies supporting early clinical evaluation, and clinical trial data that led to product approval in 2006.

1.2. RECEPTOR TYROSINE KINASE SIGNALING AFFECTS MULTIPLE AND DIVERSE CANCER PROCESSES

In the mid-to-late 1980s through the early 1990s, advances in molecular biology and DNA cloning techniques resulted in the discovery and functional characterization of genes involved in the etiology and progression of human cancer. During this period the identification of oncogenes capable of transforming healthy cells to malignant cells provided new understanding of the encoded proteins critical to signal transduction pathways and the mechanisms promoting tumor progression. The comprehensive characterization of these oncoproteins identified protein tyrosine kinases and receptor tyrosine kinase (RTK) families (Manning et al., 2002).

RTK signaling is normally tightly regulated and is critically important in processes, such as cell proliferation and survival, migration, and metabolism (Schlessinger, 2000). To date, at least 60 RTK transmembrane signaling proteins have been identified. Each RTK is characterized by an extracellular domain that functions as a binding site for a specific polypeptide ligand, a cytoplasmic kinase catalytic domain, and additional regulatory sequences that facilitate downstream signal transduction. The stimulation of RTK catalytic activity in response to ligand binding initiates the transfer of ATP gamma-phosphate to tyrosine residues on target proteins. This phosphorylation initiates a downstream intracellular signaling cascade.

The dysregulation of RTK signaling caused by a mutation, ectopic receptor, or ligand expression has been implicated in aspects of tumor progression including cell proliferation, survival, angiogenesis, and tumor dissemination (Blume-Jensen and Hunter, 2001). The characterization and expression of tyrosine kinases at the RNA and protein levels indicated that these tyrosine kinases were often highly expressed in tumor tissue relative to normal or surrounding adjacent tissues. The early protein tyrosine kinase drug targets were mostly RTKs associated with epithelial-derived cancers. Drug discovery research efforts in human cancer revolved around these early drug targets such as the epidermal growth factor receptor (EGFR, erbB1, HER1), epidermal growth factor receptor 2 (HER2, erbB2, neu), fibroblast growth factor receptor 1 (FGFR1), VEGFR, PDGFR, insulin-like growth factor receptor-1 (IGF-R1), and c-src, a cytoplasmic membrane-associated tyrosine kinase.

1.3. ROLE OF RECEPTOR TYROSINE KINASES IN PATHOLOGIC TUMOR ANGIOGENESIS

It has long been known that neoplasms are often accompanied by an increased and unique vascularity; however, the molecular mechanisms responsible for these vascular changes in tumor tissue were not well understood and remained elusive for over 50 years (Lewis 1927; Tannock 1968). In 1971 Judah Folkman and colleagues introduced the concept of neoangiogenesis as a critical mechanism by which neoplasms secrete a "tumor angiogenic factor or TAF" in order to recruit vascular supply and gain access to nutrients and oxygen (Folkman et al., 1971). The field gained further, newfound attention in the mid-1980s through the early 1990s when a series of soluble factors and their receptors were implicated in endothelial cell function and angiogenesis. Some of the initial factors shown to regulate endothelial cell function, angiogenesis, and vascular permeability included peptide growth factors, such as vascular permeability factor (VPF) (Senger et al., 1983) also known as vascular endothelial growth factor (VEGF) (Ferrara and Henzel, 1989), basic and acidic fibroblast growth factors (bFGF and aFGF) (Maciag et al., 1984; Shing et al., 1984), angiogenin (Fett et al., 1985), and platelet-derived growth factor (PDGF) (Folkman, 1995). When vascular permeability factor (VPF) was first identified, studies by Senger and Dvorak showed that when partially purified as a protein factor it was able to induce vascular leakage (Senger et al., 1983). Ferrara and colleagues cloned a gene product that functioned as a diffusible, soluble, and selective endothelial cell mitogen, which they termed vascular endothelial growth factor (VEGF) (Ferrara and Henzel, 1989). Subsequent cloning and characterization by multiple laboratories and investigators suggested that this factor existed in several low molecular weight species (i.e., 121, 165, and 189 amino acids) and that VPF and VEGF were determined to be the same protein (Ferrara, 2004). Efforts to identify receptors for VEGF resulted in the cloning and identification of two receptor tyrosine kinases termed vascular endothelial growth factor receptor 1 (VEGFR1, FLT1) and factor 2 (VEGFR2, KDR) in 1992 (deVries et al., 1992; Terman et al., 1992). Both receptors could bind to VEGF with high affinity, were expressed predominantly in endothelial cells, and mediated its known biological effects in endothelial cell lines. When VEGF or VEGF receptor gene loci were disrupted in mice, findings suggested that these genes were required for mammalian development and for normal embryonic vascular development, thus providing evidence of their important role as key regulators of angiogenesis (Fong et al., 1995; Carmeliet et al., 1996; Ferrara et al., 1996).

Following the discovery and characterization of VEGFs and VEGFRs, a number of studies further supported the importance of VEGF and VEGFR in tumor angiogenesis. A group of studies in 1992 reported that VEGF was highly expressed in glioblastoma multiforme and that under hypoxic conditions, VEGF could be induced. This concept was found to be common to many tumor types (Shweiki et al., 1992; Plate et al., 1992). Subsequently, the overexpression of VEGF was noted in a variety of tumor types as well as identified as an independent prognostic factor (Folkman, 1995). Additional mechanistic studies demonstrated that stable transfection of nontumorigenic cell lines with VEGF allowed these cell lines to grow with vasculature as tumor xenografts in athymic mice despite having no effect on tumor growth properties in vitro (Claffey et al., 1996; Ferrara et al., 1993). Subsequent critical experiments were designed to address whether inhibiting the function of VEGF or VEGFRs could inhibit the progression of experimental tumors. The neutralization of soluble VEGF with monoclonal antibodies demonstrated the ability to inhibit tumor growth in a variety of tumor xenograft models despite having no effect on the growth properties of the respective cell lines in vitro (Kim et al., 1993). Similarly, dominant-negative Flk1 (the mouse ortholog of VEGFR2) retrovirus was used to inhibit Flk1/VEGFR2 activity and function in mouse endothelial cells in the setting of experimental tumor models. The Flk1 dominant-negative retrovirus inhibited angiogenesis and tumor growth in several experimental tumor models and represented early data that inhibition of VEGFR2 signaling may be a viable cancer treatment strategy (Millauer et al., 1994, 1996).

The discovery of multiple and distinct RTKs important in tumorigenesis and tumor angiogenesis prompted identification of monoclonal antibodies and specific chemicals that could inhibit protein function and cell signaling. Initial nonclinical data and proven clinical utility of therapeutic monoclonal antibodies, including trastuzamab, helped foster increased interest in RTK drug discovery. Similarly, initial nonclinical studies with VEGF-neutralizing antibodies helped build confidence in the targeting of this pathway to inhibit tumor angiogenesis and delay tumor progression. The identification of mono-clonal antibodies that interrupt RTK signaling in animal cancer models has been reviewed elsewhere. With respect to chemical inhibition, initial approaches to identify chemicals that interrupted protein kinases began with natural product chemistry related to staurosporine and genistein and focused on enzyme catalytic function that could be purified from membrane prepara-tions. These first chemicals from natural sources were found to be nonselec-tive inhibitors of protein kinases but served as a starting point for novel synthetic chemistry. With the advent of DNA cloning and recombinant protein production, systematic drug design approaches were used to identify chemotypes that could interrupt protein kinase function. High-throughput screening and medicinal chemistry approaches using synthetic chemical tem-plates such as the quinazolines, quinoxalines, and pyrimidines were the first to be evaluated. The initial protein kinase drug targets were Raf, p38, EGFR, PDGFR, and c-src protein kinases. In this regard, sunitinib evolved as the first small-molecule RTK inhibitor leading to the inhibition of tumor angiogenesis.

1.4. SU5416: DISCOVERY OF FIRST-GENERATION VEGFR RTK INHIBITORS

In 1994, the drug discovery program targeting tumor angiogenesis by inhibit-ing VEGFR catalytic activity was initiated at Sugen, Inc. A high-throughput screen identified the indolin-2-one chemotype with a biochemical PDGFR protein kinase assay. Among various hit chemotypes, indolin-2-ones demon-strated relative specificity in cells comparing VEGF to FGF signaling in cul-tured human umbilical vein endothelial cells (HUVECs) and comparing

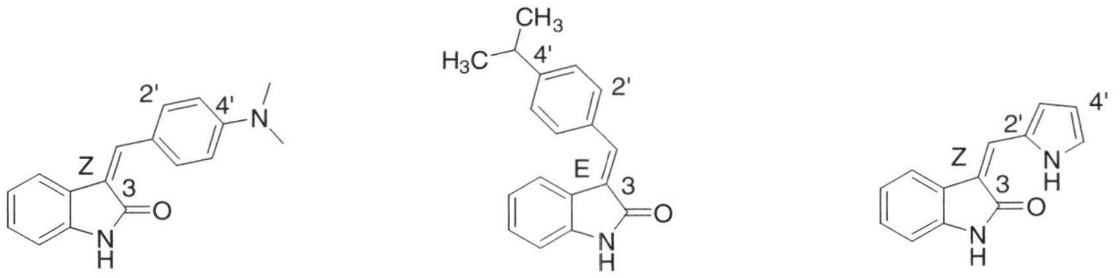

Compound	Inhibition of Cellular Tyrosine Kinase Activity (IC$_{50}$, µM)				
ID	PDGF	FLK1	EGFR	HER2	IGFR
1	19.4	0.8	>100	>100	>100
2	24.2	5.2	18.5	16.9	10.0
3	12.0	0.39	>100	>100	>100

Figure 1.1. Structures and biological evaluations of the three lead 3-substituted indolin-2-ones (Sun et al., 1998).

PDGF to EGF signaling in cultured fibroblasts. Three indolin-2-ones were identified as initial hits that exhibited inhibitory properties against various RTKs (**1–3**, Figure 1.1). Both **1** and **3** were found to be potent and selective inhibitors of VEGFR, whereas **2** was found to be nonselective for RTK inhibition.

Comparisons of these compounds suggested connections between chemical structure and the ability to modulate potency and specificity toward members of type III RTKs including PDGFR, FGFR, SCFR, and VEGFR. Compound **1** contains a dimethylamino substitution attached to the C-4′ position of the phenyl at the C-3 position of the indolin-2-one, whereas **2** contains an isosteric isopropyl moiety. Proton NMR analysis of these compounds indicated differences in *E* and *Z* isomer populations. Both **1** and **3** existed predominantly as the *Z* isomers and were relatively potent and selective inhibitors of VEGFR2 compared with other type III RTKs. Compound **2** adopted predominantly the *E* isomeric form and showed lower potency and selectivity toward VEGFR2 versus the other type III RTKs. This preliminary analysis suggested that the relative potency and selectivity of these compounds for inhibition of VEGFR2 may be sensitive to the *E/Z* configuration, which was determined by the nature of substitutions at C-3 position of the indolin-2-ones. The association of these inhibitory activities with the *Z* isomeric forms was also found to be in agreement with co-crystal studies using **4** and SU5402 bound in the ATP-binding site of the FGFR1 (Mohammadi et al., 1997), which shares high amino acid sequence homology for the ATP-binding pocket with VEGFR2 (Figure 1.2). In this study, the binding configurations for both **4** and SU5402 were found to be the *Z* isomer form even though compound **4** existed as *E* isomer and

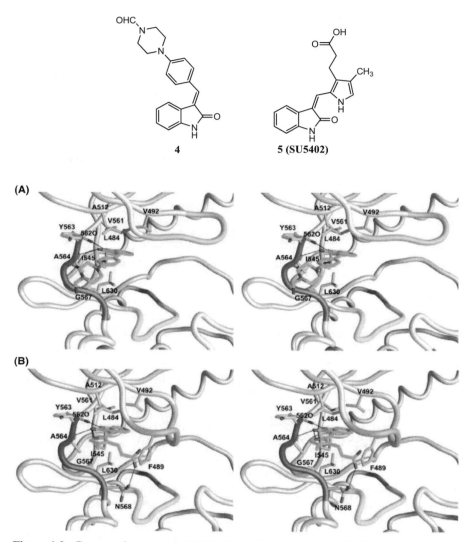

Figure 1.2. Co-crystal structure of SU5402 and compound 4 in FGFR1 kinase domain (Mohammadi et al., 1997). Stereoviews of the inhibitor binding sites. The side chains of residues that interact with the inhibitors are shown. Carbon atoms of the inhibitor and FGFR1K are green and orange, respectively; oxygen atoms are red and nitrogen atoms are blue. Selected hydrogen bonds are shown as black lines. (**A**) FGFR1K-4. (**B**) FGFR1K-SU5402. (See color insert.)

SU5402 as Z isomer in NMR solution (Sun et al., 1998). These structural studies demonstrated the probable molecular mechanism of action for this type of molecule as an ATP-competitive inhibitor and provided additional binding site information for lead optimization.

The initial efforts to establish structure–activity relationships (SARs) for this chemical series led to the identification of highly selective VEGFR2 inhibitors. A diverse set of substituted indolin-2-ones were designed and shown to modulate potency and specificity for all of the type III RTKs including PDGFR, FGFR, and VEGFR at the enzyme and cellular level (Sun et al., 1998, 1999). Of particular interest, indolin-2-ones with a C-3 pyrrole substitution demonstrated a better in vitro profile than corresponding compounds with aryl or heteroaryl substitutions. Among the initial set of pyrrol-substituted compounds, SU5416 (Figure 1.3) demonstrated potent and selective in vitro inhibitory activity toward VEGFR2 (Table 1.1) and broad spectrum of antitumor activity after daily intraperitoneal administration (Table 1.2) (Fong et al., 1999). This was consistent with previous observations with VEGFR2 dominant-negative mutants (Millauer et al., 1996).

Further study on the mechanisms underlining the in vivo antitumor effect of SU5416 revealed that it had no effect in vitro when evaluated with various tumor cell lines used in the tumor efficacy studies in vivo (Table 1.2). Interestingly, some tumor xenografts treated with SU5416 indicated an apparent lack of blood vessels compared to control tumors (Figure 1.4) (Fong et al., 1999). SU5416 also demonstrated the ability to inhibit tumor vascular density and vascular leakage (Figure 1.5) (Vajkoczy et al., 1999). All these findings suggested an antiangiogenesis mechanism rather than direct growth inhibition on tumor cells was responsible for the broad antitumor activity of SU5416.

The novel mechanism of action and substantial nonclinical efficacy coupled with a favorable toxicity profile of SU5416 prompted Sugen to move forward

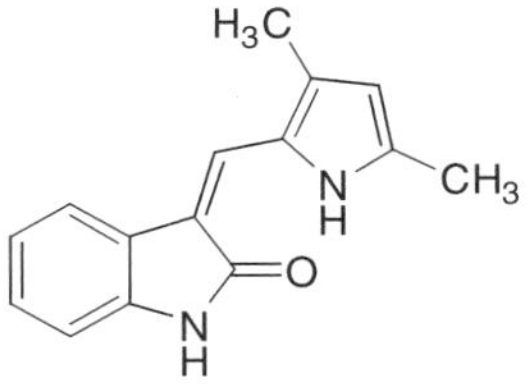

Figure 1.3. SU5416 structure.

TABLE 1.1. Inhibition of Ligand-Dependent Cellular Activities of SU5416

Ligand-Dependent Phosphorylation of RTKs in NIH 3T3 Cells IC$_{50}$ (µM)			
Flk1	PDGFR	FGFR	EGFR or IGF-R1
1.04 ± 0.53	20.26 ± 5.2	>100	>100

Ligand-Dependent Mitogenesis of HUVEC IC$_{50}$ (µM)	
VEGFR	FGFR
0.04 ± 0.02	50

Source: Fong et al. (1999).

TABLE 1.2. Efficacy of SU5416 in Solid Tumor Xenografts in Mice[a]

Cell Line	Tumor Type	Implant ×10⁶ Cells/Animal	Prcentage Inhibition @ (days)	P
A375 (human)	Melanoma	3	85 (38)	0.0005
A431 (human)	Epidermoid carcinoma	2.5	62 (20)	0.0006
Calu-6 (human)	Lung carcinoma	7.5	52 (25)	0.031
C6 (rat)	Glioma	0.5	54 (18)	0.001
LNCAP (human)	Prostatic carcinoma	3	62 (43)	0.01
EPH4-VEGF (murine)	Mammary carcinoma	0.5	44 (21)	0.00001
3T3HER2 (murine)	Fibrosarcoma	5	32 (23)	0.046
488G2M2 (murine)	Fibrosarcoma	5	71 (13)	0.0004
SF763T (human)	Glioma	0.5	23 (21)	NS[b]
SF767T (human)	Glioma	0.5	0 (21)	NS

[a]Various tumor cells were implanted subcutaneously in the hind flank region of 8–12 week-old BALB/c *nu/nu* female mice. Animals were treated once daily with a 50 µL IP bolus injection of SU5416 at 25 mg/kg/day in DMSO or DMSO alone for the indicated number of days (in parentheses) beginning 1 day after implantation. Tumor growth during the treatment period was monitored by measuring the tumor mass on the animals using venier calipers. Tumor volumes were calculated as the product of length × width × height. The percentage of inhibition of tumor growth compared with the vehicle-treated control group was calculated on the indicated days after implantation. P values were calculated by comparing mean tumor size of the treated group against mean tumor size of the vehicle control group using Student's *t* test.
[b]NS, not significant.
Source: Fong et al. (1999).

with the agent for clinical proof-of-concept in 1997. As the first antiangiogenic small molecule to enter the clinic, SU5416 was developed as an intravenous product and demonstrated clinical evidence of antiangiogenesis in von Hippel–Lindau (VHL) retinal angiogenesis (Aiello et al., 2002) and Kaposi sarcoma (Arastéh and Hannah, 2000; Giles et al., 2003; Fiedler et al., 2003). However, limitations in pharmacokinetics and solubility restricted further development of the compound.

1.5. SU6668: INHIBITOR OF PDGFR AND VEGFR TYROSINE KINASES

Early compounds like SU5416, a highly selective VEGFR inhibitor, delayed tumor growth. To enhance antitumor activity, it was hypothesized that the simultaneous inhibition of multiple RTKs critical to the regulation of both

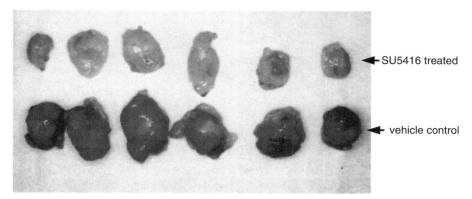

Figure 1.4. Antiangiogenesis effects of SU5416 on rat C6 glioma xenograft model (Fong et al., 1999). Rat C6 glioma cells were surgically implanted (0.5×10^6 cells/animal) under the serosa of the colon in BALB/c *nu/nu* mice. Beginning 1 day after implantation, animals were treated once daily with a 50 µL IP bolus injection of either SU5416 at 25 mg/kg/day in DMSO or DMSO alone for 16 days. On day 16 after implantation, animals were euthanized, and their local tumors in the colon were first quantitated by measurement using venier calipers and then harvested. A 73% decrease in tumor volume was recorded in the drug-treated group ($P < 0.00001$) and was calculated by comparing mean tumor size of the treated groups versus mean tumor size of the vehicle control group using Student's *t* test. Representative tumors from SU5416-treated (*top*) and DMSO-treated (*bottom*) animals are shown.

tumor cell proliferation and tumor angiogenesis may result in additive effects leading to tumor regression. As described previously, dysregulation of endothelial VEGFR1 and VEGFR2 RTKs and secretion of their cognate ligand VEGF by tumor cells was implicated in tumor-dependent angiogenesis (Ferrara, 2004). PDGFRs were expressed on both endothelia and perivascular endothelia (pericytes) and implicated as critical regulators of tumor angiogenesis (Pietras et al., 2003). Strong evidence existed that PDGFRs were critical for pericyte recruitment to nascent vessels during neoangiogenesis resulting in formation of mature and stable vasculature (Pietras et al., 2003). In addition to VEGFRs' and PDGFRs' involvement in tumor angiogenesis, selected solid tumor types directly expressed constitutively active RTKs due to mutation or autocrine stimulation by cognate ligands leading to dysregulation of cancer cell mitogenesis and survival. KIT (SCFR) genes were found to be mutated and implicated in the pathogenesis of GIST and selected melanoma subtypes. The PDGFRα gene locus was amplified in glioblastoma (Heinrich et al., 2002; Pietras et al., 2003). Direct expression of VEGFR1, VEGFR2, KIT, PDGFRα, and PDGFRβ by tumor cells along with their cognate ligands implicated RTKs in the regulation of tumor cell growth and survival (Cherrington et al., 2000; Heinrich et al., 2002; Pietras et al., 2003). Collectively, the dysregulation of these RTKs present among multiple tumor types was compelling and provided

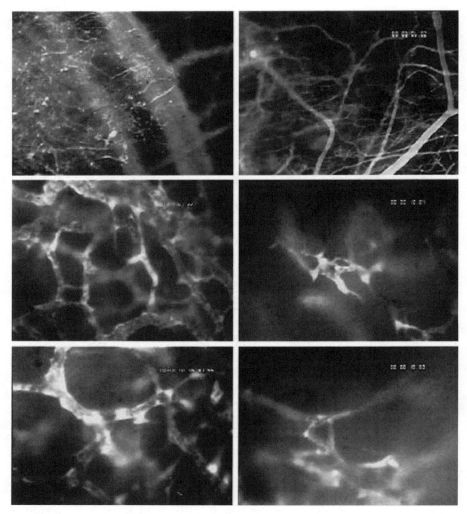

Figure 1.5. Inhibition of tumor-induced vascularity by SU5416 (Vajkoczy et al., 1999). C6 glioma microvasculature in animals treated with DMSO 50 μL/d, IP (left row) or SU5416 25 mg/kg/day, IP (right row) on day 6 (*top panels*) and 18 (*middle* and *bottom panels*) after glioma cell implantation. Intravital multifluorescence videomicroscopy, contrast enhancement with 2% FITC-dextran$_{150}$ IV.

the rationale to pursue an indolin-2-one having optimal pharmaceutical properties and an expanded RTK target profile.

To expand the target profile of the indolin-2-ones to include PDGFRβ and improve their pharmaceutical properties, second-generation indolin-2 -ones were designed and synthesized using the information deduced from co-crystallization and homology models. SU5402 (Figure 1.2), co-crystallized with FGFR1, was shown to perturb the conformation of the adenine binding pocket due to coordination of Asn568 to C-3′ propionic acid side chain substituent on the pyrrole ring. This distortion of the nucleotide-binding loop may explain the compound's increased potency for FGFR1 compared with compounds such as SU5416, where such substituent was absent. SU5402 also had potent inhibitory activity toward VEGFR2 having the same asparagine residue in the corresponding sugar-binding region as FGFR1. Unlike FGFR1 and VEGFR2, PDGFRβ contains an aspartic acid in the corresponding position of sugar-binding region. In addition, PDGFRβ also had a basic arginine residue in proximity to the C-4′ position on the pyrrole ring of SU5402. Thus in order to enhance PDGFRβ inhibitory activities, the propionic acid side chain was incorporated to the C-4′ position of the pyrrole ring to interact with the arginine residue in ATP-binding pocket. To maintain VEGFR2 inhibitory activity, the structural feature (3,5-dimethyl pyrrole) of SU5416 was incorporated into a new series. The combination of each of these small-molecule structural features resulted in the identification of SU6668, which achieved the goals of expanding the RTK target profile to include both VEGFRs and PDGFRs (Laird et al., 2000). (See Table 1.3.)

The co-crystal structure of SU6668 with FGFR1 confirmed that the ligand was localized in the ATP-binding site of the FGFR1 catalytic core (Figure 1.6) as in the case of SU5402. A homology model built for PDGFR catalytic domain with SU6668 docked into the ATP-binding site provided rationale for the high affinity of SU6668 toward PDGFR. Given the solubility limitations of SU5416, SU6668 was a more soluble and orally bioavailable product candidate that may provide more convenient dosing regimens. Unlike SU5416, which demonstrated cytostatic properties in models of tumor xenografts, SU6668 showed evidence of tumor regression in animal models, which supported the original hypothesis to inhibit both PDGFR and VEGFR activity (Figure 1.7). SU6668 was introduced into the clinic in 1999 as an oral compound that selectively inhibited PDGFR and retained inhibitory activity toward VEGFR.

TABLE 1.3. K_i and K_m Values of SU6668 Versus Flk1, FGFR1, and PDGFRβ

Flk1 Trans- phosphorylation	FGFR1 Trans- phosphorylation	PDGFRβ Autophosphorylation	EGFR, IGF-1R, Met, Src, Lck, Zap70, Abl, CDK2
$K_i = 2.1$	$K_i = 1.2$	$K_i = 0.008$	$K_i > 10$
Endothelial Cell Proliferation IC$_{50}$ (µM)			
VEGF Induced	FGF Induced	Tumor Cell Proliferation IC$_{50}$ (µM)	
0.34 ± 0.05	9.6 ± 0.4	>15	

Source: Laird et al. (2000).

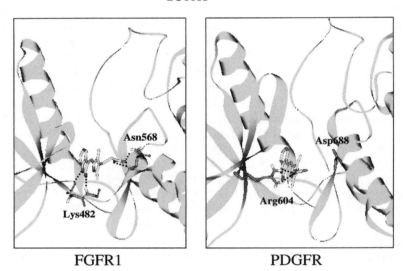

SU6668

FGFR1   PDGFR

Figure 1.6. Co-crystal structure of SU6668 in FGFR1 kinase domain (Laird et al., 2000). Crystal structure of SU6668 in FGFR1 (*left panel*) and homology model of SU6668 in PDGFR (*right panel*). (*Left panel*) The region of the SU6668/FGFR1 co-crystal structure corresponding to the ATP-binding site is shown. The receptor is represented by turquoise ribbons. The backbone/side chains of residues of particular interest with respect to their interaction with SU6668 (Asn568 and Lys482) are shown as stick figures with carbon atoms colored gray. SU6668 is also shown in stick representation, with carbon atoms colored yellow. Hydrogen bonds/close contacts between SU6668 and FGFR1 are indicated by dotted lines. (*Right panel*) SU6668 docked into a homology model of the ATP-binding site of PDGFR. Representation and color schemes are the same as those described previously for the left panel. The interaction between the terminal carboxylate of the propionic acid side chain of SU6668 and Arg-604 of PDGFR is highlighted. The position of the side chain of Asp688, the residue corresponding to Asn568 in FGFR1, is also indicated.

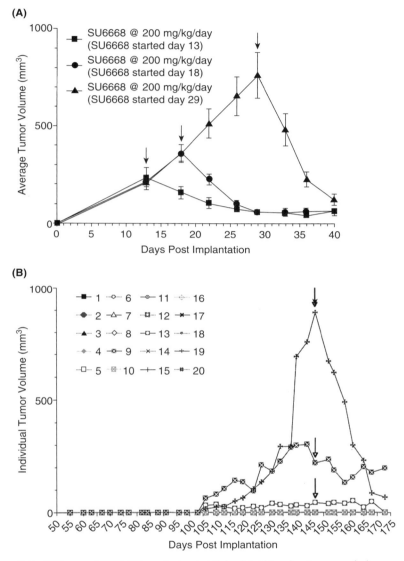

Figure 1.7. Efficacy of SU6668 against established A431 subcutaneous (sc) xenografts in athymic mice (Laird et al., 2000). Efficacy of SU6668 against established A431 sc xenografts in athymic mice. (**A**) SU6668 regresses established tumors in athymic mice. A431 cells (5×10^6) were implanted subcutaneously into the hind flank of female athymic mice on day 0. Daily oral administration of SU6668 at 200 mg/kg/day in a cremophor-based formulation was initiated for groups of animals as they attained average tumor sizes of approximately 200 (day 13; $n = 10$), 400 (day 18; $n = 10$), or 800 (day 29; $n = 19$) mm³. All animals received either SU6668 or the cremophor-based vehicle alone from day 13 onward until SU6668 treatment began. (**B**) Tumor regression was sustained in 17 of 20 mice with completely regressed tumors in the absence of further treatment. (*Arrows*) Resumption of treatment in three mice at day 147. Tumor growth was measured using vernier calipers, and tumor volumes were calculated as the product of length × width × height. Values plotted are mean tumor volume ± SE.

1.6. DESIGN, DISCOVERY, AND DEVELOPMENT RATIONALE FOR SU11248

Following the initial success with developing VEGFR and PDGFR inhibitors, efforts were focused on broadening the kinase selectivity spectrum of indolin-2-one to encompass additional class III and V RTKs. Diversification at the C-4′ position on the pyrrole ring of SU5416 was explored further. We learned from the previous SAR analysis that modifications at the C-4′ position could lead to compounds with different kinase inhibition profiles for the VEGFR2 and PDGFRβ RTKs. In this regard, the neutral SU5416 (Fong et al., 1999) was a potent and selective inhibitor for VEGFR2 while acidic SU6668 (Laird et al., 2000) also inhibited PDGFRβ. The co-crystal structure of SU6668 in the catalytic domain of the FGFR1 kinase (Laird et al., 2000) revealed that the substitution at the C-4′ position on the pyrrole ring was positioned close to the opening of the binding pocket and could be exposed to solvent. Thus substitution at this position might serve as a handle for improving pharmaceutical properties of the indolin-2-ones. Based on this analysis, various basic side chains were introduced at the C-4′ position of SU5416. Among these new analogs, SU11248 (Figure 1.8) (Sun et al., 2003) was identified and exhibited the most optimal overall profile in terms of potency for the intended receptor tyrosine kinase targets, solubility, protein binding, in vivo pharmacokinetic properties, and antitumor efficacy.

Critical limitations of the SU5416 clinical development program included (1) poor solubility, (2) an inability to administer the intravenous agent with the frequency to inhibit the VEGFR target in order to maximize its antitumor activity, (3) the lack of a translational biomarker to demonstrate the pharmacological impact of the compound on the target mechanism of action and, lastly, (4) an inappropriate selection of solid tumor patient populations to achieve proof-of-concept clinical activity and efficacy. To address lessons learned from the SU5416 program, the nonclinical discovery and early clinical development program of SU11248 was designed to address the limitations of SU5416 and was directed toward establishing a pharmacokinetic/pharmacodynamic

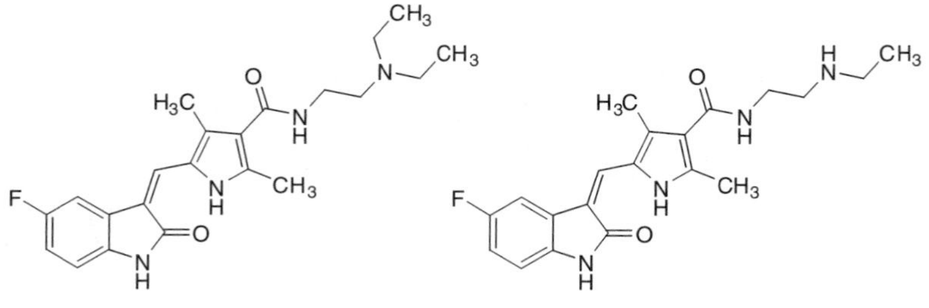

SU11248 (sunitinib)   SU12662 (metabolite of SU11248)

Figure 1.8. Structure of SU11248 and its metabolite SU12662.

(PK/PD) relationship of RTK target inhibition to plasma concentration in order to guide appropriate dose and schedule. In addition, the validation of biomarker endpoints to establish effects on targets and mechanism along with a rational selection of patient populations based on the understanding of dysregulation of RTK targets in the clinical setting was pursued with SU11248.

1.7. SU11248 IN VITRO PROTEIN KINASE TARGET PROFILE

Initial in vitro biochemical kinase screening assays using recombinant proteins demonstrated that SU11248 was a potent inhibitor of VEGFRs (VEGFR1, 2, and 3) and PDGFRβ, with K_i values ranging from 0.002 to 0.017 μM (Mendel et al., 2003). In addition, SU11248 kinase inhibitory activity was measured in broad panels of biochemical assays eventually including more than 250 tyrosine kinases or serine–threonine protein kinases. These collective studies demonstrated that SU11248 was generally selective for the class III and V RTKs compared with other protein kinase families. Since class III and V RTKs comprised the major subset of targets that were inhibited by SU11248 in biochemical assays, they were the focus of most of the pharmacological characterization of this compound. Such targets included VEGFRs 1, 2, and 3, PDGFRs α and β, KIT (SCFR), glial cell-line derived neurotrophic factor receptor (REarranged during Transfection; RET), FMS-like tyrosine kinase 3 (FLT3) and the receptor for macrophage colony-stimulating factor (CSF1R). In addition, SU12662 (Figure 1.8), a major metabolite of SU11248 in animal experiments, and in clinical studies, was found to be a potent inhibitor of the same RTKs as the parent compound SU11248 (Table 1.4). Consequently, this metabolite was included in all subsequent pharmacokinetic and pharmacodynamic characterizations of SU11248 in order to provide a more complete analysis of pharmacologic effects.

While some protein kinase targets in addition to the class III and V RTKs were inhibited by SU11248 in initial biochemical screens, subsequent cell-based assays against intended sunitinib targets and potential off-target kinase hits suggested that the pharmacologic activity of SU11248 is mediated predominantly by these RTKs. Cellular kinase assays were utilized to inhibit ligand-dependent RTK phosphorylation in cells expressing these RTK targets. Results are summarized in Table 1.4. It is important to note that SU11248 strongly inhibited VEGF-stimulated VEGFR2 phosphorylation and PDGF-stimulated PDGFRβ phosphorylation in NIH-3T3 cells expressing these targets.

SU11248 was also evaluated to determine the relative inhibitory properties of mutated RTKs with constitutive kinase activity compared to their wild-type counterparts. In these experiments, SU11248 inhibited constitutive kinase activity associated with mutant forms of KIT or PDGFRα. This was of particular interest since more than 85% of GIST cases exhibited mutated and constitutively active forms of KIT or PDGFRα receptors, which are believed to be

TABLE 1.4. Inhibition of Target Receptor Tyrosine Kinases by SU11248

Tyrosine Kinase	Biochemical[a] K_i (µM)	Cellular IC_{50} (µM)	
		RTK Phosphorylation[b]	Cell Proliferation[d]
VEGFR1	0.002	ND	ND
VEGFR2	0.009 (Flk1)	0.004 (KDR)	0.004 (KDR)
		0.01 (Flk1)[c]	
VEGFR3	0.017	ND	ND
PDGFRα	ND	ND	0.069
PDGFRβ	0.008	0.004, 0.01[c]	0.039
KIT	ND	0.001–0.01,[c] 0.013	0.002
FLT3-WT	ND	0.25[c]	0.01
FLT3-ITD	ND	0.05[c]	0.001–0.01
RET	ND	0.05[c]	0.05
CSF1R	ND	0.05–0.1[c]	ND

Abbreviations: ND = not determined; WT = wild type; ITD = internal tandem duplication; KDR = human ortholog of VEGFR2; Flk1 = mouse ortholog of VEGFR2.
[a]Values were determined in biochemical kinase assays using recombinant enzymes.
[b]Values were determined by measuring intrinsic or ligand-stimulated kinase activity (phosphorylation) in cell lines expressing a given target RTK by immunoblot or ELISA assay.
[c]Values (or value ranges) were estimated from immunoblot analysis of RTK phosphorylation over a range of concentrations.
[d]Values were determined by measuring intrinsic or ligand-stimulated cell proliferation in cell lines expressing a given target RTK.
Source: Mendel et al. (2003).

key factors in the pathogenesis of these tumors (Heinrich et al., 2003). In addition, initial sensitivity to imatinib is influenced by selected primary mutant variants of KIT and the acquisition of secondary KIT mutations were associated with acquired imatinib resistance (Heinrich et al., 2003). Evaluation of SU11248 determined that it potently inhibited KIT autophosphorylation in isolated GIST cells or cells engineered to express constitutively active KIT exon 9 and exon 11 mutants commonly found in imatinib-naive GIST (Heinrich et al., 2003; Prenen et al., 2006). More recently, SU11248 potently inhibited exon 13 and exon 14 mutant variants of KIT (i.e., V654A and T670I), which were associated with reduced binding affinity and resistance to imatinib (Prenen et al., 2006; Liegl et al., 2008). Evaluation of SU11248 against additional mutated RTK targets indicated that it inhibited constitutive FLT3 phosphorylation in MV4-11 AML cells expressing FLT-ITD and constitutive RET phosphorylation in TT human medullary thyroid carcinoma cells expressing the RET C634W mutant (O'Farrell et al., 2003a; Christensen, 2007). Collectively, the ability of SU11248 to inhibit mutant variants of its target RTKs supported the concept of pursuing SU11248 in clinical populations in which these mutations are important in tumor pathogenesis and progression.

1.8. SIMULTANEOUS INHIBITION OF VEGFR, PDGFR, AND KIT (SCFR) RTKs ESTABLISHED A UNIQUE MECHANISM OF ACTION FOR SU11248

The development of SU11248 as a therapeutic agent served to address the hypothesis that simultaneous inhibition of multiple RTKs critical to the regulation of both tumor cell proliferation and survival as well as tumor angiogenesis would cooperate to produce cytoreductive antitumor efficacy. An early experiment in this regard (Bergers et al., 2003) demonstrated that addition of VEGFR and PDGFR kinase inhibitors together showed profound differences of effect compared with either inhibitor alone (Figure 1.9). In this case, addition of either SU5416 with SU6668 or SU5416 with imatinib resulted in more substantial effects on large tumors in the RIP1-Tag2 murine pancreatic model than any of the agents on their own. This was hypothesized to involve an effect of PDGFR on the perivascular endothelial cell population, which supports newly formed vessels. Studies in colon cancer models (Reinmuth et al., 2001) also substantiated this hypothesis. In this latter case, SU6668 was used to inhibit PDGFR and VEGFR signaling in cells derived from blood vessels supporting an effect on both pericytes and endothelial cells.

Additional studies were initiated to determine the relative contributions of individual RTK targets (Potapova et al., 2006) to the antitumor efficacy of SU11248. This was accomplished by investigating the antiangiogenic and antitumor effects of other inhibitors that more selectively target VEGFR, PDGFR, and KIT. In the case of Potapova et al. (2006), the reduction of microvessel density and antitumor efficacy of an indolin-2-one analog (SU10944 in Figure 1.10: selective VEGFR inhibitor) combined with imatinib was similar to that of single-agent SU11248 and was greatly superior to that of each compound alone (Figure 1.11). Together, these data suggested that simultaneous inhibition of VEGFR, PDGFR, and KIT contribute in a cooperative fashion to the antitumor and antiangiogenic effects of SU11248, at least in the five tumor models examined. A recent nonclinical study by Yao and co-workers (2006) also supported the conclusion that dual inhibition of VEGFR and PDGFR with SU11248 was associated with greater antiangiogenic effects than selective inhibition of VEGFR or PDGFR alone by comparing the effects of SU11248, AG-028262 (a selective VEGFR inhibitor), and CP-673,451 (a selective PDGFR inhibitor). In this case, tumor endothelial cells or pericytes in pancreatic islet tumors from RIP1-Tag2 transgenic mice were evaluated at dose levels associated with complete inhibition of the intended targets. In these studies, SU11248 treatment was associated with a 75% reduction in the density per unit area of endothelial cells and a 63% reduction in that of pericytes (Figure 1.12) (Yao et al., 2006). In contrast, AG-028262 alone reduced the tumor endothelial cell density (−61%) but had no effect on the tumor pericyte population (+0.6%), while CP-673,451 alone reduced pericyte density (−50%) but had no effect on endothelial cells (−5%). The combination of AG-028262 with

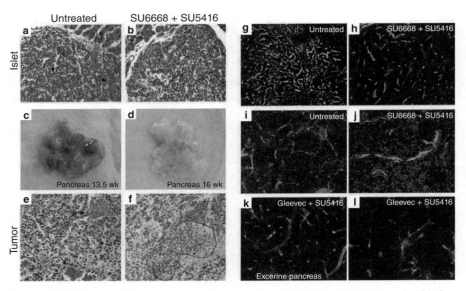

Figure 1.9. Effects of the combined therapy using SU5416 + SU6668 or SU5416 + imatinib. Hematoxylin and eosin staining of islets from (**a**) untreated and (**b**) SU6668 + SU5416 treated transgenic mice at 10.5 weeks in a prevention trial. Gross pathology of dissected pancreata from (**c**) untreated and (**d**) SU5416 + SU6668 treated mice in a 4 week regression trial targeting late-stage disease. Hematoxylin and eosin staining of tumors from (**e**) untreated and (**f**) SU5416 + SU6668 treated mice. Arrows indicate hemorrhage formation, and dotted area confines necrotic region. Comparison of the functional vasculature in (**g**) control and (**h**) SU5416 + SU6668 treated mice from a regression trial. Mice were injected intravenously with FITC-labeled tomato lectin (*Lycopersicon esculentum*) to stain blood vessels in green, and then heart perfused with 4% PFA, followed by immunohistochemical staining with Cy3-labeled desmin Ab to label desmin-expressing perivascular cells in red. Apoptotic cells in tumors of (**i**) control and (**j**) SU6668 + SU5416 treated mice were detected by TUNEL staining with fluorescent visualization (red), and the vasculature was revealed as above by intravenous FITC-lectin perfusion before sacrifice. Mice were treated with SU5416 + imatinib in the regression trial, and blood vessels and perivascular cells of (**k**) exocrine pancreas and (**l**) adjacent islet tumors were visualized with FITC-lectin and a Cy3-labeled desmin Ab. (See color insert.)

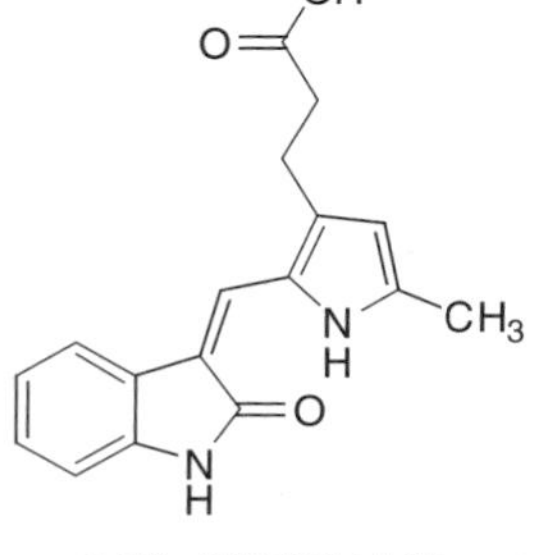

Figure 1.10. SU10944 Structure.

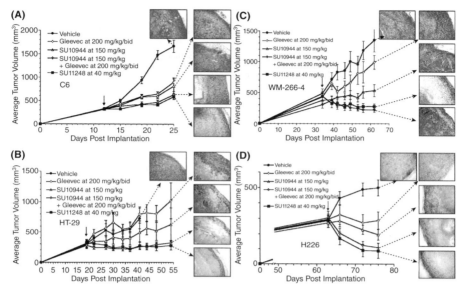

Figure 1.11. Combined administration of SU10944 and imatinib recapitulates the antitumor effect of SU11248 (Potapova et al. 2006). (**A**) C6 rat glioma, (**B**) HT-29 human colon carcinoma, (**C**) WM-266-4 human melanoma, and (**D**) H226 lung carcinoma tumor xenografts were established in athymic mice. Oral administration of indicated compounds was initiated (*arrows*) when tumors reached an average size of 320 mm³ (*C6*), 300 mm³ (*HT-29*), 410 mm³ (*WM-266-4*), and 290 mm³ (*H226*) and was continued through the end of the experiment. *Points*, mean tumor volume for groups of 8–10 (treated) or 16–20 (vehicle control) mice; *bars*, ±SE. A representative H&E-stained tumor tissue section taken at the end of the experiment for each treatment group (original magnification, 200×; connected with the efficacy plot by a dotted line to indicate the treatment group from which it originated).

CP-673,451 led to treatment that had comparable effects to SU11248 on both endothelial cells and pericytes (Yao et al., 2006).

In summary, these data supported the hypothesis that simultaneous inhibition of multiple critical targets such as VEGFR, PDGFR, and KIT resulted in robust antitumor activity and may recapitulate the cumulative antitumor efficacy of multiple single-target inhibitors given simultaneously.

1.9. SU11248 PKPD STUDIES ESTABLISHED THE OPTIMAL DOSING PARAMETERS

SU11248 demonstrated favorable oral bioavailability and plasma exposure (Mendel et al., 2003). Fluoro substitution at the C-5 position of SU11248 contributed to metabolic stability of SU11248 since it prevented metabolic hydroxylation at this position. The major metabolite of SU11248 (SU12662)

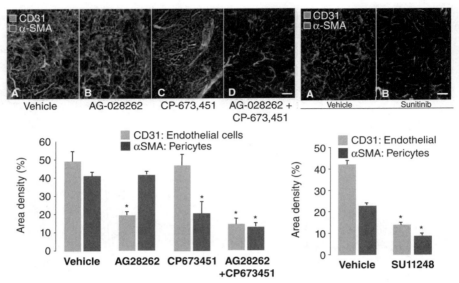

Figure 1.12. Effects of SU11248, a selective VEGFR inhibitor, or a selective PDGFR inhibitor on density of CD31 positive microvessels or α-SMA positive perivascular endothelia in RIP1-Tag2 islet cell tumors (Yao et al. 2006). (*Top left panel*) Large islet tumors from RIP1-Tag2 mice treated with: (**A**) vehicle, (**B**) AG-028262, (**C**) CP-673,451, or (**D**) AG-028262 + CP-673,451 for 7 days. Significant regression of pericytes (α-SMA, red) after treatment with CP-673,451 or AG-28262 + CP-673,451, whereas vessels (CD31, green) in CP-673,451 treated tumors were not significantly affected. Scale bar in (**D**) applies to all panels, 106 μm. (*Top right panel*) Islet tumors from RIP-Tag2 mice treated with (**A**) vehicle or (**B**) SU11248 for 7 days show decreased vessel (CD31, green) and pericyte (SMA, red) area densities. Scale bar in (**B**) applies to all panels, 47 μm. (*Bottom panels*) Quantification of CD31 and α-SMA area densities from 3 mice per group, 5–7 tumors per mouse (AG28262, CP-673,451) or 5 mice per group, 5 tumors per mouse (SU11248). *ANOVA Bonferroni test of significance of CD31 and α-SMA to corresponding vehicle values, where $P < 0.01$. (See color insert.)

demonstrated comparable in vitro and in vivo antitumor properties. SU11248 demonstrated a broad antitumor spectrum in vivo. Tumor regression was observed at relatively low dose levels in some tumor xenografts treated with SU11248 (Table 1.5). Since SU11248 exhibited the desired pharmaceutical properties (i.e., oral bioavailability, solubility, stability) and the desired class III and V split RTK target profile, efforts were initiated to characterize its potential as a product candidate.

Experiments were performed to establish the pharmacokinetic–pharmacodynamic (PK–PD) relationship between RTK target inhibition and plasma concentration in order to guide appropriate dose and schedule in the clinic. Several approaches evaluated the extent and duration of inhibition of key SU11248 RTK targets. Multiple approaches were initiated to assess target inhibition and establish a PK–PD relationship including (1) VEGFR2

TABLE 1.5. SU11248 Treatment Effectively Inhibits the Growth of Established Tumor Xenografts[a]

Cell Line	Tumor Type	Initial Tumor Volume (mm³)	Dose (mg/kg/day)	Growth Inhibition (%)	Regression (%)
HT-29	Colon	360	40		62 (d74)
A431	Epidermoid	400	80		30 (d40)
			40	93 (d36)	
			20	65 (d36)	
Colo205	Colon	250	80		38 (d35)
			40		13 (d35)
			20	55 (d35)	
H460	NSCLC	300	80	84 (d25)	
SF763T	Glioma	550	80	79 (d30)	
C6	Rat glioma	330	80	88 (d25)	
			40	82 (d25)	
		110	40	72 (d25)	
			20	41 (d25)	
A375	Melanoma	230	40	64 (d74)	
MDA-MB-435	Breast	150	80	71 (d73)	
			20	11 (d73)	

[a]Tumors were established by subcutaneous (sc) xenografts. Number of cells implanted per animal: SF763T and C6, 3×10^6; MDA-MB-435, 1×10^7; all other tumors, 5×10^6. Once daily treatment with oral SU11248 was initiated at the indicated dosages, when tumors had reached the indicted sizes. Percentage of growth inhibition values relative to vehicle-treated controls are indicated for cases in which overall effect was growth inhibition; maximum regression relative to tumor size at which treatment was initiated is indicated for cases in which overall effect was regression.

Source: Mendel et al. (2003).

phosphorylation in A375 xenografts directly expressing this target, (2) VEGF-dependent vascular permeability in mouse skin, (3) PDGFRβ phosphorylation in Colo205 xenografts expressing PDGFRβ in stroma, (4) KIT phosphorylation in NCI-H526 xenografts expressing KIT, (5) KIT-dependent hair pigmentation, or FLT3 phosphorylation in MV4-11 AML cells, and (6) AML xenografts expressing the FLT3-ITD mutant variant (Abrams et al., 2003; Mendel et al., 2003; Moss et al., 2003; O'Farrell et al., 2003a). To fully understand the relationship of the extent and duration of target inhibition to antitumor efficacy, SU11248 was evaluated in selected animal tumor models over a range of dose levels and schedules. A selected set of these data are illustrated in Table 1.5. The comparison of dose-dependent inhibition of SU11248 on RTK targets and antitumor efficacy are described next (Mendel et al., 2003).

The extent of tumor growth inhibition or tumor regression and pharmacologic modulation of RTKs was evaluated for SU11248 using administration schedules that varied between 10 and 80 mg/kg/day and given once daily or twice daily (Figure 1.13). Inhibition of VEGFR2 and PDGFRβ in tumors was observed for at least half of the dosing interval (12 hours) at 40 mg/kg/day and

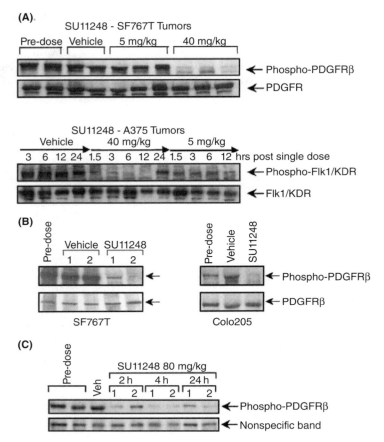

Figure 1.13. SU11248 treatment causes dose- and time-dependent inhibition of Flk1/KDR and PDGFRβ phosphorylation in vivo (Mendel et al., 2003). SF767T, A375, or Colo205 cells (5×10^6 cells/mouse) were implanted subcutaneously into the hind flank region of athymic mice. Mice bearing established (300–500 mm³) tumors were treated with a single oral dose of SU11248 at the indicated dose or vehicle alone. Each lane represents a separate animal. (**A**) Mice bearing SF767T tumors were sacrificed 2 h after dosing. PDGFRβ was immunoprecipitated from tumor lysates, and Western blots probed for phosphotyrosine (*Phospho-PDGFR*β) or total PDGFRβ (*PDGFR*β). Alternatively, mice bearing A375 tumors were sacrificed at the indicated times after treatment with SU11248. Total phosphotyrosine-containing proteins were immunoprecipitated from tumor lysates and Western blots probed for Flk1/KDR. Total Flk1/KDR was determined in a second sample of the same lysate. (**B**) PDGFRβ was immunoprecipitated from tumor lysates prepared 4 h after oral administration of an 80 mg/kg dose of SU11248 to mice bearing SF763T tumors, which express PDGFRβ on the tumor cells, or Colo205 tumors, which do not express PDGFRβ. Phospho-PDGFRβ and total PDGFRβ were detected as described above. (**C**) SF767T tumors were resected at the indicated time after oral administration of SU11248 at 80 mg/kg. In this experiment phosphotyrosine-containing proteins were immunoprecipitated from tumor lysates, and Western blots probed for PDGFRβ. Each lane represents a single animal, and the data shown are representative of at least two experiments.

for the full dosing interval (24 hours) at 80 mg/kg/day. At 20 mg/kg/day, the extent of tumor growth inhibition was to a lesser degree comparable with 40 mg/kg/day and, in most models, the inhibition of VEGFR2 and PDGFRβ in tumors was observed for 6–8 hours. At 20 mg/kg twice daily, the extent of tumor growth inhibition or tumor regression was comparable with 40 or 80 mg/kg administered once daily in the Colo205 model. Since 40–80 mg/kg/day was the fully efficacious dose in repeat dose studies (and more effective than 20 mg/kg/day), it was concluded that inhibition of target RTKs (VEGFR, PDGFRβ) for at least half of the dosing interval and the full dosing interval in selected models was required at a minimum to achieve full efficacy.

The above findings were related to the combined plasma concentration for the SU11248 and its major metabolite (SU12662) in order to establish pharmacodynamic inhibition of VEGFR2 and PDGFRβ and to determine the optimal target plasma concentration. In target modulation studies, it was observed that substantial inhibition of PDGFRβ and VEGFR2 phosphorylation and vascular permeability occurred at doses and time points where the total plasma concentration was 50 ng/mL or greater (Mendel et al., 2003). Taken together, the combined data generated from target modulation studies and antitumor efficacy studies indicated that inhibition of target RTKs resulting from ≥50 ng/mL in the plasma for at least half of the daily dosing interval was required to achieve full efficacy (Figure 1.14). Dose schedule studies investigating administration of a suboptimal dose more frequently (i.e., 20 mg/kg twice daily) also supported the conclusion that maintenance of a minimal effective plasma concentration would be necessary for achieving efficacy of SU11248 (Mendel et al., 2003). Similar studies investigating inhibition of other RTK targets suggested that minimal effective plasma concentrations would be similar for KIT and slightly lower for FLT3 (≥30 ng/mL). The above experiments concluded that SU11248 should achieve at least 50 ng/mL at 12 hours and this could serve as a guide for dose and schedule selection for SU11248 clinical studies. It is important to note that subsequent to the animal experiments, median C_{max} plasma concentrations for SU11248 and its major metabolite in human clinical studies following oral administration at a commonly utilized clinical dose of 50 mg daily for 28 days were found to be 100–125 ng/mL (approximately 0.01 μM unbound), indicating that predicted optimal target plasma concentration derived from animal studies could be achieved in humans (Faivre et al., 2006).

1.10. SU11248 NONCLINICAL STUDIES SUPPORTED CLINICAL STRATEGY AND TUMOR INDICATION SELECTION

Another goal of the SU11248 nonclinical development program was to provide insight toward the rational selection of patient populations based on the understanding of SU11248 mechanism and dysregulation of RTK targets in the clinical setting. Efforts were initiated to study the antiangiogenic and direct antitumor mechanisms of SU11248.

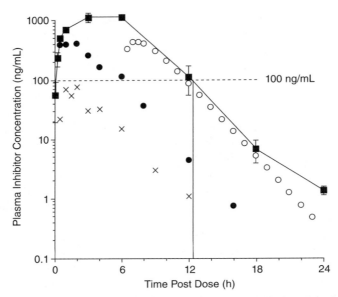

Figure 1.14. Plasma inhibitor concentration versus time profile in mice given an oral dose of SU11248 (Mendel et al., 2003). Athymic mice were given a single oral dose of SU11248. At the indicated times after dosing, plasma samples were obtained from terminal bleeds of individual mice, and the concentration of inhibitor in each sample determined by LC/MS/MS. ■, Data from PK study with mice dosed at 40 mg/kg; •, data from target modulation studies at 20 mg/kg; ○, simulated projection of expected plasma inhibitor concentrations in mice given a second 20 mg/kg dose 6 h after the first dose; x, data from target modulation studies at 5 mg/kg. For the PK study, each point represents mean for groups of three animals; *bars*, ±SE. For the target modulation studies, each point represents individual animals.

SU11248 demonstrated broad antitumor efficacy across a panel of tumor xenograft models implanted in athymic mice, transgenic models of cancer, and carcinogen-induced tumors. The models utilized represented broad histologies derived from various human tumors, including lung (NCI-H460, NCI-H226, NCI-H526, NCI-H82), colorectal (Colo205, HT-29), melanoma (A375, WM-266-4), epidermoid (A431), renal (786-O), glioblastoma (C6, SF763T), a mouse MMTV-v-Ha-ras transgenic mammary tumor model, and a DMBA-induced rat mammary carcinogenesis tumor model. In each of these models, orally administered SU11248 significantly inhibited tumor growth and/or progression of established tumors. In several of the models (Colo205, HT-29, WM-266-4, A431, 786-O, NCI-H226), SU11248 produced marked regression of large established tumors (Christensen, 2007). The ability of SU11248 to produce tumor regression suggested that initial proof-of-concept (POC) clinical trials should focus on objective response rate (ORR)-driven clinical endpoints.

The antiproliferative or pro-apoptotic effect of SU11248 on tumor cells was further profiled using anchorage-dependent and -independent conditions with a wide variety of tumor cell lines representing various histologies. Although the majority of cell lines were not directly affected by SU11248 in these studies, there were several examples of direct antiproliferative activity. SU11248 was shown to inhibit ligand-independent proliferation of primary GIST cells expressing KIT with activating mutations (Ikezoe et al., 2006; Prenen et al., 2006), MV4-11 cells expressing FLT3-ITD mutations (O'Farrell et al., 2003b), and TT human medullary thyroid carcinoma cells expressing RET (C634W) mutations (Christensen, 2007). These findings suggested the SU11248 IC_{50} values for inhibition of proliferation were similar to the IC_{50} values for inhibition of RTK autophosphorylation. More recent studies (McDermott et al., 2007) across an even broader panel of cell lines corroborate SU11248 antigrowth activity to a small subset of SU11248-sensitive cell lines. Collectively, these data suggested that SU11248 exhibits direct antiproliferative activity against a subset of tumor cells that is dependent on presence of its constitutively active or genetically altered RTK targets.

Prompted by the above findings, additional studies in animals were performed for which SU11248 demonstrated dramatic tumor regression in the MV4-11 AML xenograft model and exhibited a robust prolongation of survival in the MV4-11 AML bone marrow engraftment model (O'Farrell et al., 2003a). Similarly, SU11654 (Figure 1.15), a close structural analog of SU11248 with the same RTK target profile, showed evidence of objective tumor responses in canine mast cell tumors with KIT mutation positive (London et al., 2003). In this latter study, all local mast cell neoplasms and most lymph node positive KIT mutation positive neoplasms exhibited objective tumor responses, whereas few local mast cell neoplasms and no lymph node positive KIT-negative neoplasms exhibited objective responses. This data in animals supported the rationale for early Phase I clinical studies in AML patients and the Phase I enrichment strategy for imatinib-refractory GIST patients.

Studies were also initiated to characterize the antiangiogenic properties of SU11248. SU11248 inhibited VEGF-A stimulated proliferation of human umbilical vein endothelial cells ($IC_{50} = 0.004\,\mu M$), serum-stimulated endothelial tube formation of human microvascular endothelial cells ($IC_{50} = 0.055\,\mu M$) in vitro, and VEGF-A-stimulated vascular permeability in mouse skin in vivo when orally administered to mice (Table 1.6). The concentration range for

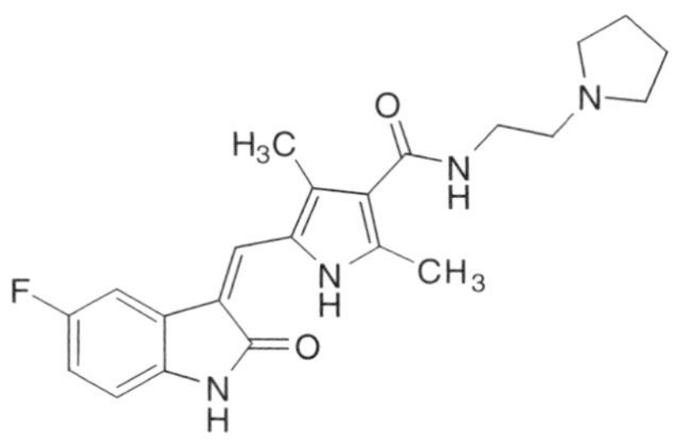

Figure 1.15. SU11654 structure.

TABLE 1.6. SU11248 Dose-Dependent Relationship of Target Modulation, Vascular Permeability, Hair Pigmentation, and Antitumor Efficacy

Dose (mg/kg)	Duration of Inhibition							Hair Pigment Inhibition	Antitumor Efficacy (% Inhibition)	
	Target Modulation (VEGFR2/PDGFRβ)			Vascular Permeability (% Inhibition)						
	8h	12h	24h	8h	12h	16h	24h	cKIT	Colo 205	A431
80	Yes	Yes	Yes	95	85	94	98	Complete	84	84
40	Yes	Yes	No	97	96	0	0	Partial	79	74
20	Yes	Slight	No	93	0	0	0	None	73	51
5	No	No	No	ND	ND	ND	ND	ND	ND	ND

Sources: Mendel et al. (2003) and Moss et al. (2003).

TABLE 1.7. Effect of SU11248 on Microvessel Density of Established Tumor Xenografts

Tumor Model[a]	Treatment Day	Vehicle MVD[b]	Sunitinib MVD	Sunitinib	P Value
SF763T glioma	13	39.3	24.2	38	0.04
C6 glioma	12	24.6	31.8	NA	NS
786-O renal	14	106.2	25.3	76	0.027
WM-266-4 melanoma	29	43.2	13.7	68	0.001
NCI-H226 lung	14	74.2	8.4	89	0.012

[a]Tumors were grown as subcutaneous xenografts in athymic mice to average sizes of 300–400 mm³. When optimal tumor size was established, daily oral administration of sunitinib was initiated at 40 mg/kg/day qd until the end of the study as indicated. At the end of each study, tumors were removed, fixed, and sectioned, and microvessels were visualized by immunohistochemical staining for CD-31 and counterstained with hematoxylin. Five fields/tumor were scored in blinded fashion at 100× magnification and the average number of mirovessels/field was calculated.
[b]MVD = average number of microvessels/100× field.
Source: Potapova et al. (2006).

inhibition of endothelial cell function in vitro and vascular permeability in vivo demonstrated a strong correlation with inhibition of VEGFR2 phosphorylation. In addition, SU11248 demonstrated a robust effect (≥70% reduction) on tumor microvessel density (MVD) in the majority of tumor xenograft models evaluated (Table 1.7). In these studies, SU11248 induced apoptosis (measured by activated caspase-3) in tumor endothelial cells within 4 hours and demonstrated a reduction of MVD as early as 2–3 days after first dose administration (Christensen, 2007). In addition, SU11248 demonstrated marked tumor regression in tumor xenograft models (e.g., HT-29 colon carcinoma, A431 epidermoid carcinoma) for which no effect was observed on tumor cell growth in vitro, suggesting a predominant antiangiogenic mechanism in these tumors (Mendel et al., 2003). Together, these studies provided the first evidence of potent antiangiogenic properties of SU11248 and provided the rationale to pursue SU11248 clinical development in tumor types with a strong angiogenic potential such as metastatic renal carcinoma.

1.11. SU11248: TRANSLATIONAL STUDIES PROVIDED A DRUG REGISTRATION PATH

Nonclinical or translational findings with SU11248 were valuable to generate hypotheses to support pharmacodynamic and biomarker endpoints useful in the identification of an appropriate dose and schedule for the clinic. Nonclinical findings were also useful to identify specific tumor types where SU11248 may be most likely to be active based on the anti-RTK and antiangiogenesis mechanism of action. The main goal of early clinical studies with SU11248 was to determine drug plasma levels and establish dose and schedules consistent with inhibition of its RTK targets. Inhibition of SU11248 RTK targets in human target tissue provided data to support targeting patient populations who may respond best to therapy. Rapid achievement of these initial goals was believed to have accelerated successful future studies with SU11248.

Furthermore, the in vivo tumor modeling studies establishing the PK–PD relationship for SU11248 previously described (Mendel et al., 2003) helped build confidence in clinical trial results. In the clinical setting, a dose-ranging pharmacokinetic trial of patients with advanced solid tumors identified 50 mg/day (administered in 6 week treatment cycles of 4 weeks on and 2 weeks off) as the recommended SU11248 dose. This was based on assessment of early clinical antitumor activity and tolerability (Faivre et al., 2006). This trial achieved a mean steady-state plasma level of 125 ng/mL and supported further studies since this plasma level exceeded the minimum target plasma levels required in animal efficacy studies.

Significant additional clinical studies focused on inhibition of RTK targets with an attempt to link target inhibition with SU11248 plasma levels. One such study was conducted in acute myelogenous leukemia (AML) cancer patients using FLT3 phosphorylation as a way to follow the pharmacodynamic effects of a single dose of SU11248. This patient population and endpoint were selected because (1) FLT3 phosphorylation could be measured in easily accessible circulating AML blasts, (2) AML with FLT3-ITD mutations exhibited a strong rationale for clinical benefit from SU11248 based on previous data, and (3) FLT3 was inhibited by SU11248 at similar concentrations compared with other target RTKs (e.g., VEGFR2, PDGFRβ, KIT). Therefore FLT3 was determined to be a potential surrogate clinical marker for inhibition of multiple RTK targets and would help strengthen studies in solid tumors, where tissue access was more difficult. In this pioneering clinical study, dose-dependent inhibition of FLT3 phosphorylation was apparent in 50% of FLT3–wild-type (WT) patients and in 100% of FLT3-mutant patients (O'Farrell et al., 2003b). Of the 16 evaluable FLT3-WT patients, 7 of 8 (87%) with a $C_{max} \geq 100$ ng/mL and only 1 of 8 (13%) with $C_{max} \geq 100$ ng/mL were inhibited. In contrast, for FLT3-ITD patients, phosphorylation was inhibited at a mean C_{max} of 34 ng/mL ($n = 3$) (O'Farrell et al., 2003b). These data suggested that a target plasma concentration of 100 ng/mL was required for strong inhibition of FLT3-WT, whereas lower concentrations still led to inhibition of FLT3-ITD, consistent with animal experiments. This AML translational study helped bridge animal models to the patient setting and provided the first evidence of inhibition of RTKs by SU11248 in a clinical setting.

Subsequent to the first clinical study in AML, repeat tumor biopsies were collected in patients during the Phase I and II studies evaluating SU11248 in GIST patients. Immunohistochemical and/or immunoblotting analyses of tumor biopsies from SU11248-treated patients in the GIST Phase I/II trial demonstrated near complete inhibition of KIT or PDGFRβ phosphorylation in multiple patients 1–2 weeks following initiation of treatment (Demetri et al., 2004; Davis et al., 2005) (Figure 1.16). In addition, selected patients treated with SU11248 exhibited evidence of patterns of hair depigmentation consistent with the 4 week on 2 week off cycle providing additional confidence that plasma levels consistent with robust inhibition of cKIT were achieved (Moss et al., 2003) (Figure 1.16).

Additional biomarker approaches integrated into clinical studies with SU11248 included functional imaging (i.e., FDG-, FLT-, or water-based PET imaging) and soluble plasma biomarker approaches where additional evidence of antitumor activity was generated. One study, utilizing serial PET images, showed that patients with advanced malignancies treated with SU11248 had >20% reductions in standard uptake values of radiolabeled glucose and water. PET tracers within the second week of treatment indicated decreased blood flow in metastases (Scott et al., 2005).

Measurements of soluble protein biomarkers in plasma were also acquired during clinical studies in order to understand the relationship between SU11248 inhibition and RTK target biology. These included VEGF-A, PlGF (placental growth factor), soluble VEGFR2 (sVEGFR2), and KIT ecto-domains. These plasma markers were selected for further study based on animal biomarker studies and plasma proteomic profiling of plasma samples from SU11248 clinical studies. All four of these biomarkers were modulated during the SU11248 treatment cycles consistent with the 4 week on 2 week off schedule. In multiple clinical studies including both RCC and GIST, both VEGFA and PlGF levels increased and sVEGFR2 and sKIT levels decreased by the end of each dosing cycle (DePrimo et al., 2006, 2007; Motzer et al., 2006). After 2 weeks following SU11248 therapy, the levels of VEGF-A, PlGF, and sVEGFR2 consistently returned to near baseline levels, whereas sKIT remained below baseline values during the 2 week off period in each study. The differences between baseline and end-of-cycle biomarker levels were statistically significant in each study. VEGF levels were known to increase in response to hypoxia and pharmacologic inhibition of angiogenesis. Additional analyses indicated that these markers correlated with trough plasma levels of SU11248 in multiple indications including GIST, RCC, neuroendocrine tumors, and breast cancer (Bello et al., 2006; DePrimo et al., 2006, 2007; Motzer et al., 2006). Furthermore, selected plasma markers correlated with selected measures of clinical benefit (e.g., response rate or progression-free survival) in Phase II studies. These studies measured reduction of sKIT in GIST and breast cancer patients, reduction of sVEGFR2 in metastatic RCC (mRCC), breast cancer patients and neuroendocrine tumors, and induction of VEGFA in mRCC (Bello et al., 2006; DePrimo et al., 2006, 2007; Motzer et al., 2006). Although the mechanism for consistent decreases in sVEGFR2 and increases in VEGFR ligands is not currently entirely understood, the consistency and high degree of correlation of sVEGFR2, sKIT, VEGF, and PlGF serum level changes to tumor response to SU11248 treatment was encouraging and prompted further investigation.

One of the most striking effects of SU11248 in the clinic was observed in Phase I studies using GIST and mRCC (metastatic renal cell carcinoma)

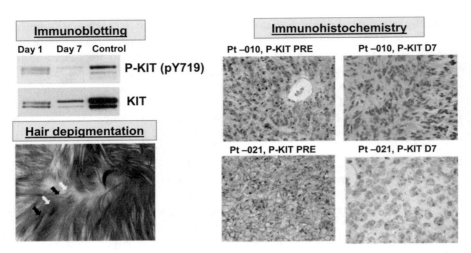

Figure 1.16. Evidence of sunitinib inhibition of KIT in repeat GIST tumor biopsies and KIT-dependent hair pigmentation (Moss et al., 2003; Demetri et al., 2004; Davis et al., 2005). (*Upper left panel*) Repeated resected biopsies (baseline and day 7 post–treatment) were obtained from a GIST patient, frozen, protein lysates were created and resolved by SDS-PAGE, transferred and immunoblots were performed utilizing total KIT and phosphorylated KIT (phosphotyrosine 719) antibodies. Results indicated a qualitative reduction in the levels of phosphorylated KIT following 7 days of sunitinib administration at 50 mg/day. (*Right panel*) Repeated biopsies (baseline and day 7 post–treatment) were obtained from 2 GIST patients (patients 010 and 021), were formalin-fixed and paraffin-embedded, and immunohistochemistry was performed utilizing a phosphorylated KIT (phosphotyrosine 719) antibody. Results indicated a qualitative reduction in the levels of phosphorylated KIT following 7 days of sunitinib administration at 50 mg/day. (*Lower left panel*) Images of study subject with metastatic synovial sarcoma undergoing treatment with SU11248. This subject received multiple 6-week cycles of treatment over a 4 week period receiving 50 mg SU11248 daily and a 2-week break from treatment. Cyclical hair depigmentation is evident that was concordant with the treatment regimen. Depigmented bands of hair grown during periods when the patient was receiving SU11248 (*white arrows*) are distinct from pigmented bands of hair grown during drug-free breaks (*black arrows*). (See color insert.)

cancer patients. The GIST study was an extension of earlier animal studies based on dysregulation of the RTK target, KIT. One particular patient population of interest was GIST patients who were imatinib refractory. SU11248 was shown to effectively bind to and inhibit mutated variants of KIT (e.g., T670I, V654A) that are associated with imatinib resistance and tumor progression (Prenen et al., 2006; Liegl et al., 2008). In the case of RCC patients, it was known that loss of VHL function was associated with high levels of HIF-1α, high levels of VEGF-A, and high microvessel density indicating that angiogenesis was highly dysregulated and may be particularly sensitive to SU11248 (Kim and Kaelin, 2006). Of the 117 patients enrolled on the initial single-agent

SU11248 Phase I clinical studies, there were a total of 16 confirmed objective partial responses including 4 in mRCC, 4 in GIST, and 2 in tumors of neuro-endocrine origin (Faivre et al., 2006; Christensen, 2007). This data was critical to select mRCC, imatinib-refractory GIST, and neuroendocrine tumors (pan-creatic islet and carcinoid) as the first three Phase II clinical studies for SU11248. This strategy and the data from these studies resulted in two regis-trational studies leading to a multinational regulatory approval of SU11248 for advanced RCC and imatinib-resistant or -intolerant GIST in 2006. Extensive clinical efforts to evaluate and understand the potential for SU11248 in other patient populations, its use in novel combination and chemotherapy scheduling strategies, as well as the exploration of potential patient selection strategies are presently ongoing.

1.12. SUMMARY

The recent success of targeted therapies for the treatment of human cancer resulted from enhanced knowledge of specific molecular targets and their association with the growth, survival, and metastatic spread of tumor cells. The identification of protein kinases, and more specifically protein tyrosine kinases, as potential drug targets prompted the pioneering research efforts in this area. SU11248 (sunitinib) emerged from a drug development program that was focused on understanding the cellular signaling mechanisms important in the development and treatment of human cancer. SU11248 resulted from many years of iterative drug design and development, as evidenced by its predeces-sors (Figure 1.17) and from collaborative efforts within the biotechnology and pharmaceutical industries and academia.

From a medicinal chemistry perspective, the indolin-2-one chemotype of SU11248 was interesting and was discovered serendipitously via random screening of chemical libraries with an enzymatic PDGF receptor protein kinase assay. The chemotype was selected primarily due to its selectivity for signaling-dependent activity in cellular systems and its potential for various levels of potency and selectivity for the individual members of class III and V receptor protein kinases. Early candidates (SU5416) effectively inhibited VEGFR in vitro and tumor angiogenesis in nonclinical models but possessed less suitable pharmaceutical properties necessary for practical use in a clinical setting. Later candidates, such as SU6668 and SU11248, were suitable for the clinic, were multitargeted, and established their antitumor activity with evidence of tumor regression as well as disruption of newly formed blood vessels (antiangiogenesis). In parallel, our understanding of the critical tyro-sine kinases (e.g., SCFR, KIT) necessary for growth and survival of selected tumor cells, such as GIST and others, was evolving. SU11248 simultaneously inactivated VEGF, PDGF, and SCF receptor tyrosine kinases and demon-strated improved solubility, bioavailability, and potency in animal model systems, which supported its transition to the clinical trial setting. Substantial

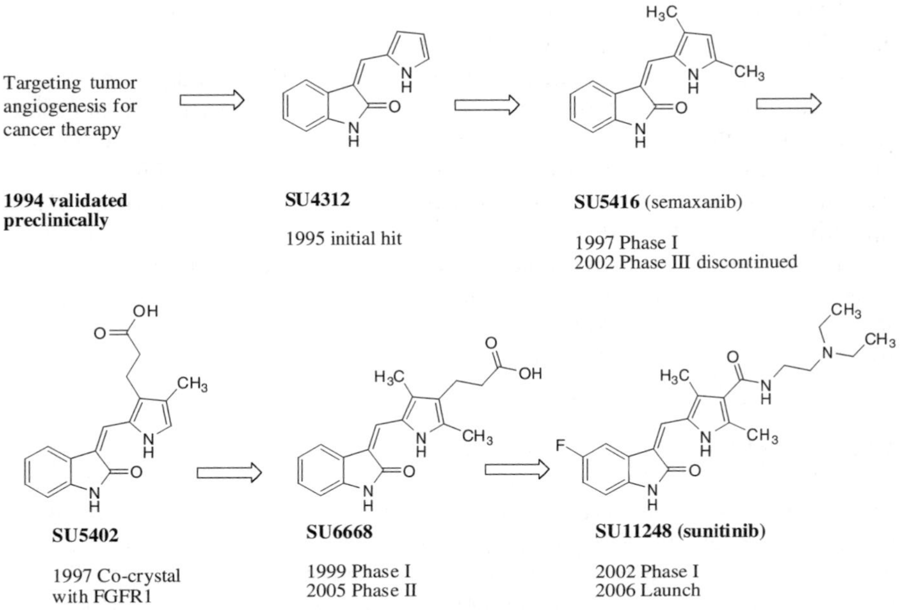

Targeting tumor angiogenesis for cancer therapy ⟹

1994 validated preclinically

SU4312

1995 initial hit

SU5416 (semaxanib)

1997 Phase I
2002 Phase III discontinued

SU5402

1997 Co-crystal with FGFR1

SU6668

1999 Phase I
2005 Phase II

SU11248 (sunitinib)

2002 Phase I
2006 Launch

Figure 1.17. Path to SU11248.

nonclinical studies were performed to establish the mechanisms of action, validate potential biomarkers, and provide the rationale for dose and patient selection. The SU11248 early clinical program established an understanding of key PK–PD relationships for selected RTK targets, supported Phase I dose selection, and demonstrated safety and antitumor activity in a variety of solid tumors. These early studies supported the registration path and eventual approval in indications where selected RTK targets were implicated such as angiogenesis in RCC or oncogenic signaling by mutated variants of KIT in GIST. Further studies evaluating sunitinib (SU11248) in other tumor types including breast cancer and non-small-cell lung cancer are ongoing.

ACKNOWLEDGMENTS

The authors would like to thank the founding scientists at Sugen, Dr. Joseph Schlessinger and Dr. Axel Ullrich, for their contributions to the understanding of signal transduction and their foresight of target protein kinases. We would also like to thank the many people who work at Sugen, Pharmacia, and Pfizer, Inc., who enabled the successful discovery, development, and commercial availability of sunitinib for use in the treatment of human cancers.

Editorial assistance was provided by Kristen Letrent of Pfizer, Inc. and by ACUMED® (Tytherington, UK) with funding from Pfizer, Inc.

REFERENCES

Abrams, T. J., Lee, L. B., Murray, L. J., et al. (**2003**). SU11248 inhibits KIT and platelet-derived growth factor receptor beta in preclinical models of human small cell lung cancer. *Mol Cancer Ther.* 2, 471–478.

Aiello, L. P, George, D. J, Cahill, M. T., et al. (**2002**). Rapid and durable recovery of visual function in a patient with von Hippel–Lindau syndrome after systemic therapy with vascular endothelial growth factor receptor inhibitor SU5416. *Ophthalmology.* 109(9), 1745–1751.

Arastéh, K., and Hannah, A. (**2000**). The role of vascular endothelial growth factor (VEGF) in AIDS-related Kaposi's sarcoma. *Oncologist.* 5 (Suppl 1):28–31.

Bello, C. L., DePrimo, S. E., Friece, C., et al. (**2006**). Analysis of circulating biomarkers of sunitinib malate in patients with unresectable neuroendocrine tumors (NET): VEGF, IL-8, and soluble VEGF receptors 2 and 3. *American Society of Clinical Oncology 42nd Annual Meeting*, Atlanta, GA, 2–6 June 2006.

Bergers, G., Song, S., Meyer-Morse, N., et al. (**2003**), Benefits of targeting both pericytes and endothelial cells in the tumor vasculature with kinase inhibitors. *J Clin Invest.* 111(9), 1277–1295.

Blume-Jensen, P., and Hunter, T. (**2001**). Oncogenic kinase signalling. *Nature.* 411, 355–365.

Carmeliet, P., Ferreira, V., Breier, G., et al. (**1996**). Abnormal blood vessel development and lethality in embryos lacking a single VEGF allele. *Nature.* 380, 435–439.

Cherrington, J. M., Strawn, L. M., and Shawver, L. K. (**2000**). New paradigms for the treatment of cancer; the role of anti-angiogenesis agents. *In:* G. Klein and G. F. Vande Woude (eds.), *Advances in Cancer Research*, Vol. 79, pp. 1–38. San Diego, CA: Academic Press.

Christensen, J. G. (**2007**). A preclinical review of sunitinib, a multitargeted receptor tyrosine kinase inhibitor with anti-angiogenic and antitumour activities. *In:* K. Fizazi (ed.), *A Multitargeted Approach: Clinical Advances in the Treatment of Solid Tumours*, Vol. 18 S10, Annals of Oncology, pp. 3–10.

Claffey, K. P., Brown, L. F., del Aguila, L. F., et al. (**1996**). Expression of vascular permeability factor/vascular endothelial growth factor by melanoma cells increases tumor growth, angiogenesis, and experimental metastasis. *Cancer Res.* 56, 172–181.

Davis, D. W, Heymach, J. V., McConkey, D. J., et al. (**2005**). Receptor tyrosine kinase activity and apoptosis in gastrointestinal stromal tumours: a pharmacodynamic analysis of response to sunitinib malate (SU11248) therapy. *Eur J Cancer Suppl.* 3, 203.

Demetri, G. D., Desai, J., Fletcher, J., et al. (**2004**). SU11248, a multi-targeted tyrosine kinase inhibitor, can overcome imatinib (IM) resistance caused by diverse genomic mechanisms in patients (pts) with metastatic gastrointestinal stromal tumor (GIST). *ASCO Annual Meeting 2004*; Abstract No. 3001.

DePrimo, S. E., Friece, C., Huang, X., et al. (**2006**). Effect of treatment with sunitinib malate, a multitargeted tyrosine kinase inhibitor, on circulating plasma levels of VEGF, soluble VEGF receptors 2 and 3 and soluble KIT in patients with metastatic breast cancer. *American Society of Clinical Oncology 42nd Annual Meeting*, Atlanta, GA, 2–6 June 2006.

DePrimo, S. E., Bello, C. L., Smeraglia, J., et al. (**2007**). Circulating protein biomarkers of pharmacodynamic activity of sunitinib in patients with metastatic renal cell carcinoma: modulation of VEGF and VEGF-related proteins. *J Translational Med.* 5, 32.

de Vries, C., Escobedo, J. A., Ueno, H., et al. (**1992**). The FMS-like tyrosine kinase, a receptor for vascular endothelial growth factor. *Science.* 255, 989–991.

Faivre, S., Delbaldo, C., Vera, K., et al. (**2006**). Safety, pharmacokinetic, and antitumor activity of SU11248, a novel oral multitarget tyrosine kinase inhibitor, in patients with cancer. *J Clin Oncol.* 24, 25–35.

Ferrara, N., and Henzel, W. J. (**1989**). Pituitary follicular cells secrete a novel heparin-binding growth factor specific for vascular endothelial cells. *Biochem Biophys Res Commun.* 161, 851–858.

Ferrara, N., Winer, J., Burton, T., et al. (**1993**). Expression of vascular endothelial growth factor does not promote transformation but confers a growth advantage in vivo to Chinese hamster ovary cells. *J Clin Invest.* 91, 160–170.

Ferrara, N., Carver-Moore, K., Chen, H., et al. (**1996**). Heterozygous embryonic lethality induced by targeted inactivation of the VEGF gene. *Nature.* 380, 439–442.

Ferrara, N. (**2004**). Vascular endothelial growth factor: basic science and clinical progress. *Endocr Rev.* 25, 581–611.

Fett, J. W., Strydom, D. J., Lobb, R. R., et al. (**1985**). Isolation and characterization of angiogenin, an angiogenic protein from human carcinoma cells. *Biochemistry.* 24, 5480–5486.

Fiedler, W., Mesters, R., Tinnefeld, H., et al. (**2003**). A Phase II clinical study of SU5416 in patients with refractory acute myeloid leukemia. *Blood.* 102(8), 2763–2767.

Folkman, J., Merler, E., Abernathy, C., and Williams, G. (**1971**). Isolation of a tumor factor responsible for angiogenesis. *J Exp Med.* 133, 275–288.

Folkman, J. (**1995**). Angiogenesis in cancer, vascular, rheumatoid and other disease. *Nat Med.* 1, 27–31.

Fong, G. H., Rossant, J., Gertsenstein, M., et al. (**1995**). Role of the Flt-1 receptor tyrosine kinase in regulating the assembly of vascular endothelium. *Nature.* 376, 66–70.

Fong, T. A. T., Shawver, L. K., Sun, L., et al. (**1999**). SU5416 is a potent and selective inhibitor of the vascular endothelial growth factor receptor (Flk-1/KDR) that inhibits tyrosine kinase catalysis, tumor vascularization, and growth of multiple tumor types. *Cancer Res.* 59(1), 99–106.

Giles, F. J., Stopeck, A. T., Silverman, L. R., et al. (**2003**). SU5416, a small molecule tyrosine kinase receptor inhibitor, has biologic activity in patients with refractory acute myeloid leukemia or myelodysplastic syndromes. *Blood.* 102(3), 795–801.

Heinrich, M. C., Blanke, C. D., Druker, B. J., et al. (**2002**). Inhibition of KIT tyrosine kinase activity: a novel molecular approach to the treatment of KIT-positive malignancies. *J Clin Oncol.* 20, 1692–1703.

Heinrich, M. C., Corless, C. L., Demetri, G. D., et al. (**2003**). Kinase mutations and imatinib response in patients with metastatic gastrointestinal stromal tumor. *J Clin Oncol.* 2, 4342–4349.

Ikezoe, T., Yang, Y., Kentaro, B., et al. (**2006**). Effects of SU11248, a class III and V receptor tyrosine kinase inhibitor, on GIST-T1 cells: enhancement of growth inhibition via inhibition of PI3K/Akt/mTOR signaling. *Cancer Sci.* 97, 945–951.

Kim, K. J., Li, B., Winer, J., et al. (**1993**). Inhibition of vascular endothelial growth factor-induced angiogenesis suppresses tumor growth in vivo. *Nature.* 362, 841–844.

Kim, W. Y., and Kaelin, W. G. Jr. (**2006**). Molecular pathways in renal cell carcinoma—rationale for targeted treatment. *Semin Oncol.* 33, 588–595.

Laird, A. D., Vajkoczy, P., Shawver, L. K., et al. (**2000**). SU6668 is a potent anti-angiogenic and anti-tumor agent that induces regression of established tumors. *Cancer Res.* 60, 4152–4160.

Lewis, W. H. (**1927**). The vascular pattern of tumors. *Johns Hopkins Hosp Bull.* 41, 156–162.

Liegl B., Kepten I., Le C., et al. (**2008**). Heterogeneity of kinase inhibitor resistance mechanisms in GIST. *J Pathol.* 216, 64–74.

London, C. A., Hannah, A. L., Zadovoskaya, R., et al. (**2003**). Phase I dose-escalating study of SU11654, a small molecule receptor tyrosine kinase inhibitor, in dogs with spontaneous malignancies. *Clin Cancer Res.* 9, 2755–2768.

Maciag, T., Mehlman, T., Friesel, R., and Schreiber, A. B. (**1984**). Heparin binds to endothelial cell growth factor, the principal endothelial cell mitogen in bovine brain. *Science.* 225, 932–935.

Manning, G., Whyte, D. B., Martinez, R., et al. (**2002**). The protein kinase complement of the human genome. *Science.* 298, 1912–1934.

McDermott, U., Sharma, S. V., and Dowell, L. (**2007**). Identification of genotype-correlated sensitivity to selective kinase inhibitors by using high-throughput tumor cell line profiling. *Proc Natl Acad Sci USA.* 104, 19936–19941.

Mendel, D. B., Laird, A. D., Xin, X., et al. (**2003**). In vivo anti-tumor activity of SU11248, a novel tyrosine kinase inhibitor targeting vascular endothelial growth factor and platelet-derived growth factor receptors: determination of a pharmaco-kinetic/pharmacodynamic relationship. *Clin Cancer Res.* 9, 327–337.

Millauer, B., Shawver, L. K., Plate, K. H., et al. (**1994**). Glioblastoma growth inhibited in vivo by a dominant-negative Flk-1 mutant. *Nature.* 367, 576–579.

Millauer, B., Longhi, M. P., Plate, K. H., et al. (**1996**). Dominant-negative inhibition of Flk-1 suppresses the growth of many tumor types in vivo. *Cancer Res.* 56, 1615–1620.

Mohammadi, M., McMahon, G., Sun, L., et al. (**1997**). Structures of the tyrosine kinase domain of fibroblast growth factor receptor in complex with inhibitors. *Science.* 276, 955–960.

Moss, K. G., Toner, G. C., Cherrington, J. M., et al. (**2003**). Hair depigmentation is a biological readout for pharmacological inhibition of KIT in mice and humans. *J Pharmacol Exp Ther.* 307, 476–480.

Motzer, R. J., Michaelson, M. D., Redman, B. G., et al. (**2006**). Activity of SU11248, a multitargeted inhibitor of vascular endothelial growth factor receptor and platelet-derived growth factor receptor, in patients with metastatic renal cell carcinoma. *J Clin Oncol.* 24, 16–24.

O'Farrell, A. M., Abrams, T. J., Yuen, H. A., et al. (**2003a**). SU11248 is a novel FLT3 tyrosine kinase inhibitor with potent activity in vitro and in vivo. *Blood.* 101, 3597–3605.

O'Farrell, A. M., Foran, J. M., Fiedler, W., et al. (**2003b**). An innovative Phase I clinical study demonstrates inhibition of FLT3 phosphorylation by SU11248 in acute myeloid leukemia patients. *Clin Cancer Res.* 9, 5465–5476.

Pietras, K., Sjoblom, T., Rubin, K., et al. (**2003**). PDGF receptors as cancer drug targets. *Cancer Cell*. 3, 439–443.

Plate, K. H., Breier, G., Weich, H. A., et al. (**1992**). Vascular endothelial growth factor is a potential tumour angiogenesis factor in human gliomas in vivo. *Nature*. 359, 845–848.

Potapova, O., Laird, A. D., Nannini, M., et al. (**2006**). Contribution of individual targets to the anti-tumor efficacy of the multi-targeted receptor tyrosine kinase inhibitor SU11248. *Mol Cancer Ther*. 5, 1280–1289.

Prenen, H., Cools, J., Mentens, N., et al. (**2006**). Efficacy of the kinase inhibitor SU11248 against gastrointestinal stromal tumor (GIST) mutants refractory to imatinib mesylate. *Clin Cancer Res*. 12, 2622–2627.

Reinmuth, N., Liu, W., Jung, Y. D., et al. (**2001**). Induction of VEGF in perivascular cells defines a potential paracrine mechanism for endothelial cell survival. *FASEB J*. 15(7), 1239–1241.

Schlessinger, J. (**2000**). Cell signaling by receptor tyrosine kinases. *Cell*. 103, 211–225.

Scott, A. M., Mitchell, P., O'Keefe, G., et al. (**2005**). Tumor perfusion as assessed by (oxygen-15)-water PET imaging during treatment with sunitinib malate (SU11248) in patients with advanced malignancies. Presented at the International Conference on Molecular Targets and Cancer Therapeutics. Philadelphia, PA, November 2005.

Senger, D. R., Galli, S. J., Dvorak, A. M., et al. (**1983**). Tumor cells secrete a vascular permeability factor that promotes accumulation of ascites fluid. *Science*. 219, 983–985.

Shing, Y., Folkman, J., Sullivan, R., et al. (**1984**). Heparin affinity: purification of a tumor derived capillary endothelial cell growth factor. *Science*. 223, 1296–1298.

Shweiki, D., Itin, A., Soffer, D., et al. (**1992**). Vascular endothelial growth factor induced by hypoxia may mediate hypoxia-initiated angiogenesis. *Nature*. 359, 843–845.

Sun, L., Tran, N., Tang, F., et al. (**1998**). Synthesis and biological evaluations of 3-substituted indolin-2-ones: a novel class of tyrosine kinase inhibitors that exhibit selectivity towards particular receptor tyrosine kinases. *J Med Chem*. 41(14), 2588–2603.

Sun, L., Tran, N., Liang, C., et al. (**1999**). Design, synthesis, and evaluations of substituted 3-[(3- or 4-carboxyethylpyrrol-2-yl)methylidenyl]indolin-2-ones as inhibitors of VEGF, FGF, and PDGF receptor tyrosine kinases. *J Med Chem*. 42(25), 5120–5130.

Sun, L., Liang, C., Shirazian, S., et al. (**2003**). Discovery of 5-[5-fluoro-2-oxo-1,2-dihydroindol-(3Z)-ylidenemethyl]-2,4-dimethyl-1H-pyrrole-3-carboxylic acid (2-diethylaminoethyl)amide, a novel tyrosine kinase inhibitor targeting vascular endothelial and platelet-derived growth factor receptor tyrosine kinase. *J Med Chem*. 46, 1116–1119.

Tannock, I. F. (**1968**). The relation between cell proliferation and the vascular system in a transplanted mouse mammary tumour. *Br. J. Cancer*. 22, 258–273.

Terman, B. I., Dougher-Vermazen, M., Carrion, M. E., et al. (**1992**). Identification of the KDR tyrosine kinase as a receptor for vascular endothelial cell growth factor. *Biochem Biophys Res Commun*. 187, 1579–1586.

Vajkoczy, P., Menger, M. D., Vollmar, B., et al. (**1999**). Inhibition of tumor growth, angiogenesis, and microcirculation by the novel Flk-1 inhibitor SU5416 as assessed by intravital multi-fluorescence videomicroscopy. *Neoplasia.* 1(1), 31–41.

Yao, V. J., Sennino, B., Davis, R. B., et al. (**2006**). Combined anti-VEGFR and anti-PDGFR actions of sunitinib on blood vessels in preclinical tumor models. *The 18th EORTC–NCI–AACR Symposium*, Prague, Czech Republic, 7–10 November 2006.

2

TYKERB DISCOVERY: A DUAL EGFR AND ERBB2 TYROSINE KINASE INHIBITOR

KAREN LACKEY AND G. STUART COCKERILL

2.1. INTRODUCTION

Most cells in the human body use a system of communication that involves signal cascades connecting the messages from outside the cells to the nucleus largely through growth factors, cytokines, and hormones. Cell proliferation signaling is initiated upon ligand-induced dimerization of growth factor receptors via formation of hetero- and homodimers with members of the Type I receptor kinase family, which includes EGFR (erbB1), erbB2 (HER2), the tyrosine kinase inactive erbB3, and erbB4 (Yarden and Sliwkowski, 2001). Aberrant signaling from overexpression or constitutive activation has been associated with tumor growth in certain solid tumors, which include a subset of breast, non-small-cell lung cancer (NSCLC), gastric, colon, head and neck, and ovarian cancer (Klapper et al., 2000) GlaxoSmithKline scientists discovered an orally available, potent, reversible, small-molecule tyrosine kinase inhibitor of both EGFR and erbB2 activity. With over 500 different kinases in human cells that are used in every biological process, it is a major challenge to design selective inhibitors, where the compounds bind to the ATP site of specific kinases preferentially, avoiding kinases that could result in side effects or toxicity, and modulate the signal in the cell milieu that contains naturally high concentrations of ATP.

Well-known examples of potent EGFR TK inhibitors currently in clinical trials or used for anticancer therapy are shown in Figure 2.1 (Baselga and

Kinase Inhibitor Drugs. Edited by Rongshi Li and Jeffrey A. Stafford
Copyright © 2009 John Wiley & Sons, Inc.

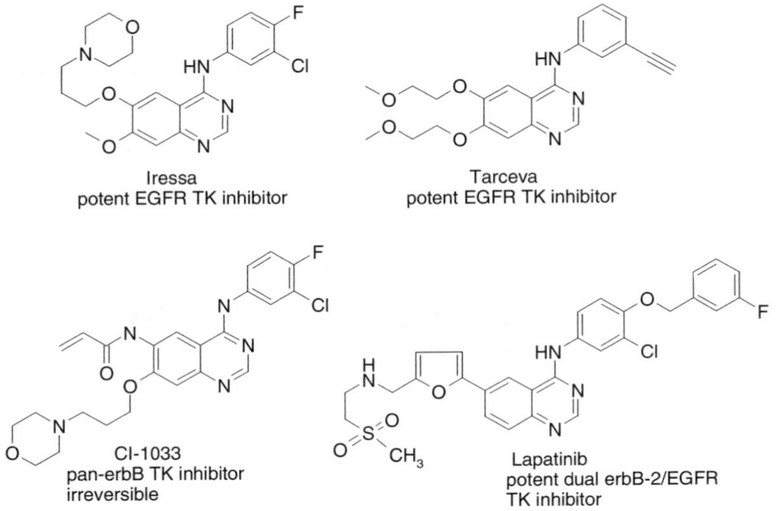

Figure 2.1. Potent erbB family TK inhibitors with cancer clinical trial results.

Averbuch, 2000; de Bono and Rowinsky, 2002; Tiseo et al., 2004). While there are clearly similarities in structure for the leading compounds in the field, there are differences in the kinase inhibition profiles, mechanisms of inhibition, in vivo properties, and more. Rather than cover them here, there are several published reviews covering small-molecule Type I receptor inhibitors that provide excellent information regarding the current state of the art in this class of drug candidates (Ranson, 2004). A range of results for signaling inhibitors are emerging from clinical trials and a review by Pearson and Fabbro (2004) summarizes the key issues and strategies used to address the drug development of kinase inhibitors.

Successful drug discovery is always worth reviewing and analyzing, if only for the question "Why did that project produce a drug?" The history of the discovery of the target often provides an answer and the erbB2/EGFR story is a useful exemplar. The erbB oncogene family was revealed by characterization of the erbB1 gene (EGFR) in 1984 (Downward et al., 1984) and erbB2 followed a year later (Semba et al., 1985). The oncogene identifications were further validated as viable drug targets by a clinical link to cancer progression in 1987 (Sainsbury et al., 1987). The outstanding molecular oncology discoveries that occurred during this period of time have led ultimately to many of the current signaling drug intervention points being pursued in the drug discovery industry today. How Tykerb was discovered and brought to the clinic in the following twenty years is a journey through company mergers and scientific strategies, a journey guided by people committed to the project and to the purpose of finding medicines for unmet medical needs. The Tykerb story shows that the two key ingredients in the discovery of worthwhile new treatments are commitment and excellence in science.

2.2. EARLY EFFORTS ESTABLISHED THE FEASIBILITY OF INHIBITING ERBB2 AND EGFR TYROSINE KINASE ACTIVITY AS A DRUG INTERVENTION APPROACH

The Wellcome Foundation had initiated an interest in the erbB2 receptor as a cancer target for several years in the 1980s due to the clinical influence of the oncogene on the disease-free and overall survival of breast cancer patients (Sainsbury et al., 1987). A general scheme for the signaling pathway is shown in Figure 2.2. While the overall protein structure is similar, the four members of the erbB family display differences in the autophosphorylation docking sites, in substrate specificity, and in the potency of the kinase activity. By way of example, erbB3 lacks kinase activity and erbB-2 has no known ligand, but has the highest transforming capability (Alroy and Yarden, 1997). These erbB family receptors are membrane spanning with a cysteine-rich extracellular ligand binding domain, a hydrophobic membrane-spanning region, and an intracellular domain containing the kinase function (Riese and Stern, 1998). The homo- or heterodimerization of erbB receptors after specific extracellular ligand binding leads to the activation of the intrinsic tyrosine kinase activity via autophosphorylation, or heterodimerization and transactivation-autophosphorylation of erbB2. The formation of the erbB family dimers activates downstream Erk1/2 MAP kinases and PI3K/AKT kinase survival pathways (Riese and Stern, 1998; Moghal and Sternberg, 1999).

The Wellcome Foundation in Beckenham in Kent increased its interest in the erbB/EGFR family of tyrosine kinases in the early 1990s. The interest was

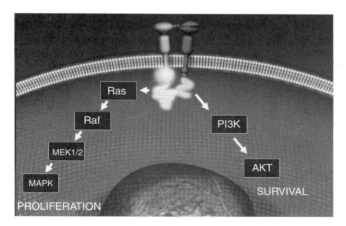

Figure 2.2. Schematic rendition of the erbB family signaling pathway. (See color insert.)

focused on both EGFR and the lesser characterized erbB2. Initial studies with EGFR were carried out using receptor/kinase isolated from EGFR overexpressing A-431 cell preparations utilizing a radiometric measure of autophosphorylation. The oncology research team at Beckenham was able to clone and express a partial construct of the erbB2 receptor. Since the construct contained the intracellular kinase portion of the receptor and had functional activity, the team was able to specifically target the protein with small molecules by means of a radiometric substrate phosphorylation assay. Several cell line clones were established so that compounds could be assessed for their specific intracellular mechanistic inhibition of erbB2 autophosphorylation as opposed to other downstream kinase inhibition. These cell lines were engineered from a human breast line and were designated as HB4a.c5.2, an erbB2 overexpressing line, and HB4.c4.2, which contained mutant *ras* (downstream of the desired signal inhibition) thus serving as a pathway selectivity control. While this work was ongoing, further target validation was added to the scientific literature by Brandt and colleagues (1995), describing the prognostic relevance of erbB oncogenes in several cancers. Screening in the early part of the drug discovery program was done in a modest and focused manner. Screening of a variety of known kinase chemotypes, both available commercially and derived from other projects within the company, for example, staurosporines, their aglycones, bis-indolylmaleimides, and coumarin analogs, had provided some level of activity against both kinases. Establishment of a project screening cascade enabled the start-up of a full chemistry research optimization effort by mid- to late 1994. The landmark discovery of PD153035, wherein selective EGFR activity was demonstrated for the first time, provided the project with a fresh impetus (Fry et al., 1994).

In light of the anilinoquinazoline EGFR activity, sets of compounds were synthesized based on this substructure. Initial examples contained either an unsubstituted quinazoline or the 6,7-dimethoxy variant as shown in Figure 2.3. Multiple variations of substitutions on the aniline were prepared, where the compound design was based largely on intermediate availability and synthetic accessibility due to scant structure–activity relationship (SAR) data and no protein crystal structure. While several years in advance of Lipinski's guidelines (Lipinski et al., 1997) and the advent of ligand efficiency design principles (Hopkins et al., 2004), compounds synthesized at this stage were low molecular weight (<400 Da) with appropriate $c \log P$ values allowing room for elaboration in lead optimization. In addition, all compounds synthesized for the inhibition of the target, including intermediates, were screened in the enzyme and cellular assays.

Trends observable among this group of compounds was that potency in both the erbB2 assay and EGFR assays was much enhanced with the 6,7-dimethoxy substitution. The aniline substitution pattern provided a more subtle set of relationships and the SAR remained consistent through the entire duration of the drug discovery effort. For example, substituents like halogens and methoxy, particularly in the 3-position of the aniline, **2** in Figure 2.3,

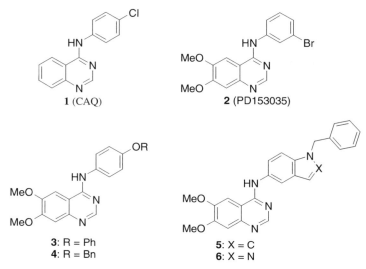

Figure 2.3. Early potent erbB family TK inhibitors.

provided modest EGFR and erbB2 activity, but the erbB2 potency could be improved significantly by the inclusion of a larger substituent such as the 4-benzyloxy as shown for **4** (Brignola et al., 2002). Other similar substituents like 4-phenoxy aniline **3** provided good activity although also had generally poorer kinase selectivity. Notable among other modifications of this larger substituent were the "tied back" versions like 4-(N-benzyl indol-5-yl) quinazoline **5** and 4-(N-benzylindazol-5-yl) quinazoline **6**. These findings were important in staying focused on discovering a drug with potent erbB2 inhibition, the key target identified in the molecular oncology studies to date. At this point, the known literature from competitor companies only described examples of selective EGFR inhibitors that contained the smaller halogen or acetylene substituted anilines.

It was important to establish that inhibiting the desired target(s) led to an efficacious response in an animal model. Human xenograft mouse models using relevant cell lines whose growth was driven by erbB family signaling were chosen at the time due to the lack of other viable ways to test multiple compounds in an antitumor activity assay. Early human tumor xenograft mouse studies were performed for **4** and **6** because their cell activity in EGFR and erbB2 driven lines, albeit not very potent, was consistent with the desired mechanism. The in vivo efficacy evaluation strategy was biased toward erbB2 by utilizing the N87 gastric cell line, which was driven predominantly by erbB2, dosing at 10 mg/kg bid in 25% β-cyclodextrin sulfobutyl ether. Inhibition of tumor growth could be observed in this higher throughput, rapidly growing xenograft and the better compounds were progressed into the slower, more difficult to maintain, erbB2 driven, BT-474 breast cell line xenograft model. In both tumor models, indazolyl quinazoline **6** was shown to be superior to the simpler aniline-quinazoline **4**. A benefit of the corporate merger between Glaxo and Burroughs Wellcome was the increased kinase profiling capacity of Glaxo Wellcome. Anilinoquinazoline **4** was shown to be a selective inhibitor of the erbB family kinases across a panel of over 30 kinases, including c-src, c-Raf1, VEGFR2, TIE2, and CDK2. By combining the data for the lead compounds' kinase profile with the cell activity in relevant tumor lines, the dual EGFR/erbB2 tyrosine kinase inhibition concept proved feasible. This tool compound, **4**, served a valuable purpose for establishing the in vivo models and confidence to move forward into a lead optimization phase and as such became a high priority project for the oncology research area at Glaxo Wellcome.

2.3. LEAD OPTIMIZATION EFFORTS PRODUCED TWO DRUG CANDIDATES WITH THE DESIRED MECHANISM OF ACTION: GW2974 AND GW0277

Modifications to the central core quinazoline became a feature of the medicinal chemistry campaign to search for potency and SAR, but also as an approach to reducing log P and perhaps improving physicochemical characteristics. A range of heteroatoms was investigated in order to provide alternatives to the phenyl ring of the quinazoline. Among these were thienopyrimidines exemplified by **7** shown in Figure 2.4 and regioisomers of the pyridopyrimidine system. The most interesting quinazoline alternative from these core quinazoline change studies was the pyrido[3,4-*d*]pyrimidine exemplified by **8**.

Initial data from this series were encouraging as compound **8** had a bioavailability of 37% in rats and represented an improvement over quinazoline analogs. The synthesis of these compounds, outlined in Figure 2.5, allowed the team to scale up intermediates and synthesize a large number of analogs to fully probe the SAR (Cockerill et al., 2001). The versatility of the reaction sequences proved invaluable as larger amounts of materials were needed for in vivo studies and toxicology evaluations.

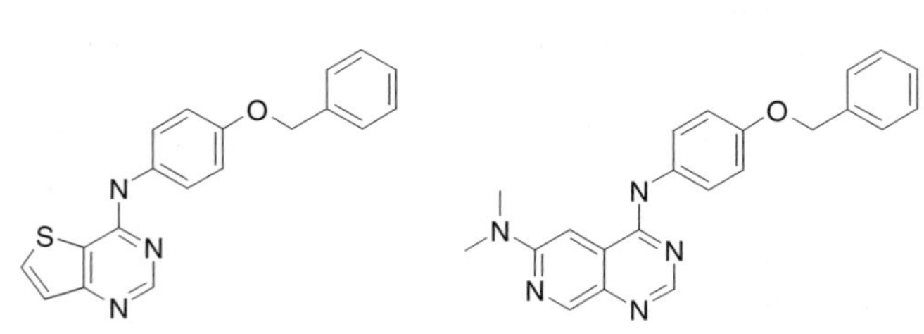

Figure 2.4. Core quinazoline changes designed to improve compound properties.

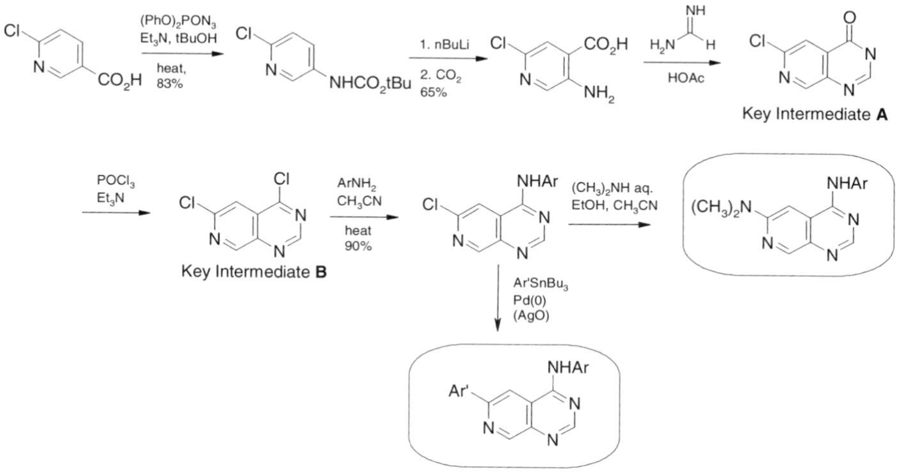

Figure 2.5. General synthesis for pyridopyrimidine scaffold.

The program strategy utilized several assays in parallel, thus requiring the chemists to make sufficient quantity of the first batch of each novel compound in order to perform enzyme, cell, and pharmacokinetic evaluations. Since the team lacked access to a raft of in vitro permeability, stability, and solubility assays, an LCMS based in vivo cassette pharmacokinetic rat assay assumed a primary testing position (Shaffer et al., 1999). Flexibility on the exact criteria for enzyme potency and kinase selectivity was employed, so that compounds that met basic, nominal erbB2-driven cell activity (<500 nM) and PK criteria ($F > 10\%$, plasma concentrations >500 nM at $t = 8$ h) were progressed into the human xenograft mouse models. It is fair to say that the cell assays were the key decision-making assays, dramatically overshadowing the kinase enzyme activities. Criteria as described above were not rigidly enforced and during this phase of the project compounds were often progressed into in vivo studies. A "criteria test mentality" was a key part of the project ethos.

The leading compound to appear from this exercise was the benzyl indazole **9** (GW2974) shown in Figure 2.6 (Cockerill et al., 2001). It was one of the first compounds to exhibit an IC_{50} value under 100 nM in the HB4a.c5.2, the c-erbB2 overexpressing cell line, and appeared potent (IC_{50} ~250 nM) in three relevant tumor cell lines: BT474 breast cancer cell line, CaLu3 lung line, and HN5 head and neck tumor line. Another characteristic of **9**, and indeed the series, was its selectivity for the erbB family of kinases as no appreciable activity was observed for the c-src, MAPK, and CDK families. Cell selectivity was good as measured by comparing the *erbB*-driven versus the *ras*-driven HB4a results. Compound **9** exhibited moderate clearance in rats, marmosets, and dogs; a variable intravenous (IV) half-life in these species (18–44 minutes); and a moderate volume of distribution equivalent to or slightly in excess of whole

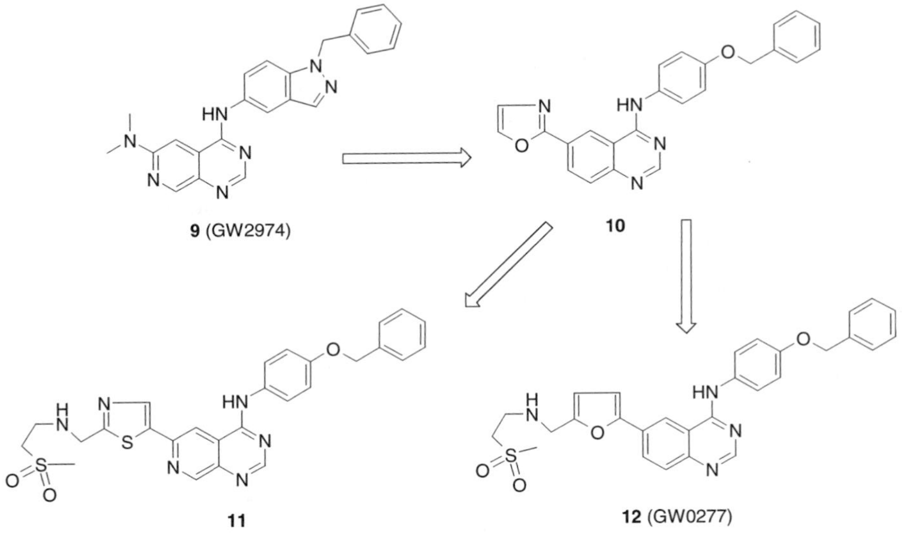

Figure 2.6. Advanced EGFR/erbB2 tyrosine kinase inhibitors.

body volume. Mean plasma levels on repeat dosing in rats and mice showed that levels above the IC_{50} for the compound could be maintained at doses of 20 mg/kg bid. At a dose of 10 mg/kg, complete inhibition of tumor growth was observed for **9** in the BT474 xenograft mouse model and >85% inhibition of tumor growth was observed in the Calu3 and HN5 model (Rusnak et al., 2001a,b). These results were better than expected from the exposure data from the pharmacokinetic studies. When the dose was increased to 50 mg/kg, irreversible tumor regression was observed (Cockerill et al., 2001). Based on the efficacy and mechanism of action of **9**, it was progressed into preclinical development. Several issues were uncovered at this stage. The pharmacokinetics were evaluated more extensively and found to be nonlinear and **9** had a saturation of metabolism effect that occurred at higher doses, presumably associated with N-demethylation. Variably active metabolites formed, and the inherent insolubility of **9** was found difficult to work with. Finally, a number of hematological and lymphoid effects precluded the initial definition of a no effect level. GW2974 could have been a first-generation, effective dual erbB2/EGFR TK inhibitor for a selective set of advanced cancer patients whose tumors are driven by this mechanism. Although the issues could have been addressed, the further development of **9** was halted, as the strategy was taken to deliver a dual inhibitor that possessed an improved therapeutic index.

Dual erbB2/EGFR potency, good rat pharmacokinetic properties, and cellular activity were discovered in the 6-heteroaryl quinazolines (**10**) and 6-heteroaryl pyridopyrimidines. When this 6-heteroaryl-containing core was combined with the moderately basic methylsulfonylethyl-aminomethylene side chain, potent compounds like GW0277 (**12**) were identified and provided the basis for the subsequent medicinal chemistry strategy to achieve the desired product profile. An immense amount of work is summarized in Figure 2.6, which omits dead ends and an intensive investigation of solubilizing side chains. Lead compounds from this effort were thiazole pyridopyrimidine **11** and furan quinazoline **12**. Compound **11** exhibited good linear, multispecies pharmacokinetics but only moderate cell potencies. Subsequently, moderate animal model efficacy was achieved. Compound **12** exhibited very good cell efficacy but only very moderate pharmacokinetics in rats. Despite this seemingly inadequate PK, compound **12** demonstrated good activity in mouse xenograft models. Although not understood at the time, perhaps some correlation can now be drawn (in hindsight) with efficacy not dependent on assumed plasma coverage. The high protein binding of the compound seemed to conclusively preclude any free fraction argument.

2.4. DATA REANALYSIS AND MIX-AND-MATCH STRATEGY LEAD TO TYKERB

The project had reached a critical decision point because several viable drug candidates had been discovered, each with the desired novel mechanism of action, but each had a feature preventing development. There remained bias in the scientific community regarding the feasibility of discovering a selective, and therefore presumed nontoxic kinase inhibitor. Considerable resource had been dedicated to the dual erbB2/EGFR TK inhibitor project, so we needed a way to determine if a drug could be discovered that met the desired product profile. At this point in the drug discovery efforts, we did not have access to a crystal structure of EGFR, as is currently state-of-the art in the field (Stamos et al., 2002). Earlier design work was guided by using p38 crystal structures as a surrogate for the creation of a docking model for the quinazoline and pyridopyrimidine series with a binding mode that did not correlate to the enzyme SAR.

All of the data generated to date in the project was compiled together and reanalyzed. A calculated index for the SAR of dual inhibition or pan-erbB family inhibition was created to combine multiple parameters into one value for rapid analysis of general trends and was used for kinase enzyme and cellular proliferation assay data (Lackey, 2006). Data for more than 3000 compounds were included and there was an apparent lack of correlation between the enzyme profile and the desired cellular activity. A subset of compounds was tested in multiple developability assays (e.g., solubility in multiple solvents, cell permeability assays, protein binding measures, in vitro metabolic stability) and the physical properties of the compounds could not explain the apparent lack of correlation between the cellular and enzyme activity. The data were parsed and only the trends from the subset of compounds with a reasonable correlation between the cell and enzyme values were studied for determining the preferred groups.

TABLE 2.1. Summary of Primary Assays Used in the Lead Optimization Phase

In Vitro Assays	Cell Panel	In Vivo Assays
Purified, catalytic EGFR, erbB2, and erbB4/ peptide substrate	Normal control line: HFF (normal fibroblast)	Limited pharmacokinetic analyses
Mixed binding and catalytic kinase panel of assays	Tumor lines: BT474 (breast) erbB2+++ NH5 (head/neck) EGFR+++ N87 (gastric) erbB2+++/ EGFR+	Tumor xenograft assays: BT474 HN5
Variety of developability assays such as solubility, permeability, and p450	Transform lines: HB4a r4.1 (Ha-*ras*) HB4a c5.2 (c-*erbB2*)	In vivo kinase inhibition

The compound evaluation pathway summarized in Table 2.1 was revamped, but it is important to note that the general principles of using the cellular panel of assays and pharmacokinetic evaluations remained the same. In the early stages of the drug discovery program, an unpurified version of the assay system was used and was able to determine active EGFR and erbB2 inhibitors, but the SAR interpretations were less robust. Different catalytic properties and substrate kinetics exist for the three kinase active members of the erbB family (Brignola et al., 2002). By purifying the enzymes and optimizing the biochemical and kinetic parameters, accurate SAR comparisons from the EGFR, erbB2, and erbB4 assay results could be made. The cell-based assay included HN5 and BT474, as described earlier, with the addition of a gastric carcinoma line N87 with overexpression of both erbB2 and EGFR (Pasleau et al., 1993; Modjtahedi et al., 1998). A control cell line, derived from human foreskin fibroblasts (HFF), was used to assess the selectivity for tumor cells versus normal cells. To further confirm that the compounds were active and selective due to their inhibition of erbB2, the transfected cell system in which proliferation is driven by either *erbB2* (HB4a c5.2) or mutant Ha-*ras* (HB4a r4.1) continued to be used to ensure that the compound effects were not due to inhibition of downstream members of the signal cascade (Harris et al., 1999).

Two of the tumor lines, BT474 and HN5 (EGFR), were grown as subcutaneous human tumor xenograft models and compounds were evaluated in each model at two doses (30 and 100 mg/kg bid, 21 days) after the tumors reached a standard size in duplicate experiments with 8 animals per study group (Rusnak et al., 2001a). After the 21 days of dosing, tissue samples were saved for clinical chemistry parameters and liver, gastrointestinal, kidney, and cardiac pathology. An in vivo kinase inhibition assay was established to correlate the observed tumor growth inhibition to the inhibition of receptor TK phosphorylation without affecting the protein expression level. Animals were treated

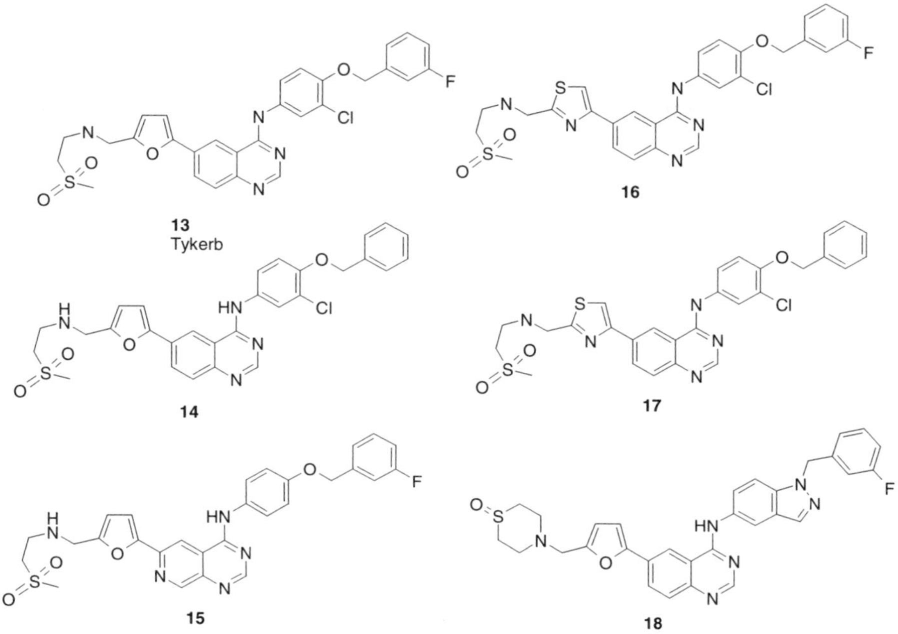

Figure 2.7. Top six derivatives evaluated for drug candidate selection.

orally for five doses (twice daily) and the treated tumors were excised and the inhibition of phophorylated tyrosine levels were measured compared with the tumors of the untreated animals. A limited PK protocol was developed to assess the compounds in a standardized procedure to understand some SAR in the pharmacokinetic properties. A truncated protocol of using four time points and two animals per time point predicted a full pharmacokinetic profile for oral dosing. The calculated values for the area under the curve (AUC) for the plotted data were used to assess the compounds, and trends for improved oral bioavailability could be seen even with relatively small numbers of compounds.

Approximately 70 compounds were synthesized in this phase of the project, and 6 highly functionalized quinazolines and pyridopyrimidine compounds shown in Figure 2.7 were chosen for early toxicity studies. Twenty-two distinguishing candidate selection criteria included efficacy parameters (cellular and in vivo), biometabolism parameters (time of drug exposure over IC_{50} or IC_{90} levels, percent oral bioavailability, p450 enzymes), toxicity measurements (cellular, cardiovascular, 7 day rat studies, Ames test), and chemical issues (cost of goods, scalability). Blood samples were collected at the end of 21 day dosing from all of the animals receiving 100 mg/kg bid of compound in our antitumor evaluations for the following clinical chemistry parameters: hemolysis, albumin, alkaline phosphatase, serum glutamic-oxaloacetic transaminase, blood urea nitrogen, cholesterol, total protein, glucose, sodium, potassium, and chloride (Keith et al., 2001). While the general appearance and lack of body weight loss demonstrated that the top six compounds were well tolerated, varied results were obtained in the clinical chemistry analysis, and only compounds with no effects on these selected clinical chemistry parameters were considered for drug development.

2.5. DRUG CANDIDATE SELECTION

Lapatinib is potent on two of the erbB family members with enzymatic IC_{50} values against erbB2 and EGFR receptor tyrosine kinases of 9 and 10 nM, respectively, with greater than an order of magnitude loss in activity for erbB4 (Rusnak et al., 2001b). A small-molecule kinase interaction map was created for lapatinib (GW2016) by Ambit researchers using an ATP site-dependent competition binding assay in a panel of 119 kinases and demonstrated a very clean profile (Fabian et al., 2005). The average range of IC_{50} values obtained for lapatinib in tumor cell lines that had Type I receptor expression was ~50–125 nM with an average cellular selectivity of 100-fold.

Lichtner and co-workers (2001) reported the cellular effects of quinazolines and 4,5-dianilinophthalimides, two classes of potent EGFR TK inhibitors, and found that the quinazoline's cellular efficacy was due to a novel mode of action even though both classes of compounds bind in the ATP site with similar potency. The quinazoline inhibitors affected the ligand binding properties by stabilizing the ligand/receptor/inhibitor complex resulting in potent cellular activity, while the dianilinopthalimides did not. Studies were performed with lapatinib to determine if there was a similar explanation for its effectiveness in the preclinical models. The inhibitor off-rates were evaluated using an EGFR enzyme reactivation procedure and Tarceva™ was found to have a rapid off-rate ($t_{1/2} < 10$ minutes) whereas after preincubation with lapatinib, there was a significantly slower off-rate ($t_{1/2} = 300$ minutes) (Wood et al., 2004). A similar dissociation rate was observed with lapatinib using erbB2. The crystal structure of EGFR bound to lapatinib revealed an inactive-like conformation in contrast to the published active-like structure with Tarceva (Stamos et al., 2002). The differences in the ligand-bound structures included the shape of the ATP site (closed versus open conformation), the position of the C helix (large back pocket versus intact Glu738–Lys721 salt bridge), the conformation of the COOH-terminal tail (partially blocking the ATP cleft versus poorly defined), the conformation of the activation loop (A-loop similar to ones found in inactive structures versus ones found for active structures), and the hydrogen bonding pattern with quinazoline scaffold (water-mediated interaction with Thr830 versus Thr766). To determine if the kinetics affected cellular activity, HN5 tumor cells were treated for 4 hours with lapatinib, and the receptor phosphorylation was analyzed at multiple time points after washout. The slow off-rate found for lapatinib in the enzyme reaction correlated with the observed, prolonged signal inhibition in tumor cells based on receptor tyrosine phosphorylation measurements. Lapatinib not only inhibits baseline activation of both erbB2 and EGFR but also interrupts downstream activation of Erk1/2 MAP kinases and AKT (Xia et al., 2002). The inhibition of AKT by lapatinib was associated with a 23-fold increase in apoptosis compared with vehicle controls. Lapatinib was also found to inhibit the signal transduction in the presence of saturating concentrations of epidermal growth factor (EGF), in tumor cell lines that overexpress Type I receptors as well as stimulated tumor lines that do not overexpress EGFR by measuring the p-Tyr, p-ERK, and p-AKT levels. Many more cellular activity and mechanism of action evaluations were done to understand the scope of a dual erbB2/EGFR TK inhibitor. We were confident that lapatinib had the desired in vitro properties of efficacy and selectivity.

Lapatinib demonstrated reproducible tumor growth inhibition of $34 \pm 28\%$ (30 mg/kg bid) and $101 \pm 20\%$ (100 mg/kg bid), in the HN5 xenograft model with regression (defined as >25% reduction in tumor volume) in 33% of the treated animals (Rusnak et al., 2001b). In the BT474 model, inhibition of $42 \pm 35\%$ (30 mg/kg bid) and $94 \pm 18\%$ (100 mg/kg bid) was observed with 10% of the treated animals with regressions. The level of erbB2 phosphotyrosine in tumor excised after therapy in the 100 mg/kg treatment was reduced by 93% in the BT474 model and 85% in the HN5 model and occurred in a dose-dependent manner for other treatment groups. Lapatinib was not toxic at this dose and activity/safety profiles observed in the xenograft models suggested that lapatinib could also be safely combined with standard chemotherapy (Mullin, 2003). We focused on the correlation of efficacy and mechanism of action and disregarded the high doses needed in the xenograft models due to the inherent limitations of the system.

Safety and tolerability was demonstrated in Phase I and Phase II human clinical studies, with healthy volunteers as well as cancer patients (Bence et al., 2005). The safety studies were designed to prepare for the long-term usage anticipated in early disease and cancer preventive settings, thus the need for a drug candidate with a large therapeutic window. Clinical responses were observed in heavily pretreated Phase I patients with metastatic diseases in both EGFR-driven and erbB2 overexpressing solid tumors in several cancer types, which included breast, non-small-cell lung, bladder, and head and neck (Spector et al., 2005). Biomarkers of signal inhibition were used throughout the drug discovery program to determine maximal biological effects and patient selection.

Lapatinib (also known as GW572106, GW2016, Tykerb, and Tyverb) has an impressively selective kinase enzyme profile and has been independently reported to be the most selective kinase inhibitor among 37 marketed or late-stage kinase inhibitors (Karaman et al., 2008). Lapatinib inhibits the proliferation of EGFR and/or erbB2 overexpressing cells with a selectivity of greater than 80-fold over normal cells. It blocks receptor autophosphorylation in preclinical and clinical settings to demonstrate the mechanism of action for the observed efficacy, which allows for careful and appropriate patient selection and treatment. The enzyme binding kinetics of lapatinib feature a remarkably slow off-rate potentially leading to higher receptor occupancy and longer signal inhibition (Wood et al., 2004). Ligand-bound protein crystal structure studies confirmed a unique conformational change that supported the kinetic mechanism of inhibition. Following positive Phase III results in breast cancer indications, lapatinib (generic name) launched in the United States in March 2007 as Tykerb™ and continues to be extensively studied in more than 55 ongoing clinical trials with approvals in 23 different countries thus far.

REFERENCES

Alroy, I., and Yarden, Y. (**1997**). The erbB signaling network in embryogenesis and oncogenesis: signal diversification through combinatorial ligand–receptor interactions. *FEBS Lett.* 410, 83–86.

Baselga, J., and Averbuch, S. G. (**2000**). ZD1839 ("Iressa") as an anticancer agent. *Drugs.* 60(Suppl. 1), 33–40.

Bence, A. K., Anderson, E. B., Halepota, M. A., et al. (**2005**). Phase I pharmacokinetic studies evaluating single and multiple doses of oral GW572016, a dual EGFR-ErbB-2 inhibitor, in healthy subjects. *Invest New Drugs.* 23(1), 39–49.

Brandt, B., Vogt, U., Sclotter, C. M., et al. (**1995**). Prognostic relevance of aberrations in the erbB oncogenes from breast, ovarian, oral and lung cancers: double-differential polymerase chain reaction (ddPCR) for clinical diagnosis. *Gene.* 159, 35–42.

Brignola, P. S., Lackey, K., Kadwell, S. H., et al. (**2002**). Comparison of the biochemical and kinetic properties of the type 1 receptor tyrosine kinase intracellular domains: demonstration of differential sensitivity to kinase inhibitors. *J Biol Chem.* 277(2), 1576–1585.

Cockerill, G. S., Stubberfield, C., Stables, J., et al. (**2001**). Indazolylamino quinazolines and pyridopyrimidines as inhibitors of the EGFr and c-erbB-2. *Bioorg Med Chem Lett.* 11(11), 1401–1405.

de Bono, J. S., and Rowinsky, E. K. (**2002**). The ErbB receptor family: a therapeutic target for cancer. *Trends Mol Med.* 8(4), S19–S26.

Downward, J., Yarden, Y., Mayes, E., et al. (**1984**). Close similarity of epidermal growth factor receptor and v-erbB oncogene protein sequences. *Nature.* 307, 521–527.

Fabian, M. A., Biggs, W. H., Treiber, D. K., et al. (**2005**). A small molecule-kinase interaction map for clinical kinase inhibitors. *Nat Biotechnol.* 23(3), 329–336.

Fry, D. W., Kraker, A. J., McMichael, A., et al. (**1994**). A specific inhibitor of the epidermal growth factor receptor tyrosine kinase. *Science.* 265(5175), 1093–1095.

Harris, R. A., Eichholtz, T. J., Hiles, I. D., et al. (**1999**). New model of erbB-2 over-expression in human mammary luminal epithelial cells. *Int J Cancer.* 80(3), 477–484.

Hopkins, A. L., Groom, C. R., and Alex, A. (**2004**). Ligand efficiency: a useful metric for lead selection. *Drug Discov Today.* 9(10), 430–431.

Karaman, M. W., Herrgard, S., Treiber, D. K., et al. (**2008**). A quantitative analysis of kinase inhibitor selectivity. *Nat Biotechnol.* 26(1), 127–132.

Keith, B. R., Allen, P. P., Alligood, K. J., et al. (**2001**). Anti-tumor activity of GW2016 in the erbB-2 positive human breast cancer xenograft, BT474. *Proceedings of the American Association of Cancer Research 92nd Annual Meeting.*

Klapper, L. N., Kirschbaum, M. H., Sela, M., and Yarden, Y. (**2000**). Biochemical and clinical implications of the erbB/HER signaling network of growth factor receptors. *Adv Cancer Res.* 77: 25–79.

Lackey, K. E. (**2006**). Lessons from the drug discovery of lapatinib, a dual ErbB1/2 tyrosine kinase inhibitor. *Curr Topics Med Chem.* 6(5), 435–460.

Lichtner, R. B., Menrad, A., Sommer, A., et al. (**2001**). Signaling-inactive epidermal growth factor receptor/ligand complexes in intact carcinoma cells by quinazoline tyrosine kinase inhibitors. *Cancer Res.* 61, 5790–5795.

Lipinski, C. A., Lombardo, F., Dominy, B. W., and Feeney, P. J. (**1997**). Experimental and computational approaches to estimate solubility and permeability in drug discovery and development settings. *Adv Drug Delivery Rev.* 23(1–3), 3–25.

Modjtahedi, H., Affleck, K., Stubberfield, C., and Dean, C. (**1998**). EGFR blockade by tyrosine kinase inhibitor or monoclonal antibody inhibits growth, directs terminal differentiation and induces apoptosis in the human squamous cell carcinoma HN5. *Int J Oncol.* 13, 335–342.

Moghal, N., and Sternberg, P. W. (**1999**). Multiple positive and negative regulators of signaling by the EGF-receptor. *Curr Opin Cell Biol.* 11(2), 190–196.

Mullin, R. J. (**2003**). Discovery and profile of GW572016, a dual reversible EGFR/ErbB-2 tyrosine kinase inhibitor. *Abstracts of Papers, 226th ACS National Meeting,* New York.

Pasleau, F., Grooteclaes, M., and Gol-Winkler, R. (**1993**). Expression of the c-erbB-2 gene in the BT474 human mammary tumor cell line: measurement of c-erbB-2 mRNA half-life. *Oncogene.* 8, 849–854.

Pearson, M. A., and Fabbro, D. (**2004**). Targeting protein kinases in cancer therapy: a success? *Exp Rev Anticancer Ther.* 4(6), 1113–1124.

Ranson, M. (**2004**). Epidermal growth factor receptor tyrosine kinase inhibitors. *Br J Cancer.* 90(12), 2250–2255.

Riese, D. J., and Stern, D. F. (**1998**). Specificity within the EGF family/ErbB receptor family signaling network. *BioEssays.* 20(1), 41–48.

Rusnak, D. W., Affleck, K., Cockerill, S. G., et al. (**2001a**). The characterization of novel, dual ErbB-2/EGFR, tyrosine kinase inhibitors: potential therapy for cancer. *Cancer Res.* 61(19), 7196–7203.

Rusnak, D. W., Lackey, K., Affleck, K., et al. (**2001b**).The effects of the novel, reversible EGFR/ErbB-2 tyrosine kinase inhibitor, GW2016, on the growth of human normal and tumor-derived cell lines *in vitro* and *in vivo. Mol Cancer Ther.* 1(2), 85–94.

Sainsbury, J. R., Farndon, J. R., Needham, G. K., et al. (**1987**). Epidermal-growth-factor receptor status as predictor of early recurrence of and death from breast cancer. *Lancet.* 1398–1402.

Semba, K., Kamata, N., Toyoshima, K., and Yamamoto, T. (**1985**). A v-erbB-related protooncogene, c-erbB-2, is distinct from the c-erbB-1/epidermal growth factor-receptor gene and is amplified in a human salivary gland adenocarcinoma. *Proc Natl Acad Sci USA*. 82, 6497–6501.

Shaffer, J. E., Adkison, K. K., Halm, K., et al. (**1999**). Use of "*N*-in-one" dosing to create an in vivo pharmacokinetics database for use in developing structure–pharmacokinetic relationships. *J Pharm Sci*. 88(3), 313–318.

Spector, N. L., Xia, W., Burris, H., et al. (**2005**). Study of the biologic effects of lapatinib, a reversible inhibitor of ErbB1 and ErbB-2 tyrosine kinases, on tumor growth and survival pathways in patients with advanced malignancies. *J Clin Oncol*. 23(11), 2502–2512.

Stamos, J., Sliwkowski, M. X., and Eigenbrot, C. (**2002**). Structure of the EGF receptor kinase domain alone and in complex with a 4-anilinoquinazoline inhibitor. *J Biol Chem*. 277, 46265–46272.

Tiseo, M., Loprevite, M., and Ardizzoni, A. (**2004**). Epidermal growth factor receptor inhibitors: a new prospective in the treatment of lung cancer. *Curr Med Chem Anticancer Agents*. 4(2), 139–148.

Wood, E. R., Truesdale, A. T., McDonald, O. B., et al. (**2004**). Unique structure for epidermal growth factor receptor bound to GW572016 (lapatinib): relationship between protein conformation, inhibitor off-rate, and receptor activity in tumor cells. *Cancer Res*. 64(18), 6652–6659.

Xia, W., Mullin, R. J., Keith, B. R., et al. (**2002**). Anti-tumor activity of GW572016: a dual tyrosine kinase inhibitor blocks EGF activation of EGFR/erbB-2 and down-stream Erk1/2 and AKT pathways. *Oncogene*. 21(41), 6255–6263.

Yarden, Y., and Sliwkowski, M. X. (**2001**). Untangling the erbB signaling network. *Nature Rev*. 2, 127–137.

3

DISCOVERY OF PAZOPANIB: A PAN VASCULAR ENDOTHELIAL GROWTH FACTOR KINASE INHIBITOR

PHILIP A. HARRIS AND JEFFREY A. STAFFORD

3.1. INTRODUCTION

The mainstay of cancer therapy over the past 30 years has been surgical excision and/or the killing of cancer cells with radiation and chemotherapy (Chabner and Longo, 2005). Cancer chemotherapy has provided good efficacy for hematological tumors, for example, certain leukemias and lymphomas, and some relatively uncommon solid tumors, but the treatment of major epithelial-derived solid tumors remains challenging for chemotherapeutic approaches. In several of the more prevalent solid tumors, chemotherapy is used following surgical resection in order to prevent disease recurrence, so-called adjuvant therapy. These chemotherapeutic agents were discovered by their ability to kill proliferating cells, usually in vitro, with limited understanding of their mechanisms of action. Although this approach bore fruit in the past, it is unlikely to provide new breakthrough therapies in the future.

With the advent of molecular targeted therapy, highlighted by the introduction of the Bcr-Abl kinase inhibitor Gleevec in 2001, oncology care continues to switch to newer agents reflecting deeper understanding of cancer biology and selective targeting in areas such as cell signaling, angiogenesis, and immunology. These agents are expected to be more efficacious than cytotoxics

Kinase Inhibitor Drugs. Edited by Rongshi Li and Jeffrey A. Stafford
Copyright © 2009 John Wiley & Sons, Inc.

although with a narrower spectrum of antitumor activity, have minimal or manageable side effects, and be amenable for oral delivery.

The growth of solid tumors depends on the supply of nutrients and oxygen from newly formed capillaries sprouting from existing blood vessels. This process of new vessel growth is known as angiogenesis (Folkman, 2007). Tumors induce angiogenesis by secretion of a number of endogenous proteins, notably vascular endothelial growth factor (VEGF), which binds to one of three transmembrane tyrosine kinase receptors, VEGFR1–3, on nearby endothelial cells (Veikkola et al., 2000). Data supporting the notion that inhibiting tumor angiogenesis would "starve" a tumor and thus inhibit growth began to emerge in the mid-1990s, leading to the anticipation that a VEGFR inhibitor could be effective in a broad number of tumors. Another advantage for inhibiting angiogenesis as an anticancer therapy is that the genetically stable endothelial cells are unlikely to develop mutation-based resistance to a drug, which is in stark contrast to therapies that target genetically unstable tumor cells that are undergoing rapid cell division. It should also be noted that, with the potential for angiogenesis inhibitors to be used as monotherapy in the early disease setting, manageable or negligible side effects are anticipated.

Based on the hypothesis that inhibition of this angiogenesis should block tumor growth, much effort has gone into inhibiting the VEGF pathway by small-molecule kinase inhibitors, receptor or ligand antibodies, or soluble decoy receptors (Baka et al., 2006). The late Judah Folkman and co-workers described the anticancer efficacy of the endogenous angiogenesis-inhibiting proteins angiostatin and endostatin in animal models, stimulating a great deal of interest in the scientific community in antiangiogenesis as a new approach to targeting solid tumors (O'Reilly et al., 1997). The first clinical validations to this approach came in 2004 from bevacizumab (Avastin™), a monoclonal antibody to VEGF, which is now approved for treatment of metastatic colorectal cancer in combination with 5-fluorouracil, non-small-cell lung cancer in combination with carboplatin and paclitaxel, and metastatic breast cancer in combination with paclitaxel (Caprioni and Fornarini, 2007; Ramalingam and Belani, 2007). More recently, the small-molecule multikinase inhibitors sorafenib (Nexavar™) and sunitinib (Sutent™), both of which inhibit the VEGF and PDGF receptor kinases (among others), have been approved for the treatment of advanced renal cancer, with additional indications of liver cancer for sorafenib and gastrointestinal stromal tumors for sunitinib (Kane et al., 2006; Chow and Eckhardt, 2007).

At GlaxoSmithKline (GSK), our interest in developing an antiangiogenic cancer therapy targeting VEGFR2 began in the late 1990s, around the time that Folkman published his pioneering experiments using angiostatin and endostatin. We had recently set up a research group focused on the development of small-molecule kinase inhibitors using a systems-based approach to drug discovery, and VEGFR2 as a kinase target was viewed as a perfect fit for this approach.

3.2. EARLY VEGFR2 KINASE INHIBITOR LEAD STRUCTURES

A compound screening campaign against VEGFR2 kinase was conducted using kinase-focused screening sets comprised of compounds from (1) prior and ongoing kinase programs, (2) literature-based kinase chemotypes, and (3) chemotypes that originated through structure-based design. The most potent hits that we uncovered from the initial screen were thiazolo- and pyridyl-fused indolinone derivatives, as exemplified by **1** and **2** in Figure 3.1, that were originally prepared as part of the CDK2 kinase program (Bramson et al., 2001). By varying the aromatic ring we were able to observe good potencies against VEGFR2 with IC$_{50}$ values between 10 and 100 nM, and corresponding cellular activities in the range of 200–500 nM for the more potent compounds, as demonstrated by inhibition of VEGF-induced proliferation of human umbilical vein endothelial cells (v-HUVEC). Interestingly, these inhibitors were structurally similar to SU5416 (later known as semaxanib, Figure 3.1), which was discovered at Sugen, Inc. SU5416 showed moderate in vitro potency in our assays, with VEGFR2 and v-HUVEC IC$_{50}$ values of 350 nM and 950 nM, respectively. SU5416 became the first small-molecule VEGFR2 inhibitor to enter clinical trials and was evaluated against multiple cancer types in combination with cytotoxics (Carter, 2000). The development of SU5416 was eventually discontinued due to lack of clinical efficacy (Fong et al., 1999). Ultimately, we discontinued our own efforts to advance the indolinone series due to overall poor developability properties of members of this class, in particular, low solubility.

An alternative starting point, also identified from screening, was the triazole **3**, which showed modest enzyme inhibition but failed to show effects in cell-based assays (Figure 3.2). Replacement of the triazole heterocycle with

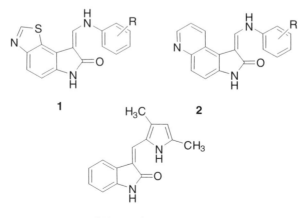

SU5416 (semaxanib)

Figure 3.1. Chemical structures of indolinones **1** and **2** and SU5416.

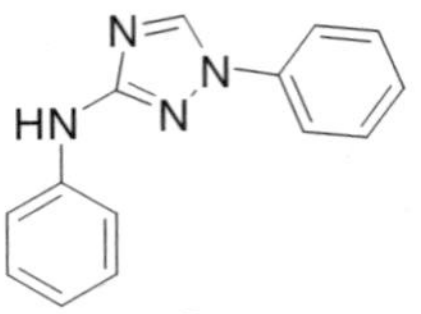

Figure 3.2. Chemical structures of triazole **3** and oxazoles **4** and **5**.

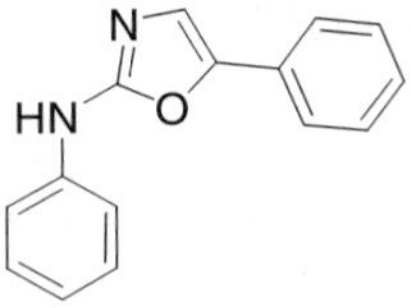

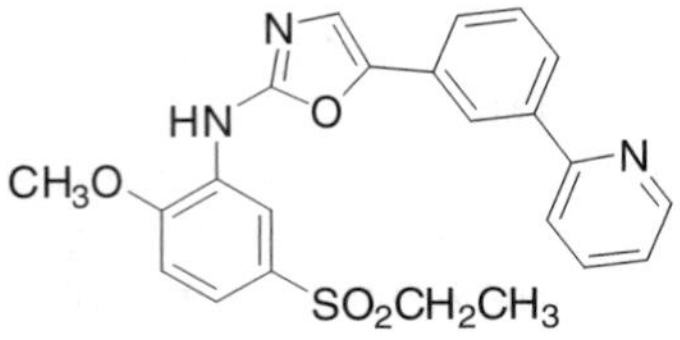

an oxazole core successfully introduced cell-based activity to this class. 2-Anilino-5-phenyloxazole (**4**) inhibited the enzymatic VEGFR2 and cellular v-HUVEC assays with IC_{50} values of 1.2 and 3 μM, respectively. Lead optimization of this oxazole involved a series of SAR iterations that ultimately led to the identification of oxazole **5**, a compound with improved VEGFR2 potency of 22 nM and v-HUVEC cellular activity of 370 nM (Harris et al., 2005). With the addition of the basic pyridine ring in **5**, we were able to prepare a stable bis-mesylate salt, resulting in enhanced aqueous solubility over its free base. The improved solubility of the bis-mesylate translated to an eight-fold higher oral AUC, which allowed for an evaluation of its in vivo efficacy in a mouse model of cancer. Oxazole **5**, dosed orally once per day at either 30 or 100 mg/kg to mice bearing implanted human HT-29 colon carcinoma cells, provided tumor growth inhibition of 43% and 55% in the two dose groups, respectively. As support that the observed inhibition of xenograft growth was working through an antiangiogenic mechanism rather than by direct effects on the implanted tumor cell, it was confirmed that oxazole **5** fails to inhibit the proliferation of cultured HT-29 cells. Although compounds from the oxazole series showed excellent in vitro properties that were consistent with the target research profile, most notably in the area of cell-based potency and selectivity, only a small handful of these compounds were demonstrating favorable in vivo pharmacokinetic profiles, a prerequisite for advancement to efficacy studies. In addition, the synthetic chemistry to generate analogs was lower-throughput than desired. A decision was made at this stage to halt further lead optimization work on the oxazole class and to focus the medicinal chemistry resources on an alternative series, the indazolylaminopyrimidines, which, while progressing in parallel, had advanced further and appeared to offer greater promise to deliver a clinical candidate from the program.

3.3. SCREENING HITS AND STRUCTURE-BASED DESIGN

The initial pyrimidine that we identified from screening was $N2,N4$-bis(3-bromophenyl)-5-fluoro-2,4-pyrimidinediamine (**6**), which had a VEGFR2 IC_{50} value of 400 nM. A separate screening hit, 4-(4-methyl-3-hydroxyanilino)-6,7-dimethoxyquinazoline (**7**), was found to be more potent than **6** against VEGFR2 with an IC_{50} value of 6 nM, and we recognized an opportunity to apply structure-based design in the optimization of **6**. Since crystallography data on VEGFR2 were not available at the time, a homology model of the kinase domain was created by using atomic coordinates, either publicly available from the RCSB or from in-house structures, for tyrosine kinases including c-FMS, Tie2, FGFR2, and insulin receptor. This model was then used to predict the binding mode of each screening hit. Examination of their respective binding modes indicated the pyrimidine and the quinazoline bound similarly in the ATP binding site. The pyrimidine N-1 and the C-2 anilino N-H were predicted to make the canonical hydrogen acceptor and donor bonds with the "hinge" residue Cys919, respectively, while the quinazoline N-1 was predicted to make a hydrogen bond accepting interaction with Cys919, along with the quinazoline C-2 hydrogen making an aromatic CH···O=C interaction to Glu917. In these conformations, the arylamino substituents at the C-4 pyrimidine and C-4 quinazoline, respectively, overlay to suggest the synthesis of N-(3-bromophenyl)-N'-(4-methyl-3-hydroxyphenyl)-2,4-pyrimidinediamine (**8**). The predicted binding mode of **8** overlaid with **7** is shown in Figure 3.3.

Pyrimidine **8** inhibited VEGFR2 with an IC_{50} of 6.3 nM, representing almost a hundred-fold improvement in binding compared to **6**, with a corresponding cell-based v-HUVEC potency of 540 nM. This dramatic increase in binding affinity was attributed to the key predicted hydrogen bond interaction between the phenol OH and the NH of Asp1046 in the protein backbone (Figure 3.3). As an indicator of growth factor inhibition selectivity, we measured each test

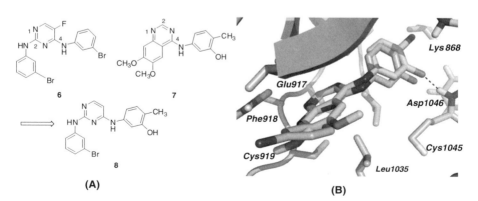

Figure 3.3. (**A**) The binding modes of screening hits **6** and **7** suggested the synthesis of pyrimidine **8**. (**B**) Pyrimidine **8** is overlaid with quinazoline **7**, revealing an identical interaction to the Asp1046 NH by both hydroxyaniline OH groups. (See color insert.)

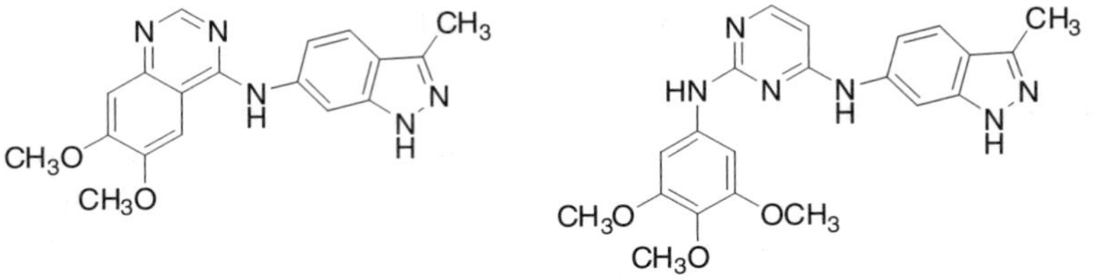

Figure 3.4. Chemical structures of quinazoline **9** and pyrimidine **10**.

compound's ability to inhibit proliferation of HUVECs whose growth was also stimulated by basic fibroblast growth factor, bFGF (b-HUVEC). In contrast to the v-HUVEC assay, the b-HUVEC assay should be unaffected by a selective VEGFR2 inhibitor. In this assay pyrimidine **8** has an IC_{50} value of 3.5 μM, demonstrating at least a sixfold selectivity for VEGFR2 over the other angiogenic growth factor, bFGF.

Although introduction of the 4-methyl-3-hydroxy aniline at the pyrimidine C-4 position imparted excellent in vitro potency, the pharmacokinetic profiles of compound **8** and other meta-hydroxyanilinopyrimidines were poor. In general, we observed low oral bioavailabilities (<11%) and moderate to high clearances in the mouse (28–83 mL/min/kg), presumably due to rapid phase II glucuronidation or sulfation reactions of the phenol functionality. At this stage, further screening of in-house kinase inhibitor libraries identified the quinazoline **9** with excellent potency against VEGFR2 with an IC_{50} of 1.7 nM (Figure 3.4). The 3-methylindazole appeared to be an equipotent replacement of the 4-methyl-3-hydroxyphenyl, having, we surmised, a reduced potential for glucuronidation. Subsequent to this work, researchers from GlaxoSmithKline's UK group engineered a similar replacement of a phenol to an indazole in the context of an Lck inhibitor program (Bamborough et al., 2007). Incorporation of the 3-methylindazole heterocycle into the pyrimidine series yielded the indazolylaminopyrimidine **10**, which possessed good potency against both VEGFR2 enzyme (IC_{50} = 8 nM) and v-HUVECs (IC_{50} = 180 nM), with ~20-fold selectivity over the b-HUVECs. Importantly, we observed improved pharmacokinetics with lowered clearance (16 mL/min/kg) and an oral bioavailability of 85% at a dose of 10 mg/kg in the rat.

The predicted binding mode of **10** shows the 3-methylindazole occupying the same hydrophobic backpocket as the 4-methyl-3-hydroxyphenyl group as shown in Figure 3.5. The model suggests a π-cation interaction between the indazole ring of the 3-methylindazole and the epsilon amino group of Lys868, as opposed to the hydrogen bond interaction predicted between the phenol OH of pyrimidine **8** and the NH of Asp1046. Given the relatively similar potencies of the 3-methylindazole versus the phenol, the current hypothesis is that the Lys868–indazole π-cation interaction is energetically comparable to that of the Asp1046–phenol OH interaction. Importantly, the isosteric

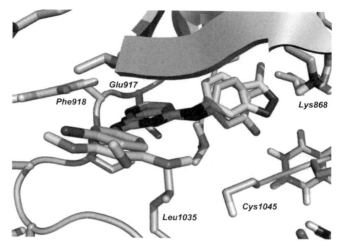

Figure 3.5. Computational overlay of pyrimidine **8** with GW2286 (**10**). The model of GW2286 suggests an important π-cation interaction between Lys868 and the heterocycle.

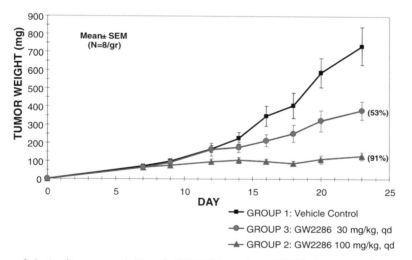

Figure 3.6. Antitumor activity of GW2286 against HT-29 human colon tumor xenografts in nude mice.

replacement of the phenolic hydroxyl in **8** was effectively achieved with the indazole, and we were able to begin evaluation of test compounds in animal models of cancer and angiogenesis. In an in vivo efficacy study using HT-29 human colon tumor xenografts, pyrimidine **10** dosed orally once per day at 30 and 100 mg/kg for a period of 3 weeks resulted in tumor growth inhibition of 53% and 91%, respectively, compared to vehicle control (Figure 3.6). This compound, known as GW612286 (or GW2286 for short), enjoyed several attributes of a "lead compound" and its promising activities were highlighted in a poster presentation at the 2001 Annual Meeting of the American Association of Cancer Research (AACR). Superior pharmacokinetic properties, good in vivo efficacy, and ease of synthesis of pyrimidine **10** compared to oxazole **5** were the key areas of differentiation that supported our decision to focus chemistry efforts on the indazolylaminopyrimidines.

3.4. MEDICINAL CHEMISTRY STRATEGY AND SYNTHETIC ROUTE

With GW2286 serving as the lead molecule in the program, the medicinal chemistry strategy focused on optimizing the biochemical potency and cell-based selectivity of the pyrimidine scaffold, while simultaneously improving the pharmacokinetic profile to support a once-daily oral therapy. As summarized in Figure 3.7, GW2286 (**10**) was sectioned into three regions for SAR development: replacement of the aniline group that points toward the solvent exposed region, replacement of the core that interacts with the hinge, and replacement of the heterocycle motif that addresses the backpocket of the binding site. In addition, alkylation at the linker nitrogen at C-4 of the pyrimidine was also investigated to introduce conformational restraint, remove an H-bond donor, and increase potential hydrophobic interactions in the binding pocket.

Compounds were prepared according to the synthetic sequence outlined in Figure 3.8. Thus o-ethylaniline (**11**) was nitrated to yield 2-ethyl-5-nitroaniline (**12**), and this underwent cyclization with isoamyl nitrite in acetic acid to give 3-methyl-6-nitroindazole (**13**). Reduction with tin(II) chloride gave 6-amino-3-methylindazole (**14**) and condensation with 2,4-dichloropyrimidine using basic conditions in THF and ethanol yielded the indazolylaminopyrimidine (**15**). Finally, a second condensation with substituted anilines was accomplished using acidic conditions to yield the desired pyrimidines (**16**).

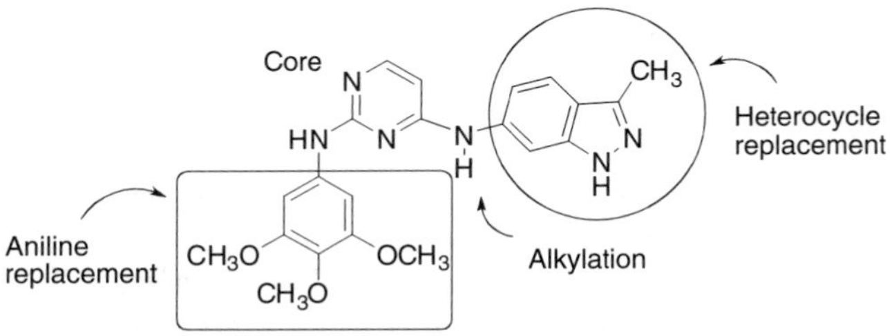

Figure 3.7. Medicinal chemistry strategy for lead optimization of GW2286 (**10**).

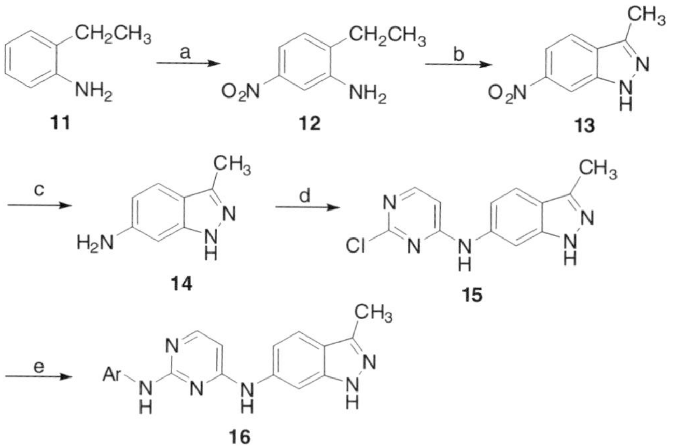

Figure 3.8. Synthetic route to the indazolylaminopyrimdines. Reagents and conditions: (a) Fuming HNO_3, conc. H_2SO_4, 6%; (b) isoamyl nitrite, AcOH, 98%; (c)$SnCl_2$, conc. HCl, glyme, 92%; (d) 2,4-dichloropyrimidine, $NaHCO_3$, EtOH, THF, rt, 89%; (e) $ArNH_2$, iPrOH, HCl, 80 °C, 66–92%.

3.5. STRUCTURE–ACTIVITY RELATIONSHIP OF INDAZOLYLAMINOPYRIMIDINES

3.5.1. Aniline Replacement

Keeping the 3-methylindazole constant, a survey of substituted anilines at the C-2 position of the pyrimidine revealed the 3,4,5-trimethoxy aniline-substituted pyrimidine **10** among the most potent inhibitors, with the majority of other anilines having diminished activity compared to this starting point. However, a modest increase in potency could be achieved by combination of a 2′-methoxy group with 5′-sulfonyl-containing group, either as a sulfonamide or a sulfone. For example, pyrimidine **17** was found to have excellent potency against VEGFR2, with an IC_{50} value of 2 nM, and promising cellular potency and selectivity in VEGF- and bFGF-driven HUVECs, with IC_{50} values of 130 and 13000 nM, respectively. In the rat, plasma clearance (40 mL/min/kg) and oral bioavailability (28%) were viewed as potential areas for improvement. Compound **17** followed from an SAR trend also observed in the oxazole series (e.g., compound **5**). Molecular modeling, later supported by crystallographic data, suggested that the methoxy group of **17** sits in a lipophilic pocket and acts to orient the sulfone group to interact with the side chain of Asn923 as shown in Figure 3.9.

3.5.2. Alkylation

To examine the potential for substitution at the C-4 amino nitrogen of the pyrimidine, a number of alkylated derivatives were examined. We observed

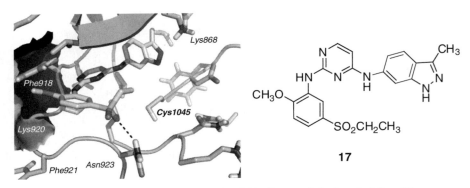

Figure 3.9. Chemical structure and binding model of pyrimidine **17**.

that small alkyl groups were well tolerated, but groups larger than ethyl resulted in loss of potency. At this stage in the program we became enabled with X-ray crystal structures of our inhibitors bound to the VEGFR2 active site, and the structure of GW2286 (**10**) confirmed its binding within the ATP site, with the pyrimidine N-1 and the C-2 anilino N-H making hydrogen acceptor and donor interactions with the peptide backbone of Cys919 (Figure 3.10A). Unexpectedly, however, the electron density map indicated that the indazole heterocycle could populate two alternative pockets, resulting in an "S-shaped" conformation with the indazole projected into the back lipophilic pocket as in the previously described model, or a "U-shaped" conformation with the indazole projected out into the ATP binding pocket. A crystal structure of the N-methylated analog, pyrimidine **18**, reveals that the inhibitor favors an extended S-shaped conformation (Figure 3.10B). It also suggests that the N2-H tautomer of **18** is donating an H bond to Glu883. This "induced fit" indazole tautomerization provides added rationale for the apparent mismatched donor–acceptor relationships between the 3-methylindazole and their 3-hydroxyaniline precursors. Additional crystal structures of indazolylaminopyrimidines reinforced the trend that N-unalkylated derivatives displayed U-shaped binding conformations, while N-alkylated derivatives displayed S-shaped conformations. The Schrodinger modeling package was used to explore the conformational space of truncated forms of **10** and **18**. As might be expected from the crystal structure data, the two distinct conformations for **10** are calculated to be close in energy, with the U-shaped conformation favored by only 0.22 kcal/mol over the S-shaped conformer. In the case of the N-methylated compound **18**, the S-shaped conformation is preferred by 1.10 kcal/mol, most likely to avoid an unfavorable steric interaction between the N-methyl group and the pyrimidine C-5 hydrogen (Figure 3.10C).

The attributes of the 5′-sulfonyl group on the aniline and the N-methylation were combined in pyrimidine **19** (Figure 3.11), a potent inhibitor of VEGFR2

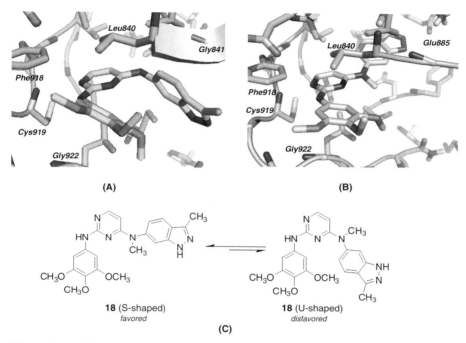

Figure 3.10. (**A**) X-ray crystal structure of pyrimidine **10** with U-shaped conformation in VEGFR2. (**B**) X-ray crystal structure of pyrimidine **18** with S-shaped conformation in VEGFR2. (**C**) Conformational equilibrium of pyrimidine **18**.

kinase (IC_{50} < 10 nM) with good cell-based potency in the endothelial cell assay (110 nM). This compound exhibited improved oral bioavailability in both rat and dog (65% and 54%, respectively) over its unalkylated analog. We reasoned that this improved profile may result from removal of an H-bond donor from the inhibitor, since the presence of multiple H-bond donors is known to be detrimental to absorption and introduces potential sites of metabolism (Veber et al., 2002). It was generally observed that pyrimidines containing the 3-methylindazole heterocycle and methylated at the C-4 amino nitrogen possessed both good in vitro and in vivo cross-species pharmacokinetic profiles, and except for its P450 inhibition profile, pyrimidine **19** and its near analogs possessed all the desired attributes of a clinical candidate. The complete in vivo and in vitro profiles of pyrimidine **19**, known within the project team as GW654652, were disclosed in several poster presentations at the 94th Annual Meeting of the AACR (Kumar et al., 2003; Dev et al., 2004). In addition to its in vivo characterization at GSK, studies conducted in Dr. Jeffrey Green's lab at the National Institutes of Health (NIH) revealed that GW654652 significantly inhibited mammary cancer growth and improved survival in a C3(1)/Tag transgenic mouse model

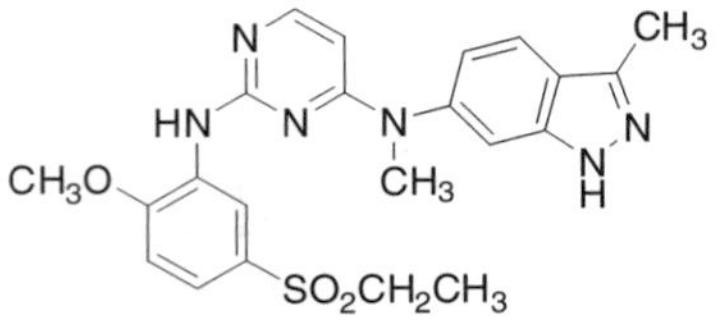

19 (GW654652)

Figure 3.11. Chemical structure of pyrimidine **19** (GW654652).

through antiangiogenic mechanisms (Huh et al., 2005). Notwithstanding the considerable attributes of GW654652, the VEGFR2 research team felt the need to modulate its P450 inhibition profile.

3.5.3. Heterocycle Replacement

It was hypothesized that the molecular mechanism for P450 inhibition elicited by GW654652 and related members in the class was a result of the indazole N2 nitrogen interacting with the heme iron of the CYP enzyme. A scenario to disrupt this interaction would be to add steric hindrance to the heterocycle ring (Rogerson et al., 1977). Subsequent to this work at GlaxoSmithKline, and within the context of a p38 kinase inhibition program, researchers at Takeda modulated the CYP3A4 inhibition profiles by adding a substituent ortho to a pyridyl nitrogen (Miwatashi et al., 2005). In this example, the Takeda group found that both electronic and steric factors played a role in modulating the inhibitory activity.

Our first approach was to synthesize a methylated form of the indazole heterocycle in **19**. Under basic conditions methylation of an intermediate indazole provided a mixture of N-methyl regioisomers, the major isomer being N1-methylated, and the minor isomer methylated at N2. We were gratified to discover that the P450 inhibition profiles of the N2-methylated indazoles, in accordance with our hypothesis, were generally improved over their unmethylated counterparts (data not shown). Indeed, the composite profiles of the methylated analogs, including cell-based potency and pharmacokinetic disposition, pointed to the 2,3-dimethylindazole (N2-methylated isomer) as the preferred heterocycle. With this result, it was immediately evident that the project team had taken another step closer to identifying a clinical candidate. With the modified 2,3-dimethylindazole heterocycle now installed, we carried out a final focused aniline survey examining first the optimum meta-substituted sulfonamide and sulfone substitutions. This led to the preparation of indazolylaminopyrimidine **20** (code name: GW786034), a compound that brought together a unique and attractive combination of in vitro, in vivo, and developability profiles. (See Figure 3.12.)

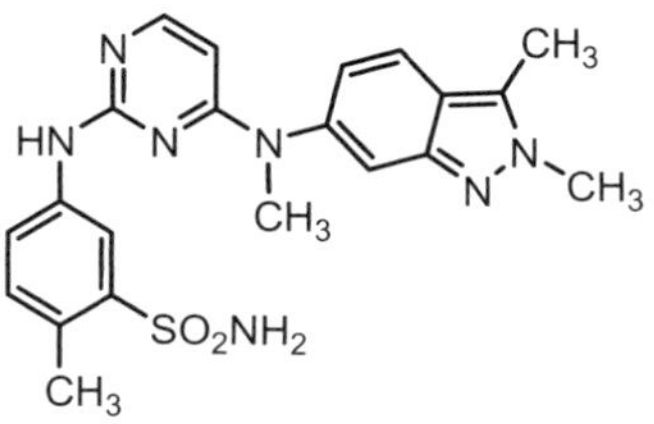

20 (GW786034)

Figure 3.12. Chemical structure of GW786034 (20).

3.6. PROPERTIES OF PAZOPANIB (GW786034)

3.6.1. Structural, Biochemical, and Cellular Profiles

It is interesting to consider the binding mode of the N2-methylated indazole in GW786034 (**20**). In the co-complex structure of pyrimidine **20** we observe that the conserved Asp-Phe-Gly (DFG) motif is in a so-called DFG-out conformation (Pargellis et al., 2002), allowing access to the backpocket and the C-helix. As earlier described in the model of pyrimidine **10**, a π cloud-cation interaction between Lys868 and the indazole moiety may also be contributing to its affinity (Figure 3.13). With N2 methylated, **20** makes the indazole N1 available as an acceptor to make an interaction with the backbone NH of Asp1046 of the DFG loop, either water-mediated or directly. However, the structure reveals an N-NH distance that is significantly longer than one would expect for an optimal H bond. The methyl group on the linker N between the indazole and pyrimidine rings may also be enjoying a favorable herringbone-type arrangement with Phe1047 of the DFG loop. Based on the observation that the biochemical potency of **20** is approximately 10-fold less than its unmethylated isomer **21**, we can attribute the diminished affinity primarily to the loss of the NH interaction with Glu885 (Figure 3.14). Other interactions that have been described are presumed to be intact. Although less active against the enzyme, **20** showed a sevenfold greater inhibition of v-HUVEC proliferation over pyrimidine **21**, a general trend observed for N2-methylated indazoles when compared to their unmethylated analogs, which can be attributed to the removal of an H-bond donor, a property commonly associated with improved transport across cell membranes and epithelial layers.

GW786034, as predicted from the binding mode and confirmed by crystallography, is an ATP-competitive inhibitor of VEGFR2 with a K_i of 24 nM. It is a potent pan inhibitor against members of the VEGFR kinase family, as well as inhibiting the closely related tyrosine receptor kinases PDGFRβ and c-Kit (Table 3.1). Ambit Biosciences (San Diego, CA) subsequently profiled GW786034 in an in vitro competition binding assay against 317 kinases, which include more than half of the total predicted human protein kinases (Karaman et al., 2008). From this extensive cross-screening only a few additional potent kinase inhibitions were revealed in addition to those from our limited in-house

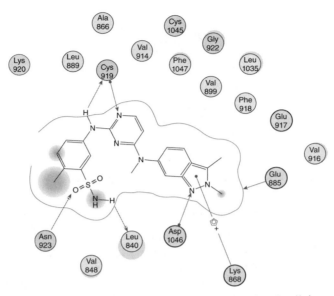

Figure 3.13. Binding mode of pazopanib. (See color insert for details.)

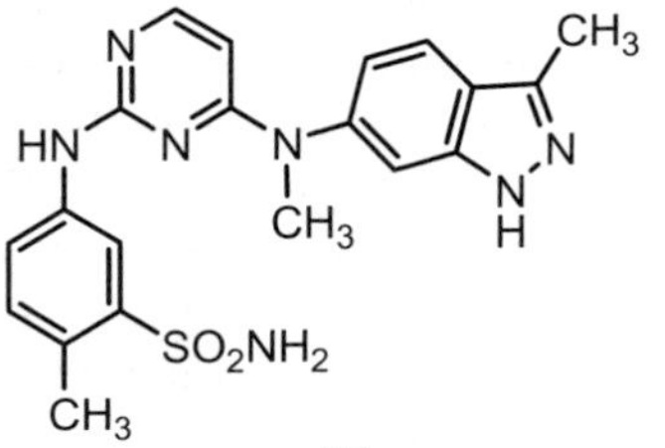

21

Figure 3.14. Chemical structure of pyrimidine **21**.

set of kinase assays. For example, DDR1, DDR2, and STK10 were inhibited with IC50 values between 50 and 100 nM. In cellular assays, GW786034 inhibited proliferation of VEGF-driven HUVEC with an IC_{50} of 21 nM, with a 35-fold selectivity over bFGF-induced HUVEC proliferation (Figure 3.15). In addition, GW786034 potently inhibited VEGF-induced phosphorylation of VEGFR2 in HUVEC with an IC_{50} of ~8 nM as determined by Western blotting. The inhibition of VEGF-induced HUVEC proliferation was greater than 1400-fold more selective than that observed for inhibition of proliferation of a variety of tumor cells and greater than 48-fold for fibroblasts.

TABLE 3.1. Inhibition of Protein Kinases by GW786034[a]

Enzyme	Kinase IC_{50} (μM)	Enzyme	Kinase IC_{50} (μM)
Human VEGFR1	0.010	FAK	0.80
Human VEGFR2	0.030	P38α	1.1
Human VEGFR3	0.047	Abl1	2.0
Mouse VEGFR2	0.042	JNK1	2.5
PDGFRα	0.071	Ret	2.8
PDGFRβ	0.084	Src	3.1
c-Kit	0.074	GSK3	3.5
FGFR1	0.14	JNK3	341
FGFR3	0.13	ALK6	4.3
FGFR4	0.80	Tie-2	4.5
c-fms	0.15	Met	6.0
LCK	0.41	IGF-1R	8.0
ITK	0.43	JNK2	10

[a]Activity was greater than 20 μM for Akt3, CDK1, CDK2, EphB4, ErbB1, ErbB2, ErbB4, Flt3, INS-R, PLK1, PLK3, PKC-β1, PKC-β2, Syk, and Wee1.

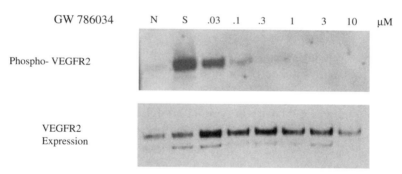

Figure 3.15. HUVECs were treated with the indicated concentration (μM) of GW786034, followed by VEGF stimulation. After treatments, lysates were prepared and analyzed by SDS-PAGE and immunoblotting. Lysates were initially probed by an anti-phosphotyrosine antibody (*top blot*) and subsequently reprobed using an antibody directed against VEGFR2 to visualize the receptor levels (*bottom blot*). S and N refer to lysates prepared from untreated HUVECs with or without VEGF stimulation, respectively.

3.6.2. Pharmacokinetic Properties

Several pharmacokinetic studies with GW786034 were performed. These studies included evaluation of oral exposure of the mono-HCl, di-HCl (amorphous), and the free base of GW786034 with various formulations (data not shown). Summaries of the PK parameters and oral bioavailability of GW786034 in rat, dog, and monkey are shown in Table 3.2. Both volume of distribution and plasma clearance were low across the three species, consistent with its high protein binding. An in vitro study using human liver microsomes showed that

TABLE 3.2. Pharmokinetic Profile of GW786034

Parameter	Rat	Dog	Monkey
$T_{1/2}$ (IV, h)	3.6	2.2	4.7
MRT_{0-t} (h)	4.4	3.4	43.0
CL (mL/min/kg)	1.7	1.4	1.6
Vdss (mL/kg)	478	297	283
Oral bioavailabilities (%)			
Solution dose (rat/dog/monkey: 10/1/5 mg/kg)	72	47	65
Suspension dose (50 mg/kg)	36	12	30

oxidative metabolism is primarily mediated by CYP3A4 with minor contributions from CYP1A2 and CYP2C8. GW786034 inhibits the CYP enzymes 1A2, 3A4, 2B6, 2C8, 2C9, 2D6, and 2E1 with a range from 7.9 to 18 μM. After in vitro incubation of ^{14}C-GW786034 with hepatocytes and liver microsomes from mouse, rat, dog, monkey, and humans, the primary metabolites were mono-oxygenation, di-oxygenation, and possibly oxidation to a carboxylic acid. There were no human-specific phase I metabolites in human microsomal or hepatocyte incubations, but a single phase II metabolite, a glucuronide potentially derived from a carboxylic acid, was observed only in human hepatocytes. The mono-HCl salt of GW786034 was selected due to its superior solid state and solution stability versus the di-HCl and free base, and this compound was later named pazopanib.

3.6.3. Antiangiogenic Activity in Animal Models

As a measure of its ability to inhibit angiogenesis in vivo, pazopanib was examined in the mouse matrigel plug assay (Kumar et al., 2007). In this assay a gel plug of extracellular matrix containing bFGF, which gives a more robust angiogenic response than VEGF in this assay format, is implanted subcutaneously to stimulate vascularization inside the plug. The plug is then removed after 5 days and the vascularization of this plug is estimated by determination of the hemoglobin content. Following once-daily oral administration of pazopanib, angiogenesis was inhibited in a dose-dependent manner as shown in Table 3.3. The oral exposure increased in a dose-proportional manner in going from a 10 to 30 mg/kg dose, with a more modest increase in exposure observed from the 30 to 100 mg/kg dose level. Pazopanib was also examined in a second animal model of angiogenesis, the mouse corneal micropocket assay, in which ocular angiogenesis is induced by implantation of slow-release pellets of VEGF into the mouse cornea. Treatment of mice with 100 mg/kg of pazopanib twice daily orally for 5 days resulted in significant inhibition in the degree of vascularization as measured by reduced blood vessel growth along the cornea periphery as well as smaller maximum vessel lengths.

The antitumor efficacy of pazopanib was examined in mice bearing established human xenografts using HT-29 (colon carcinoma), A375P (melanoma),

TABLE 3.3. Mouse Oral Exposures and Xenograft Tumor Growth Inhibition by Pazopanib

Dose (mg/kg)	AUC_{0-inf} ($\mu g \cdot h/mL$)	Plasma Concentration @ 12h (ng/mL)	Inhibition of Angiogenesis (Matrigel Plug Assay, %)	Tumor Model (% Inhibition)[a] HT-29	A375P	HN5
10	220	6,320	0	32	16	99
30	657	24,831	57	59	35	102
100	1,141	38,538	83	69	55	110

[a]Inhibition of tumor growth compared to vehicle-treated mice after daily dosing for 21 days.

and HN5 (head and neck carcinoma) tumors following once-daily oral dosing and a 3-week course of therapy. The HN5 and HT-29 xenografts responded better at all doses compared to the A375P model, which we found in general to be more resistant to VEGFR2 inhibitors (Table 3.3). As further evidence that the observed inhibition of xenograft growth is not acting through a direct anti-tumor mechanism, no antiproliferative activity was observed below $10\,\mu M$ for these human tumor lines (HT-29, HN5, A375P) growing in serum-containing media. No significant effect on the body weight of mice was observed, and the animals appeared healthy and active throughout the study duration.

With the efficacy of pazopanib established in human xenograft models, a final remaining hurdle was to demonstrate that VEGFR2 phosphorylation was inhibited in an in vivo setting and to establish a PK–PD correlation. The effect of pazopanib on VEGF-induced VEGFR2 phosphorylation in vivo was evaluated in mouse lungs, which were chosen due to their high endothelial cell content (Kumar et al., 2007). A single oral dose of 30 mg/kg pazopanib inhibited phosphorylation for more than 8 hours, corresponding to $>40\,\mu M$ of drug plasma concentration. Mean drug plasma concentrations of 153.9, 47.5, 41.1, 17.4, and $4.3\,\mu M$ were achieved at 1, 4, 8, 16, and 24 hours, respectively. At 16 and 24 hours, the plasma concentration dropped below $40\,\mu M$ and the inhibition of VEGFR2 phosphorylation was minimal, if any, indicating a $\geq 40\,\mu M$ steady-state concentration of pazopanib is required for optimal in vivo activity. The discrepancy between the in vivo required concentration and in vitro potency against v-HUVEC can be attributed to the high protein binding for pazopanib of >99.9% as measured by equilibrium dialysis.

3.7. NONCLINICAL TOXICOLOGY

Based on a favorable pharmacokinetic profile, antitumor efficacy, demonstration of in vivo antiangiogenic effects, and a PK–PD correlation, pazopanib was progressed into preclinical development. In toxicology studies, pazopanib was well tolerated in rats at repeat oral doses up to 300 mg/kg/day for 29 days. Drug-related findings included mild liver enzyme increases in individual animals at doses of >100 mg/kg/day; however, there were no liver histopathology findings. Additional target organ findings were observed in bone, bone marrow, testes, and ovary, some of which can be attributed to the pharmacological inhibition of VEGFR2. All drug-related effects had reversed or were progressing to recovery by the end of the 6 week recovery period. The no observable adverse effect level (NOAEL) in rats was determined to be 30 mg/kg/day. There were no toxic effects observed in monkeys given 500 mg/kg/day of pazopanib for 28 days, establishing this as the NOAEL. Pazopanib was also found to be nonmutagenic and nonclastogenic when tested in a range of genetic toxicity assays.

3.8. CLINICAL STUDIES

A Phase I study was conducted to evaluate safety and tolerability and assess early indications of clinical efficacy, as well as to characterize the pharmacokinetic profile of pazopanib (Hurwitz et al., 2005). Patients were enrolled at doses ranging from 50 mg three times per week to 2000 mg daily. The mean half-life of pazopanib was approximately 35 hours and the maximal exposure with mean trough concentrations over 15 μg/mL at 24 hours was observed after daily doses of 800 mg or more. The most common adverse events were nausea, diarrhea, anorexia, hypertension, fatigue, hair depigmentation, and vomiting; a maximum tolerated dose (MTD) was not achieved. The outcome of this study was a recommended Phase II dose of 800 mg daily.

A number of Phase II trials of pazopanib are ongoing or have recently been completed in patients with renal, ovarian, breast, and cervical cancers, soft tissue sarcoma, non-small-cell lung cancer (NSCLC), malignant glioblastomas, and myeloma. A Phase II study that evaluated 225 patients with advanced renal cell carcinoma receiving 800 mg of pazopanib once daily was recently completed (Hutson et al., 2008). Although initially designed as a randomized discontinuation trial, the study was modified based on a positive interim analysis after 12 weeks to an open-label, single-arm study with all patients receiving pazopanib. Overall, the percentage of patients who responded to treatment was 35% and stable disease was achieved in 45% of patients. Responses were durable with median duration of 68 weeks and an estimated median progression free survival of 11.9 months. A Phase II study was carried out in 141 patients with advanced and/or metastatic soft tissue sarcoma who had relapsed following standard therapies or for whom no therapy options exist (Sleijfer et al., 2007). Patients received 800 mg of pazopanib once daily and were assessed for the primary endpoint of progression-free survival (PFS) at 12 weeks with an observed activity of PFS in 34–44% of patients with leiomyosarcoma, synovial sarcoma, and other less common forms, but not in liposarcoma. Another Phase II study was designed to assess the efficacy of pazopanib as a neoadjuvant presurgical treatment for patients with stage 1 or 2 NSCLC. Preliminary results from this study were presented at ASCO 2008 (Altorki et al., 2008). After an initial biopsy, 35 eligible treatment-naïve patients received 800 mg of pazopanib daily for between 2 and 6 weeks, with a median treatment of 16 days, followed by a treatment-free period of 1 week prior to surgery to allow pazopanib to be eliminated from the body. High-resolution computed tomography scans pre- and post-treatment measuring tumor size showed 30 patients (86%) had experienced a tumor volume reduction, with overall changes ranging from a reduction of 86% to an increase in 17%. In an Phase II open-label study evaluating pazopanib in patients with ovarian cancer who had failed standard platinum-based therapy (Friedlander et al., 2007), biological activity measured as a decrease in CA-125, a biologic marker of clinical activity, was seen in 9 of 22 evaluable patients (41%) with relapsed disease. A number of Phase I trials are also ongoing, which are investigating the combination of pazopanib with lapatanib, which targets EGFR and ErbB2 receptor tyrosine kinases, in subjects with locally advanced or metastatic breast cancer, malignant glioblastomas, and other solid tumors (Sorbera et al., 2006; Sonpavde and Hutson, 2007). An eye-drop formulation of pazopanib is also in Phase II development for the treatment of neovascular age-related macular degeneration, a form of vision loss due to abnormal blood vessel growth, which has been shown to respond to antiangiogenic treatment as demonstrated by the VEGF antibody fragment ranibizumab (Lantry, 2007).

ACKNOWLEDGMENTS

A great many people contributed to the discovery of pazopanib. The authors wish to acknowledge first the dedication and leadership of Diedre Luttrell, who skillfully guided the program from the beginning through to its early stage of clinical development. Other GSK scientists who played a role in the discovery and development of pazopanib are the following: Amogh Boloor, Mui Cheung, Ronda Davis-Ward, Robert Mook, Matthew Brown, Robert Hunter, Kevin Hinkle, Jerzy Szewczyk, James Veal, Robert Nolte, Rakesh Kumar, Greg Miller, Stephen Frye, Nelson Johnson, Andrea Epperly, Emile Chen, Stephanie Harrelson, Anne Truesdale, Christopher Laudeman, Christopher Terry, Sharon Rudolph, Victoria Knick, Jennifer Johnson, Renae Crosby, Douglas Jones, Philip Ertel, Ben Suttle, Neil Spector, Michael McGuire, Jennifer Johnson, Renae Crosby, Inderjit Dev, Laura Harrington, James Onori, Teresa Hopper, Robert Mullin, Tona Gilmer, Michelle Rizzolio, Tony Tong, John Gleason, Ken Batchelor, and Allen Oliff. There are undoubtedly others who have been inadvertently omitted, and the authors apologize for any oversight. The authors also thank James Veal, Robert Nolte, and David Lawson for helpful discussions during the writing of this chapter.

REFERENCES

Altorki, N., Guarino, M., Lee, P., et al. (**2008**). Preoperative treatment with pazopanib (GW786034), a multikinase angiogenesis inhibitor in early-stage non-small cell lung cancer (NSCLC): a proof-of-concept Phase II study. *J Clin Oncol.* 26, May 20 suppl; abstr 7557.

Baka, S., Clamp, A. R., and Jayson, G. C. (**2006**). A review of the latest clinical compounds to inhibit VEGF in pathological angiogenesis. *Expert Opin Ther Targets.* 10, 867–876.

Bamborough, P., Angell, R. M., Bhamra, I., et al. (**2007**). N-4-pyrimidinyl-1H-indazol-4-amine inhibitors of Lck: indazoles as phenol isosteres with improved pharmacokinetics. *Bioorg Med Chem Lett.* 17(15), 4363–4368.

Bramson, H. N., Corona, J., Davis, S. T., et al. (**2001**). Oxindole-based inhibitors of cyclin-dependent kinase 2 (CDK2): design, synthesis, enzymatic activities, and X-ray crystallographic analysis. *J Med Chem.* 44, 4339–4358.

Caprioni, F., and Fornarini, G. (**2007**). Bevacizumab in the treatment of metastatic colorectal cancer. *Future Oncol.* 3, 141–148.

Carter, S. K. (**2000**). Clinical strategy for the development of angiogenesis inhibitors. *Oncologist.* 5(Suppl. 1), 51–54.

Chabner, B. A., and Longo, D. L., Eds. (**2005**). *Cancer Chemotherapy and Biotherapy: Principles and Practice,* 4th Edition. Philadelphia: Lippincott Williams & Wilkins.

Chow, L. Q. M., and Eckhardt, S. G. (**2007**). Sunitinib: from rational design to clinical efficacy. *J Clin Oncol.* 25, 884–896.

Dev, I. K., Dornsife, R. E., Hopper T. M., et al. (**2004**). Antitumor efficacy of VEGFR2 tyrosine kinase inhibitor correlates with expression of VEGF and its receptor VEGFR2 in tumor models. *Br J Cancer.* 91, 1391–1398.

Folkman, J. (**2007**). Angiogenesis: an organizing principle for drug discovery? *Nat Rev Drug Discov.* 6, 273–286.

Fong, T. A. T., Shawver, L. K., Sun, L., et al. (**1999**). SU5416 is a potent and selective inhibitor of the vascular endothelial growth factor receptor (Flk-1/KDR) that inhibits tyrosine kinase catalysis, tumor vascularization, and growth of multiple tumor types. *Cancer Res.* 59, 99–106.

Friedlander, M., Hancock, K. C., Benigno, B., et al. (**2007**). Pazopanib (GW786034) is active in women with advanced epithelial ovarian, fallopian tube and peritoneal cancers: initial results of a Phase II study. *J Clin Oncol.* 25(18S), 5561.

Harris, P. A., Cheung, M., Hunter, R. N. III, et al. (**2005**). Discovery and evaluation of 2-anilino-5-aryloxazoles as a novel class of VEGFR2 kinase inhibitors. *J Med Chem.* 48, 1610–1619.

Huh, J.-I., Calvo, A., Stafford, J., et al. (**2005**). Inhibition of VEGF receptors significantly impairs mammary cancer growth in C3(1)/Tag transgenic mice through antiangiogenic and non-antiangiogenic mechanism. *Oncogene.* 24, 790–800.

Hutson, T. E., Davis, I. D., Machiels, J. H., et al. (**2008**). Biomarker analysis and final efficacy and safety results of a Phase II renal cell carcinoma trial with pazopanib (GW786034), a multi-kinase angiogenesis inhibitor. *J Clin Oncol.* 26, May 20 suppl; abstr 5046.

Hurwitz, H., Dowlati, A., Savage, S., et al. (**2005**). Safety, tolerability and pharmacokinetics of oral administration of GW786034 in pts with solid tumors. *J Clin Oncol.* 23(16S), 3012.

Kane, R. C., Farrell, A. T., Saber, H., et al. (**2006**). Sorafenib for the treatment of advanced renal cell carcinoma. *Clin Cancer Res.* 12, 7271–7278.

Karaman, M. W., Herrgard, S., Treiber, D. K., et al. (**2008**). A quantitative analysis of kinase inhibitor selectivity. *Nat Biotechnol.* 26, 127–132.

Kumar, R., Miller, C. G., Johnson, J. H., et al. (**2003**). Discovery and biological evaluation of GW654652: A pan inhibitor of VEGF receptors. *Proc Amer Assoc Cancer Res.* 44, 9 (abstract #39).

Kumar, R., Knick, V. B., Rudolph, S. K., et al. (**2007**). Pharmacokinetic–pharmacodynamic correlation from mouse to human with pazopanib, a multi-kinase angiogenesis inhibitor with potent antitumor and antiangiogenic activity. *Mol Cancer Ther.* 6, 2012–2021.

Lantry, L. E. (**2007**). Drug evaluation: ranibizumab, a mAb against VEGF-A for the potential treatment of age-related macular degeneration and other ocular complications. *Curr Opin Mol Ther.* 9, 592–602.

Miwatashi, S., Arikawa, Y., Kotani, E., et al. (**2005**). Novel inhibitor of p38 MAP kinase as an anti-TNFα drug: discovery of N-[4-[2-ethyl-4-(3-methylphenyl)-1,3-thiazol-5-yl]-2-pyridyl]benzamide (TAK-715) as a potent and orally active anti-rheumatoid arthritis agent. *J Med Chem.* 48, 5966–5979.

O'Reilly, M. S., Boehm, T., Shing, Y., et al. (**1997**). Endostatin: an endogenous inhibitor of angiogenesis and tumor growth. *Cell.* 88, 277–285.

Pargellis, C., Tong, L., Churchill, L., et al. (**2002**). Inhibition of p38 MAP kinase by utilizing a novel allosteric binding site. *Nat Structural Biol.* 9(4), 268–272.

Ramalingam, S., and Belani, C. P. (**2007**). Role of bevacizumab for the treatment of non-small-cell lung cancer. *Future Oncol.* 3, 131–139.

Rogerson, T. D., Wilkinson, C. F., and Hetarski, K. (**1977**). Steric factors in the inhibitory interaction of imidazoles with microsomal enzymes. *Biochem Pharmacol.* 26, 1039–1042.

Sleijfer, S., Papai, Z., Cesne, A. Le, et al., (**2007**). Phase II study of pazopanib (GW786034) in patients (pts) with relapsed or refractory soft tissue sarcoma (STS): EORTC 62043. *J Clin Oncol.* 25(18S), 10031.

Sorbera, L. A., Bolos, J., and Serradell, N. (**2006**). Pazopanib hydrochloride. Oncolytic, angiogenesis inhibitor, VEGFR-2 tyrosine kinase inhibitor. *Drug Future.* 31, 585–589.

Sonpavde, G., and Hutson, T. E. (**2007**). Pazopanib: a novel multitargeted tyrosine kinase inhibitor. *Curr Oncol Rep.* 9, 115–119.

Veber, D. F., Johnson, S. R., Cheng, H.-Y., et al. (**2002**). Molecular properties that influence the oral bioavailability of drug candidates. *J Med Chem.* 45, 2615–2623.

Veikkola, T., Karkkainen, M., Claesson-Welsh, L., et al. (**2000**). Regulation of angiogenesis via vascular endothelial growth factor receptors. *Cancer Res.* 60, 203–212.

4

ROAD TO ABT-869: A MULTITARGETED RECEPTOR TYROSINE KINASE INHIBITOR

MICHAEL MICHAELIDES AND DANIEL H. ALBERT

4.1. INTRODUCTION

Targeting angiogenesis as a means of treating cancer became a major focus of research for the academic community and the pharmaceutical industry in the mid-1990s. Angiogenesis—the process by which new blood vessels are formed from preexisting vessels—is essential for primary tumor growth and metastatic progression. However, angiogenesis is highly regulated in adult humans and is restricted to physiological processes such as wound healing and menstruation. Thus inhibition of angiogenesis held great promise as a novel and relatively nontoxic anticancer therapy (Folkman, 1995).

The proangiogenic factor most commonly implicated in tumor progression is vascular endothelial growth factor (VEGF). Its angiogenic responses are primarily the result of signaling through the VEGFR2 (KDR) receptor tyrosine kinase. KDR is a member of the VEGF receptor family, which also includes the FLT1 (VEGFR1) and FLT4 (VEGFR3) kinases. Many different cell types are able to produce VEGF, but its biological activity is limited predominantly to the vasculature by way of the endothelial-cell selective expression of KDR (Ferrara et al., 2003).

Based on the key role of the VEGF/KDR axis as a mediator of angiogenesis, a program targeting selective inhibition of KDR was initiated in the late 1990s at the BASF Bioresearch Center in Worcester, Massachusetts, which was a division of Knoll Pharmaceutical and subsequently became a part of Abbott

Kinase Inhibitor Drugs. Edited by Rongshi Li and Jeffrey A. Stafford

Laboratories. The initial focus of this program was on KDR selective agents as this was thought to minimize the potential for toxicity. Minimizing toxicity was an important goal since it was widely believed that targeted antiangiogenic therapies would have significantly larger therapeutic windows than classical cytotoxic agents. One anticipated potential problem was activity against members of the platelet-derived growth factor receptor (PDGFR) tyrosine kinases, the subfamily of RTKs closest to the VEGFR kinase family on the phylogenetic tree.

The PDGFR family consists of PDGFRα and PDGFRβ, CSF1R, cKIT, and FLT3 and has been shown to mediate hematopoiesis. For example, cKIT promotes the survival of early hematopoietic progenitor cells and is important for the growth and differentiation of mast cells (Lyman and Jacobsen, 1998). Also, PDGF is a growth factor for marrow stromal fibroblasts, which in turn are important for the formation of a productive hematopoietic microenvironment in bone marrow. Finally, FLT3 plays an important role in the development of hematopoietic stem cells, dendritic cells, and natural killer cells (McKenna et al., 2000). Thus nonselective agents targeting both VEGFR and PDGFR kinases were expected to potentially cause bone marrow toxicity.

4.2. EARLY LEAD SERIES

The project team pursued multiple chemotypes before ultimately arriving at the aminoindazole series and the clinical compound ABT-869. During the early stages of the project the bulk of the medicinal chemistry effort was directed at optimizing two high-throughput screening hits: the tricyclic pyrazole **1** and the indolinone **2** (Figure 4.1). Optimization of the pseudo C2-symmetric tricyclic pyrazole HTS hit **1** proved to be particularly difficult and time consuming, partly due to the lengthy synthetic schemes. This series was also intermittently plagued with any of the following liabilities: high clearance, low oral bioavailability, low aqueous solubility, and significant hERG channel affinity. We were eventually able to prepare compounds that overcame these liabilities as described in several publications (Dinges et al., 2006a, b, 2007; Akritopoulou-Zanze et al., 2007). However, this was only a Pyrrhic victory as none of the optimized compounds ultimately were superior to ABT-869.

The indolinone SU11248-like HTS hit **2** yielded two novel chemotypes through manipulation of the indolinone hinge binding core: namely, the ring-expanded 6,6 bicyclic benzothiazinones (**2a**) (Rafferty et al., 2000) and the monocyclic C3-aryl substituted pyrazolinones (**2b**) (Moset Marina et al., 2001; Cusack et al., 2004). In general, the benzothiazinones exhibited poor KDR cellular activity. The pyrazolinones were potent against KDR and active in tumor growth inhibition models but exhibited poor selectivity against members of the PDGFR family. An advanced compound from this series with potent dual inhibitory activity (KDR IC_{50} = 70 nM, cKIT IC_{50} = 60 nM) was found to

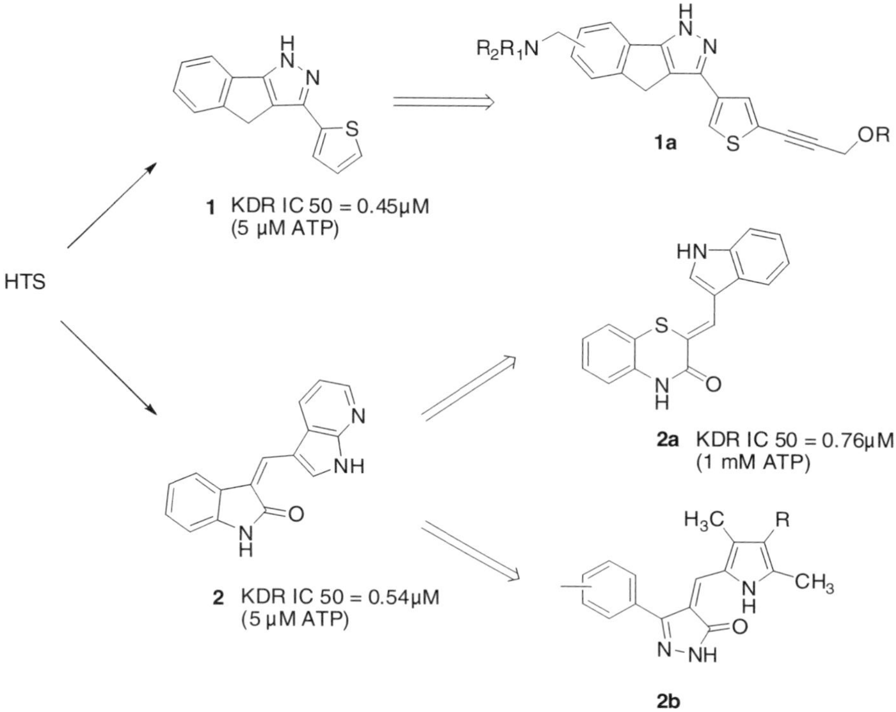

Figure 4.1. HTS hits to early lead series.

cause bone marrow hypocellularity at doses similar to those that produced robust efficacy in tumor growth models, thus seemingly confirming the notion that KDR selectivity would be essential for an acceptable therapeutic window.

At the same time, a separate kinase inhibitor project at BASF Bioresearch was exploring a series of phenoxyphenyl pyrazolopyrimidines (**5a**) (Figure 4.2) as inhibitors of the cytosolic src-family lymphoid T-cell protein tyrosine kinase (Lck) (Arnold et al., 2000). This series of compounds was a hybrid of the screening hit **3** and the well-known src inhibitor PP1 (**4**) (Figure 4.2). In an attempt to optimize selectivity for Lck, a variety of different groups in place of the oxygen linking the two phenyls occupying the back hydrophobic pocket were prepared and counterscreened against the available receptor tyrosine kinases. The nature of the Ph-X-Ph linker dictated the potency and selectivity for Lck and KDR with a urea moiety introducing KDR activity (**5b** IC$_{50}$ = 260 nM) (Burchat et al., 2002). Interestingly, a sulfonamide linker resulted in compounds with potent Tie-2 activity (**5c**). Tie-2 is another RTK involved in angiogenesis and, in fact, was the subject of a separate cancer drug discovery project. The boost in KDR inhibitory activity associated with diaryl ureas ultimately led to the discovery of ABT-869, as described next.

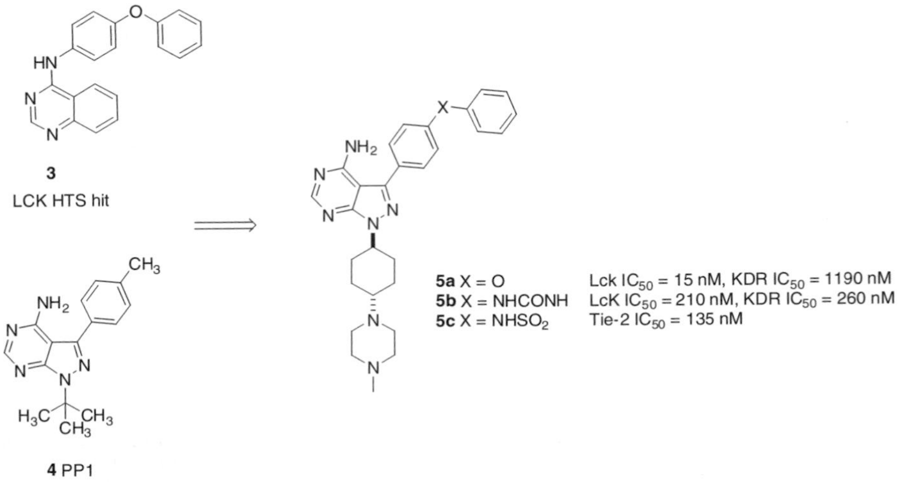

Figure 4.2. From Lck to KDR inhibitors.

4.3. DRUG DISCOVERY FUNNEL

Project compounds were characterized and prioritized based on a testing scheme that reflected KDR inhibitory activity at the enzymatic, cellular, and in vivo level. We employed the same general assays throughout the course of the project, although adjustments were made to reflect the different stages of the project as it matured toward the selection of a clinical candidate.

The primary project testing strategy is depicted in Figure 4.3. Compounds were first assessed in parallel for their enzymatic potency and selectivity, testing against a panel of kinases using high-throughput automated homogeneous time-resolved fluorescence (HTRF) based assays at a high (1 mM) physiologically relevant concentration of ATP. The use of high concentrations of ATP proved useful as it predicted cellular responses quite well and was ideal for the lead optimization stage of a project. The selectivity panel initially consisted of the human intracellular domain of KDR along with Tie-2, Lck, and cKIT and was later expanded to include FLT3, CSF1R, and FLT1. Compounds with an IC_{50} value of less than 100 nM were progressed to a KDR ELISA-based cellular assay, evaluating inhibition of VEGF-stimulated KDR receptor phosphorylation in 3T3 murine fibroblasts transfected with human KDR.

In vivo tumor growth inhibition experiments are time and compound intensive and consequently are very low throughput. Thus there was a critical need to develop a rapid in vivo assay that would allow us to efficiently triage compounds. To that end, we adapted an acute in vivo assay that exploits the ability of VEGF to induce vascular permeability (Ma et al., 2001; Sengupta et al., 2003). In this model, female mice are primed with pregnant mare's serum gonadotropin, then treated with 17β-estradiol, resulting in an upregulation of

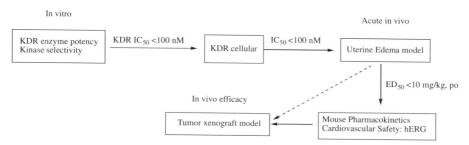

Figure 4.3. Primary project testing strategy.

VEGF and subsequent uterine edema, via ligand interaction with KDR. Test compounds administered prior to estradiol injection that are active as KDR inhibitors block the uterine edema. A comparison of the uteri weights in treated versus control animals, sacrificed 3 hours after estradiol injection provided a rapid and convenient method of measuring acute in vivo VEGF inhibition. The route of administration, screening dose, and timing of test compound administration changed over the course of the project, gradually becoming more stringent. Specifically, the route of administration changed from intraperitoneal to oral, the screening dose was decreased from 100 to 30 and finally to 10 mg/kg, while the time period between compound and estradiol administration was increased from 30 min to 2 h. These changes were made in an effort to select for potent, oral, and long-lived compounds. The high-throughput nature of this model and small amount of compound required (<15 mg) allowed us to rapidly screen multiple compounds per week, in excess of our PK capabilities. Importantly, triaging compounds based on in vivo activity was more relevant than selecting compounds based on oral exposure, since in vivo activity does not simply correlate with plasma levels but rather reflects multiple parameters such as on–off rates, plasma binding, and distribution.

Compounds that were active in the uterine edema model (>50% inhibition) at the screening dose were then evaluated for a dose response in order to determine an ED_{50} value. The ED_{50} values were then used to prioritize the compounds for further pharmacokinetic evaluation (intravenous and oral administration in mice) and cardiovascular safety characterization (primarily dofetilide binding). Compounds with an ED_{50} of less than 10 mg/kg, po in the uterine edema model were typically advanced into the human fibrosarcoma (HT1080) xenograft tumor growth model. During the early stages of the program compounds were screened at 30 and 100 mg/kg dosed for 2 or 3 weeks; however, once potent compounds such as ABT-869 were identified screening doses were reduced to 10 and 30 mg/kg.

4.3.1. Optimization of Thienopyrimidine Series

Based on the KDR activity of the pyrazolopyrimidine diaryl urea **5b**, we investigated the replacement of the pyrazolopyrimidine template with

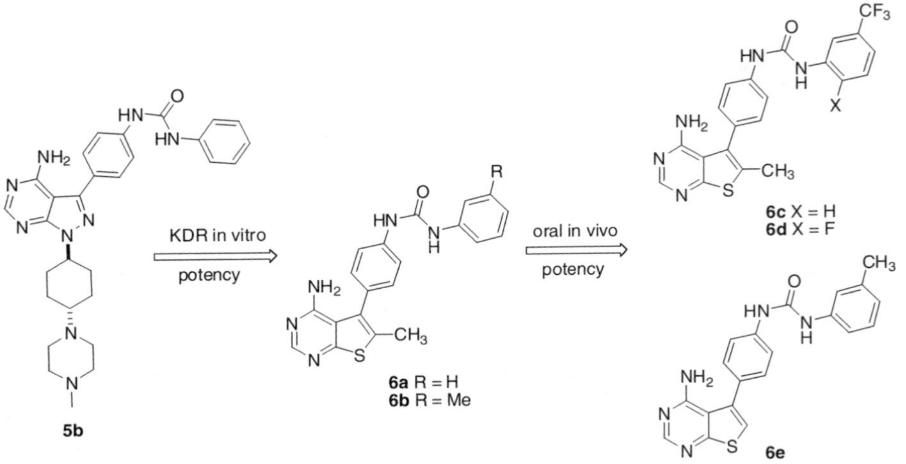

Figure 4.4. Thienopyrimidine series optimization.

alternate five-membered heterocycle-fused pyrimidines. The first heterocycle prepared was the thienopyrimidine **6a** (Figure 4.4) (Dai et al., 2005). Gratifyingly, the compound displayed potent inhibition of KDR with an IC_{50} value of 36 nM, representing a ninefold boost in potency relative to **5b**, and a significant increase in ligand efficiency, given the removal of the large N1 substituent. Furthermore, the compound is highly selective over Lck (Lck $IC_{50} = 30,800$ nM vs. 210 nM for **5b**), suggesting that the large cyclohexylpiperazine solubilizing group makes productive interactions with Lck, but not with KDR. Standard SAR studies around the terminal phenyl substituent led to a further sixfold boost in activity with the *meta*-methyl substituted urea **6b** (KDR: enzyme $IC_{50} = 6$ nM, cell $IC_{50} = 10$ nM). However, the compound was inactive in the uterine edema model, which is not surprising given its high clearance (6.6 L/h/kg) and poor oral bioavailability ($F = 10\%$) in mice. We speculated that the poor exposure was due to metabolism of one or both methyl groups. Thus we prepared the *meta*-trifluoromethyl analogs **6c** and **6d** and the 2-des-methyl analog **6e**, among others. This approach was successful as the compounds were active in the uterine edema model with ED_{50} values of 19, 5, and 5 mg/kg (after oral administration) for **6b**, **6d**, and **6e**, respectively. However, these compounds did not meet our goal of KDR selectivity since they were potent inhibitors of all members of the VEGFR and PDGFR families (e.g., **6e**: CSF1R, cKIT, FLT3 $IC_{50} = 2$–6 nM; PDGFRβ $IC_{50} = 48$ nM). Nonetheless, in light of their impressive oral activity in the uterine edema model, compounds from this series were advanced to in vivo tumor studies, a decision that proved critical to the success of this project. Several compounds were impressively efficacious in tumor xenograft models, at least in the eyes of the authors whose previous experience in oncology was with matrix metalloproteinase and histone deacetylase inhibitors. For example, **6e** inhibited the

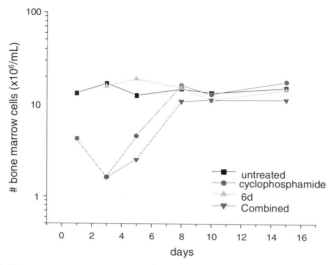

Figure 4.5. Bone marrow recovery following cyclophosphamide ablation dose. Cyclophosphamide dosed at 300 mg/kg; **6d** dosed at 25 mg/kg/day, bid, orally ($n = 3$/ time point).

growth of a fibrosarcoma HT1080 cell line implanted subcutaneously into the flank of SCID-beige mice by at least 76% at a dose of 25 mg/kg/day, administered twice daily.

One concern with this series of compounds was the possibility of bone marrow effects due to their nonselective kinase inhibitory profile. This led us to perform histopathology on femurs from mice treated with **6e**. Gratifyingly, only minimal hypocellularity was observed at the preclinically effective doses. In order to further address the effects of this series of compounds on bone marrow function, several compounds were tested in a bone marrow repopulation study. In one such experiment with compound **6d** BALB/c female mice were divided into four groups (Figure 4.5) (Bousquet, 2002). Group 1 received no treatment; Group 2 received a bone marrow ablating dose of cyclophosphamide; Group 3 received **6d** at a dose of 25 mg/kg/day, bid (a dose that produced 75% inhibition of tumor growth in the HT1080 xenograft model); and Group 4 received both cyclophosphamide and **6d** (25 mg/kg/day, bid). Bone marrow (femur) was then harvested at multiple time points as indicated in Figure 4.5 ($n = 3$/time point). Cyclophosphamide treatment reduced bone marrow cellularity by about 85% on day 3. Repopulation of the marrow occurred in the cyclophosphamide-treated animals by day 8. Fortunately, bone marrow recovery was not significantly blocked in animals treated with **6d** during the repopulation phase. Likewise **6d** itself did not have an effect on bone marrow cellularity. Additionally, these data appeared to be in agreement with emerging clinical findings from compounds that inhibited the PDGFR family. For example, bone marrow suppression was not reported as a dose-limiting toxicity with either Gleevec™ (cKIT inhibitor) or SUGEN's investigational multitargeted inhibitor SU11248 (later approved as Sutent™).

4.3.2. Shift to Multitargeted Inhibitors

Our discovery of the multitargeted thienopyrimidines as potent in vivo antitumor agents coincided with a renewed emphasis by the development team on compounds with the potential for a strong early signal of efficacy. The costly industry failure of large Phase III trials with cytostatic agents, such as matrix metalloproteinase inhibitors, highlighted the difficulty of designing clinical trials with agents having "subtle" antitumor effects. Also, during this time (2002 through 2003), the benefits of multitargeted inhibitors in terms of improved efficacy began to be better appreciated, since multiple biological pathways are typically dysregulated in cancer. For example, while VEGF is clearly a dominant mediator of tumor angiogenesis, it is not the only factor capable of supporting tumor vascularity (Folkman, 1996). In fact, tumors are capable of secreting multiple angiogenic factors, which play various roles in tumor growth at different stages of progression (Bergers et al., 1999; Carmeliet, 2003). VEGF causes a large increase in blood vessel formation, yet these vessels are immature and leaky. The formation of thicker, more stable vessels requires encapsulation by pericytes that is driven by PDGFRβ signaling. Thus PDGFRβ inhibition results in microvessels lacking pericyte coverage, which regress upon deprivation of VEGF signaling. Synergistic antiangiogenic effects were thought to be possible by targeting not only endothelial cells but also the supporting perivascular cells (Bergers and Benjamin, 2003; Gerber and Ferrara, 2003). Indeed, Bergers et al. (2003) showed that therapeutic regimes combining a VEGFR inhibitor with a PDGFR inhibitor were more efficacious against all stages of islet carcinogenesis than either agent alone and the combination regressed late-stage tumors. The authors concluded: "In the longer term, a new generation of RTKI with dual specificity against VEGF and PDGFRs have similar potential to significantly impact treatment of well-established solid tumors."

The discovery that the tumor microenvironment actively participates in tumor progression provides another reason to pursue agents capable of blocking multiple VEGF and PDGF receptor family members. Tumor-associated fibroblasts that express PDGFRβ are functionally distinct from normal fibroblasts and are thought to foster tumor cell invasion and metastasis through the release of growth factors and proteases (Camps et al., 1990). FLT1 and CSF1R regulate the production and activation of tumor-associated macrophages that hasten breakdown of the extracellular matrix by triggering gelatinase A expression. KIT-expressing inflammatory mast cells have been implicated as accessory cells in tumor angiogenesis.

In addition to blocking host-derived kinases, multitargeted VEGF/PDGF RTK inhibitors can also produce direct effects on cancer cells, whose proliferation is reliant either on a mutant such as FLT3 mutations in acute myelogenous leukemia (AML) patients or cKIT-activating mutations in gastrointestinal

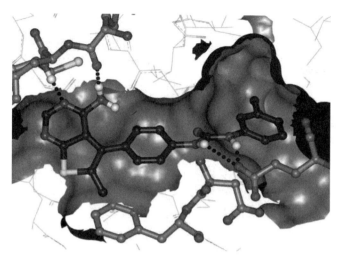

Figure 4.6. Model of **6b** bound to KDR kinase. Hydrogen bonds in black are shown between the urea NHs and Glu885 carboxylate, between the exocyclic amine and Glu917 backbone carbonyl, and between the ring nitrogen and Cys919 N-H. Also in thick bond are residues Asp1046-Phe1047 of the "DFG" motif in the "inactive" conformation ("DFG-out"). Reprinted with permission from *J Med Chem.* **2005**, 48, 6066–6083. Copyright © 2005 American Chemical Society. (See color insert.)

stromal tumors or an overexpressed kinase such as high expression of KIT in small cell lung cancer (SCLC). Indeed, the clinical efficacy of Gleevec in gastrointestinal stromal tumor patients is attributed to its cKIT kinase activity.

4.3.3. Diaryl Urea Mode of Binding

Introduction of the diaryl moiety was critical to potent KDR inhibition in the thienopyrimidine series. However, the thienopyridine diaryl ureas exhibited very low aqueous solubility (a fact not left unnoticed by the project biologists) and high plasma binding. Additionally, the team was concerned about possible metabolism of the urea to a potentially toxic aniline metabolite. Thus considerable efforts were made to identify suitable urea replacements. As depicted in the model of **6b** bound to KDR (Figure 4.6) the urea unit accesses the back hydrophobic pocket adjacent to the ATP binding site, which is available only when KDR is in an inactive kinase conformation. The carbonyl oxygen of the urea is within H-bonding distance of the backbone N-H of Asp 1046 (of the DFG motif), while both urea N-H groups project toward the side chain carboxylate of Glu885, with the external N-H forming a more optimal H-bonding interaction. Consistent with this model, the effect of urea N-methylation was more dramatic for the external NH (310-fold loss in activity) than for the internal NH (9-fold loss). Homologated amides resulting from replacement of the internal NH with a methylene were tolerated although generally these compounds were less active in vivo. All attempts at replacing the urea with groups such as amides, sulfonamides, aminobenzoxazoles, and 3,4-diaminocyclobutene diones led to loss of activity. Since we failed to identify urea replacements, we then focused our attention on identifying replacements for the thienopyrimidine core as described next.

4.3.4. Extension of Diaryl Ureas to Other Chemotypes

Encouraged by the potent antitumor in vivo efficacy and lack of bone marrow effects of the thienopyrimidine diaryl urea series, we sought to investigate additional scaffolds that could serve as hinge binders in parallel to the optimization of the thienopyrimidines. The team began with conservative changes to the thienopyrimidine core, maintaining the hinge binding pyrimidine portion intact and investigating other five-membered heterocycle analogs in place of the thiophene portion, such as isothiazole (**7a**), furan (**7b**), and isoxazole (**7c**) (Figure 4.7) (Ji et al., 2006). Generally, the isothiazolo and isoxazolopyrimidines were potent in vitro inhibitors but had modest pharmacokinetic profiles. The furo analogs were active in both in vitro and in vivo models but did not offer any advantages over the thienopyrimidine lead series. Scientists at GSK have also extensively investigated this series (Miyazaki et al., 2005, 2007b). The ring-expanded diazepine analogs (**7d**) maintained potent in vitro activity but were inferior in terms of in vivo efficacy as measured in the uterine edema model (Gracias et al., 2008). We briefly investigated a 4-aminopyrrolotriazine core (**7e**), a close analog of the 4-anilinopyrrolotriazines, which were originally developed by BMS scientists as an alternative to the well-studied quinazoline core. However, this series was quickly terminated when we realized that Bayer scientists were also active in this area (Dixon et al., 2005).

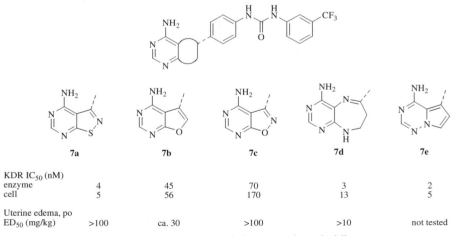

KDR IC$_{50}$ (nM)	7a	7b	7c	7d	7e
enzyme	4	45	70	3	2
cell	5	56	170	13	5
Uterine edema, po ED$_{50}$ (mg/kg)	>100	ca. 30	>100	>10	not tested

Figure 4.7. Alternate bicyclic heterocyclopyrimidines.

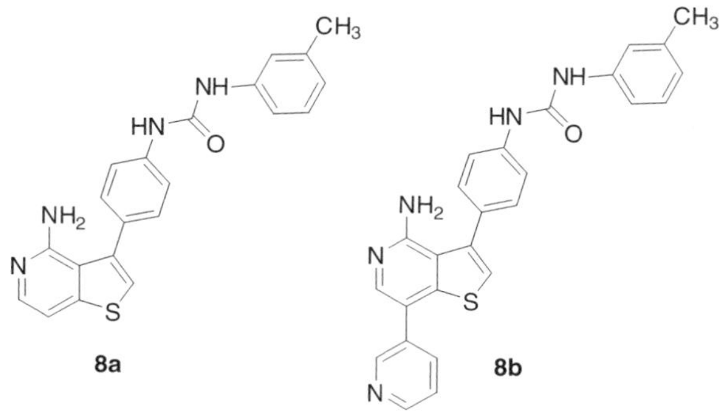

Figure 4.8. Thienopyridine diaryl ureas.

As shown in Figure 4.6, the pyrimidine portion of the molecule interacts with the hinge region of KDR through the classic binding motif of a pair of hydrogen bond donor/acceptor interactions between (1) the exocyclic amine and the backbone carbonyl of Glu 917 and (2) the proximal ring nitrogen and the backbone N-H of Cys 919. Therefore we expected that replacement of the N1 nitrogen with carbon would be tolerated, although we were uncertain if the H-bond strength would be affected by the change in electron density. The thienopyridine analog **8a** (Figure 4.8) was prepared and found to be a potent multitargeted inhibitor in both enzymatic and cellular assays (KDR: enzyme IC_{50} = 9 nM, cell IC_{50} = 32 nM; cKIT IC_{50} = 2 nM) (Heyman et al., 2007). This model also suggested that substituents at the now accessible C7 position would project away from the active site toward solvent, thus providing a convenient means to modulate the physiochemical properties of this series. Consistent with this hypothesis introduction of heterocycles such as pyridine provided analogs (e.g., **8b**) that were equipotent with **8a**. This series along with the corresponding furopyridines have been independently evaluated as KDR and Tie-2 inhibitors by scientists at GSK (Miyazaki et al., 2007a).

Recognizing the need to maximize structural diversity, we concurrently explored more drastic template changes. We investigated alternate bicyclic systems that would satisfy the two critical design requirements of (1) ability to form hydrogen bond interactions with the hinge region and (2) providing an appropriate attachment vector for the diaryl urea. The first template investigated was an isoindolinone, as exemplified by **9a** (Figure 4.9) (Curtin et al., 2004). Although the isoindolinone diaryl series was discontinued due to low oral exposure, we were satisfied that we could apply the diaryl motif to templates other than fused pyrimidines and maintain potent enzymatic and cellular activity (e.g., **9a**: KDR cell IC_{50} = 65 nM). We thus continued our investigation of alternate 5–6 systems by preparing the 3-aminoindazole **9b** (Dai et al., 2007). As shown in Figure 4.10, there is an almost ideal overlap between the aminoindazole **9b** and the thienopyridine **6b**, particularly regarding the hinge and urea H-bond interaction elements. The aminoindazole **9b** is

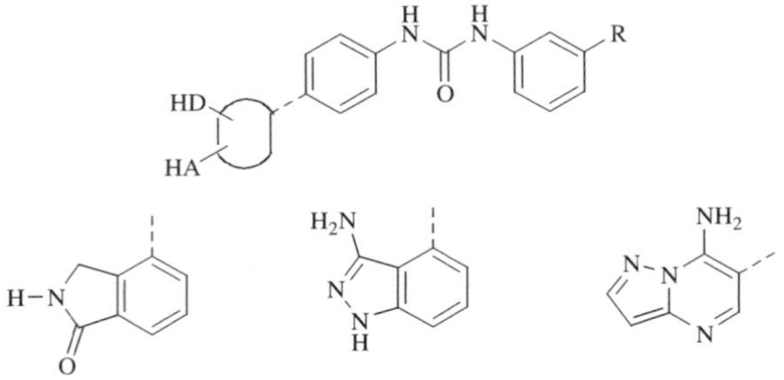

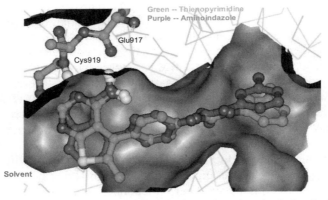

Figure 4.9. Alternate diaryl urea chemotypes.

	9a R= CF$_3$	**9b R = CH$_3$**	**9c R = CF$_3$**
KDR IC$_{50}$ (nM)			9
enzyme	7	3	35
cell	65	13	
Uterine edema, po ED$_{50}$ (mg/kg)	>100	4	>10

Figure 4.10. Overlap of thienopyrimidine **6b** (green) and aminoindazole **9b** (purple) bound to KDR kinase. (See color insert.)

in fact a potent KDR inhibitor with an IC$_{50}$ value of 3 nM. A close analog of **9b**, ABT-869, was ultimately developed as a clinical candidate, as shown next. A third structurally distinct series developed after the discovery of ABT-869 was the 7-aminopyrazolopyrimidine (**9c**) wherein the hinge binding exocyclic amine and diarylurea attachment points are on adjacent atoms as opposed to the usual 1,3 arrangement in the other series (Frey et al., 2008). Optimization led to compounds with potent in vitro and acute in vivo efficacy; however tumor growth inhibition was inferior to ABT-869.

4.3.5. Aminoindazole Optimization: Discovery of ABT-869

The first aminoindazole urea prepared was the *meta*-methyl substituted urea **9b**. This compound had an unusually favorable overall profile with good

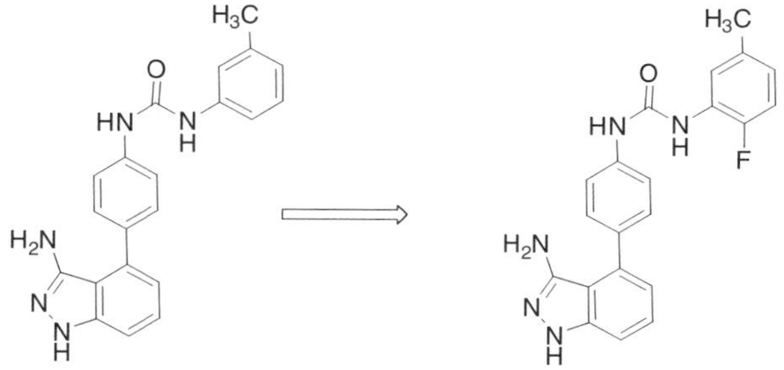

9b

KDR cell IC_{50} = 13nM
Uterine Edema, ED_{50} (po) = 4 mg/kg
oral bioavailability (mouse) = 38%
dofetilide binding IC_{50}>10 μM

ABT-869

KDR cell IC_{50} = 3nM
Uterine Edema, ED_{50} (po) = 0.5 mg/kg
oral bioavailability (mouse) > 50%
dofetilide binding IC_{50}>10 μM

Figure 4.11. Discovery of ABT-869.

efficacy in the uterine edema model, good oral bioavailability, and low affinity for the hERG channel (as measured by dofetilide binding) suggesting that this series might require minimal optimization (Figure 4.11). This proved true, as ABT-869 was one of the first twenty compounds synthesized. These early compounds were designed based on our in vitro and in vivo findings on the thienopyrimidine series, which were found to be predictive for the aminoindazole series. A large number of aminoindazoles progressed rapidly through our testing funnel exhibiting potent oral activity in the uterine edema model. The compounds were differentiated based on xenograft tumor growth inhibition studies. ABT-869 distinguished itself as the most potent compound with the broadest spectrum of activity across multiple models as will be described in detail. Importantly, ABT-869 also had a favorable safety pharmacology profile with no QT signal, as accessed in the hERG patch clamp, dog Purkinje fiber, and anesthetized dog cardiovascular assays as well as minimal inhibition of any of the cytochrome P450 isoforms tested (3A4, 2D6, 2C9, 2C19, 1A2, 2A6: $IC_{50} > 30\,\mu M$).

Optimization of the aminoindazole series was facilitated by an efficient and versatile synthesis, which allowed for the relatively rapid preparation of multiple analogs in significant (1–2 g) amounts, thus expediting compound characterization (Figure 4.12). The key 4-iodo-3-aminoindazole intermediate (**12d**) was prepared in good overall yield starting with a substituted 1-fluoro-3-iodobenzene (**12a**). Fluoride-directed lithiation and subsequent reaction with CO_2 provided the acid **12b**, which was converted to the nitrile **12c** via the corresponding amide. Reaction of **12c** with hydrazine gave **12d** in high yield. The final compounds were then prepared via a Suzuki reaction of **12d** with diaryl urea boronates, easily prepared via the reaction of aniline boronates with the corresponding aryl isocyanates.

The general SAR trends observed in the aminoindazole series are depicted in Figure 4.13. SAR of the urea terminal phenyl was consistent with the

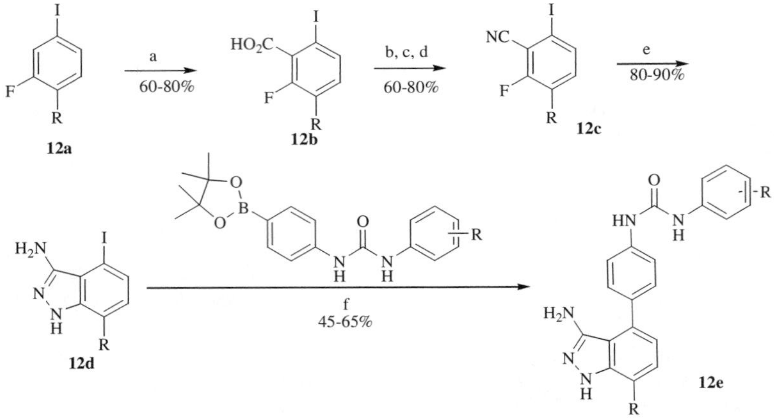

Figure 4.12. General synthesis of 3-aminoindazoles. (a) 1. LDA/THF, $-78\,^{\circ}$C; 2. CO_2 (60–80%); (b) $SOCl_2$, reflux; (c) NH_4OH; (d) $SOCl_2$, DMF, $115\,^{\circ}$C; (e) $NH_2NH_2 \cdot H_2O$, n-BuOH, $110\,^{\circ}$C; (f) Pd(dppf)Cl_2, Na_2CO_3/DME/H_2O, $85\,^{\circ}$C, 16 h.

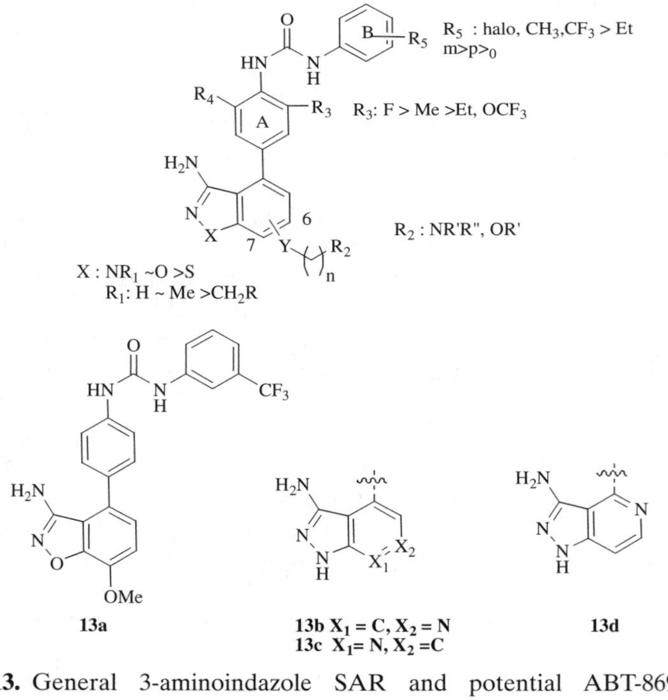

Figure 4.13. General 3-aminoindazole SAR and potential ABT-869 backup compounds.

thienopyrimidine series, with *meta*-substitution being optimal for KDR inhibitory activity. We investigated substitutions on the internal urea aryl (A ring) in the hope that this would lead to improved solubility through disruption of intermolecular forces. However, substitution with groups other than fluoro had a detrimental effect on activity. Disubstitution, in particular (R_3,R_4 = Me), led to a complete loss of activity. N-methylation of the endocyclic indazole NH (X) was tolerated, confirming that there is no direct hydrogen bonding interaction between the NH and the enzyme. Similarly, replacement of the same nitrogen with oxygen afforded largely equipotent compounds. Conversely, replacement with the larger sulfur atom was less tolerated. Considerable effort was made to optimize the isoxazole analogs of ABT-869 leading to orally bioavailable compounds with potent in vivo antitumor efficacy (Ji et al., 2008). For example, **13a** exhibited 81% inhibition of tumor growth in the HT1080 model at 10 mg/kg/day, bid; however, none of the compounds offered any advantage relative to ABT-869.

4.3.6. Attempts to Identify ABT-869 Backup Compounds with Improved Water Solubility

Although the poor water solubility of ABT-869 did not limit its oral bioavailability, we were concerned that its high lipophilicity ($c\log P$ = 4.2) coupled with its low aqueous solubility (27 ng/mL at pH 7.2) might present formulation challenges. Therefore backup or replacement compounds with improved physiochemical properties were rigorously pursued. Kinase inhibitors are generally more lipophilic than other classes of compounds and this has presented solubility challenges to multiple medicinal chemistry kinase groups. The standard approach has been to introduce water-solubilizing groups at positions that project toward solvent and therefore do not compromise inhibitory potency. Examining the mode of binding of the aminoindazoles to the KDR ATP binding site revealed that the optimal positions for introducing hydrophilic groups were the benzo positions at C6 and C7 (Figures 4.10 and 4.13). In the event, introduction of typical solubilizing groups such as morpholine, piperazine, piperidine, and acyclic tertiary amines tethered by 1, 2, or 3 atom spacers was well tolerated in terms of enzymatic and cellular activity. However, introduction of these amines did not overcome the inherent poor solubility of the diaryl urea, particularly at neutral pH. Additionally, the compounds were inactive in the uterine edema model after oral administration. Consistent with this inactivity, pharmacokinetic evaluation of select compounds revealed high clearance and low oral exposure presumably due to rapid metabolism of the amine moieties. In an effort to maintain the favorable pharmacokinetic profile of the aminoindazole series, while also improving solubility, we prepared the more basic azaindazole core analogs (**13b–d**). The 6- and 7-aza analogs were equipotent with the parent compounds, whereas the 5-aza analogs (**13d**) had weaker activity (Dai et al., 2008). These findings were consistent with the binding model, which suggested that the 5-position projects to a hydrophobic region comprised of Phe1047 of the DFG motif. An improvement in solubility (2–10 μM vs. 0.07 μM for ABT-869) was noted, albeit solubility was still lower than desired.

A recent paper by Bergström et al. (2007) analyzed poorly soluble but successfully marketed oral drugs. The authors concluded that these oral drugs display solvation-limited solubility. Solvation-limited compounds are lipophilic compounds that have poor water solubility because of an inability to form bonds with water, as opposed to compounds that have poor water solubility because of strong intermolecular bonds leading to stable crystals. Therefore compounds with poor water solubility but good lipid solubility can successfully be formulated using lipids and other excipients. Additionally, bile salts in intestinal fluids can improve the solubility of highly lipophilic compounds. The lipid solubility of ABT-869 is consistent with the above profile, since it is significantly more soluble in simulated intestinal fluid (10 and 43 μg/mL fasted and fed, respectively), and in various organic and lipid vehicles with excipient and complexation agents (2 to >200 mg/mL). This profile opened the door to the lipid-based formulations successfully used in its initial clinical development.

4.4. CHARACTERIZATION OF ABT-869 AND ADVANCEMENT TO CLINICAL TRIALS

4.4.1. Kinase Inhibition Profile and Cellular Activity

ABT-869 has been evaluated for effects on both the primary enzyme targets (VEGF and PDGF receptors) as well as a number of structurally related receptor tyrosine kinases, cytosolic tyrosine kinases, and serine/threonine kinases. As shown in Table 4.1, ABT-869 exhibits IC_{50} values under 100 nM for all members of the VEGF and PDGF receptor families. It has some enzyme activity against the Tie-2 and RET receptors, but is much less active against

TABLE 4.1. Inhibition of VEGF and PDGF Family Receptor Tyrosine Kinases

Kinase	IC_{50} (nM)[a]
KDR	4
FLT1	3
FLT4	40
PDGFRβ	66
CSF1R	3
KIT	14
FLT3	4

[a]IC_{50} values determined at an ATP concentration of 1 mM.

Source: Adapted from Albert et al. (2006) and Guo et al. (2006).

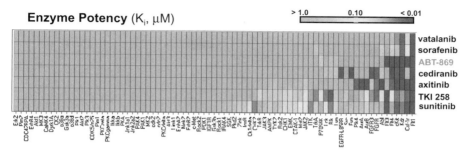

Figure 4.14. Kinase inhibition profile. (See color insert.)

nonrelated tyrosine kinases. Assessment of ABT-869 inhibitory activity against a broader representation of the kinome (80 kinases) revealed activity (IC_{50} values between 0.075 and 1 μM) for only seven additional kinases: Aurora1, Aurora2, Mst2, P70S6K, Rock1, Rock2, and Rsk2 (Figure 4.14). The modest potency for these serine/threonine kinases likely represents an overestimation of physicologically relevant activity, as these IC_{50} values were determined at an ATP concentration (5 μM) that was 200-fold lower than the 1 mM concentration—more reflective of cellular ATP—that was used for the tyrosine kinase assays discussed previously.

The potency of ABT-869 against enzyme preparations is reflected in receptor-mediated responses to VEGF at the cellular level. Phosphorylation of KDR induced by VEGF is potently inhibited by ABT-869 (IC_{50} values of 2–4 nM) in human endothelial cells and murine fibroblasts engineered to express human KDR (Table 4.2). Phosphorylation of other primary kinase targets of ABT-869 (i.e., PDGFRβ, KIT, CSF1R, and FLT3) are also potently inhibited in cell-based assays, with IC_{50} values of 1–31 nM (Table 4.2).

A potentially challenging feature of ABT-869 is the high degree of plasma protein binding exhibited across several species. As shown in Table 4.3, values of percent bound range from 96% to >99% depending on the species and analytical method utilized. Given this high level of protein binding, it is perhaps not surprising that the cellular potency of ABT-869 is affected by serum protein. The presence of 50% mouse or human plasma increased the IC_{50} value for inhibiting KDR phosphorylation by a magnitude (80- and 113-fold, Table 4.2) that closely approximates the free fraction predicted by the protein binding of ABT-869 in serum (1.8% and 1.0%, respectively, based on the ultracentrifugation results). A similar effect of serum proteins is observed when monitoring FLT3 phosphorylation. These results suggest that potency determined in serum-free settings, such as those used to assess enzyme activity, may be shifted as much as 85-fold in the presence of physiologically relevant protein concentrations. However, the high level of protein binding exhibited by ABT-869 did not substantially diminish its in vivo potency, since ABT-869 exhibits profound activity in the mechanism-based and tumor growth models discussed later.

TABLE 4.2. Activity of ABT-869 in Cellular Receptor Phosphorylation Assays

Cell	Receptor	Ligand	Protein	IC_{50} (nM)
HUAEC	KDR[a]	VEGF	—	2
3T3	KDR	VEGF	50% Mouse	3
transfectants			plasma	240
			50% Human	340
			plasma	
MG63	PDGFRβ	PDGF-BB	—	31
3T3	KIT	VEGF	—	48
transfectants				
3T3	CSF1R	CSF1	—	24
transfectants				
3T3	FLT3	Autoactivation		13
transfectants				
3T3	TIE2	Autoactivation	—	3,500
transfectants				
MV-4 11	FLT3 (ITD)	Autoactivation	—	1
			Human	100
			blood	

[a]Assay done using immunoprecipitation and Western blot techniques. All others done by ELISA.
Source: Adapted from Albert et al. (2006).

TABLE 4.3. Plasma Protein Binding

Assay Method/ Concentration	Protein Binding (%)				
	Mouse	Rat	Dog	Monkey	Human
Ultracentrifugation/ 5 μM	98.2	99.1	98.9	96.8	99.0
Ultrafiltration[a]/ 0.3–8 μM	99.8	99.8	99.9	99.9	99.9

[a]Determined with [³H]ABT-869.
Source: Mandli et al. (2006).

Inhibition of kinase activation translates into antiproliferative activity if the cell population is dependent for survival on the targeted kinase pathway (Stirewalt and Radich, 2003). ABT-869 is a potent inhibitor of proliferation of endothelial cells, a cell type long known to be dependent on the mitogenic signaling of VEGF (Leung et al., 1989), and this activity is presumably the primary basis for the antiangiogenic effects of this class of kinase inhibitors. In general, ABT-869 is a potent antiproliferative agent only toward cell populations that are dependent on the mitogenic signaling pathways of the kinases targeted by ABT-869. Thus ABT-869 exhibits only weak antiproliferative activity (IC_{50} values > 1000 nM) for cell lines derived from solid tumors and from factor-independent hematopoietic tumor cell lines (Table 4.4). In contrast,

TABLE 4.4. Inhibition of Cell Proliferation[a]

Cell Type	Source	Growth Factor[b]	IC_{50} (nM)	Reference
Endothelial	HUAEC	VEGF	0.2	Albert et al. (2006)
Colon carcinoma	HT-29	FBS	1,300	Albert et al. (2006)
Fibrosarcoma	HT1080	FBS	6,800	Albert et al. (2006)
Epidermoid carcinoma	A431	FBS	3,200	Albert et al. (2006)
Breast carcinoma	MDA-435	FBS	2,400	Albert et al. (2006)
Breast carcinoma	MDA-231	FBS	>10,000	Albert et al. (2006)
SCLC	H526	FBS	4,500	Albert et al. (2006)
Colon carcinoma	DLD-1	FBS	>10,000	Albert et al. (2006)
Rat glioma	9L	FBS	270	Albert et al. (2006)
B-cell (FLT3-WT)	BAF3[c]	FBS	~70	Glaser (2008)
B-cell (FLT3-ITD)	BAF3[c]	FBS	~7	Glaser (2008)
Mast cell (KIT V560G)	M-07e[d]	FBS	~20	Glaser (2008)
AML (FLT3-ITD)	MV-4-11	FBS	4–6	Shankar et al. (2007), Zhou et al. (2008a, c)
AML (FLT3-ITD) ABT-869 resistant	MV-4-11-R	FBS	52	Zhou et al. (2009)
AML–FLT3-ITD	MOLM-13	FBS	6	Shankar et al. (2007)
AML–FLT3-ITD	MOLM-14	FBS	10	Zhou et al. (2008c)
AML–FLT3-ITD	TF1-ITD	FBS	4	Zhou et al. (2008c)
AML–ETO (SCF-KIT loop; KIT N822K)	Kasumi-1	FBS	16	Shankar et al. (2007)
Factor-independent AML	RS4;11	FBS	4,100	Shankar et al. (2007)
AML–wt-FLT3 (FGF-FGFR loop)	KG-1	FBS	>100	Shankar et al. (2007)
ALL-FLT3 negative	Jurkat	FBS	4,200	Shankar et al. (2007)
APL-FLT3 negative	HL-60	FBS	~8,000	Shankar et al. (2007)
APL-PML-RARα	NB4	FBS	>10,000	Shankar et al. (2007)
CML–Bcr-Abl-FLT3 negative	K562	FBS	>5,000	Shankar et al. (2007)

[a]Cells were incubated with ABT-869 for 72 hours.
[b]VEGF: 10 ng/mL; FBS: 10% fetal bovine serum.
[c]B-cell line transfected with either FLT-WT or FLT-ITD.
[d]Mast cell line, M-07e, transfected with KIT V560G.

ABT-869 potently inhibits (IC_{50} values < 20 nM) the proliferation of tumor cells expressing constitutively active forms of FLT3 (FLT3-ITD) and KIT (V560G mutation) receptors and, to a lesser extent (IC_{50} values 20–70 nM), cells over-expressing either wild-type or mutant FLT3 or KIT receptors. ABT-869 does not have a significant effect on the proliferation and differentiation of human bone marrow cells up to a concentration of 1 μM (Shankar et al., 2007).

Tumor cells that have a profound survival dependence on growth factor signaling can over time lessen their dependence on the mitogen and acquire resistance to the effects of growth factor inhibitors (Gorre et al., 2001; Weisberg et al., 2002). In the case of FLT3-ITD AML, MV-4-11 cells in culture become resistant to ABT-869 and other FLT3 inhibitors through activation of STAT pathways and overexpression of survivin (Zhou et al., 2009). Further studies are needed to define possible resistance strategies across multiple tumor types but these initial reports suggest that the STAT and anti-apoptotic pathways are potential targets for reducing resistance developed in patients receiving FLT3 inhibitors.

4.4.2. Preclinical Pharmacokinetics

The pharmacokinetics of ABT-869 has been evaluated in CD-1 mouse, Sprague–Dawley rat, beagle dog, and cynomolgus monkey (Marsh, 2003). Plasma elimination half-lives following intravenous dosing range from 1.7 hours in the mouse to 3.6 hours in the rat (Table 4.5, Figure 4.15). Equilibrium volume of distribution values (V_{ss}) were fairly constant across species, with values ranging from 1.0 L/kg in rat to 2.2 L/kg in monkey. Plasma clearance values were low in all species, with the highest values in mouse (0.85 L/h·kg) and the lowest values in the rat (0.20 L/h·kg). Bioavailability was modest (11%) when dosed as a suspension but was significantly improved when dosed as a solution or as an amorphous solid dispersion. This preclinical pharmaco-kinetic profile was the basis for predicting, using allometric scaling and scaling based on in vitro turnover in human microsomes, an average human oral clear-ance of 13 L/h and a terminal phase half-life of 13–18 hours—a profile consis-tent with once-daily dosing (Marsh, 2003).

Given the extremely low aqueous solubility of ABT-869, formulation for preclinical in vivo studies represented a significant challenge. However, surface-active excipients improve the aqueous solubility of ABT-869 and ABT-869 has high solubility (>200 mg/g solution) in some organic solvents. Based on these solubility properties, vehicles consisting of either PEG-400 or combinations of cosolvents (e.g., 2% EtOH, 5% Tween 80, 20% PEG400, 73% saline) were devised and proved suitable for the preclinical studies discussed later.

4.4.3. Inhibition of VEGF-Mediated Responses In Vivo

As a way of confirming mode of action, the effect of ABT-869 on the functional consequences of KDR activation (e.g., receptor phosphorylation, vascular

TABLE 4.5. Pharmacokinetic Parameters Following in Mouse, Rat, Monkey, and Dog

Species	$t_{1/2}$ (h)	V_β (L/kg)	V_{ss} (L/kg)	AUC∞ (µg·h/mL)	CL$_p$ (L/h·kg)	F (%)
Mouse	1.7	2.1	1.6	5.87	0.85	48
Rat	3.6	1.1	1.0	25.10	0.20	28–34
Monkey	3.1	2.2	2.2	5.20	0.49	11
Dog	2.0	1.3	1.2	5.83	0.43	26–60

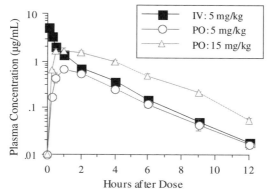

Figure 4.15. Pharmacokinetics of ABT-869 in mouse. Mean (±SEM, n = 3) plasma concentrations of ABT-869 after a single intravenous or oral dose.

permeability, and angiogenesis) have been evaluated in several in vivo settings. Effects on a surrogate tissue and lung, which expresses a high level of KDR, have been utilized to demonstrate target inhibition (Sepp-Lorenzino et al., 2004). As is shown in Figure 4.16, oral administration of ABT-869 (0.3 mg/kg) provided complete inhibition of KDR activation for up to 1 hour whereas a dose of 3 mg/kg was required to extend the inhibition to 3.5 hours post dose, a period more reflective of the duration of significant inhibition observed in a VEGF-response model after an efficacious dose of ABT-869 (see later discussion).

Further support of target inhibition was provided by observing the effects of ABT-869 on estradiol-induced edema, a hallmark of VEGF-induced vascular permeability in the uterus (Ma et al., 2001; Sengupta et al., 2003). As shown in Figure 4.17, ABT-869 given orally inhibited the edema response in a dose-dependent manner with a potency (ED$_{50}$ value of 0.5 mg/kg) that agrees well with the potency for inhibiting receptor phosphorylation of ABT-869 in lung. In addition, the plasma C_{max} value (predicted based on pharmacokinetic studies, Figure 4.15) for a 0.5 mg/kg dose (190 nM) also approximates the IC$_{50}$ value for inhibiting cellular KDR phosphorylation in the presence of mouse

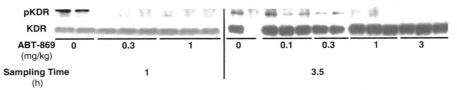

Figure 4.16. Inhibition of VEGF-induced KDR phosphorylation in mouse lung. ABT-869 was administered (orally) at the indicated dose either 1 h (*left*) or 3.5 h (*right*) prior to intravenous challenge with VEGF (3 µg). Adapted from Albert et al. (2006).

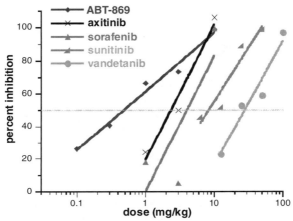

Figure 4.17. Inhibition of VEGF-induced uterine edema. Mice (6 per group) were dosed orally and challenged with estradiol 30 min later. Edema was assessed 2 h after dosing and is expressed as mean percent inhibition. Values >30% were significantly different ($p < 0.05$) from control. Adapted from Albert et al. (2006).

serum (240 nM, Table 4.2). This potency compared favorably to the potency of other known KDR inhibitors (Figure 4.17).

The acute response to estradiol challenge was used to evaluate the kinetics of inhibition of a VEGF-mediated response in the uterine edema model following a single 5 mg/kg dose of ABT-869 that is sufficient, when given twice a day, to produce 60–70% inhibition in most of the tumor growth models discussed later. Administration of this dose resulted in >50% inhibition of the VEGF response for 3–4 hours (Albert et al., 2006). This duration of activity corresponds to inhibition of VEGF-mediated responses for approximately 6–8 hours in a 24 hour period if the compound is given twice daily.

Final confirmation of target inhibition was provided by the efficacy of ABT-869 to alter angiogenesis in animal models. When given daily for 7 days, ABT-869 (7.5 and 15 mg/kg, bid) significantly ($p < 0.001$) inhibited growth factor-induced increases in vessel density in the cornea (Albert et al., 2006). Consistent with an antiangiogenic MOA, treatment with ABT-869 has also been shown to reduce tumor-associated vascular density in xenograft models (Albert et al., 2006; Jasinghe et al., 2008).

4.4.4. Activity in Tumor Growth Models

Given the intrinsic potency of ABT-869 against VEGF and PDGF receptor tyrosine kinases and its potent activity in VEGF-mediated in vivo models, there was considerable interest in evaluating ABT-869 in tumor xenografts models, particularly those that were highly vascularized and viewed as VEGF centric. One such model, based on the HT1080 human fibrosarcoma cell line, served as a workhorse for our efforts to characterize antiangiogenic agents. Tumors in the HT1080 model release impressive levels of VEGF into circulation and tumor-associated vessels appear disorganized and leaky (Figure 4.18), typical of the chaotic nature of human tumor neovasculature (Jain, 2005). As such, this model was ideal for defining potency and efficacious exposure of KDR inhibitors.

Results from a representative study with ABT-869 in the HT1080 model are shown in Figure 4.19(*left*). When given twice daily, ABT-869 produced dose-dependent and potent inhibition of tumor growth (ED_{75}: 15 mg/kg/day). A comparison of the dose-dependent effects of ABT-869 with other rival kinase inhibitors known at the time demonstrated that ABT-869 was more potent than the competitor inhibitors (Figure 4.19).

In further studies ABT-869 exhibited significant antitumor activity in a range of tumor models encompassing fibrosarcoma, breast (ED_{75}: 12 mg/kg/day), colon (ED_{75}: 9 mg/kg/day), and small cell lung (ED_{75}: 24 mg/kg/day)

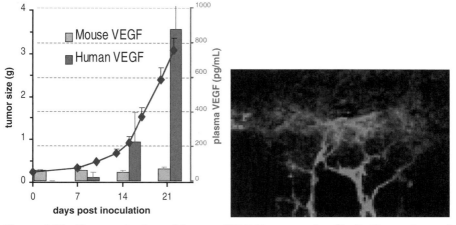

Figure 4.18. Characterization of human HT1080 xenografts. (*Left*) Comparison of tumor size (line graph) and plasma VEGF (murine and human indicated by bar) in tumor-bearing mice. (*Right*) Representative peripheral vasculature (stained with lectin-FITC) in HT1080 tumors 13 days post inoculation.

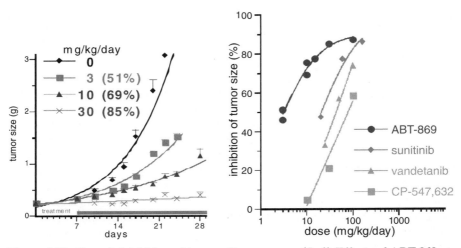

Figure 4.19. Growth inhibition of human fibrosarcoma. (*Left*) Effects of ABT-869 on the growth of HT1080 cells implanted subcutaneously in the flank of SCID-beige mice. Dosing (twice daily) started on day 7. Tumor volumes are expressed as mean ± SEM, $n = 10$ per group. Significant differences ($p < 0.05$ vs. control) in mean tumor volume were observed for all treatment groups by day 14. Dose (mg/kg/day) is given on art and percent inhibition of control (2 g) is indicated in parentheses. Adapted from Albert et al. (2006). (*Right*) Inhibition as a function of dose. Values are expressed as percent inhibition of control from five studies.

carcinoma xenograft models. In addition, the inhibitor was effective in ortho-topic models (breast, 62–70%, 25 mg/kg/day; rat glioma, 52%, 10 mg/kg/day and 67%, 20 mg/kg/day; and rat prostate, 87%, 10 mg/kg/day) and in a synge-neic murine melanoma model (74%, 25 mg/kg/day). Tumor regression was observed in an epidermoid carcinoma model and a FLT3-ITD leukemia xeno-graft model (Albert et al., 2006; Shankar et al., 2007). The profound activity and survival benefit observed in the FLT3-ITD leukemia model presumably reflects the potent antiproliferative effect of ABT-869 on FLT3-dependent cells (Table 4.4). However, interestingly, ABT-869 also reduced the leukemia burden and prolonged survival in a systemic leukemia model using cells with wild-type FLT3 (Zhou et al., 2008b). These results highlight the role of VEGFR/PDGFR in leukemia and suggest that the therapeutic potential of multitar-geted kinase inhibitors like ABT-869 may not be limited to patients with FLT3 mutations.

As an attempt to summarize the activity of ABT-869 in preclinical tumor models, the effect of treatment on tumor volume (percent of vehicle-treated control) at a fixed dose (25 mg/kg/day, bid) is presented in Figure 4.20. It is apparent from the tumor growth inhibition summary plot that ABT-869 is efficacious (<50% of control) in most of the tumor models evaluated, although there is variation in sensitivity to treatment among and within tumor types.

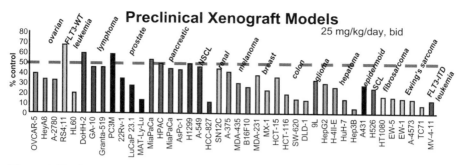

Figure 4.20. Summary of the effects of ABT-869 in preclinical xenograft models. (See color insert.)

The fibrosarcoma, hepatocellular carcinoma, and colon tumor models evaluated are exceptionally responsive to ABT-869 treatment, whereas the pancreatic and lymphoma models are relatively resistant to therapy. Variation within tumor type is most evident among the ovarian tumor models, where two of the three tumor lines evaluated were responsive and the third resistant. Variation in response is perhaps not surprising, given the complexity of the host–tumor interaction and the multiplicity of activities of the kinase inhibitor. Thus while these results provide compelling evidence of the overall potential antitumor efficacy of ABT-869, additional data, such as gene expression and kinase activation status profiling, will be needed to support the analysis necessary to accurately identify optimal patient populations for clinical studies.

Although ABT-869 exhibits notable monotherapy activity in preclinical models, its ultimate fate in the clinic may depend on dosing compatibility in combination with existing standard-of-care therapies. In the preclinical setting, ABT-869 has demonstrated a capacity to be coadministered with cancer therapies, including carboplatin, cisplatin, docetaxel, gemcitabine, irinotecan, paclitaxel, rapamycin, TMZ, and Ara-C (Albert et al., 2006; Li et al., 2006; Jasinghe et al., 2008; Zhou et al., 2008c). As illustrated in Figure 4.21, the typical combination response is approximately additive in efficacy (combination better than either monotherapy) with no observable increase in overall toxicity. In the studies illustrated, combination therapies were dosed concurrently. However, sequence of administration can be important, as has been observed in studies with FLT3-ITD leukemia cells. In that case, simultaneous combination with ABT-869 and Ara-C produced an additive effect on cell survival in culture that was recapitulated in an in vivo model where pretreatment with Ara-C followed by ABT-869 resulted in a synergistic effect. In contrast, pretreatment with ABT-869 followed by Ara-C yielded an antagonistic effect. These results, coupled with their observation of an ABT-869-induced G1-phase cell cycle arrest, prompted the authors to conclude that chemotherapy followed by ABT-869 is the sequence of choice for combination therapy in FLT3-dependent AML (Zhou et al., 2008c).

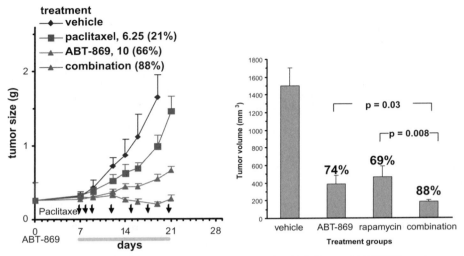

Figure 4.21. Examples of combination studies. (*Left*) Effects of ABT-869 on the growth of HT1080 cells implanted subcutaneously in the flank of SCID-beige mice. Dosing (twice daily) started on day 7. Tumor volumes are expressed as mean ± SEM, *n* = 10 per group. Significant differences (*p* < 0.05 vs. control) in mean tumor volume were observed for all treatment groups by day 14. Dose (mg/kg/day) is given on art and percent inhibition of control (2 g) is indicated in parentheses. (*Right*) Inhibition of the growth of Sk-hep-1 HCC tumors. Adapted from Jasinghe et al. (2008).

4.4.5. Efficacious Drug Levels

In an effort to relate efficacy to drug exposure and to provide exposure targets for preclinical safety and potential clinical studies, the presence of ABT-869 was assayed in plasma samples obtained over a 12 hour period after the last dose at the completion of xenograft efficacy studies. The results of this analysis for a representative HT1080 study with ABT-869 are shown in Figure 4.22 (blue line). The dose from the illustrated study provided plasma levels of ABT-869 that exceeded the cellular IC_{50} value for KDR in the presence of mouse plasma (240 nM) for only approximately 3.5 of the 12 hours in the twice daily dosing cycle. Treatment with this dose in a tumor growth study results in approximately 70% inhibition in tumor size; thus continuous exposure above the plasma binding corrected IC_{50} threshold value is not required for robust inhibition of tumor growth. The extent of time above the plasma IC_{50} value correlates well with the duration of >50% inhibition of receptor phosphorylation (~4 h, Figure 4.22, red line) and provides the basis for defining a time over threshold value of 8 hours per day as a target for subsequent clinical studies. The targeted human threshold, based on cellular KDR inhibition potency in the presence of human plasma, was 130 ng/mL (340 nM, Table 4.2).

In addition to plasma level and time over threshold values, overall exposure (i.e., AUC_{24}) was a useful pharmacokinetic parameter to define efficacious exposure targets. The relationship between terminal drug exposure achieved

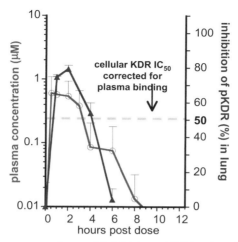

Figure 4.22. Plasma concentration and inhibition of KDR phosphorylation following an efficacious dose of ABT-869. Adapted from Albert et al. (2006).

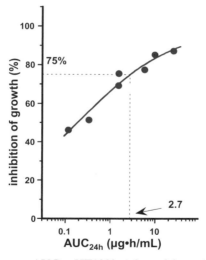

Figure 4.23. TGI versus AUC_{24h} HT1080. Adapted from Albert et al. (2006).

at different doses and efficacy in the HT1080 xenograft is illustrated in Figure 4.23. Based on this relationship, an AUC_{24} value of $2.7\,\mu g \cdot h/mL$ was predicted to produce growth inhibition of approximately 75%. This estimate is model dependent: analysis of other tumor models indicates they vary in sensitivity to treatment with ABT-869, ranging from highly responsive (A431) to relatively resistant (OVCAR-5) (Figure 4.20). In the face of this variability, we viewed the HT1080 model as representative and used the AUC_{24} value of $2.7\,\mu g \cdot h/mL$ as the basis for estimating the potential therapeutic window of ABT-869.

4.4.6. Preclinical Safety Pharmacology and Toxicity Profile

ABT-869 cleared standard safety pharmacology hurdles. It was tested in a battery of receptor binding, CNS, cardiovascular, cardiac electrophysiological, and gastrointestinal assays and was found to be inactive (<50% inhibition of binding a concentration of $10\mu M$) in all 75 receptor assays. In CNS tests, the compound produced no changes in a functional observational battery, stimulation and sedation in the rat, motor coordination, hypnotic potentiation, pro- or anticonvulsant effects in the mouse, or analgesic effects in either mouse or rat. As discussed previously, the preclinical cardiovascular profile of ABT-869 also was acceptable, although ABT-869 did produce a modest increase (6% above baseline) in mean arterial pressure and a compensatory reduction in cardiac output at fourfold the predicted efficacious concentration. The effect on blood pressure was consistent with an increased incidence of hypertension associated with anti-VEGF therapies (Gordon et al., 2001; Tolcher et al., 2002) and was not viewed as detrimental to clinical development.

In preclinical toxicity studies, ABT-869 produced compound-related changes associated with inhibition of angiogenesis in rats. Reversible proteinuria was identified as dose limiting in rats at an exposure (AUC) greater than eightfold the efficacious exposure in mice. In 2 week multiple-dose studies, ABT-869 produced no adverse findings in dogs at exposures fourfold above the efficacious exposure in mice.

4.4.7. Human Pharmacokinetics

The pharmacokinetic profile of ABT-869 has been evaluated in Phase I clinical studies in adult patients receiving 10 mg ABT-869 once daily. Oral plasma clearance averaged from 3.3 to 4.6 L/h in Asian and Caucasian populations with a corresponding half-life of 14.8 and 13.4 h, respectively. Exposures (AUC from 0 to 24 h) were also similar between Asian and Caucasian populations (2.7 vs. 2.3 µg·h/mL, respectively). In both populations mean ABT-869 plasma concentration was >130 ng/mL for at least 6 h after dosing (Gupta et al., 2007a). These pharmacokinetic parameters, which were similar whether the drug was dosed as an oral solution or as a Meltrex® tablet formulation (Gupta et al., 2007b), met the exposure targets derived from preclinical efficacy studies discussed earlier and paved the way for future Phase II studies in patients with advanced nonhematologic malignancies.

4.5. SUMMARY

The discovery of ABT-869 and the advancement of this compound into clinical trials for the treatment of cancer was the culmination of a multiyear effort by several research groups at multiple sites within the Abbott organization. The discovery of new therapeutic agents is an exceedingly difficult process as has been amply documented over the last few years. There is neither a general "road map" nor a universal set of solutions that can guide all drug discovery projects. Instead, each project faces a unique set of problems requiring unique solutions. Nevertheless, it is instructive to review projects, independent of their outcome, and identify keys to success and lessons learned. Looking back at this project, several factors were critical in the discovery of ABT-869.

1. *Question Project Assumptions.* The original project goal was to develop KDR inhibitors with selectivity over the PDGFR family, since we believed that this would be necessary for an acceptable therapeutic window. However, prompted by the impressive in vivo efficacy of non-selective compounds, we decided to take an empirical approach and challenge the selectivity hypothesis. This proved to be a turning point in the project's history. Optimizing and extensively characterizing nonselective agents in both efficacy and safety studies disproved our working hypothesis and demonstrated that multitargeted VEGFR/PDGFR inhibitors can have acceptable therapeutic windows.

2. *Rapid In Vivo Evaluation.* The availability of the mouse uterine edema model of acute in vivo VEGF inhibition was critical to our ability to rapidly investigate and optimize a large number of compounds from different structural classes. This model had several attractive features that were especially useful in a testing scheme: (a) relatively high throughput with rapid turnaround time; (b) minimal compound requirements; (c) dosing versatility regarding timing and route of administration; and (d) readout closely tied to biological efficacy.

3. *Multiple Chemotypes.* The advantages of pursuing multiple chemotypes as a means of addressing the numerous ADME and safety problems that can derail a compound are self-evident. Additionally, multiple series are required as insurance against the ever-present threat of patent interference, especially in a highly competitive area such as the kinase field. We were often surprised at the types of structural series that were either pursued or conversely not pursued by other groups. Thus our crystal ball looking past the 18 month period from filing to patent publication was cloudy at times.

4. *Lipid Versus Water Solubility.* Lipid-based formulations can provide an attractive path forward for compounds that have poor water solubility but good lipid solubility. Lipid solubility should therefore be assessed early on, especially when working with highly lipophilic compounds. Arguably, water-soluble compounds provide the easiest path forward for development. We invested considerable resources toward improving the aqueous solubility of our compounds, but our strategy of introducing basic water-solubilizing groups was not sufficient to overcome the inherently poor aqueous solubility of the core diaryl ureas. In retrospect, these resources might have been better utilized investigating more speculative non diaryl urea-based chemotypes.

5. *Kinase Platform.* Given the structural similarity among the various kinase catalytic sites, it is not surprising that kinase inhibitors can have significant cross-reactivity. Screening of compounds prepared for different kinase programs has been a rich source of leads for other kinase programs. In our experience, the spectrum of inhibition cannot be predicted based on a simple phylogenetic tree or homology modeling. Thus a broad kinase panel is essential in a modern kinase program.

6. *Commitment.* The drug discovery process is characterized by a series of peaks and valleys, with frequent and unexpected pitfalls. In most cases, progress does not follow a predetermined timeline but is based on intermittent breakthroughs that drive the project forward. It is therefore important that project teams and management remain committed, particularly in terms of resources, throughout the unavoidable low points of any project.

ACKNOWLEDGMENTS

The work described in this chapter was the result of the dedicated efforts of numerous individuals from several departments and sites within the Abbott organization, under the leadership of Lee Arnold, who initiated the project and guided it through its early phases, and Steve Davidsen, who drove the project to ABT-869.

REFERENCES

Akritopoulou-Zanze, I., Albert, D. H., Bousquet, P. F., et al. (**2007**). Synthesis and biological evaluation of 5-substituted 1,4-dihydroindeno[1,2-*c*]pyrazoles as multitargeted receptor tyrosine kinase inhibitors. *Bioorg Med Chem Lett.* 17(11), 3136–3140.

Albert, D. H., Tapang, P., Magoc, T. J., et al. (**2006**). Preclinical activity of ABT-869, a multitargeted receptor tyrosine kinase inhibitor. *Mol Cancer Ther.* 5(4), 995–1006.

Arnold, L. D., Calderwood, D. J., Dixon, R. W., et al. (**2000**). Pyrrolo[2,3-*d*]pyrimidines containing an extended 5-substituent as potent and selective inhibitors of Lck I. *Bioorg Med Chem Lett.* 10(19), 2167–2170.

Bergers, G., and Benjamin, L. E. (**2003**). Tumorigenesis and the angiogenic switch. *Nat Rev Cancer.* 3(6), 401–410.

Bergers, G., Javaherian, K., Lo, K. M., et al. (**1999**). Effects of angiogenesis inhibitors on multistage carcinogenesis in mice. *Science.* 284(5415), 808–812.

Bergers, G., Song, S., Meyer-Morse, N., et al. (**2003**). Benefits of targeting both pericytes and endothelial cells in the tumor vasculature with kinase inhibitors. *J Clin Invest.* 111(9), 1287–1295.

Bergström, C. A., Wassvik, C. M., Johansson, K., et al. (**2007**). Poorly soluble marketed drugs display solvation limited solubility. *J Med Chem.* 50(23), 5858–5862.

Bousquet, P. F. (**2002**). Bone marrow recovery following cyclophosphamide ablation. (Unpublished results.)

Burchat, A. F., Calderwood, D. J., Friedman, M. M., et al. (**2002**). Pyrazolo[3,4-*d*] pyrimidines containing an extended 3-substituent as potent inhibitors of Lck—a selectivity insight. *Bioorg Med Chem Lett.* 12(12), 1687–1690.

Camps, J. L., Chang, S. M., Hsu, T. C., et al. (**1990**). Fibroblast-mediated acceleration of human epithelial tumor growth in vivo. *Proc Natl Acad Sci USA.* 87(1), 75–79.

Carmeliet, P. (**2003**). Angiogenesis in health and disease. *Nat Med.* 9(6), 653–660.

Curtin, M. L., Frey, R. R., Heyman, H. R., et al. (**2004**). Isoindolinone ureas: a novel class of KDR kinase inhibitors. *Bioorg Med Chem Lett.* 14(17), 4505–4509.

Cusack, K. P., Arnold, L. D., Barberis, C. E., et al. (**2004**). A 13C NMR approach to categorizing potential limitations of alpha,beta-unsaturated carbonyl systems in drug-like molecules. *Bioorg Med Chem Lett.* 14(22), 5503–5507.

Dai, Y., Guo, Y., Frey, R. R., et al. (**2005**). Thienopyrimidine ureas as novel and potent multitargeted receptor tyrosine kinase inhibitors. *J Med Chem.* 48(19), 6066–6083.

Dai, Y., Hartandi, K., Ji, Z., et al. (**2007**). Discovery of *N*-(4-(3-amino-1H-indazol-4-yl) phenyl)-*N*′-(2-fluoro-5-methylphenyl)urea (ABT-869), a 3-aminoindazole-based orally active multitargeted receptor tyrosine kinase inhibitor. *J Med Chem.* 50(7), 1584–1597.

Dai, Y., Hartandi, K., Soni, N. B., et al. (**2008**). Identification of aminopyrazolopyridine ureas as potent VEGFR/PDGFR multitargeted kinase inhibitors. *Bioorg Med Chem Lett.* 18(1), 386–390.

Dinges, J., Akritopoulou-Zanze, I., Arnold, L. D., et al. (**2006a**). Hit-to-lead optimization of 1,4-dihydroindeno[1,2-*c*]pyrazoles as a novel class of KDR kinase inhibitors. *Bioorg Med Chem Lett.* 16(16), 4371–4375.

Dinges, J., Ashworth, K. L., Akritopoulou-Zanze, I., et al. (**2006b**). 1,4-Dihydroindeno[1,2-*c*]pyrazoles as novel multitargeted receptor tyrosine kinase inhibitors. *Bioorg Med Chem Lett.* 16(16), 4266–4271.

Dinges, J., Albert, D. H., Arnold, L. D., et al. (**2007**). 1,4-Dihydroindeno[1,2-*c*]pyrazoles with acetylenic side chains as novel and potent multitargeted receptor tyrosine kinase inhibitors with low affinity for the hERG ion channel. *J Med Chem.* 50(9), 2011–2029.

Dixon, J. A., Brennan, C., Miranda, K., et al. (**2005**). Bayer Pharmaceuticals Corporation, assignee. Preparation of pyrrolotriazine urea derivatives useful for treating hyperproliferative disorders and diseases associated with angiogenesis. WO2005121147. 22 December 2005.

Ferrara, N., Gerber, H. P., and LeCouter, J. (**2003**). The biology of VEGF and its receptors. *Nat Med.* 9(6), 669–676.

Folkman, J. (**1995**). Angiogenesis in cancer, vascular, rheumatoid and other disease. *Nat Med.* 1(1), 27–31.

Folkman, J. (**1996**). Angiogenesis and angiogenesis inhibition: an overview. *In*: I. D. Goldberg and E. M. Rosen (eds.) *Regulation of Angiogenesis*, pp. 1–8. Basel, Switzerland: Birkhauser Verlag.

Frey, R. R., Curtin, M. L., Albert, D. H., et al. (**2008**). 7-Aminopyrazol[1,5-a]pyrimidines as potent multitargeted receptor tyrosine kinase inhibitors. *J Med Chem.* 51(13), 777–3787.

Gerber, H.-P., and Ferrara, N. (**2003**). The role of VEGF in normal and neoplastic hematopoiesis. *J Mol Med.* 81(1), 20–31.

Glaser, K. (**2008**). Effect of ABT-869 on the proliferation of mast and B cells expressing FLT3-WT or mutated FLT3. (Unplublished results.)

Gordon, M. S., Margolin, K., Talpaz, M., et al. (**2001**). Phase I safety and pharmacokinetic study of recombinant human anti-vascular endothelial growth factor in patients with advanced cancer. *J Clin Oncol.* 19(3), 843–850.

Gorre, M. E., Mohammed, M., Ellwood, K., et al. (**2001**). Clinical resistance to STI-571 cancer therapy caused by BCR-ABL gene mutation or amplification. *Science.* 293(5531), 876–880.

Gracias, V., Ji, Z., Akritopoulou-Zanze, I., et al. (**2008**). Scaffold oriented synthesis. Part 2: Design, synthesis and biological evaluation of pyrimido-diazepines as receptor tyrosine kinase inhibitors. *Bioorg Med Chem Lett.* 18(8), 2691–2695.

Guo, J., Marcotte, P. A., McCall, J. O., et al. (**2006**). Inhibition of phosphorylation of the colony-stimulating factor-1 receptor (c-Fms) tyrosine kinase in transfected cells by ABT-869 and other tyrosine kinase inhibitors. *Mol Cancer Ther.* 5(4), 1007–1013.

Gupta, N., Goh, B.-C., Soo, R., et al. (**2007a**). Pharmacokinetic comparison of multiple receptor tyrosine kinase inhibitor ABT-869 in Asian and Caucasian populations. *In: AACR-NCI-EORTC International Conference on Molecular Targets and Cancer Therapeutics: Discovery, Biology, and Clinical Applications*, San Francisco, CA, p. C148.

Gupta, N., Goh, B.-C., Soo, R., et al. (**2007b**). Relative bioavailability study of multiple receptor tyrosine kinase inhibitor ABT-869 for comparison of oral solution and Meltrex® tablet formulations. *In: AACR-NCI-EORTC International Conference on Molecular Targets and Cancer Therapeutics: Discovery, Biology, and Clinical Applications*, San Francisco, CA, p. C149.

Heyman, H. R., Frey, R. R., Bousquet, P. F., et al. (**2007**). Thienopyridine urea inhibitors of KDR kinase. *Bioorg Med Chem Lett.* 17(5), 1246–1249.

Jain, R. K. (**2005**). Normalization of tumor vasculature: an emerging concept in antiangiogenic therapy. *Science.* 307(5706), 58–62.

Jasinghe, V. J., Xie, Z., Zhou, J., et al. (**2008**). ABT-869, a multi-targeted tyrosine kinase inhibitor, in combination with rapamycin is effective for hepatocellular carcinoma (HCC) in vivo. *J Hepatol.* 49(6), 985–997.

Ji, Z., Ahmed, A. A., Albert, D. H., et al. (**2006**). Isothiazolopyrimidines and isoxazolopyrimidines as novel multi-targeted inhibitors of receptor tyrosine kinases. *Bioorg Med Chem Lett.* 16(16), 4326–4330.

Ji, Z., Ahmed, A. A., Albert, D. H., Bouska, J. J., et al. (**2008**). 3-Amino-benzo[*d*] isoxazoles as novel multitargeted inhibitors of receptor tyrosine kinases. *J Med Chem.* 51(5), 1231–1244.

Leung, D. W., Cachianes, G., Kuang, W. J., et al. (**1989**). Vascular endothelial growth factor is a secreted angiogenic mitogen. *Science.* 246(4935), 1306–1309.

Li, L., Lin, X., Shoemaker, A. R., et al. (**2006**). Hypoxia-inducible factor-1 inhibition in combination with temozolomide treatment exhibits robust antitumor efficacy in vivo. *Clin Cancer Res.* 12(15), 4747–4754.

Lyman, S. D., and Jacobsen, S. E. W. (**1998**). c-kit ligand and Flt3 ligand: stem/progenitor cell factors with overlapping yet distinct activities. *Blood.* 91(4), 1101–1134.

Ma, W., Tan, J., Matsumoto, H., et al. (**2001**). Adult tissue angiogenesis: evidence for negative regulation by estrogen in the uterus. *Mol Endocrinol.* 15(11), 1983–1992.

Mandli, M., and Darbyshire, J. (**2006**). Protein binding of [3H]A-741439 to mouse, rat, dog, monkey and human plasma. (Unpublished results.)

Marsh, K. C. (**2003**). Preclinical pharmacokinetics of ABT-869. (Unpublished results.)

McKenna, H. J., Stocking, K. L., Miller, R. E., et al. (**2000**). Mice lacking flt3 ligand have deficient hematopoiesis affecting hematopoietic progenitor cells, dendritic cells, and natural killer cells. *Blood.* 95(11), 3489–3497.

Miyazaki, Y., Matsunaga, S., Tang, J., et al. (**2005**). Novel 4-amino-furo[2,3-d]pyrimidines as Tie-2 and VEGFR2 dual inhibitors. *Bioorg Med Chem Lett.* 15(9), 2203–2207.

Miyazaki, Y., Nakano, M., Sato, H., et al. (**2007a**). Design and effective synthesis of novel templates, 3,7-diphenyl-4-amino-thieno and furo-[3,2-c]pyridines as protein kinase inhibitors and in vitro evaluation targeting angiogenetic kinases. *Bioorg Med Chem Lett.* 17(1), 250–254.

Miyazaki, Y., Tang, J., Maeda, Y., et al. (**2007b**). Orally active 4-amino-5-diarylurea-furo[2,3-d]pyrimidine derivatives as anti-angiogenic agent inhibiting VEGFR2 and Tie-2. *Bioorg Med Chem Lett.* 17(6), 1773–1778.

Moset Marina, M., Berlanga, J. M. C., Fernandez, I. F., et al. (**2001**). BASF Aktiengesellschaft, assignee. Preparation of 2-pyrazolin-5-ones as inhibitors of serine/threonine and tyrosine kinase activity. WO01009121. 8 February 2001.

Rafferty, P., Calderwood, D., Arnold, L. D., et al. (**2000**). BASF Aktiengesellschaft, assignee. Preparation and effects of benzothiazinones and benzoxazinones as protein kinase inhibitors. WO00/075139. 14 December 2000.

Sengupta, K., Banerjee, S., Saxena, N., et al. (**2003**). Estradiol-induced vascular endothelial growth factor-A expression in breast tumor cells is biphasic and regulated by estrogen receptor-alpha dependent pathway. *Int J Oncol.* 22(3), 609–614.

Sepp-Lorenzino, L., Rands, E., Mao, X., et al. (**2004**). A novel orally bioavailable inhibitor of kinase insert domain-containing receptor induces antiangiogenic effects and prevents tumor growth in vivo. *Cancer Res.* 64(2), 751–756.

Shankar, D. B., Li, J., Tapang, P., et al. (**2007**). ABT-869, a multitargeted receptor tyrosine kinase inhibitor: inhibition of FLT3 phosphorylation and signaling in acute myeloid leukemia. *Blood.* 109(8), 3400–3408.

Stirewalt, D. L., and Radich, J. P. (**2003**). The role of FLT3 in haematopoietic malignancies. *Nat Rev Cancer.* 3(9), 650–665.

Tolcher, A. W., O'Leary, J. J., DeBono, J. S., et al. (**2002**). A Phase I and biologic correlative study of an oral vascular endothelial growth factor receptor-2 (VEGFR-2) tyrosine kinase inhibitor, CP-547,632, in patients (pts) with advanced solid tumors. *Proc Am Soc Clin Oncol.* 21 Abstract #334.

Weisberg, E., Boulton, C., Kelly, L. M., et al. (**2002**). Inhibition of mutant FLT3 receptors in leukemia cells by the small molecule tyrosine kinase inhibitor PKC412. *Cancer Cell.* 1(5), 433–443.

Zhou, J., Bi, C., Janakakumara, J. V., et al. (**2009**). Enhanced activation of STAT pathways and overexpression of survivin confer resistance to FLT3 inhibitors and could be therapeutic targets in AML. *Blood*. 113(7), 4052–4062.

Zhou, J., Khng, J., Jasinghe, V. J., et al. (**2008b**). In vivo activity of ABT-869, a multi-target kinase inhibitor, against acute myeloid leukemia with wild-type FLT3 receptor. *Leuk Res*. 32(7), 1091–1100.

Zhou, J., Pan, M., Xie, Z., et al. (**2008c**). Synergistic antileukemic effects between ABT-869 and chemotherapy involve downregulation of cell cycle-regulated genes and c-Mos-mediated MAPK pathway. *Leukemia*. 22(1), 138–146.

5

DISCOVERY OF MOTESANIB

Andrew S. Tasker and Vinod F. Patel

5.1. INTRODUCTION

Pathological angiogenesis is associated with a variety of disease states, including psoriasis (Detmar, 2000), diabetic retinopathy (Adamis et al., 1993), rheumatoid arthritis (Giatromanolaki et al., 2001), and cancer (Carmeliet and Jain, 2000). In cancer, tumor development beyond a certain size gives rise to a hypoxic state as passive diffusion fails to keep pace with the tumor's growing demand for oxygen. In response, the tumor initiates an angiogenic program transcribing a multitude of cytokines, one of which is the vascular endothelial growth factor or VEGF, whose mitogenic signaling in endothelial cells is conveyed through the receptor tyrosine kinase VEGFR2 (Dvorak, 2002). An increasing body of evidence indicates that the expression and action of VEGF is critical for tumor angiogenesis; anti-ligand (Hurwitz et al., 2004) and anti-receptor (Witte et al., 1998) antibodies, in addition to chemical inhibitors (Hurwitz et al., 2005; Ryan et al., 2005; Strumberg et al., 2005; Motzer et al., 2006; Drevs et al., 2007) of the kinase activity have been shown to ablate neovascularization in preclinical models of angiogenesis and in tumor xenografts, and have entered clinical trials. Bevacizumab, a recombinant humanized monoclonal antibody directed against VEGF, is approved (Cohen et al., 2007) for first or second line treatment of patients with metastatic carcinoma of the colon or rectum and for patients with advanced nonsquamous non-small-cell lung cancer (Sandler et al., 2006). Sunitinib is approved (Goodman et al., 2007) for the treatment of renal cell carcinoma (RCC) and imatinib-resistant gastrointestinal stromal tumors (GIST). Sorafenib is approved for RCC and hepatocellular carcinoma (HCC) (Zhu, 2008). By targeting the genetically

Kinase Inhibitor Drugs. Edited by Rongshi Li and Jeffrey A. Stafford
Copyright © 2009 John Wiley & Sons, Inc.

stable vascular system wherein mutations rarely occur, therapy-induced resistance is expected to be minimal. VEGF, however, is known to mediate endothelium-dependent vasorelaxation in a signaling event also driven through VEGFR2 (Li et al., 2002); thus inhibition of this signaling pathway may potentially lead to an on-mechanism hypertensive side effect. With the exception of this possible side effect, one would anticipate a substantial therapeutic index in a nondeveloping state for a selective agent exploiting this approach. In this chapter we review the discovery of motesanib, a novel, oral inhibitor of angiogenesis with direct antitumor activity that selectively inhibits vascular endothelial growth factor receptors (VEGFR) 1, 2, and 3; platelet-derived growth factor receptor (PDGFR); and stem cell factor receptor (cKit).

5.2. BACKGROUND AND LEAD OPTIMIZATION STRATEGY

Upon binding of VEGF to the extracellular domain of its cognate receptor, the intrinsic activity of the associated kinase domain is increased by transphosphorylation. This event initiates a divergent signal through both the mitogen activated protein kinase pathway (Ras-Raf-ERK) and cell survival (Akt) pathway leading to a proliferative response in endothelial cells. The mitogen basic fibroblast growth factor (bFGF) signals in an analogous fashion to VEGF by transmitting a bifurcated signal through ERK and Akt, but utilizes its cognate receptor tyrosine kinase. With a multitude of protein kinases of high homology involved in the signal transduction, the potential exists for a nonselective ATP-competitive kinase inhibitor to interdict these pathways at a number of locations. For this reason, the use of cell-based proliferation assays requires rigorous interpretation; thus we coupled proliferation assays driven by VEGF or bFGF with a direct measure of target modulation and monitored protein autophosphorylation. We also employed extensive biochemical counterscreening across the gene family to provide further evidence of on-target activity. Increased understanding of inhibitor binding to the kinase garnered through iterative X-ray crystallography, both on- and off-target, assisted in narrowing choices during structure–activity investigation. Early pharmacokinetic assessment aided in further refining promising agents. Finally, a robust acute pharmacodynamic assessment monitoring VEGF-induced vascular permeability in vivo enabled selection of mechanism-based inhibitors prior to evaluation in models of disease.

5.2.1. Lead Generation

We were intrigued by the phthalazine CGP 79787D (compound **1**, Figure 5.1) (Bold et al., 2000). In the ground state, this compound likely exists in an extended conformation where the chloroaniline and the benzenoid ring of the phthalazine are anti-coplanar and the pyridylmethane lies in a plane perpendicular to the central ring system. The investigators report critical reliance on

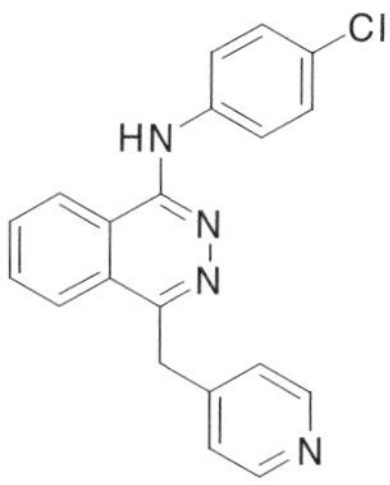

Figure 5.1. CGP 79787D (**1**).

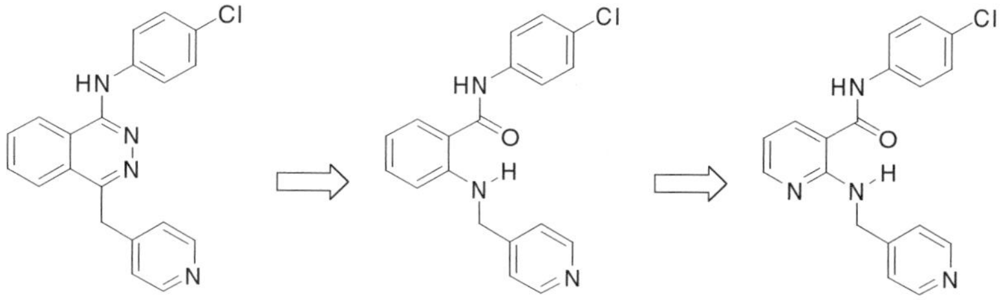

Figure 5.2. Evolution of design from CGP 79787D (**1**) to anthranilide **2** to prototypical nicotinamide **3**.

the 4-pyridylmethane moiety for inhibitory activity; for example, the 2-pyridyl and 3-pyridyl analogs showed greatly diminished potency on VEGFR. The published model (Bold et al., 2000), however, depicts the hinge region (Cys919) unsatisfied and the pyridine exposed to the hydrophilic surface of the protein. Therefore the published binding mode is not supported by the reported SAR (Bold et al., 2000) around the pyridine ring, as one would expect positional modifications to a solvent exposed moiety to have little impact on activity.

Based on the published SAR data, we postulated that the pyridylmethane is likely the hinge-binding element, although it was unclear how the remainder of the molecule would be accommodated within the binding pocket. For our own efforts, in the absence of co-crystal data, we proposed a molecule of more simple architecture in order to investigate further. We envisaged substituting the phthalazine with an anthranilamide (Figure 5.2, structure **2**). This internally hydrogen-bonded system retains most of the features of the phthalazine, including the extended coplanar conformation. In addition, the targets were amenable to rapid analog synthesis. Anthranilic acids are, however, characterized by poor reactivity both at the carbonyl toward nucleophiles and particularly at the amine toward electrophiles. We therefore undertook a broad approach surveying a variety of 2-amino substituted carboxamides derived from readily available starting materials. A nicotinic acid-based system (Winn et al., 1993) **3** was identified which overcame the chemical reactivity issue (Figure 5.2). Although useful in a synthetic sense, the introduction of this nitrogen atom represented a departure from the carbocyclic nature of the phthalazine. We then undertook a thorough investigation of the structure–activity relationships of this novel series (Dominguez et al., 2007).

5.2.2. Lead Optimization

The prototypical nicotinamide **3** (Figure 5.2) proved to be a potent VEGFR inhibitor in both enzymatic and cellular settings, with IC_{50} values of 13 and 70 nM, respectively. Moreover, this agent was selective against the FGF receptor and enzymes within the signaling cascade as evidenced by a lack of inhibition in the bFGF-driven proliferation assay. These results demonstrated the effective use of simple proliferation assays to measure potency on the target and simultaneously garner information around cellular selectivity and cytotoxicity. Modifications to the pyridine failed to yield improvements in either potency or selectivity; for example, substituting for 4-pyrimidinyl realized an order of magnitude loss in activity, an observation congruent with that described by Bold et al. (2000).

With a potent starting point available, structure–activity expansion at the amide was initiated. Compounds were prepared in a high-throughput library format from the penultimate carboxylic acid using routine peptide coupling methodologies. During the early phase of this endeavor one compound (derived from *p*-phenoxyaniline) yielded to crystallization with the enzyme, as depicted in Figure 5.3.

We were struck by the reorientation of the Asp1046–Phe1047–Gly1048 sequence to the so-called "DFG-out" conformation. Hitherto, the only protein known to undergo such a conformational change was the Abelson receptor tyrosine kinase complexed with an imatinib analog published six months prior (Schindler et al., 2000). The DFG-out conformation was not observed in the apo structure (McTigue et al., 1999) of VEGFR2 or in the related fibroblast growth factor receptor kinase in complex with adenylyl diphosphonate (Mohammadi et al., 1996).

The 4-pyridinylmethane engages the hinge residue Cys919 as predicted. This is the only interaction in common with ATP and explains the steep structure–activity at this site; for example, substitution with 3-pyridinylmethane led to a 1000-fold loss in activity. Of note is the edge-to-face interaction of the pyridine with the phenylalanine 1047; the normally solvent exposed region of the protein now contains a hydrophobic element and explains why the pyrimidine substitution results in a tenfold decline in potency. A 180° rotation of the pyrimidine C(4)–methane bond to reorient the ring is precluded by the loss of a van der Waals interaction of C(5) with the gatekeeper residue valine 916. Thus in either conformer the pyrimidine analog is expected to suffer a loss of productive interactions with the protein. The amide linker passes in proximity to the catalytic lysine (K868), accepting a hydrogen bond from Asp1046 on the DFG loop

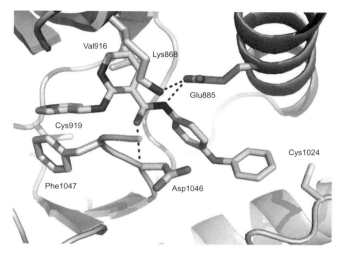

Figure 5.3. Active site of VEGFR2 kinase with bound *p*-phenoxyaniline analog (PDB code 2P2I). Construct: E815 through D1171 with a C-terminal His-tag. Mutations: C817A; E990V; kinase insert domain (T940–E989) deleted. Resolution: 2.4 Å. Reprinted from Dominguez et al., Discovery of *N*-phenyl nicotinamides as potent inhibitors of Kdr. *Bioorg Med Chem Lett.* 17(21), 6003–6008. Copyright © 2007, with permission from Elsevier.

and donating a hydrogen bond to the conserved Glu885 on helix C. Carbons 4–6 on the nicotinyl ring engage the protein in a van der Waals interaction. The phenoxyaniline ring reaches into an extended hydrophobic pocket normally occupied by the activation loop phenylalanine when the protein is phosphorylated.

A closer inspection of the newly opened hydrophobic pocket reveals an expanse of unoccupied volume bordered by a small cysteine residue (C1024) in the outermost region. This observation was in accord with the structure–activity information gathered from the library synthesis (Dominguez et al., 2007); thus analogs bearing *meta*- or *para*-substituents that could exploit this hydrophobic pocket were clearly superior to either *ortho*- or unsubstituted variants. There is some divergence among protein kinases at this site, notably p38 and Lck, wherein this residue is isoleucine (I146) or tyrosine (Y360), respectively. Therefore the distal subspace seemed a fruitful area to improve kinase selectivity and potency for this series of inhibitors.

Increasing the steric bulk in the *para* position from chloro to trifluoromethyl or isopropyl afforded an order of magnitude gain in potency with a minimal cellular shift (9 and 2 nM VEGFR2; 12 and 11 nM VEGF-driven HUVEC proliferation, respectively). While the location of the *para* substituent with reference to the protein was unambiguous, given their degenerate symmetry, the *meta*-substituted compounds either could orient with the substituent occupying a hydrophobic subpocket or, if simply too large, rotate and face the solvent. A

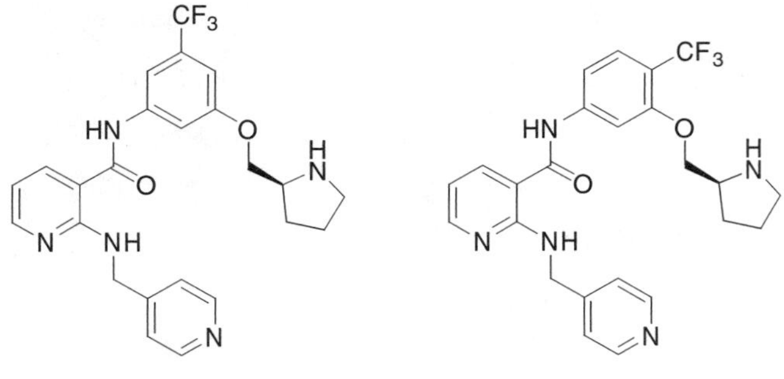

Figure 5.4. Proline-derived inhibitors with increased aqueous solubility.

3,5-bis-trifluoromethyl congener was prepared to address this question; with now degenerate symmetry one of the substituents would be required to face the protein. This compound was equipotent to the monosubstituted congener and suggested that indeed the trifluoromethyl group occupied a hydrophobic cleft in the protein. While potent on the enzyme, this compound was somewhat weaker in the cellular context, likely a consequence of an increase in log P of two units. Broad biochemical counterscreening of this series across both serine/threonine and the more related receptor tyrosine kinase family revealed selectivity in excess of 1000-fold. Noteworthy exceptions were limited to cKit and PDGF receptors. With little to differentiate the most potent derivatives in the molecular and cellular pharmacology setting, attention was directed toward identifying analogs with the most desirable pharmacokinetic properties.

In a standard pharmacokinetic testing paradigm, compounds were evaluated through in vitro metabolism screens and panels of cytochrome P450 enzymes prior to advancement to an in vivo assay. Despite bearing a sterically unencumbered pyridine moiety, these agents possessed only modest cytochrome inhibitory activities. Oral bioavailability was, however, disappointingly poor especially in higher species. Working on the assumption that poor absorption was the result of poor physicochemical properties, we sought to improve intrinsic aqueous solubility by appending a basic amino group positioned based on information garnered from X-ray crystallography. Understanding that the *meta*-trifluoromethyl substituent faced the protein, it seemed reasonable to access free solvent with an amine of appropriate chain length tethered to the opposing *meta* position. In an analogous fashion, the *para*-trifluoromethylated series could be elaborated by extending from the adjacent carbon. Discipline and caution were exercised in carrying out this endeavor given that the additional group increased both molecular weight and log P. Accordingly, we carried out Mitsunobu-type alkylations of either 3-nitro-5-trifluoromethylphenol or 3-nitro-6-trifluoromethylphenol with *N-t*-butyloxycarbonylprolinol and subsequently elaborated to yield compounds **4** and **5**, respectively (Figure 5.4).

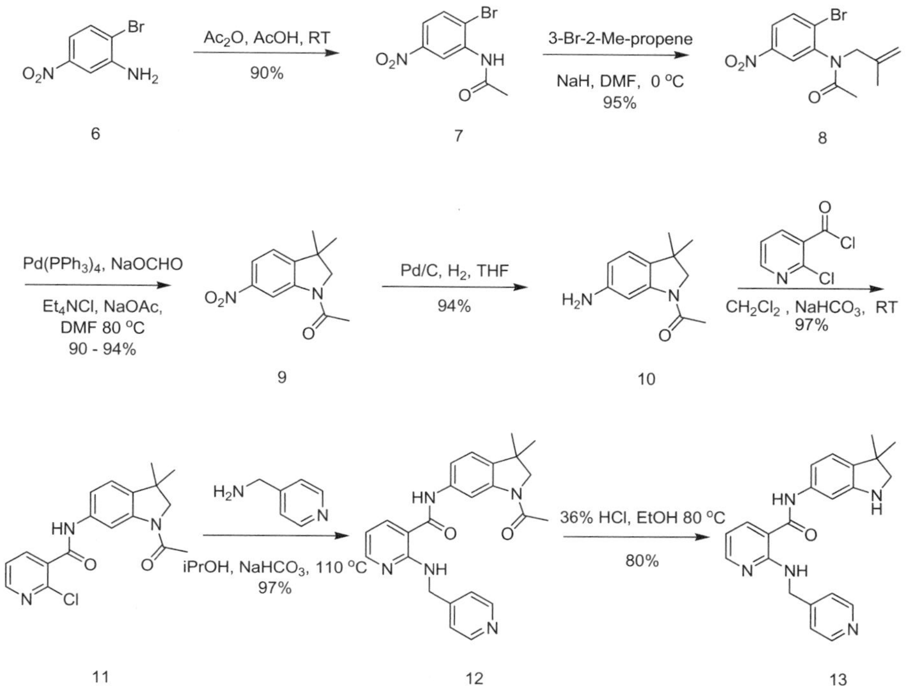

Figure 5.5. Synthesis of indoline analog **13**.

While alkylation of the *meta*-trifluorophenol proceeded uneventfully, the corresponding *ortho*-substituted analogs proved troublesome. The poor reactivity of the *ortho* analogs was attributed to steric crowding and the electron withdrawing capacity of the adjacent trifluoromethyl group. Given the synthetic challenges encountered in preparing compounds such as **5**, an alternative approach was explored (Liu et al., 2007) wherein the *para*-isopropyl substituted analog described previously was modified to form an indoline ring (i.e., compound **13**, Figure 5.5). The geminal methyl groups mimicked the isopropyl group and the open valance on the nitrogen was available for further elaboration.

2-Bromo-5-nitroaniline (**6**) was acetylated and the resultant amide (**7**) was alkylated with methallyl bromide to yield the bromo-olefin (**8**). The olefin underwent a reductive Heck-type reaction (Larock and Babu, 1987) to provide the 3,3-dimethylindoline (**9**). Reduction of the nitro group provided the novel indolinylaniline (**10**), which was reacted with chloronicotinoyl chloride to afford amide (**11**). Subsequent displacement of the remaining chlorine atom provided **12**, which upon acid hydrolysis yielded compound **13**.

The proline-derived inhibitors **4** and **5** were potent in cellular assays (5 and 10 nM, respectively). The improvement in aqueous solubility and consequent increase in oral bioavailability to 50% was accompanied by the introduction of a number of undesirable properties, including increased activity on the FGF receptor kinase, cytochrome P450 inhibition, clearance in the rat in excess of liver blood flow, and antagonism of the cardiac hERG potassium channel. In contrast, the dimethylindoline **13** was found to possess more favorable properties. This agent inhibited VEGFR2 kinase with an IC_{50} of 3 nM, was potent in VEGF-driven proliferation (10 nM), and highly selective against FGF. Broad kinase screening revealed activity against only four other enzymes: VEGFR1 (2 nM), VEGFR3 (6 nM), cKit (8 nM enzyme; 37 nM, SCF-driven cellular autophosphorylation), and PDGFR (207 nM, PDGF-induced proliferation of normal human dermal fibroblasts).

The requirement to occupy a hydrophobic subpocket in the enzyme is illustrated in Table 5.1. N-Methylation of **13** to yield **14** afforded no advantage, supporting the notion that this part of the inhibitor was solvent exposed, an observation also supported by the dihydrobenzofuran derivative **15**, where the ether oxygen is able to interact with bulk solvent. While this agent (**15**) was potent, it possessed poor pharmacokinetic properties. Removal of the geminal dimethyl groups as exemplified by the indoline **16** and the unsaturated indole congener **17** resulted in close to a 20-fold loss in potency in both enzymatic and cellular settings. Appending a basic moiety illustrated by piperidine **18** resulted in the introduction of off-target activities as assessed by inhibition of bFGF-driven proliferation. Finally, a ring expansion to the dimethyltetrahydroquinoline **19** satisfied both the hydrophobic subpocket and bulk solvent. Seemingly an agent on par with **13** in on-target measures, compound **19** proved to be more susceptible to oxidative metabolism. The relative metabolic stability of **13** is presumably due to the geminal dimethyl groups crowding C(2).

An X-ray co-crystal of **13** with VEGFR2 kinase domain reveals the presence of a water molecule tightly associated with the NH of the indoline (Figure 5.6). With the geminal dimethyls occupying a hydrophobic subpocket, the indoline, in conjunction with the remainder of the inhibitor, makes productive use of the hydrophilic and hydrophobic regions of the protein without recourse to excessive molecular weight. Lastly, polarity distributed throughout the molecule affords desirable physicochemical properties and good oral bioavailability in the absence of a basic amine. In summary, the introduction of a single nitrogen atom with its free NH reduced the log P to 3.5, and the accompanying improvement in physicochemical properties improved oral bioavailability in the dog from $F = 4\%$ for the *para*-trifluoromethyl analog to 43% for the indoline variant (**13**). Compound **13** was formulated as the diphosphate salt and renamed motesanib.

5.3. PHARMACOLOGY

Our approach toward characterizing the in vivo pharmacological properties of motesanib relied on assessing activity along the VEGF–VEGFR signaling pathway and ultimately connecting the mechanism-based efficacy to disease-based efficacy. The desired correlation was established using an appropriately

TABLE 5.1. Bicyclic Inhibitors

Entry	Anilino	IC$_{50}$ (μM) Enzyme VEGFR2	HUVEC Proliferation VEGF	bFGF
13	(structure)	0.003	0.01	>1.1
14	(structure)	0.006	0.02	>1.1
15	(structure)	0.003	0.008	>1.1
16	(structure)	0.050	0.185	>1.1
17	(structure)	0.062	0.210	>1.1
18	(structure)	0.025	0.025	0.300
19	(structure)	0.003	0.007	>1.1

selected set of in vivo biological systems (Polverino et al., 2006). The effects of motesanib were examined in an animal model of vascular permeability conducted as a function of time. A single dose of drug given 24 hours after injection of VEGF-transfected or vector control cells inhibited VEGF-induced vascular permeability in a time-dependent fashion (Figure 5.7). Motesanib rapidly and significantly ($P = 0.0022$) inhibited VEGF-induced vascular

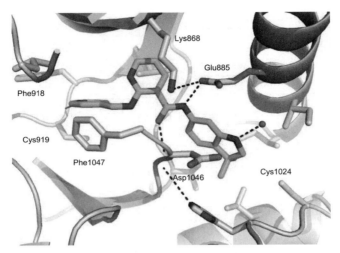

Figure 5.6. Active site of VEGFR2 kinase with bound motesanib. The red sphere is a tightly bound water molecule (PDB code 3EFL). Construct: E815 through D1171 with a C-terminal His-tag. Mutations: C817A; E990V; kinase insert domain (T940–E989) deleted. Resolution: 2.2 Å. (See color insert.)

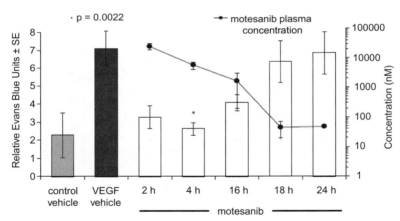

Figure 5.7. Inhibition of VEGF-induced vascular permeability in mice treated with motesanib. HEK 293 cells transfected with murine VEGF or vector control were mixed with Matrigel and injected subcutaneously into CD-1 *nu/nu* mice. A single dose of motesanib was given by oral gavage (100 mg/kg) 24 h after implantation of cells. At various time points after administration, plasma was obtained for pharmacokinetic measurement, and vascular permeability in the skin overlying the Matrigel plug was measured by quantitation of extravasation of Evans blue dye. *Columns,* relative Evans blue units (*n* = 5 per group); *bars,* SE. *$P < 0.0022$, significant difference from VEGF plus vehicle-injected control mice. Reproduced with permission from Polverino et al. (2006).

permeability, which was maintained, although not significantly, for up to 16 hours. The effect correlated with maintenance of free drug plasma levels above the measured HUVEC IC_{50}.

VEGF is a potent mitogen for endothelial cells; it is possible in an in vivo setting to use VEGF to induce the proliferation and migration of these cells to form new vasculature. This is best accomplished in a normally avascular tissue typified by corneal epithelium. The rat corneal angiogenesis assay represented a mechanism-based system to assess the antiangiogenic potential of motesanib in vivo. A nylon disk previously soaked with human VEGF was surgically implanted in the corneal stroma of rats precisely 1.8 mm from blood vessels of the lateral limbus. After 7 days, the study was terminated and the corneas were photographed, as described. For each corneal image, the number of blood vessels intersecting the midpoint between the implanted disk and the limbus was measured. All analysis was performed in a blinded fashion. As shown in Figure 5.8, motesanib given orally for 7 days at 10 mg/kg twice daily significantly reduced the vessel count with respect to control.

The rat corneal experiment was repeated as a dose response on either a once (qd) or twice daily (bid) oral dosing regimen (Figure 5.9). Motesanib given twice daily suppressed VEGF-induced angiogenesis with an estimated ED_{50} of 2.4 mg/kg, wherein the AUC_{0-24} was 4.8 μM·h, and the C_{max} was 0.62 μM. Once-daily dosing produced significant reduction in blood vessel formation, with an estimated ED_{50} of 4.9 mg/kg, wherein the AUC_{0-24} was 13.4 μM·h and C_{max} was 5.6 μM.

Motesanib was evaluated in a disease model using A431 human epidermoid tumor xenografts. This cell line was found to be insensitive to motesanib in

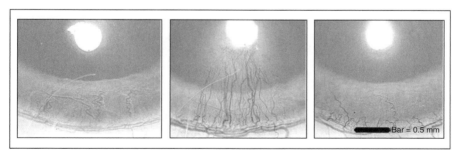

0.1% BSA in disk + vehicle   VEGF in disk + vehicle   VEGF in disk + motesanib

Figure 5.8. The effect of motesanib on blood vessel formation stimulated by VEGF in rat cornea. Angiogenesis was induced by implanting a VEGF-soaked or bovine serum albumin control-soaked nylon disk into the corneal stroma ($n = 8$ per group). For each corneal image, the number of vessels intersecting the midpoint between the disk and the limbus was measured. Motesanib was given orally twice daily for 7 days (10 mg/kg/day). *Bar* = 0.5 mm. (*Left panel*) 0.1% BSA in disk + vehicle; (*center panel*) VEGF in disk + vehicle; and (*right panel*) VEGF in disk + motesanib.

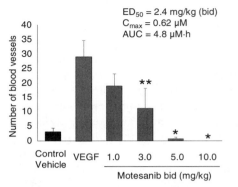
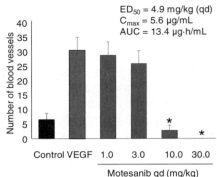

Figure 5.9. Impact of motesanib on corneal angiogenesis in rats as a dose response. Angiogenesis was induced by implanting a VEGF-soaked or bovine serum albumin control-soaked nylon disk into the corneal stroma ($n = 8$ per group). For each corneal image, the number of vessels intersecting the midpoint between the disk and the limbus was measured. Motesanib was given orally twice daily (bid) for 7 days (1, 3, 5, or 10 mg/ kg/day) or once daily (qd) for 7 days (1, 3, 10, or 30 mg/kg/day). *Columns*, mean; *bars*, SE. *$P < 0.004$; **$P < 0.018$, significant difference from VEGF plus vehicle-treated animals. Reproduced with permission from Polverino et al. (2006).

culture. The A431 cell line was previously characterized as one that expressed VEGF at high levels. Ten days post subcutaneous injection of A431 cells into nude mice, an established tumor (~125 mm³) had formed and motesanib was administered orally twice daily (bid) at 10, 30, and 100 mg/kg. Motesanib caused a dose-dependent inhibition of tumor growth after 24 days of treatment (day 34) (Figure 5.10). At the 10 and 30 mg/kg doses, there was a delay prior to tumor impact, while at 100 mg/kg, effect on tumor growth was observed almost immediately. Statistically significant tumor regression was noted at 100 mg/kg after only 7 days of treatment (day 17). In this group, 4 of 10 mice were judged to have no measurable tumor mass at the end of the study on day 24. To further explore the utility of motesanib from both an efficacy and safety perspective, when tumor mass reached 450 mm³ (day 24) six of the animals from the vehicle-treated control group were crossed over to treatment with motesanib at 100 mg/kg bid for an extended period of time (57 days). A rapid reduction in volume of these large tumor masses was observed with the loss of two animals (day 32, day 46) and the remaining 6 of 6 mice subsequently achieving complete response by day 85. Overall, the drug was generally well tolerated throughout the study, body weights being consistently maintained across all groups at greater than 90% of control.

To probe the mechanism of motesanib-induced A431 tumor regression, a study was conducted where large, established (1 cm³) A431 tumors were treated with drug at 75 mg/kg bid, po. Prior to treatment the tumors were highly vascularized with extensive blood vessel networks visible throughout the tumor mass (Figure 5.11). Tumor-associated vascular loss and disease

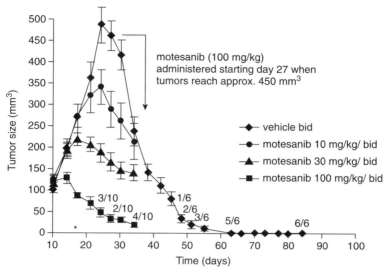

Figure 5.10. Antitumor effect of motesanib on established A431 tumors in nude mice. Inhibition and regression of A431 tumor xenograft growth by motesanib. Response of mice with intermediate (~125 mm³) and large (>400 mm³) A431 tumor xenografts to treatment with motesanib. Female athymic *nu/nu* mice ~5–6 weeks of age were injected with 1×10^7 A431 cells on day 0. Treatment with motesanib (10, 30, or 100 mg/kg/dose bid) was begun on day 10 when tumors were ~125 mm³. Six of ten mice initially treated with vehicle began treatment with motesanib on day 27. The remaining four animals were sacrificed for histochemical analysis. *Fractions*, number of mice with no measurable tumor over the total number of animals in the group. *Points*, mean (*n* = 10 per group); *bars*, SE. *$P < 0.05$, statistically significant difference from day 10 values. Reproduced with permission from Polverino et al. (2006).

regression was evident as early as 3 days after treatment with motesanib commenced. By day 5 the tumors displayed a blanched appearance, indicative of an almost complete loss of tumor vasculature. Continued treatment resulted in the physical collapse of the tumor assessed by volume and the appearance of necrotic tissue.

To investigate further the mechanism of action of motesanib, A431 xenografts from either treated or controls were examined by histology as a function of time. Quantitative histomorphometry allowed a determination of blood vessel area. Double immunostaining for CD31 and TUNEL and counterstaining with Hoechst nuclear dye allowed assessment of endothelial cell apoptosis. Finally, we measured cleaved caspase-3 in the tumor itself. A significant increase ($P < 0.026$) in endothelial cell apoptosis accompanied by a decrease ($P < 0.0005$) in blood vessel density were the first temporal events noted following drug treatment. Subsequent to these phenomena, a significant increase ($P < 0.009$) in tumor cell apoptosis was observed at 48 hours after the commencement of therapy. Taken together, these observations are consistent

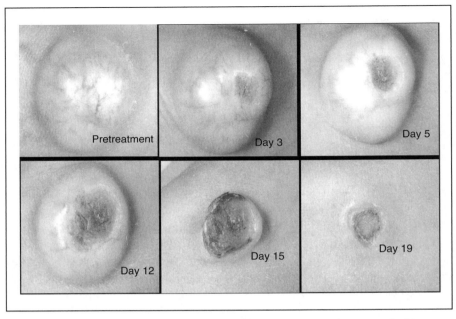

Figure 5.11. Blanching and regression of A431 xenografts in mice treated with mote-sanib. Female CD-1 *nu/nu* mice with large, established (1 cm³) A431 tumor xenografts were dosed with motesanib (75 mg/kg/dose bid) by oral gavage. A representative animal illustrates the time-dependent blanching and regression of disease associated with continued treatment. Reproduced with permission from Polverino et al. (2006).

with targeting of the tumor-associated endothelial cells and vasculature as the primary mechanism of the antitumor effect of motesanib in this model.

The broad antitumor activity of motesanib in breast cancer xenografts was recently reported (Coxon et al., 2009). In summary, the data showed that treatment with motesanib resulted in a significant, dose-dependent inhibition of tumor growth in xenografts derived from human luminal (MCF-7), mesenchymal (MDA-MB-231), and basal (Cal-51) breast cancer cell lines. Furthermore, treatment with motesanib in combination with the cytotoxic chemotherapy agent docetaxel or with the estrogen receptor modulator tamoxifen resulted in a significantly greater reduction in tumor volume than treatment with either agent alone. The data suggested broad applicability of motesanib treatment alone or in combination with chemotherapy in the management of different breast cancer subtypes, and supported further development of these treatment regimens in clinical studies.

5.3.1. Preclinical Safety Assessment

The in vitro safety profile of motesanib was determined in a standard suite of drug discovery assays. Motesanib did not interact with a panel of ion channel,

GPCR, and enzyme targets, tested at a concentration of $10\,\mu M$ and was found to be negative in an Ames screening assay. To evaluate the potential for motesanib to cause acquired long QTc prolongation syndrome, the inhibition of the hERG potassium channel was measured in an electrophysiology patch clamp assay yielding an IC_{50} of $10\,\mu M$. In vivo, no QTc prolongation was detected in anesthetized dogs when motesanib was administered as a $30\,mg/kg$ single dose ($C_{max} > 70\,\mu M$ total drug).

5.3.2. First in Human Experience

A Phase I, open label, sequential dose-ranging study (Rosen et al., 2007) was conducted to evaluate the pharmacokinetics, pharmacodynamics, safety, and tolerability of motesanib in patients with histologically documented refractory advanced solid tumors. A total of 71 patients were enrolled in small cohorts and evaluated sequentially on one of two dosing schedules: (1) intermittent (administration on days 1 to 21, followed by 7 treatment-free days) or (2) continuous (once-daily dosing for 28 days). No dose-limiting toxicities occurred in either 50 or 100 mg once-daily intermittent cohorts. Six patients were subsequently enrolled in a 175 mg once-daily intermittent cohort, half of whom experienced grade 3 dose-limiting toxicities (i.e., fatigue, hyperbilirubinemia, and encephalopathy), all of which were resolved upon discontinuation of drug. Because 175 mg once-daily exceeded the maximum tolerated dose, a 125 mg intermittent cohort was enrolled. In this cohort, one patient experienced grade 3 hyponatremia and elevated serum creatinine; both symptoms resolved upon treatment withdrawal. Six additional patients were enrolled in a 125 mg once-daily continuous administration study; no dose-limiting toxicities were observed and this particular study served to define the maximum tolerated dose (MTD). Following this dosing regimen, the cohort was expanded to 28 patients for additional safety and pharmacokinetic evaluations.

All 71 patients encountered at least one adverse event, mostly grade 1 or 2, and reversible upon drug withdrawal. The most common grade 3 event was hypertension and, as suggested previously, this event was likely pharmacologically mediated. Several reported clinical trials of angiogenesis inhibitors have noted similar incidences of hypertension (16–61%). In this study, the observed hypertension was manageable with blood pressure monitoring and antihypertensive therapy. Hematological toxicities have been observed with other antiangiogenic multikinase inhibitors, exemplified by sunitinib (Faivre et al., 2006) and vatalanib (Thomas et al., 2005). For these agents, grade 3 neutropenia was reported in up to 18% of patients dosed to their respective MTDs, and grade 3 or 4 thrombocytopenia in 20% of patients treated with sunitinib. These findings were conspicuous by their absence in patients treated with motesanib; only 3% and 1% of patients developed grade 3 or 4 neutropenia and thrombocytopenia, respectively. This improvement in safety is likely a function of motesanib's selectivity profile within the protein kinase family.

The pharmacokinetics of motesanib was approximately dose proportional, measured by either C_{max} or area under the curve (AUC). The agent was absorbed rapidly with a median T_{max} of approximately 0.6–2 h, and the mean terminal phase elimination half-life was 4.5–7.7 hours. At trough, a 125 mg dose provided continuous coverage over the preclinically determined IC_{50} value for VEGF-driven HUVEC proliferation. Upon repeat administration, no accumulation was observed as determined by trough measurements on day 21 versus day 1. These data also showed that motesanib did not induce its own metabolism. In a drug–drug interaction study, motesanib caused a modest (less than twofold) increase in the AUC of midazolam, indicating that a clinically significant drug–drug interaction would not be anticipated.

In this extensively pretreated patient population, five patients treated with motesanib were classified as partial responders. Of these patients, three had thyroid malignancies (follicular, medullary, and papillary carcinoma). Therapy lasted between 482 and 564 days in this group. The remaining partial responders had renal cell carcinoma and leiomyosarcoma. Thirty-seven treated patients were classified as having stable disease.

In summary, oral administration of motesanib in a Phase I study to patients with advanced disease was tolerable with dosing through 914 days. The pharmacokinetic behavior and antitumor activity data supported further investigation of this agent as a daily therapy, alone or in combination with cytotoxic agents or other targeted therapies.

5.4. SUMMARY

This chapter describes a structure-based design approach to motesanib, a potent, selective, and orally available inhibitor of VEGR, cKit, and PDGF receptor tyrosine kinases. Motesanib demonstrates utility in a range of preclinical models of disease, both as monotherapy, where we demonstrate that antitumor efficacy is realized by an on-mechanism inhibition of angiogenesis, and in combination with other chemotherapeutic agents. Motesanib is tolerable clinically and shows single-agent efficacy in refractory patients with advanced disease. In 2007, enrollment began for a Phase III study in non-small-cell lung cancer (NSCLC). Additionally, motesanib is being studied in a Phase II trial head-to-head versus bevacizumab in the treatment of metastatic breast cancer and NSCLC. Phase Ib combination studies are ongoing.

ACKNOWLEDGMENTS

The authors wish to thank Glenn Begley, Angela Coxon, Elizabeth Doherty, Anthony Polverino, and Ryan White for critical reading of this chapter.

REFERENCES

Adamis, A.P., Shima, D.T., Yeo, K.T., et al. (**1993**). Synthesis and secretion of vascular permeability factor/vascular endothelial growth factor by human retinal pigment epithelial cells. *Biochem Biophys Res Commun.* 193(2), 631–638.

Bold, G., Altmann, K.-H., Frei, J., et al. (**2000**). New anilinophthalazines as potent and orally well absorbed inhibitors of the VEGF receptor tyrosine kinases useful as antagonists of tumor-driven angiogenesis. *J Med Chem.* 43(12), 2310–2323.

Carmeliet, P., and Jain, R.K. (**2000**). Angiogenesis in cancer and other diseases. *Nature.* 407, 249–257.

Cohen, M. H., Gootenberg, J., Keegan, P., et al. (**2007**). FDA drug approval summary: bevacizumab plus FOLFOX4 as second-line treatment of colorectal cancer. *Oncologist.* 12, 356–361.

Coxon, A., Bush, T., Saffran, D., et al. (**2009**). Broad antitumor activity in breast cancer xenografts by motesanib, a highly selective, oral inhibitor of VEGF, PDGF, and kit receptors. *Clin Cancer Res.* 15(1), 110–118.

Detmar, M. (**2000**). The role of VEGF and thrombospondins in skin angiogenesis. *J Dermatol Sci.* 24, S78–S84.

Dominguez, C., Smith, L., Huang, Q., et al. (**2007**). Discovery of *N*-phenyl nicotinamides as potent inhibitors of Kdr. *Bioorg Med Chem Lett.* 17(21), 6003–6008.

Drevs, J., Siegert, P., Medinger, M., et al. (**2007**). Phase I clinical study of AZD2171, an oral vascular endothelial growth factor signaling inhibitor, in patients with advanced solid tumors. *J Clin Oncol.* 25(21), 3045–3054.

Dvorak, H. F. (**2002**). Vascular permeability factor/vascular endothelial growth factor: a critical cytokine in tumor angiogenesis and a potential target for diagnosis and therapy. *J Clin Oncol.* 20(21), 4368–4380.

Faivre, S., Delgaldo, C., Vera, K., et al. (**2006**). Safety, pharmacokinetic, and antitumor activity of SU11248, a novel oral multitarget tyrosine kinase inhibitor, in patients with cancer. *J Clin Oncol.* 24(1), 25–35.

Goodman, V. L., Rock, E. P., Dagher, R., et al. (**2007**). Approval summary: sunitinib for the treatment of imatinib refractory or intolerant gastrointestinal stromal tumors and advanced renal cell carcinoma. *Clin Cancer Res.* 13, 1367–1373.

Giatromanolaki, A., Sivridis, E., Athanassou, N., et al. (**2001**). The angiogenic pathway "vascular endothelial growth factor/flk-1(KDR)-receptor" in rheumatoid arthritis and osteoarthritis. *J Pathol.* 194(1), 101–108.

Hurwitz, H., Fehrenbacher, L., Novotny, W., et al. (**2004**). Bevacizumab plus irinotecan, fluorouracil, and leucovorin for metastatic colorectal cancer. *N Engl J Med.* 350(23), 2335–2342.

Hurwitz, H., Dowlati, A., Savage, S., et al. (**2005**). Safety, tolerability, and pharmacokinetics of oral administration of GW786034 in patients with solid tumors. *J Clin Oncol.* 23(16S), 3012.

Larock, R. C., and Babu, S. (**1987**). Synthesis of nitrogen heterocycles via palladium-catalyzed intramolecular cyclization. *Tetrahedron Lett.* 28(44), 5291–5294.

Li, B., Ogasawara, A. K., Yang, R., et al. (**2002**). KDR (VEGF receptor 2) is the major mediator for the hypotensive effect of VEGF. *Hypertension.* 39, 1095–1100.

Liu, P., Huang, L., Lu, Y., et al. (**2007**). Synthesis of heterocycles via ligand-free palladium catalyzed reductive Heck cyclization. *Tetetrahedron Lett.* 48(13), 2307–2310.

McTigue, M. A., Wickersham, J. A., Pinko, C., et al. (**1999**). Crystal structure of the kinase domain of human vascular endothelial growth factor receptor 2: a key enzyme in angiogenesis. *Structure.* 7(3), 319–330.

Mohammadi, M., Schlessinger, J., and Hubbard, S. R. (**1996**). Structure of the FGF receptor tyrosine kinase domain reveals a novel autoinhibitory mechanism. *Cell.* 86, 577–587.

Motzer, R. J., Michaelson, M. D., Redman, B. G., et al. (**2006**). Activity of SU11248, a multitargeted inhibitor of vascular endothelial growth factor receptor and platelet-derived growth factor receptor, in patients with metastatic renal cell carcinoma. *J Clin Oncol.* 24(1),16–24.

Polverino, A., Coxon, A., Starnes, C., et al. (**2006**). AMG 706, an oral, multikinase inhibitor that selectively targets vascular endothelial growth factor, platelet-derived growth factor, and kit receptors, potently inhibits angiogenesis and induces regression in tumor xenografts. *Cancer Res.* 66(17), 8715–8721.

Rosen, L. S., Kurzrock, R., Mulay, M., et al. (**2007**). Safety, pharmacokinetics, and efficacy of AMG 706, an oral multikinase inhibitor, in patients with advanced solid tumors. *J Clin Oncol.* 25(17), 2369–2376.

Ryan, C., Stadler, W. M., Roth, B. J., et al. (**2005**). Safety and tolerability of AZD2171, a highly potent VEGFR inhibitor, in patients with advanced prostate adenocarcinoma. *J Clin Oncol.* 23(204S), 3049.

Sandler, A., Gray, R., Perry, M. C., et al. (**2006**). Paclitaxel–carboplatin alone or with bevacizumab for non-small-cell lung cancer. *N Engl J Med.* 355, 2542–2550.

Schindler, T., Bornmann, W., Pellicena, P., et al. (**2000**). Structural mechanism for STI-571 inhibition of Abelson tyrosine kinase. *Science.* 289, 1938–1942.

Strumberg, D., Richly, H., Hilger, R. A., et al. (**2005**). Phase I clinical and pharmacokinetic study of the novel Raf kinase and vascular endothelial growth factor receptor inhibitor BAY 43-9006 in patients with advanced refractory solid tumors. *J Clin Oncol.* 23(5), 965–972.

Thomas, A. L., Morgan, B., Horsfield, M. A., et al. (**2005**). Phase I study of the safety, tolerability, pharmacokinetics, and pharmacodynamics of PTK787/ZK 222584 administered twice daily in patients with advanced cancer. *J Clin Oncol.* 23(18), 4162–4171.

Winn, M., De, B., Zydowsky, T. M., et al. (**1993**). 2-(Alkylamino)nicotinic acid and analogs. Potent angiotensin II antagonists. *J Med Chem.* 36(18), 2676–2688.

Witte, L., Hicklin, D. J., Zhu, Z., et al. (**1998**). Monoclonal antibodies targeting the VEGF receptor-2 (Flk1/KDR) as an anti-angiogenic therapeutic strategy. *Cancer Metastasis Rev.* 17, 155–161.

Zhu, A. X. (**2008**). Development of sorafenib and other molecularly targeted agents in hepatocellular carcinoma. *Cancer.* 112, 250–259.

6

DISCOVERY OF BRIVANIB ALANINATE: A DUAL VASCULAR ENDOTHELIAL GROWTH FACTOR AND FIBROBLAST GROWTH FACTOR RECEPTOR INHIBITOR

Rajeev S. Bhide and Joseph Fargnoli

6.1. INTRODUCTION

Angiogenesis, the development of new blood vessels from the endothelium of preexisting vasculature, is a critical process required by tumors to support their growth and dissemination (Carmeliet and Jain, 2000). In 1971 Judah Folkman proposed that tumor growth and metastasis are angiogenesis dependent, and thereby blocking angiogenesis may be a viable strategy to arrest tumor growth and metastases (Folkman, 1971). This proposal stimulated the search for pro- and antiangiogenic molecules, and it was subsequently shown that cells in a premalignant tissue acquire an angiogenic capacity on their way to becoming malignant (Gullino, 1978). The concept of an angiogenic switch has been proposed, in which the tumor initiates recruitment of its own blood supply by shifting the balance of angiogenesis inhibitors and stimulators in favor of endothelial cell proliferation (Hanahan and Folkman, 1996).

Regulation of angiogenesis appears to be controlled by a variety of activators and inhibitors (Table 6.1). These pro- and antiangiogenic molecules originate from cancer cells, endothelial cells, multiple types of stromal cells, blood, and the extracellular matrix, although their relative contributions are thought

Kinase Inhibitor Drugs. Edited by Rongshi Li and Jeffrey A. Stafford
Copyright © 2009 John Wiley & Sons, Inc.

TABLE 6.1. Angiogenesis Activators and Inhibitors

Activator	Function	Inhibitor	Function
VEGF family members	Stimulate angiogenesis, permeability, leukocyte adhesion	VEGFR1, soluble VEGFR1, soluble NRP-1	Sink for VEGF, VEGF-B, PlGF
VEGFR, NRP-1	Integrate angiogenic and survival signals	Ang2	Antagonist of Ang1
Ang1 and Tie2	Stabilize vessels, inhibit permeability	TSP-1, -2	Inhibit endothelial cell migration, growth, adhesion and survival
PDGF-BB and receptors	Recruit smooth muscle cells	Angiostatin and related plasminogen kringles	Suppress tumor angiogenesis
TGF-β1, endogen TGF-β receptors	Stimulate extracellular matrix production	Endostatin (collagen XVIII fragment)	Inhibit endothelial cell survival and migration
FGF, HGF, MCP-1	Stimulate angio/arteriogenesis	Vasostatin, calreticulin	Inhibit endothelial cell growth
Integrins $\alpha_v\beta_3$ $\alpha_v\beta_5$ $\alpha_5\beta$	Receptors for matrix molecules and proteinases	Platelet factor 4	Inhibit binding of FGF2 and VEGF
VE-cadherin, PECAM (CD31)	Endothelial cell junction molecules	TIMPs, MMP inhibitors, PEX	Suppress pathological angiogenesis
Ephrins	Regulate arterial venous specification	Meth-1, Meth-2	Inhibitors containing MMP, TSP, and disintegrin domains
Plasminogen activators, MMPs	Remodel matrix, release and activate growth factors	IFN-α, -β, -γ, IP-10, IL-4, IL-12, IL-18	Inhibit endothelial cell migration, downregulate FGF2

PAI-1	Stabilize nascent cells
NOS, COX-2	Stimulate angiogenesis and vasodilation
AC133	Regulate angioblast differentiation
Chemokines	Pleiotropic role in angiogenesis
Id1/Id3	Determine endothelial cell plasticity
Prothrombin kringle-2, antithrombin III fragment	Suppress endothelial cell growth
Prolactin	Inhibit VEGF/FGF2
VEGI	Modulate cell growth
Fragment of SPARC	Inhibit endothelial cell binding and activity of VEGF
Osteopontin fragment	Interfere with integrin signaling
Maspin	Protease inhibitor
Canstatin, proliferin-related protein	Mechanisms unknown

Ang1, angiopoietin 1; COX-2, cyclooxygenase 2; FGF, fibroblast growth factor; Id1, inhibitor of DNA binding 1; IFN, interferon; IL, interleukin; IP, inducible protein; MMP, matrix metalloproteinase; NOS, nitric oxide synthases; NRP-1, neuropilin 1; PAI-1, plasminogen activator inhibitor 1; PDGF-BB, platelet-derived growth factor-BB; PECAM, platelet/endothelial cell adhesion molecule; PlGF, placental growth factor; SPARC, secreted protein acidic and rich in cysteine; TGF, tumor growth factor; Tie2, tyrosine kinase receptor 2; TIMP, tissue inhibitor of metalloproteinases; TSP, thrombospondin; VE, vascular endothelial; VEGF, vascular endothelial growth factor; VEGI, vascular endothelial growth inhibitor; VEGFR, vascular endothelial growth factor receptor.

to differ between tumor types and sites (Ramanujan et al., 2000). Furthermore, their contribution is likely to change with tumor growth, regression, and relapse. Although various signals that can initiate this angiogenic switch have been characterized, including metabolic stress, hypoxia, mechanical stress and interstitial pressure, immune/inflammatory response, and genetic mutations (Kerbel, 2000), it is not clear how the interaction between these environmental and genetic mechanisms ultimately influences tumor angiogenesis and growth. Regardless of these limitations, agents that inhibit the process of angiogenesis represent a promising therapeutic strategy for a variety of tumor types (Ferrara and Kerbel, 2005) based on recent clinical approval of several antiangiogenic agents. Inhibition of tumor-induced angiogenesis can theoretically prevent not only the growth of tumors but also the dissemination of tumor cells that ultimately leads to metastatic disease, a process dependent on neovascularization (Folkman, 1971). Different types of tumors use distinct molecular strategies to activate the angiogenic switch, suggesting that a selection of therapeutic agents will need to be developed to treat all tumor types (Ferrara and Kerbel, 2005). Furthermore, as tumors grow they begin to produce a wider array of proangiogenic molecules. Therefore if only one proangiogenic molecule or pathway is blocked, tumors may switch to another, and a successful antiangiogenic approach will need to inhibit a number of molecular targeted pathways.

Vascular endothelial growth factor (VEGF) has been shown to be one of the most potent and pleiotropic proangiogenic molecules. It is implicated in several steps throughout the angiogenesis process. Many agents that target the VEGF signaling pathway are currently in development, for example, anti-VEGF antibodies such as bevacizumab that target VEGF, and small molecules that target the VEGF receptors (VEGFR) directly, for example, kinase inhibitors such as sorafenib, sunitinib, and brivanib (Table 6.2). In addition to targeting the VEGF signaling pathway, a number of these agents modulate other signaling pathways, including epidermal growth factor (EGF), platelet-derived growth factor (PDGF), and fibroblast growth factor (FGF).

Bevacizumab, a humanized monoclonal antibody directed against VEGF, was the first clinically available agent in the United States targeting the VEGF signaling pathway. It is currently approved in the United States for the treatment of colorectal carcinoma, non-small-cell lung carcinoma, and breast cancer when used in combination with standard chemotherapy. It is under investigation for use in a variety of other tumor types. Another class of antiangiogenic agents is the small-molecule tyrosine kinase inhibitors (TKIs) such as sunitinib, sorafenib, vandetanib, cediranib, brivanib, and TKI-258 (Table 6.2). In addition to targeting the VEGF pathway, these agents target a number of other pathways that are thought to be involved in angiogenesis. Brivanib alaninate is a dual inhibitor of the VEGFR and FGF receptor (FGFR) pathways. The significance of these two receptor pathways in angiogenesis and tumorigenesis is further discussed next.

TABLE 6.2. VEGF-Targeted Therapies Currently Approved

Compound	Clinical Development	VEGF	PDGFR	FGFR	EGFR	Raf	c-kit	flt-3
Bevacizumab (Avastin®)	Marketed for CRC, NSCLC, and breast cancer	X						
Sorafenib (Nexavar®)	Marketed for RCC and HCC	X	X			X	X	X
Sunitinib (Sutent®)	Marketed for RCC and GIST	X	X		X		X	X

CRC, colorectal carcinoma; EGFR, epidermal growth factor receptor; FGFR, fibroblast growth factor receptor; flt3, fms-related tyrosine kinase 3; GIST, gastrointestinal stromal tumor; HCC, hepatocellular carcinoma; NSCLC, non-small-cell lung cancer; PDGFR, platelet-derived growth factor receptor; RCC, renal cell carcinoma; VEGF, vascular endothelial growth factor.

6.2. VEGFR AND FGFR AS ANGIOGENESIS TARGETS

6.2.1. VEGFR

Antiangiogenesis therapy, initially based on inhibition of the VEGF pathway, is now firmly established in the treatment of a growing number of tumor types and has been successful in delaying tumor progression and extending survival. Among the known angiogenic growth factors implicated in the modulation of angiogenesis, the VEGF family (VEGF-A, -B, -C, and -D) and their corresponding cell surface receptors (VEGFR1 [flt1], VEGFR2 [KDR/flk1], and VEGFR3 [flt4]) play a major role in multiple facets of the angiogenic and lymphangiogenic processes (Carmeliet and Jain, 2000). Evidence indicates that expression and signaling of VEGF are critical for tumor angiogenesis as antibodies against VEGF (Kim et al., 1993) and VEGFR (Witte et al., 1998) as well as small-molecule VEGFR inhibitors (Fong et al., 1999; Drevs et al., 2000; Wedge et al., 2002) have been shown to inhibit angiogenesis in a variety of tumor xenograft models based on decreased blood flow and blood vessel density as well as induction of tumor growth stasis. VEGFR2 is the principal receptor through which VEGFs exert their mitogenic, chemotactic, and vascular permeabilizing effects on the host vasculature (Ferrara and Davis-Smyth, 1997; Korpelainen and Alitalo, 1998; Neufeld et al., 1999; Kerbel and Folkman, 2002). Indeed, increased expression of VEGFs by tumor cells and VEGFR2 and VEGFR1 in the tumor vasculature is a hallmark of a variety of human and animal tumors in vivo and correlates with tumor growth rate, microvessel density/proliferation, tumor metastatic potential, and poorer patient prognosis in a variety of malignancies (Ferrara and Davis-Smyth, 1997; Korpelainen and Alitalo, 1998; Neufeld et al., 1999; Carmeliet and Jain, 2000; Griffioen and Molema, 2000; Cristofanilli et al., 2002; Kerbel and Folkman, 2002). Despite its high VEGF binding affinity, the VEGFR1 receptor does not appear to direct a mitogenic response in endothelial cells or transfected fibroblasts, but instead plays an important role in modulating the activities of VEGFR2 (Aiello et al., 1995; Gille et al., 2000; Hiratsuka et al., 2001) and levels of circulating VEGF (Hiratsuka et al., 2001).

6.2.2. FGFR

In addition to VEGF, it is increasingly apparent that FGF signaling pathways have a significant role in tumor development and progression. Basic fibroblast growth factor (bFGF) or FGF2 was identified as the first proangiogenic molecule in the 1980s by Shing et al. (1984) who reported that FGF2 isolated from a chondrosarcoma could function as a tumor-derived capillary growth factor and stimulate angiogenesis in various models. Subsequently, FGF2 was shown to have angiogenic activity in different experimental models in vivo (Folkman and Klagsbrun, 1987) and is thought to have effects on both tumor cell growth and angiogenesis, such that it may enhance the malignancy of a variety of cancers such as hepatocellular carcinoma (HCC), pancreatic cancer, prostate cancer, and bladder cancer. FGFs, of which there are many types, are expressed in almost all tissues and play important roles in a variety of normal and patho- logical processes, including embryonic development, wound healing, and neo- plastic transformation. FGFs are considered to be pleiotropic mitogens, which are involved in diverse cellular processes, including chemotaxis, cell migration, differentiation, and cell survival (Hazan et al., 2000; Katoh and Katoh, 2006; Zittermann and Issekutz, 2006). The potential of FGFs to promote tumor progression is highly dependent on specific FGFR signaling, highlighting its importance as a target for antitumor activity. FGF1 and FGF2 and their receptors promote autocrine and paracrine regulation of malignant tumors (Takahashi et al., 1992). In general, while FGF expression is associated with tumor progression, FGFR expression is more selective; FGFR1 expression is associated with tumorigenesis, while FGFR2 expression is associated with decreased tumor progression in some tumors (Fujisawa et al., 1999; Naimi et al., 2002; Kondo et al., 2007) and early tumor development in others (Vairaktaris et al., 2006; Grose et al., 2007).

Endothelial cells have been shown to express FGFR1, and sometimes FGFR2, but have not been found to express FGFR3 or FGFR4 (Bastaki et al., 1997; Dell'Era et al., 2001; Javerzat et al., 2002). FGF has a direct effect on tumor angiogenesis by promoting proliferation in FGFR-expressing endo- thelial cells (Giavazzi et al., 2001). In addition, an intimate cross-talk exists between FGF2 and different members of the VEGF family during angiogen- esis, lymphangiogenesis, and vasculogenesis. Several studies suggest the pos- sibility that FGF2 induces neovascularization indirectly by activation of the VEGF/VEGFR pathway. In one study, simultaneous expression of FGF2 and VEGF resulted in rapid growing tumor xenografts in nude mice, which were characterized by high blood vessel density, patency, and permeability (Giavazzi et al., 2003). A further study showed that VEGFR2 antagonists inhibit both VEGF- and FGF2-induced angiogenesis in vitro and in vivo (Tille et al., 2001). In an implant mouse model of angiogenesis, VEGFR2 inhibitors were shown to completely inhibit VEGF-induced growth of vascularized tissue, and also FGF2-induced growth to some extent. In addition, the same VEGFR2 inhibi- tors were shown to inhibit VEGF- and FGF2-induced bovine endothelial cell invasion. Furthermore, both endogenous and exogenous FGF2 were shown to modulate VEGF expression in endothelial cells (Seghezzi et al., 1998). These activities suggest that suppression of the FGF pathway may have a major impact on cancer therapy by inhibiting both tumor growth and host angiogenesis.

6.2.3. Resistance to Anti-VEGF Therapy

Both intrinsic and acquired resistance to antiangiogenic therapies such as anti-VEGF/VEGFR agents is a clinically significant issue. Even though block- ing the VEGF pathway has been shown to prevent tumor progression in the short term, eventual progression of disease in the presence of VEGF/VEGFR therapies has been observed in clinical studies (Kerbel et al., 2001; Miller et al., 2003, 2005).

Intrinsic anti-VEGF resistance has been shown to be associated with infiltration of the tumor tissue by bone marrow–derived cells (CD11b$^+$Gr1$^+$ myeloid suppressor cells) (Shojaei et al., 2007). In this preclinical study, an anti-VEGF antibody-resistant tumor cell line was shown to be colonized by CD11b$^+$Gr1$^+$ myeloid suppressor cells in mouse models. Furthermore, when normal tumor cells were mixed with anti-VEGF antibody-resistant cells and transplanted into mice, the transplanted tumors showed resistance to anti-VEGF antibodies. Intrinsic resistance can occur as a result of tumor cells using existing blood vessels in vasculature-rich organs (Leenders et al., 2004) or as a result of the absence of VEGF or VEGFR in metastatic tumors in certain organ sites (Karashima et al., 2007).

The regulation of angiogenesis is highly redundant and flexible, and blockade of any one pathway inevitably promotes the selection of other compensatory pathways. This may happen both through physiologic upregulation and through selection of clones in which mutations amplify alternative pathways. The most immediate mechanism of acquired resistance is therefore increased reliance on alternative proangiogenic factors that do not use the VEGF pathway. Indeed, data suggest that other proangiogenic circuits primarily serve to enhance the critical VEGFR signal in early-stage lesions, whereas in later stages of progression, they can either enhance VEGF signaling or indeed substitute for it. It has been suggested that FGF, hepatocyte growth factor (HGF), placental growth factor (PlGF), PDGF, leptin, and insulin-like growth factor (IGF) pathways, among a continually growing list of others, may have a role in angiogenic resistance.

Acquired resistance to anti-VEGFR2 antibodies was shown in one study to be caused by the redundancy of angiogenesis stimulators, demonstrated by upregulation of FGF in a pancreatic tumor after anti-VEGFR antibody treatment. This effect was suggested to be due to elevated levels of hypoxia induced by drug treatment (Casanovas et al., 2005). In clinical studies, bevacizumab was shown to increase circulating levels of PlGF (Motzer et al., 2006), while sunitinib induced high levels of VEGF and PlGF that reverted to normal levels during drug-free periods (Willett et al., 2005). FGF2 and PDGF have been shown to synergistically promote tumor angiogenesis in mouse models (Nissen et al., 2007), suggesting that two or more growth factors could act synergistically. These effects may contribute to the rapid vascular regrowth that has been observed in tumors after removal of VEGF inhibition (Mancuso et al., 2006). Rapid vascular remodeling of tumor-associated vessels is thought to be another cause of resistance. In addition, the mature remodeled vessels are resistant to antiangiogenic therapies, which usually target relatively immature or developing blood vessels (Benjamin et al., 1999). Understanding these resistance mechanisms may provide insights into predictive markers that can be used to determine which patients are most likely to benefit from a particular therapy.

6.3. DISCOVERY OF BRIVANIB ALANINATE: PRECLINICAL STUDIES

6.3.1. Background

For almost two decades there has been intensive research into the development of small-molecule kinase inhibitors. Although these kinases have a relatively highly conserved adenosine 5'-triphosphate (ATP)-binding domain, small variations of amino acid residues in the adjacent areas have been shown to translate into selectivity for a particular molecule or molecules. To achieve potency and selectivity, a typical ATP-competitive kinase inhibitor consists of a core template that binds to the hinge region, with appended substituents that make key interactions with unique amino acid residues of the "gatekeeper" site, a selectivity pocket, and a ribose binding region (Figure 6.1). Efforts to develop compounds based on this ATP-competitive kinase inhibitor model have led to the identification of a variety of core templates. Many templates, including quinazolines, indolinones, isothiazoles, phthalazines, 2-aminothiazoles, pyrazoles, benzimidazoles, and 3-cyanoquinolines, have been identified which, with appropriate substituents, have yielded selective inhibitors for various kinases. Among these, the quinazoline scaffold was recognized as a versatile template for kinase inhibitor discovery programs. Indeed, the approved tyrosine kinase inhibitors erlotinib (OSI-774) (Moyer et al., 1997), gefinitib (ZD-1839) (Barker et al., 2001), and lapatinib (GW572016), and the VEGFR2 kinase inhibitors in development such as vandetanib (ZD-6474) (Hennequin et al., 2002) and cediranib (ZD-2171) (Wedge et al., 2005), are quinazoline-based molecules (Figure 6.2).

Crystallographic studies have shown that the N-1 nitrogen of the quinazoline template binds to residues of the kinase hinge region, the substituents at C-4 extend into the hydrophobic selectivity pocket (Hennequin et al., 2002),

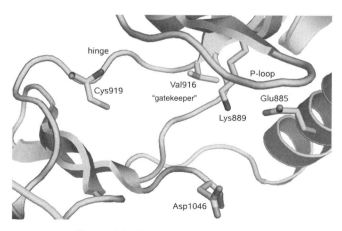

Figure 6.1. VEGFR2 kinase domain.

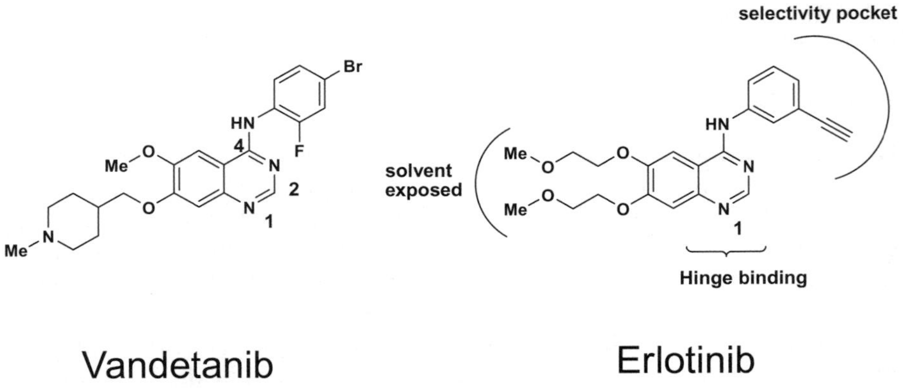

Figure 6.2. Structures of vandetanib and erlotinib.

and the substituents on the fused benzene ring orient toward the solvent exposed region. This affords opportunities to improve on the physicochemical and pharmacokinetic properties of drug candidates by substitution on the fused ring. We were intrigued by the possibility of a 5,6-fused ring system, which mandates that a nitrogen atom occupies a ring-fusion position, while maintaining the N-1 nitrogen to provide the critical hydrogen bond to the hinge region. Additionally, by replacing the six-membered fused phenyl ring with a fused five-membered ring, the appended substituents would be projected into space with different geometry. This was especially attractive because it has been observed often that even small changes in substituents and their orientation can result in dramatic changes in the kinase selectivity profile. Building on these hypotheses, the pyrrolo[2,1-*f*][1,2,4]triazine bicyclic ring system was shown to be a versatile template for designing kinase inhibitors (Hunt et al., 2004) such as potent and selective inhibitors of VEGFR2 and the EGF receptor family (HER1/HER2).

In applying the pyrrolo[2,1-*f*][1,2,4]triazine core to the discovery of VEGFR2 inhibitors, the initial structure–activity relationship (SAR) led to the identification of four series of compounds, each with a different substituted aniline at the C-4 position. These anilines accessed the selectivity pocket and made key interactions to impart selectivity for VEGFR2 and FGFR1 kinases. Based on molecular modeling, the phenol **1** (Borzilleri et al., 2005a), hydroxamate **2** (Borzilleri et al., 2005b), and the amide **3** (Cai et al., 2008) make key interactions with Asp1046, while the nitrogen of the indole **4** has key interaction with the Glu885 residue (Figure 6.3).

Compounds from all four series were tested in several in vitro assays with relevance for predicting pharmacokinetic behavior, including Caco-2 permeability, P450 enzyme inhibition, microsomal stability, and glucuronidation assays. Compounds with encouraging in vitro data were further advanced into oral bioavailability studies in mice. A 4 or 6 hour study protocol with four

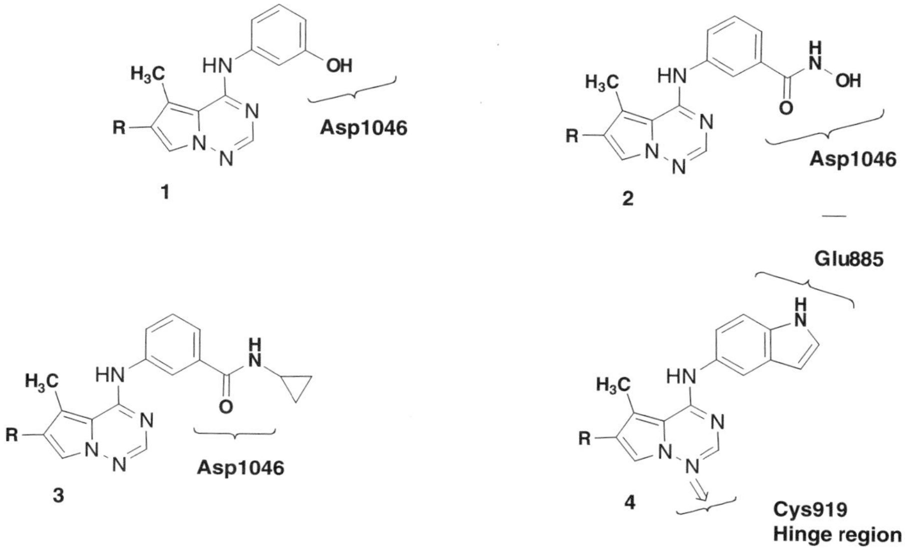

Figure 6.3. Chemical structures of pyrrolo[2,1-*f*][1,2,4]triazine based VEGFR2 inhibitors.

time-points and three mice per study was used to quickly assess many compounds. This method of testing a single compound at a time was preferred over cassette dosing of multiple compounds as a means of generating more reliable SAR data and was shown to give reliable pharmacokinetic profiles for advancing compounds into in vivo efficacy studies in cancer models. From the pharmacokinetic profile and tumor model testing, it became clear that the indole series held the most promise for drug development.

Initial SAR studies in the indole series were investigated, due to facile synthetic access, using analogs with an ester group at the 6-position. The indole ring was linked to the pyrrolotriazine core via either nitrogen or oxygen. In the nitrogen-linked series, flat SAR was observed with various changes at R^5, $R^{2'}$, and $R^{4'}$ providing little change in inhibitory activity (Table 6.3).

In the oxygen-linked series, a clear SAR was observed with respect to groups at a number of positions (Table 6.4). Similar to earlier observations in the phenol series (Borzilleri et al., 2005a), incorporation of a methyl group at the 5-position, as in compound **11**, gave optimal potency against the VEGFR2 enzyme. Although the introduction of a methyl group at the 2-position of the indole ring ($R^{2'}$) did not affect the potency against VEGFR2 (compare **11** and **14**), introduction of a fluorine group at the 4-position of indole ring ($R^{4'}$) gave a fourfold increase in potency against VEGFR2 (**15**). Substitution at the 3-position of the indole ring ($R^{3'}$) proved detrimental in both series (data not shown).

TABLE 6.3. SAR at the $R^{2'}$, $R^{4'}$, and $R^{5'}$ Positions of 3-(Piperidin-1-yl)propyl 4-(1H-indol-5-ylamino)pyrrolo[2,1-f][1,2,4]triazine-6-carboxylate

Compound	$R^{2'}$	$R^{4'}$	R^5	VEGFR2 IC_{50} (μM)
5	H	H	Et	0.104
6	Me	H	Me	0.108
7	Me	H	Et	0.087
8	H	H	i-Pr	0.144
9	Me	F	Et	0.084

TABLE 6.4. SAR at the R^5, $R^{2'}$, and $R^{4'}$ Positions of 4-(1H-indol-5-yloxy)-pyrrolo[2,1-f][1,2,4]triazine

Compound	R^1	$R^{2'}$	$R^{4'}$	R^5	VEGFR2 IC_{50} (μM)
10	Me	H	H	H	0.21
11	Et	H	H	Me	0.087
12	Et	H	H	Et	0.31
13	Et	H	H	i-Pr	0.47
14	Me	Me	H	Me	0.078
15	Me	Me	F	Me	0.017

As kinase in vitro potency did not clearly distinguish the nitrogen-linked from the oxygen-linked series with ester group at C-6, we analyzed analogs in which the ester group was converted into metabolically more stable groups. At the C-6 position, ethers, carbamates, and amides were prepared (Table 6.5). In the nitrogen-linked series, the SAR was again flat with moderate inhibition

TABLE 6.5. Comparison of Nitrogen-Linked and Oxygen-Linked Indole Series

Compound	X	R	R$^{4'}$	VEGFR2 IC$_{50}$ (μM)
16	N		H	0.28
17	N		H	0.18
18	N		H	0.18
19	O		H	0.042
20	O		H	0.084
21	O		F	>0.4
22	O	H	F	>0.4

and the most potent compound having an IC$_{50}$ value of 180 nM. In contrast, in the oxygen-linked series, ethers and amides showed greater differentiation. Thus in the oxygen-linked series, the presence of an electron acceptor group, such as ether or amide, attached to the ring at C-6 seemed to be important since both the unsubstituted compound **22** and the carbamate derivative **21** showed poor inhibitory potency. Therefore further SAR efforts were concentrated on the oxygen-linked series with amides or ethers at the C-6 position. From 4 hour exposure studies in mice, it was clear that the ether analogs had much better metabolic stability and oral exposures than the corresponding amides (unpublished data). This led to a much more focused effort on compounds with an ether-linked side chain at C-6.

Drugs with good pharmaceutical properties generally have good aqueous solubility. As such, medicinal chemists have traditionally used either an amine group or a carboxylic acid group to improve the water solubility of drug molecules. Of these, the amine group has been more successfully employed because at physiologic pH the anionic carboxylic acid group usually causes a molecule to be less penetrative through the anionic surface of a cell membrane bilayer; therefore a basic amine functionality on a tether that extends out of the kinase pocket toward solvent exposed space was introduced. As shown in Table 6.6, various amino groups and different chain lengths provided potent inhibitors against VEGFR2. These compounds were tested further in 4 hour exposure studies in mice dosed orally with a solution at 50 mg/kg in PEG400:water mixture. Some of these compounds showed acceptable area under the curve (AUC) with low C_{max} (maximum exposure) and sustained exposures (based on later long-term exposure studies of select compounds). However, these compounds also generally showed potent inhibition of CYP3A4 and the hERG ion channel using a patch-clamp assay. It was observed that incorporation of a hydroxyl group in close proximity to the amine functionality reduced the CYP3A4 and hERG channel inhibition (27). It was envisioned that these VEGFR2 inhibitors, unlike classical oncology drugs, would have to be given chronically and possibly in combination with cytotoxic drugs. Thus the aim was to minimize both the possibility of drug–drug interactions due to CYP450 inhibition and the potential for cardiac toxicity due to ion channel activity. It became clear that the in vitro profile of these amine group-containing analogs was not optimal, and that these compounds were less selective against other kinases.

In contrast, compounds **28** to **32**, which contained nonbasic polar groups, showed excellent oral exposure. Compounds **28** and **31** showed reduced CYP3A4 inhibition and hERG ion channel activity in the patch-clamp assay. Compound **28** showed better kinase selectivity, good aqueous solubility as an amorphous solid, lower human protein plasma binding (98.1%), and better oral exposures across four species when dosed as a solution. Therefore compound **28** (later named brivanib) was chosen as the development candidate.

A molecular model of brivanib bound to VEGFR2 was generated by docking the compound using the GLIDE (Schrödinger, LLC, New York) software and energy-minimizing with the CFF force field for 2000 steps of conjugate gradient minimization. As shown in Figure 6.4, the N-1 nitrogen bound to the NH group of Cys919 and the NH group of the indole nitrogen is predicted to make a critical hydrogen bond with Glu885 in the selectivity pocket.

As described later, brivanib showed potent in vivo efficacy versus H3396 and L2987 human lung carcinoma xenografts implanted in athymic mice when dosed as a solution (Bhide et al., 2006). However, in humans the preferred formulation for oral administration would be a solid dosage form using a crystalline compound. Therefore oral administration of brivanib was evaluated in rats as a micronized suspension. Suspension dosing yielded significantly lower systemic exposure levels of brivanib compared with solution

TABLE 6.6 SAR of C-6 Ethers with Amines on a Tether

Compound	R	VEGFR2 IC$_{50}$ (μM)	Mouse 4 hour Exposure (PO)		CYP3A4 IC$_{50}$ (μM)	hERG Inhibition
			AUC (μM · h)	C$_{max}$ (μM)		
23	H	0.024	0.2	0.2	ND^d	ND
24		0.017	14.0	4.2	1.0	70% @ 1μM
25		0.020	2.2	0.7	0.7	ND
26		0.020	20.5	5.9	3.4	66% @ 1μM
27		0.024	9.9	3.0	10.0	38% @ 1μM
28		0.025	136.0	41.0	18.0	IC$_{50}$ = 18μM

145

TABLE 6.6. *Continued*

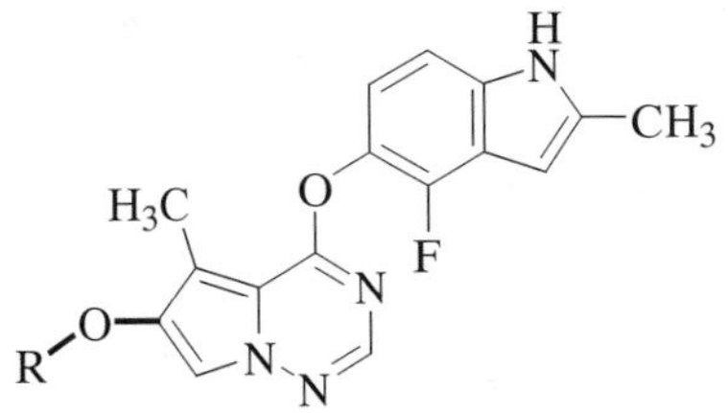

Compound	R	VEGFR2 IC$_{50}$ (µM)	Mouse 4 hour Exposure (PO)		CYP3A4 IC$_{50}$ (µM)	hERG Inhibition
			AUC (µM · h)	C$_{max}$ (µM)		
29	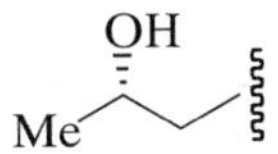 OH / Me	0.040	146.0	56.0	4.0	ND
30	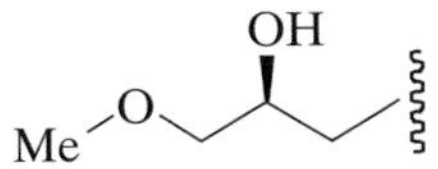 OH / Me–O	0.042	128.0	41.0	1.0	IC$_{50}$ = 18 µM
31	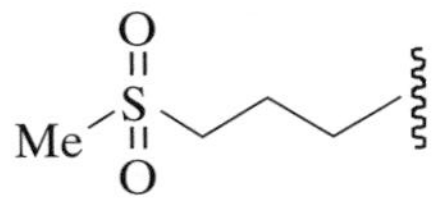 O=S=O / Me	0.070	185.0	57.0	17.0	IC$_{50}$ = 20 µM
32	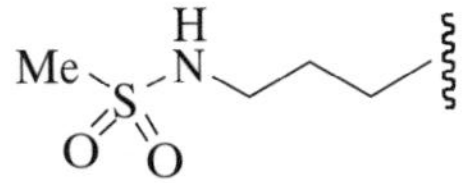 Me–S(=O)$_2$–N(H)	0.066	96.0	27.0	1.0	ND

AUC, area under the curve; *C*max, maximum plasma concentration; hERG, human ether-a-go-go-related gene; VEGFR, vascular endothelial growth factor receptor.

146

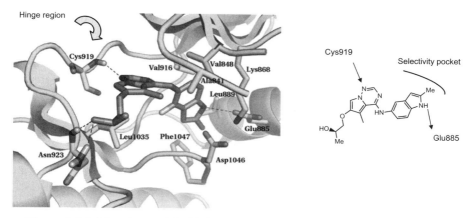

Figure 6.4. Molecular model of brivanib bound to the VEGFR2 kinase domain.

TABLE 6.7. Comparison of Pharmacokinetics of Brivanib in Mice as Solution or Micronized Suspension

	Solution[a]	Micronized Suspension[a]		
Dose (mg/kg)	25	25	100	200
C_{max} $(\mu M)^b$	6.4	0.55	2.05	1.71
AUC_{tot} $(\mu M \cdot h)^b$	13.4	3.35	8.43	7.61

[a]Vehicle for solution study was PEG400:ethanol:water (7:1:2) and for suspension study was 0.1% Tween 80 in water.
[b]$Cmax$, maximum plasma concentration; AUC, area under the curve.

formulations (Table 6.7), presumably as a result of dissolution rate-limited absorption of the compound, particularly at high doses. For a drug discovery candidate it is important to study the toxicity of the drug at high multiples of the exposures needed to produce efficacy. For brivanib, dissolution rate-limited absorption limited our ability to obtain high multiples in preclinical toxicology studies. This property also exposed the risk of not reaching efficacious exposures in humans. Efforts to improve the oral bioavailability and increase drug plasma concentrations of brivanib (**28**) at high doses using different formulation strategies were unsuccessful. As a result, a prodrug approach was investigated. A prodrug moiety has to be chosen very carefully because, upon release, it should not cause any toxicity by itself or undesirable metabolic by-products. Amino acid ester prodrugs of alcohols have been used successfully in marketed drugs to improve aqueous solubility and improve absorption (Purifoy et al., 1993). For a review on prodrugs, see reference 13 in Cai et al. (2008). Ester linkages are hydrolyzed by a number of esterases found in the stomach, intestines, liver, and plasma. It was important that the prodrug exhibit high chemical stability for ease of synthesis and long-term storage. On the other hand, it was necessary to have rapid and quantitative conversion to the parent drug to minimize unproductive metabolism of the prodrug and possible toxicity, if any, associated with the prodrug. Prodrugs of brivanib were initially evaluated to determine their stability in human and mouse liver S9 fractions and in plasma. The rate of enzymatic hydrolysis varied substantially based on the structure of the prodrug moiety, as illustrated in Table 6.8. Initial testing indicated that the ester prodrugs were moderately stable to ester cleavage in mouse plasma and very stable in human plasma. However, testing in human liver S9 fractions showed a range of conversion rates and this assay was used as the primary screening method (Moyer et al., 1997). Prodrugs based on amino acids with less hindered side chains such as **33** (glycinate), **34** (L-alaninate), **35** (D-alaninate), and **36** (L-leucinate) exhibited complete conversion to parent brivanib (**28**) in both human and mouse liver S9 fractions within the 5 minutes of incubation time, with no additional major metabolites detected (Table 6.8). Prodrugs with more hindered amino acids such as compounds **37** to **41** proved to be more stable. Similarly, benzoic acid derivatives also proved to be relatively stable.

Even though four prodrugs (**33**, **34**, **36**, and **39**) demonstrated rapid conversion to the parent drug in human and mouse liver S9 fractions, it was essential to determine how those results translate to in vivo conditions. Compounds were administered orally in mice as a 70:30 PEG:water solution at 50 and 200 mg/kg doses, and the plasma concentrations of brivanib (**28**) were determined at 0.5, 1, and 4 hour time points (Table 6.9). The parent compound **28** demonstrated almost equal systemic exposure at 50 and 200 mg/kg doses, whereas all four prodrugs produced higher exposure levels of **28**, and, importantly, the AUC increased proportionally with dose. These data demonstrated efficient in vivo conversion of these four prodrugs to the parent compound **28** in mice with no circulating prodrug in plasma for any compounds.

As compound **36** yielded the lowest levels of drug **28** concentrations in plasma, only prodrugs **33**, **34**, and **39** were further assessed in dog pharmacokinetic studies (to be published) and based on the favorable in vivo oral exposure study results in two species, **34** (brivanib alaninate) was selected as the development candidate for further pharmacokinetic, efficacy, and toxicology evaluations.

6.3.2. Synthesis

Synthesis of brivanib was conducted in a convergent fashion by synthesizing chloroimidate **47** (Godfrey et al., 2003) and 4-fluoro-2-methyl-1H-indol-5-ol **51** (Figure 6.6) separately and then reacting them in the presence of potassium carbonate in dimethylformamide (DMF) to afford fluoroindole-substituted pyrrolotriazine ester **48** (Figure 6.5) (Cai et al., 2008). Treatment of ester **48** with methyl magnesium bromide gave rise to the tertiary alcohol **49**, which was rearranged to hydroxy derivative **50** by treatment with $BF_3:OEt_2/50\%$ H_2O_2 in good yield (Kabalka et al., 1993). This approach was used as an efficient alternative to the Baeyer–Villiger reaction we had originally used to prepare the key intermediate **50** from the corresponding aldehyde (Bhide

TABLE 6.8. Prodrug Stability in Liver S9 Fraction (5 min Incubation)[a,b]

33–41   42–46

Prodrug	R^1	R^2	R^3	Prodrug: Percentage Metabolically Hydrolyzed	
				Mouse	Human
33 (gly)	H	H		100	96
34 (L-ala)	Me	H		100	100
35 (D-ala)	H	Me		100	95
36	Me	Me		100	100
37 (L-val)	*i*-Pr	H		28	64
38 (D-val)	H	*i*-Pr		14	75
39 (L-leu)	*i*-Bu	H		100	100
40 (L-ile)	*sec*-Bu	H		26	12
41 (L-phe)	Bz	H		50	56
42				9	84
43				92	84
44				27	73
45				12	42
46				18	21

[a]See Cai et al. (2008) for a description of assay conditions.
[b]Data are expressed as a mean of at least two determinations (variation < 20%).

TABLE 6.9. Oral Exposure of Various Compounds in Mice[a]

		Plasma Concentration of **1**		
Compound	Dose (mg/kg)	C_{max}[b] (μM)	AUC[b] (0–4 hour) (μM · h)	AUC Fold Increase (AUC at 200 mg/kg/AUC at 50 mg/kg)
28	50	12 ± 6	45	
	200	14 ± 10	52	1.2
33	50	21 ± 3	69	
	200	126 ± 15	303	4.4
34	50	21 ± 5	69	
	200	78 ± 20	276	4.0
36	50	15 ± 6	46	
	200	66 ± 29	213	4.6
39	50	31 ± 4	113	
	200	152 ± 17	451	4.0

[a]A mean of three female mice were evaluated for each dose group. Vehicle was PEG400:water (70%:30%).
[b]C_{max}, maximum plasma concentration; AUC, area under the curve.

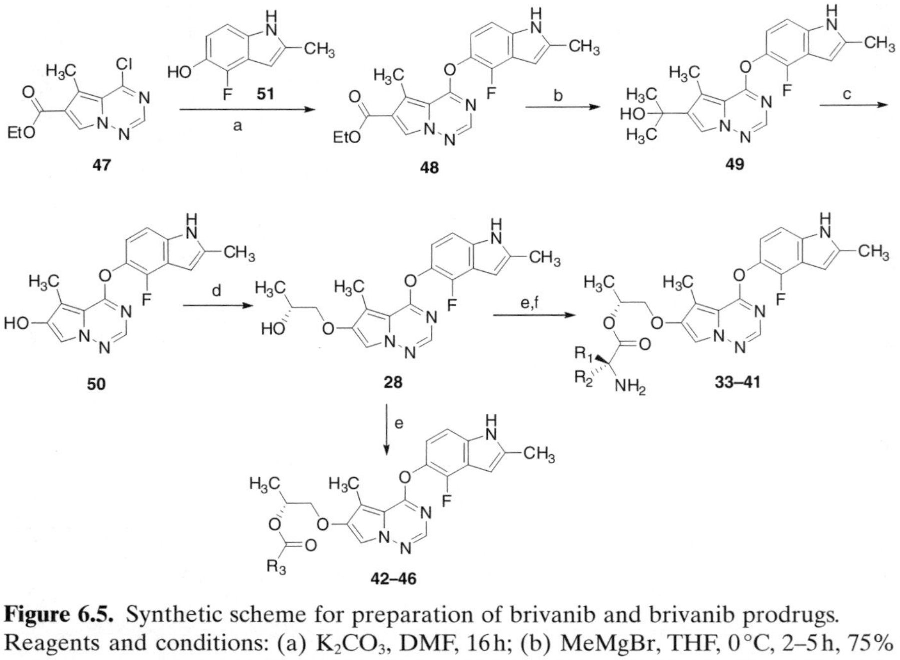

Figure 6.5. Synthetic scheme for preparation of brivanib and brivanib prodrugs. Reagents and conditions: (a) K_2CO_3, DMF, 16 h; (b) MeMgBr, THF, 0 °C, 2–5 h, 75% yield over two steps; (c) H_2O_2, BF_3:OEt_2, CH_2Cl_2, −15 to −25 °C, 1 h, 66%; (d) R-(+)-propylene oxide, LiCl, NEt₃ (cat.), EtOH, 3 h, 81%; (e) CbzNHCR₁R₂COOH (**33–41**) or R_3CO_2H (**42–46**), HATU, DIPEA, DMAP (cat.), THF, 5 h; (f) HCOO⁻NH4⁺, Pd/C, DMF.

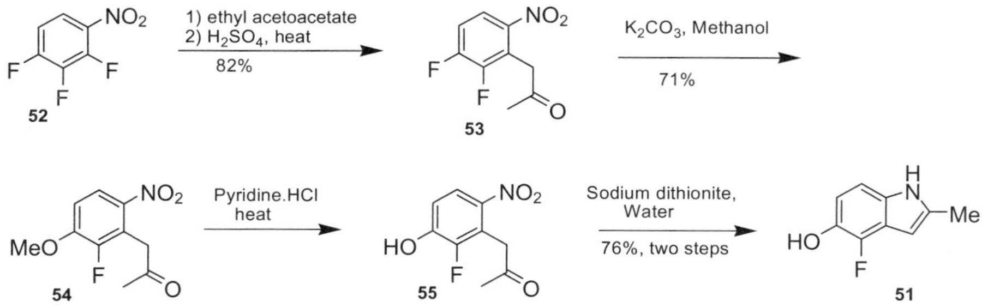

Figure 6.6. Synthetic scheme for preparation of fluoroindole **51**.

et al., 2006). Base-catalyzed epoxide opening of *R*-(+)-propylene oxide with **50** in ethanol afforded compound **28** in an enantiomeric excess of >99%. The addition of lithium chloride to the reaction mixture enhanced the rate of epoxide ring opening presumably due to chelation of the lithium ion with the epoxide oxygen. The ester prodrugs were prepared in excellent yield by coupling alcohol **28** with carbobenzyloxy (Cbz)-protected amino acids or the benzoic acids in the presence of 2-(3*H*-[1,2,3]triazol[4,5-*b*]pyridine-3-yl)-1,1,3,3-tetramethylisouronium hexafluorophosphate (HATU), diisopropylethylamine (DIPEA), and dimethylaminopyridine (DMAP) in DMF. In the case of **33–41**, the final products were obtained after deprotection of the Cbz group via a palladium-catalyzed hydrogen transfer reaction with ammonium formate. Absence of racemization of the chiral amino esters during these transformations was determined by comparing enantiomeric purities of L-alanine ester **34** and its enantiomeric isomer D-alanine ester **35** by chiral high-performance liquid chromatography (HPLC).

The fluoroindole analog **51** was prepared as shown in Figure 6.6. Commercially available **52** was reacted with ethylacetoacetate followed by acid-catalyzed decarboxylation to afford ketone **53**. The methoxy group was added regioselectively at the para position to the nitro group followed by demethylation of the methyl ether by pyrolysis with pyridine hydrochloride salt to obtain **55**. Reduction of the nitro group followed by in situ intramolecular cyclization afforded fluoroindole intermediate **51**.

6.3.3. Pharmacology

Brivanib, the parent compound of brivanib alaninate, has been shown to demonstrate selective inhibitory activity against a number of kinase families (Table 6.10). Consistent with its antiangiogenic activity, brivanib has been shown to inhibit both VEGF- and FGF2-stimulated human umbilical vascular endothelial cell (HUVEC) growth in vitro driven by either VEGF or FGF stimulation, but has no effect on EGF-stimulated HUVEC growth.

In multiple preclinical models of human xenograft tumors, both brivanib and brivanib alaninate demonstrated potent antitumor activity when dosed

TABLE 6.10. In Vitro Inhibitory Activity of Brivanib Against Various Enzymes

Biochemical	IC_{50} (nM)	Cellular	IC_{50} (nM)
VEGFR1	350	VEGF HUVEC	40
VEGFR2	25	FGF HUVEC	276
VEGFR3	10	EGF HUVEC	>2,500
FGFR1	150	L2987/H3396	>10,000
FGFR2	125		
FGFR3	68		
FGFR4	>1,000		

Enzyme	IC_{50} (nM)	Enzyme	IC_{50} (nM)
HGFR	17,600	HER1	1,970
PKC_θ	>100,000	HER2	>10,000
$PKC\alpha$	>25,000	Lck	2,730
$PKC\beta$	>25,000	Syk	>50,000
PKA	>50,000	SRC	>5,000
CDK2	>50,000	CAMK II	>50,000
EMT	>50,000	GSK-3	>50,000
IGF-R1	>50,000	JAK-3	>50,000
p38	>30,000	$PDGFR\beta$	7,460
AKT	>50,000	MEK	>25,000

CAMK, calmodulin-dependent kinase; CDK, cyclin-dependent kinase; EGF, epidermal growth factor; FGFR, fibroblast growth factor receptor; GSK, glycogen synthase kinase; HER, human epidermal growth factor receptor; HGFR, hepatocyte growth factor receptor; HUVEC, human umbilical vein endothelial cell; IGF, insulin-like growth factor; JAK, janus kinase; MEK, mitogen-activated protein kinase or extracellular signal-regulated kinase kinase; PDGFR, platelet-derived growth factor receptor; PKA, protein kinase A; PKC, protein kinase C; VEGFR, vascular endothelial growth factor receptor.

orally. Brivanib also showed potent antitumor activity against human H3396 breast cancer xenografts that had been implanted and allowed to grow for 15 days prior to treatment. The decreased tumor/control (T/C) ratios, reflecting a reduction in tumor size, were 0.70, 0.40, and 0.28 after 14 days of treatment at doses of 7.5 mg/kg bid, 15 mg/kg bid, and 30 mg/kg bid, respectively (Figure 6.7A). Tumor growth inhibition (TGI) values (see Appendix for calculation) were 30%, 37%, and 88%, respectively. Brivanib also demonstrated potent antitumor activity in paclitaxel-resistant HCT116/VM46 human colorectal carcinoma (CRC) xenografts (Figure 6.7B). Brivanib was shown to have greater inhibitory effects on tumor growth at doses of 15–45 mg/kg bid for 14 days than paclitaxel 36 mg/kg intravenously (IV) every 2 days for 10 days. Both brivanib and brivanib alaninate showed potent antitumor activity against L2987 human lung carcinoma xenografts over a variety of doses (Figure 6.7C, D). The T/C values following brivanib administration were 0.85, 0.40, and 0.36 at once-daily (qd) doses of 30 mg/kg, 60 mg/kg, and 90 mg/kg, respectively, after 9 days of treatment starting on day 17 post-implantation, while the TGI values

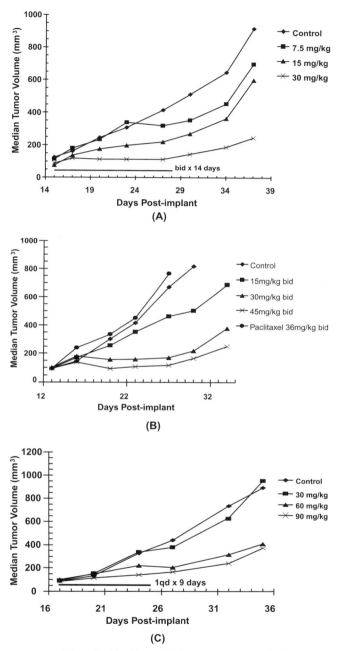

Figure 6.7. Effects of brivanib (**A–C**) and brivanib alaninate (**D**) on tumor growth rate of human H3396 breast cancer xenograft (**A**), human HCT116/VM46 colon carcinoma xenograft (**B**), and human L2987 lung cancer xenograft lines (**C**, **D**).

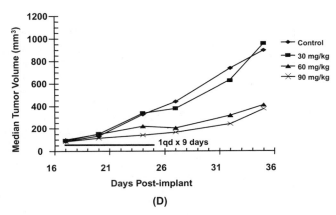

Figure 6.7. *Continued*

were 10%, 57%, and 61%, respectively. There was a similar effect on tumor growth following the administration of brivanib alaninate, with T/C ratios of 0.88, 0.40, and 0.28 at once-daily (qd) doses of 53 mg/kg, 80 mg/kg, and 107 mg/kg for 14 days starting on day 17 post-implantation. The TGI values were 34%, 85%, and 97%, respectively.

Repeated treatment with brivanib was shown to inhibit regrowth of human L2987 lung cancer xenografts, which had resumed growth following cessation of treatment (Figure 6.8). In this study, brivanib was administered at doses of 30, 60, and 90 mg/kg for 10 days to animals with tumors staged to 100 mm^3. Following cessation of treatment, tumors were allowed to regrow to approximately 400 mm^3 before reinitiating treatment for an additional 10 days. A final cycle of treatment was initiated when tumor sizes reached 800 mm^3. Induction of tumor stasis was evident with brivanib at doses of 60 and 90 mg/kg at all tumor sizes.

6.3.4. Biomarker Studies

The effect of brivanib treatment in inhibiting neovascularization but not pre-existing blood vessels is anticipated to result in tumor stasis rather than regression. As a result, brivanib, like other antiangiogenic agents, is expected to be used either in conjunction with standard chemotherapy or in an adjuvant setting. Consequently, there exists a need to identify biomarkers that can reflect both biological activity and predict efficacy at the molecular level. One approach is to use cDNA microarrays to identify novel biomarkers that correlate with response to treatment. Studies have shown that gene expression information generated by microarray analysis of human tumors can predict clinical outcome (Shipp et al., 2002; 't Veer et al., 2002; Glinksy et al., 2004). To identify such biomarkers, tumor samples from brivanib-treated and untreated athymic mice bearing L2987 lung human tumor xenografts were

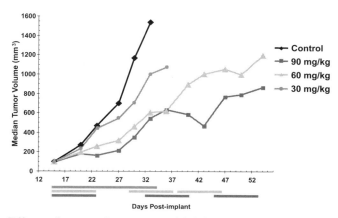

Figure 6.8. Effects of repeated treatment with brivanib on tumor regrowth of human L2987 lung cancer xenografts.

collected, and the RNA was extracted for gene expression profiling (Ayers et al., 2007). Five target genes were identified to be significantly modulated by treatment with brivanib and were chosen for validation using immunohisto-chemistry. The markers identified were tyrosine kinase receptor 1 (Tie-1), collagen IV, complement component 1 q subcomponent receptor 1 (C1QR1), angiotensin receptor-like 1 (Agtrl1), and vascular endothelial-cadherin (Cdh5). Further investigation of these markers by immunohistochemistry in L2987 (lung), HCT166/VM46 (paclitaxel-resistant CRC), and GEO (CRC) human tumor xenografts revealed that the two biomarkers that maintained the same behavior in transcriptional profiling and immunohistochemistry were collagen IV and C1QR1. Collagen IV is present in vessels and blood and has previously been implicated to play a role in angiogenesis and tumor pro-gression (Kalluri, 2003). In addition, collagen IV abnormalities including a loose association with endothelial cells and pericytes, broad extensions away from the vessel wall, and multiple layers visible by electron microscopy (Baluk et al., 2003) have been detected in the tumor microenvironment, and they may be linked to a possible mechanism of resistance for antiangiogenesis therapies by providing a scaffold for endothelial cell regrowth (Mancuso et al., 2006). Furthermore, treatment with brivanib was shown to decrease collagen IV levels. These findings support the hypothesis that collagen IV may be an important biomarker of angiogenesis in cancer and could be used as a pharmacodynamic marker of treatment response. Indeed, results from initial clinical studies have shown a reduction in collagen IV following brivanib treat-ment (see later discussion).

6.3.5. DCE-MRI

The in vivo activity of brivanib was also assessed in tumor-bearing mice using dynamic contrast-enhanced magnetic resonance imaging (DCE-MRI)

(Malone et al., 2005). Using this radiographic technique, blood flow, vessel surface area, and permeability were evaluated indirectly by assessing uptake of a contrast agent by DCE-MRI. In this study, changes in tumor microcirculation resulting from the antiangiogenic effects of VEGFR2 inhibition were measured in mice with human L2987 lung tumor xenografts by DCE-MRI. The contrast uptake in the tumor was measured as a pharmacodynamic marker of treatment response using the area under the gadolinium concentration–time curve for the first 60 seconds (AUC_{60}) after bolus injection of gadolinium DTPA using T1 weighted DCE-MRI. Reproducibility experiments conducted in the same mice 24 hours apart demonstrated that the 95% limit of change was −18% to +22% for a group of nine mice and the within-subject CV was 24%. Mice dosed orally once daily (qd) with brivanib had DCE-MRI assessments performed at 24 hours, 2 hours after the second dose and at 48 hours, 2 hours after the third dose. A dose-dependent response in blood flow and perfusion was observed at dose levels correlated with antitumor activity.

Figure 6.9 shows DCE-MRI images of blood flow in tumor tissue after administration of brivanib alaninate at 36 mg/kg and 107 mg/kg, with higher contrast uptake (associated with higher blood flow) observed in tumor following treatment with the lower dose of brivanib alaninate. A reduction in AUC_{60} of 54% and 64% was observed at 24 hours and 48 hours, respectively, in mice receiving brivanib alaninate at 107 mg/kg qd (Figure 6.10). This dose level

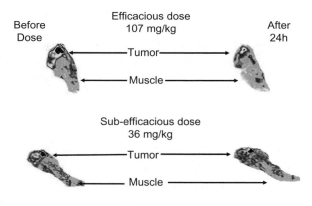

Higher contrast uptake, i.e., higher blood flow   Lower contrast uptake, i.e., lower blood flow

Figure 6.9. DCE-MRI analysis of coronal single slice images through the tumor and the muscle of the hind limb area before and 24 hours after administration of brivanib in the L2987 lung xenograft mouse model showing a markedly reduced uptake of contrast agent with brivanib 107 mg/kg compared with the 36 mg/kg dose, indicating lower blood flow to the tumor. (See color insert.)

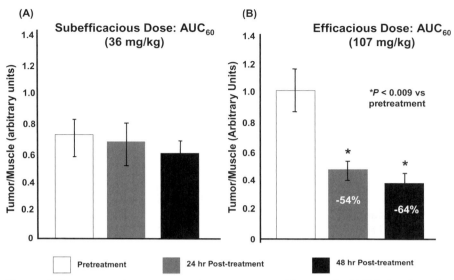

Figure 6.10. Area under concentration curve over 60 seconds (AUC$_{60}$) values for tumor/muscle ratio by DCE-MRI analysis. There was a significant reduction in AUC$_{60}$ of 54% and 64% at 24 hours and 48 hours, respectively, at the 107 mg/kg dose ($n = 9$). In contrast, there was no significant difference at the nonefficacious dose of 36 mg/kg ($n = 10$).

produced complete tumor stasis over a 10 day dosing period. In contrast, brivanib alaninate at 36 mg/kg qd led to an insignificant delay in tumor growth, with AUC$_{60}$ reductions of 6% and 18% at 24 hours and 48 hours, respectively. At an intermediate dose of 75 mg/kg, brivanib alaninate produced a significant growth delay, but not complete stasis, with reductions in AUC$_{60}$ of 27% and 44% at 24 and 48 hours, respectively. Reductions in AUC$_{60}$ of 25% at 2 hours, 29% at 4 hours, and 16% at 24 hours were observed with a single dose of brivanib alaninate at 107 mg/kg, which returned to baseline values by 48 hours. At a continuous daily dose of 107 mg/kg, brivanib alaninate treatment led to reductions in AUC$_{60}$ of 41% and 50% after 6 and 12 days, respectively. These results indicate that a marked reduction in tumor microcirculation even as early as 24 hours after brivanib treatment can be detected. In addition, gado-linium contrast agent uptake can be used as an early indicator of tumor microcirculation changes in solid tumors, and it has been incorporated into several clinical trials (Jayson et al., 2002; Galbraith et al., 2003). This prelimi-nary evidence suggests a direct correlation between changes by DCE-MRI, which are seen soon after initiation of anti-VEGFR2 therapy, and other con-ventional measures of antitumor activity such as tumor shrinkage, which may not appear until much later.

6.4. CLINICAL STUDIES

In a Phase I open-label dose escalation study conducted in 18 patients with advanced or metastatic solid tumors, the maximum tolerated dose of brivanib alaninate was established to be 800 mg qd. Dose escalation starting at a dose of 180 mg in cohorts of patients (n = 3 or 6 for 800 mg dose) on a continuous daily schedule was undertaken until dose-limiting toxicities were observed. The dose-limiting toxicities observed in two of three patients at a dose of 1000 mg were fatigue and dizziness, and altered mental status and dehydration in one patient each. Systemic exposure of the active moiety brivanib increased proportionally with increasing doses of brivanib alaninate from 180 to 1000 mg. The accumulation ratio (day 26:day 1) of C_{24h}, C_{max}, and AUC was 4.8, 2.0, and 2.1, respectively, at 1000 mg, but close to 1 at lower doses. The appropriate lower dose level of brivanib alaninate for further evaluation by DCE-MRI was established to be 320 mg (Rosen et al., 2006).

In a continuation of this Phase I study, the optimal dose or dose ranges for Phase II studies from measurement of the effects of brivanib on the DCE-MRI parameters AUC_{60} and K^{trans} on either continuous (C) daily or intermittent (I) schedules (320 mg, 800 mg continuous, 800 mg intermittent [5 days on, 2 days off], and 400 mg bid of brivanib alaninate) were investigated in patients with CRC, renal cell carcinoma (RCC), and hepatocellular carcinoma (HCC). Of the total of 68 patients included in the study, 14, 19, 12, and 13 received brivanib alaninate at doses of 320 mg, 800 mg, 800 mg, and 400 mg bid, respectively. The remaining ten patients were only evaluated in part A of the study. Most adverse events were mild with the most frequently reported being gastrointestinal (nausea, vomiting, diarrhea), fatigue, hypertension, and reversible transaminitis. The most frequently reported grade 3 to 4 toxicities were fatigue and reversible transaminitis. No grade 5 adverse events were reported, and no QTc prolongation was observed across the 180–1000 mg brivanib alaninate dose range. There was evidence of antitumor activity with two confirmed partial responses in patients receiving brivanib alaninate at ≥600 mg and 6 patients with stable disease at ≥6 months. The median time on study for all patients was 84 days. Furthermore, favorable changes in tumor size were observed in patients with a variety of tumors following brivanib alaninate treatment (Figure 6.11). The effect of brivanib on tumor perfusion as measured by DCE-MRI was related to dose and schedule of administration. The largest reduction in contrast agent occurred in patients receiving brivanib alaninate 800 mg qd and 400 mg bid. This reduction was sustained at trough on days 8 and 2; however, some recovery was observed with intermittent dosing, suggesting that continuous daily dosing is the optimum regimen. A dose response was observed with brivanib at doses of 320–800 mg in the three antiangiogenic pharmacodynamic markers (DCE-MRI, collagen IV, and soluble VEGFR2) (Jonker et al., 2007).

In a second open-label Phase I dose-escalation study, brivanib alaninate was given in combination with cetuximab to patients with advanced gastroduodenal malignancies who had failed prior therapy (Garrett et al., 2008).

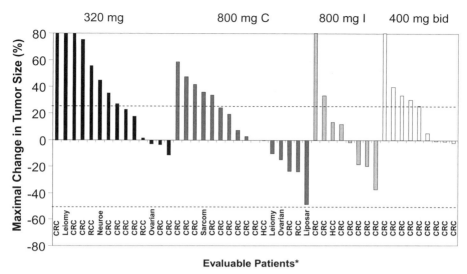

Figure 6.11. Change in patient tumor size with brivanib alaninate treatment at doses of 320 and 800 mg with varying schedules in a variety of tumor types. *Patients with available bidimensional tumor measurements.
Note: The two partial responses occurred in patients receiving brivanib at doses of 600 mg and 1000 mg (doses not shown in this figure).

Brivanib alaninate was given orally on day 1 and once daily (qd) from day 8, starting at a dose of 320 mg, and cetuximab was given intravenously on day 8 (400 mg/m^2), then weekly (250 mg/m^2). Dose escalation of brivanib continued to 800 mg qd when an expansion cohort for patients with CRC was opened for additional safety and efficacy. To date, a total of 62 patients (59 CRC, 2 esophageal, and 1 HCC) have been treated with brivanib alaninate 320, 600, or 800 mg qd in combination with cetuximab. A single dose-limiting toxicity, bilateral pulmonary emboli occurred on day 28 in a patient receiving brivanib alaninate 320 mg. There was no dose-limiting toxicity at the 800 mg dose. The combination of brivanib alaninate plus cetuximab was tolerable; adverse events included fatigue, diarrhea, dermatitis acneiform, anorexia, pyrexia, vomiting, and headache. The pharmacokinetics of brivanib was linear up to 800 mg of brivanib alaninate with no apparent effect of cetuximab or brivanib on the pharmacokinetics of either agent. A dose-dependent decline was observed in the pharmacodynamic markers, collagen IV and VEGFR2 levels, on day 29 compared with baseline. The best responses in the subset of 34 evaluable patients with colorectal cancer receiving brivanib alaninate 800 mg plus cetuximab were 6 partial responses (29%) and 11 stable disease (52%) in EGFR inhibitor-naive patients; 5 partial responses (50%) and 5 stable disease (50%) in VEGF inhibitor-naive patients; and 5 partial responses (56%) and 4 stable disease (44%) in EGFR and VEGF inhibitor-naive patients. The best antitumor activity was seen in the subset of patients who had not received either EGFR or VEGF inhibitor therapy.

Currently, additional studies are ongoing to evaluate the pharmacokinetics and pharmacodynamics of brivanib alaninate as well as the potential for drug–drug interactions. In addition, a Phase II open-label study to evaluate the effects of brivanib alaninate 800 mg on progression-free survival rate at 6 months in patients with unresectable locally advanced or metastatic HCC who have received no prior systemic therapy for HCC is ongoing.

6.5. POTENTIAL LIABILITIES OF ANTIANGIOGENIC THERAPY

Early on in the development of antiangiogenic therapy, minimal toxicity was anticipated based on the concept that only newly forming blood vessels would be affected, such as those found in the growing tumor. Recent clinical experience with the three approved antiangiogenic agents, bevacizumab, sorafenib, and sunitinib, that inhibit the VEGFR signaling pathway, however, have demonstrated overlapping as well as distinct side effects. The most common side effects have included high blood pressure, which can be managed by appropriate treatment, and possible increased risks of thromboembolic events in patients with preexisting cardiovascular disease (Pereg and Lisher, 2008). Other side effects may include excessive bleeding in surgical patients and impaired wound healing but, as a class, these agents are associated in general with manageable side effects and lower incidence of severe toxicities as experienced with classical cytotoxic therapies.

6.6. CONCLUSIONS AND FUTURE DIRECTIONS

Brivanib is a novel, oral, small-molecule dual inhibitor of VEGFR and FGFR tyrosine kinase activity, which has shown marked antitumor effects in a wide variety of preclinical xenograft tumor models. In Phase I studies, brivanib 800 mg qd has been shown to be well tolerated with evidence of antitumor activity in patients with advanced or metastatic solid tumors.

Although clinical efficacy for FGFR pathway inhibition alone is lacking, the dual inhibition of VEGFR and FGFR may provide a more effective means of sustaining antitumor activity based on the important roles that both of these signaling pathways play in tumor vascularization (Grose and Dickson, 2005). Studies by Casanovas et al. (2005) suggest the importance of blocking the FGFR signaling pathway following acquired resistance to VEGFR inhibition and that ultimately blocking multiple signaling pathways involved in tumor vascularization may provide a more durable delay to disease progression. As a result of its favorable efficacy and safety profile, brivanib continues to undergo clinical testing alone and in combination with other anticancer agents for the treatment of a variety of tumor types, including HCC and CRC.

APPENDIX: FORMULA FOR CALCULATION OF TUMOR GROWTH INHIBITION

Antitumor efficacy was expressed as percent tumor growth inhibition (%TGI) and calculated as follows:

$$\%TGI = \{1 - [(T_t - T_0)/(C_t - C_0)]\} \times 100$$

where C_t = median tumor volume (mm^3) of control (C) mice at time t; T_t = median tumor volume (mm^3) of treated mice (T) at time t; C_0 = median tumor volume (mm^3) of control mice at time 0. Tumor volume doubling time (TVDT) was measured over the linear growth range of the tumor. TGI $\geq 50\%$ over one TVDT was considered an active antitumor response.

ACKNOWLEDGMENT

The authors thank Dr. John T. Hunt for helpful suggestions in the preparation and proofreading of this chapter. Editorial support was provided by J. Fawcett, PhD, of PAREXEL and was funded by BMS.

REFERENCES

Aiello, L. P., Pierce, E. A., Foley, E. D., et al. (**1995**). Suppression of retinal neovascularization in vivo by inhibition of vascular endothelial growth factor (VEGF) using soluble VEGF-receptor chimeric proteins. *Proc Nat Acad Sci.* 92(23), 10457–10461.

Ayers, M., Fargnoli, J., Lewin, A., et al. (**2007**). Discovery and validation of biomarkers that respond to treatment with brivanib alaninate, a small-molecule VEGFR-2/FGFR-1 antagonist. *Cancer Res.* 67(14), 6899–6906.

Baluk, P., Morikawa, S., Haskell, A., et al. (**2003**). Abnormalities of basement membrane on blood vessels and endothelial sprouts in tumors. *Am J Pathol.* 163(5), 1801–1815.

Barker, A. J., Gibson, K. H., Grundy, W., et al. (**2001**). Studies leading to the identification of ZD1839 (IRESSA): an orally active, selective epidermal growth factor receptor tyrosine kinase inhibitor targeted to the treatment of cancer. *Bioorg Med Chem Lett.* 11(14), 1911–1914.

Bastaki, M., Nelli, E. E., Dell'Era, P., et al. (**1997**). Basic fibroblast growth factor-induced angiogenic phenotype in mouse endothelium: a study of aortic and microvascular endothelial cell lines. *Arterioscler Thromb Vasc Biol.* 17(3), 454–464.

Benjamin, L. E., Golijanin, D., Itin, A., et al. (**1999**). Selective ablation of immature blood vessels in established human tumors follows vascular endothelial growth factor withdrawal. *J Clin Invest.* 103(2), 159–165.

Bhide, R. S., Cai, Z. W., Zhang, Y. Z., et al. (**2006**). Discovery and preclinical studies of (*R*)-1-(4-(4-fluoro-2-methyl-1*H*-indol-5-yloxy)-5-methylpyrrolo[2,1-*f*][1,2,4] triazin-6-yloxy)propan-2-ol (BMS-540215), an in vivo active potent VEGFR-2 inhibitor. *J Med Chem.* 49(7), 2143–2146.

Borzilleri, R. M., Cai, Z. W., Ellis, C., et al. (**2005a**). Synthesis and SAR of 4-(3-hydroxyphenylamino)pyrrolo[2,1-*f*][1,2,4]triazine based VEGFR-2 kinase inhibitors. *Bioorg Med Chem Lett.* 15, 1429–1433.

Borzilleri, R. M., Zheng, X., Qian, L., et al. (**2005b**). Design, synthesis, and evaluation of orally active 4-(2,4-difluoro-5-(methoxycarbamoyl)phenylamino)pyrrolo[2,1-*f*][1,2,4]triazines as dual vascular endothelial growth factor receptor-2 and fibroblast growth factor receptor-1 inhibitors. *J Med Chem.* 48(12), 3991–4008.

Cai, Z. W., Zhang, Y. Z., Borzilleri, R. M., et al. (**2008**). Discovery of brivanib alaninate ((*S*)-((*R*)-1-(4-(4-fluoro-2-methyl-1*H*-indol-5-yloxy)-5-methylpyrrolo[2,1-*f*][1,2,4] triazin-6-yloxy)propan-2-yl) 2-aminopropanoate), a novel prodrug of dual vascular endothelial growth factor receptor-2 and fibroblast growth factor receptor-1 kinase inhibitor (BMS-540215). *J Med Chem.* 51(6), 1976–1980.

Carmeliet, P., and Jain, R. K. (**2000**). Angiogenesis in cancer and other diseases. *Nature.* 407(6801), 249–257.

Casanovas, O., Hicklin, D. J., Bergers, G., et al. (**2005**). Drug resistance by evasion of antiangiogenic targeting of VEGF signaling in late-stage pancreatic islet tumors. *Cancer Cell.* 8(4), 299–309.

Cristofanilli, M., Charnsangavej, C., and Hortobagyi, G. N. (**2002**). Angiogenesis modulation in cancer research: novel clinical approaches. *Nat Rev Drug Discov.* 1(6), 415–426.

Dell'Era, P., Belleri, M., Stabile, H., et al. (**2001**). Paracrine and autocrine effects of fibroblast growth factor-4 in endothelial cells. *Oncogene.* 20(21), 2655–2663.

Drevs, J., Hofmann, I., Hugenschmidt, H., et al. (**2000**). Effects of PTK787/ZK 222584, a specific inhibitor of vascular endothelial growth factor receptor tyrosine kinases, on primary tumor, metastasis, vessel density, and blood flow in a murine renal cell carcinoma model. *Cancer Res.* 60(17), 4819–4824.

Ferrara, N., and Davis-Smyth, T. (**1997**). The biology of vascular endothelial growth factor. *Endocr Rev.* 18(1), 4–25.

Ferrara, N., and Kerbel, R. S. (**2005**). Angiogenesis as a therapeutic target. *Nature.* 438(7070), 967–974.

Folkman, J. (**1971**). Tumor angiogenesis: therapeutic implications. *N Engl J Med.* 285(21), 1182–1186.

Folkman, J., and Klagsbrun, M. (**1987**). Angiogenic factors. *Science.* 235(4787), 442–447.

Fong, T. A., Shawver, L. K., Sun, L., et al. (**1999**). SU5416 is a potent and selective inhibitor of the vascular endothelial growth factor receptor (flk-1/KDR) that inhibits tyrosine kinase catalysis, tumor vascularization, and growth of multiple tumor types. *Cancer Res.* 59(1), 99–106.

Fujisawa, H., Kurrer, M., Reis, R. M., et al. (**1999**). Acquisition of the glioblastoma phenotype during astrocytoma progression is associated with loss of heterozygosity on 10q25-qter. *Am J Pathol.* 155(2), 387–394.

Galbraith, S. M., Maxwell, R. J., Lodge, M. A., et al. (**2003**). Combretastatin A4 phosphate has tumor antivascular activity in rat and man as demonstrated by dynamic magnetic resonance imaging. *J Clin Oncol.* 21(15), 2831–2842.

Garrett, C., Siu, L., El-Khoueiry, A., et al. (**2008**). A Phase I study of brivanib alaninate (BMS-582664), an oral dual inhibitor of VEGFR and FGFR tyrosine kinases, in combination with full dose cetuximab (BC) in patients (pts) with advanced gastrointestinal malignancies (AGM) who failed prior therapy. *J Clin Oncol.* 26(May supplement), Abstract 4111.

Giavazzi, R., Giuliani, R., Coltrini, D., et al. (**2001**). Modulation of tumor angiogenesis by conditional expression of fibroblast growth factor-2 affects early but not established tumors. *Cancer Res.* 61(1), 309–317.

Giavazzi, R., Sennino, B., Coltrini, D., et al. (**2003**). Distinct role of fibroblast growth factor-2 and vascular endothelial growth factor on tumor growth and angiogenesis. *Am J Pathol.* 162(6), 1913–1926.

Gille, H., Kowalski, J., Yu, L., et al. (**2000**). A repressor sequence in the juxtamembrane domain of Flt-1 (VEGFR-1) constitutively inhibits vascular endothelial growth factor-dependent phosphatidylinositol 3′-kinase activation and endothelial cell migration. *EMBO J.* 19(15), 4064–4073.

Glinksy, G. V., Glinskii, A. B., Stephenson, A. J., et al. (**2004**). Gene expression profiling predicts clinical outcome of prostate cancer. *J Clin Invest.* 113(6), 913–923.

Godfrey, J. D., Hynes, J., et al. (**2003**). Methods for the preparation of pyrrolotriazine compounds useful as kinase inhibitors. US patent application 2,003,186,982.

Griffioen, A. W., and Molema, G. (**2000**). Angiogenesis: potentials for pharmacologic intervention in the treatment of cancer, cardiovascular diseases, and chronic inflammation. *Pharmacol Rev.* 52(2), 237–268.

Grose, R., and Dickson, C. (**2005**). Fibroblast growth factor signaling in tumorigenesis. *Cytokine Growth Factor Rev.* 16(2), 179–186.

Grose, R., Fantl, V., Werner, S., et al. (**2007**). The role of fibroblast growth factor receptor 2b in skin homeostasis and cancer development. *EMBO J.* 26(5), 1268–1278.

Gullino, P. M. (**1978**). Angiogenesis and oncogenesis. *J Natl Cancer Inst.* 61(3), 639–643.

Hanahan, D., and Folkman, J. (**1996**). Patterns and emerging mechanisms of the angiogenic switch during tumorigenesis. *Cell.* 86(3), 353–364.

Hazan, R. B., Phillips, G. R., Qiao, R. F., et al. (**2000**). Exogenous expression of N-cadherin in breast cancer cells induces cell migration, invasion, and metastasis. *J Cell Biol.* 148(4), 779–790.

Hennequin, L. F., Stokes, E. S. E., Thomas, A. P., et al. (**2002**). Novel 4-anilinoquinazolines with C-7 basic side chains: design and structure activity relationship of a series of potent, orally active, VEGF receptor tyrosine kinase inhibitors. *J Med Chem.* 45(6), 1300–1312.

Hiratsuka, S., Maru, Y., Okada, A., et al. (**2001**). Involvement of flt-1 tyrosine kinase (vascular endothelial growth factor receptor-1) in pathological angiogenesis. *Cancer Res.* 61(3), 1207–1213.

Hunt, J. T., Mitt, T., Borzilleri, R., et al. (**2004**). Discovery of the pyrrolo[2,1-*f*][1,2,4]triazine nucleus as a new kinase inhibitor template. *J Med Chem.* 47(16), 4054–4059.

Javerzat, S., Auguste, P., and Bikfalvi, A. (**2002**). The role of fibroblast growth factors in vascular development. *Trends Mol Med.* 8(10), 483–489.

Jayson, G. C., Zweit, J., Jackson, A., et al. (**2002**). Molecular imaging and biological evaluation of HuMV833 anti-VEGF antibody: implications for trial design of antiangiogenic antibodies. *J Natl Cancer Inst.* 94(19), 1484–1493.

Jonker, D., Rosen, L. S., Sawyer, M., et al. (**2007**). A Phase I study of BMS-582664 (brivanib alaninate), an oral dual inhibitor of VEGFR and FGFR tyrosine kinases, in patients (pts) with advanced/metastatic solid tumors: safety, pharmacokinetic (PK), and pharmacodynamic (PD) findings. *J Clin Oncol.* 25(18S), 152 S [Abstract 3559].

Kabalka, G. W., Reddy, N. K., and Narayana, C. (**1993**). Sodium perborate: a convenient reagent for benzylic hydroperoxide rearrangement. *Tetrahedron Lett.* 34, 7667–7668.

Kalluri, R. (**2003**). Basement membranes: structure, assembly and role in tumour angiogenesis. *Nat Rev Cancer.* 3(6), 422–433.

Karashima, T., Inoue, K., Fukata, S., et al. (**2007**). Blockade of the vascular endothelial growth factor-receptor 2 pathway inhibits the growth of human renal cell carcinoma, RBM1-IT4, in the kidney but not in the bone of nude mice. *Int J Oncol.* 30(4), 937–945.

Katoh, M., and Katoh, M. (**2006**). FGF signaling network in the gastrointestinal tract (review). *Int J Oncol.* 29(1), 163–168.

Kerbel, R. S. (**2000**). Tumor angiogenesis: past, present and the near future. *Carcinogenesis.* 21(3), 505–515.

Kerbel, R., and Folkman, J. (**2002**). Clinical translation of angiogenesis inhibitors. *Nat Rev Cancer.* 2(10), 727–739.

Kerbel, R. S., Yu, J., Tran, J., et al. (**2001**). Possible mechanisms of acquired resistance to anti-angiogenic drugs: implications for the use of combination therapy approaches. *Cancer Metastasis Rev.* 20, 79–86.

Kim, K. J., Li, B., Winer, J., et al. (**1993**). Inhibition of vascular endothelial growth factor-induced angiogenesis suppresses tumour growth in vivo. *Nature.* 362(6423), 841–844.

Kondo, T., Zheng, L., Liu, W., et al. (**2007**). Epigenetically controlled fibroblast growth factor receptor 2 signaling imposes on the RAS/BRAF/mitogen-activated protein kinase pathway to modulate thyroid cancer progression. *Cancer Res.* 67(11), 5461–5470.

Korpelainen, E. I., and Alitalo, K. (**1998**). Signaling angiogenesis and lymphangiogenesis. *Curr Opin Cell Biol.* 10(2), 159–164.

Leenders, W. P. J., Kusters, B., Verrijp, K., et al. (**2004**). Antiangiogenic therapy of cerebral melanoma metastases results in sustained tumor progression via vessel co-option. *Clin Cancer Res.* 10(18), 6222–6230.

Malone, H., Pictroski, C., Kukral, D., et al. (**2005**). Dynamic contrast enhanced magnetic resonance imaging (DCE-MRI) tumor microcirculation studies in tumor bearing mice treated with VEGFR inhibitor BMS-582664. *Proc Am Assoc Cancer Res.* 46, 911–912.

Mancuso, M. R., Davis, R., Norberg, S. M., et al. (**2006**). Rapid vascular regrowth in tumors after reversal of VEGF inhibition. *J Clin Invest.* 116(10), 2610–2621.

Miller, K. D., Sweeney, C. J., and Sledge, G. W. Jr. (**2003**). The Snark is a Boojum: the continuing problem of drug resistance in the antiangiogenic era. *Ann Oncol.* 14, 20–28.

Miller, K. D., Sweeney, C. J., and Sledge, G. W. Jr. (**2005**). Can tumor angiogenesis be inhibited without resistance? *EXS.* 94, 95–112.

Motzer, R. J., Michaelson, M. D., Redman, B. G., et al. (**2006**). Activity of SU11248, a multitargeted inhibitor of vascular endothelial growth factor receptor and platelet-derived growth factor receptor, in patients with metastatic renal cell carcinoma. *J Clin Oncol.* 24(1), 16–24.

Moyer, J. D., Barbacci, E. G., Iwata, K. K., et al. (**1997**). Induction of apoptosis and cell cycle arrest by CP-358,774, an inhibitor of epidermal growth factor receptor tyrosine kinase. *Cancer Res.* 57(21), 4838–4848.

Naimi, B., Latil, A., Fournier, G., et al. (**2002**). Down-regulation of (IIIb) and (IIIc) isoforms of fibroblast growth factor receptor 2 (FGFR2) is associated with malignant progression in human prostate. *Prostate.* 52(3), 245–252.

Neufeld, G., Cohen, T., Gengrinovitch, S., et al. (**1999**). Vascular endothelial growth factor (VEGF) and its receptors. *FASEB J.* 13(1), 9–22.

Nissen, L. J., Cao, R., Hedlund, E. M., et al. (**2007**). Angiogenic factors FGF2 and PDGF-BB synergistically promote murine tumor neovascularization and metastasis. *J Clin Invest.* 117(10), 2766–2777.

Pereg, D., and Lisher, M. (**2008**). Bevacizumab treatment for cancer patients with cardiovascular disease: a double edged sword? *Eur Heart J.*, doi:10.1093/eurheartj/ehn384.

Purifoy, D. J. M., Beauchamp, L., De Miranda, M., et al. (**1993**). Review of research leading to new anti-herpesvirus agents in clinical development: valaciclovir hydrochloride (256u, the L-valyl ester of acyclovir) and 882c, a specific agent for varicella zoster virus. *J Med Virol Suppl.* 1, 139–145.

Ramanujan, S., Koenig, G. C., Padera, T. P., et al. (**2000**). Local imbalance of proangiogenic and antiangiogenic factors: a potential mechanism of focal necrosis and dormancy in tumors. *Cancer Res.* 60(5), 1442–1448.

Rosen, L. S., Wilding, G., Sweeney, C. J., et al. (**2006**). Phase I dose escalation study to determine the safety, pharmacokinetics and pharmacodynamics of BMS-582664, a VEGFR/FGFR inhibitor in patients with advanced/metastatic solid tumors. *J Clin Oncol.* 24(18S), Abstract 3051.

Seghezzi, G., Patel, S., Ren, C. J., et al. (**1998**). Fibroblast growth factor-2 (FGF-2) induces vascular endothelial growth factor (VEGF) expression in the endothelial cells of forming capillaries: an autocrine mechanism contributing to angiogenesis. *J Cell Biol.* 141(7), 1659–1673.

Shing, Y., Folkman, J., Sullivan, R., et al. (**1984**). Heparin affinity: purification of a tumor-derived capillary endothelial cell growth factor. *Science.* 223(4642), 1296–1299.

Shipp, M. A., Ross, K. N., Tamayo, P., et al. (**2002**). Diffuse large B-cell lymphoma outcome prediction by gene-expression profiling and supervised machine learning. *Nat Med.* 8(1), 68–74.

Shojaei, F., Wu, X., Malik, A. K., et al. (**2007**). Tumor refractoriness to anti-VEGF treatment is mediated by CD11b⁺Gr1⁺ myeloid cells. *Nat Biotechnol.* 25(8), 911–920.

Takahashi, J. A., Igarashi, K., Oda, K., et al. (**1992**). Correlation of basic fibroblast growth factor expression levels with the degree of malignancy and vascularity in human gliomas. *J Neurosurg.* 76(5), 792–798.

Tille, J. C., Wood, J., Mandriota, S. J., et al. (2001). Vascular endothelial growth factor (VEGF) receptor-2 antagonists inhibit VEGF- and basic fibroblast growth factor-induced angiogenesis in vivo and in vitro. *J Pharmacol Exp Ther.* 299(3), 1073–1085.

't Veer, L. J., Dai, H., van de Vijver, M., J., et al. (2002). Gene expression profiling predicts clinical outcome of breast cancer. *Nature.* 415(6871), 530–536.

Vairaktaris, E., Ragos, V., Yapijakis, C., et al. (2006). FGFR-2 and -3 play an important role in initial stages of oral oncogenesis. *Anticancer Res.* 26(6B), 4217–4221.

Wedge, S. R., Ogilvie, D., J., Dukes, M., et al. (2002). ZD6474 inhibits vascular endothelial growth factor signaling, angiogenesis, and tumor growth following oral administration. *Cancer Res.* 62(16), 4645–4655.

Wedge, S. R., Kendrew, J., Hennequin, L. F., et al. (2005). AZD2171: a highly potent, orally bioavailable, vascular endothelial growth factor receptor-2 tyrosine kinase inhibitor for the treatment of cancer. *Cancer Res.* 65(10), 4389–4400.

Willett, C. G., Boucher, Y., Duda, D. G., et al. (2005). Surrogate markers for antiangiogenic therapy and dose-limiting toxicities for bevacizumab with radiation and chemotherapy: continued experience of a Phase I trial in rectal cancer patients. *J Clin Oncol.* 23(31), 8136–8139.

Witte, L., Hicklin, D. J., Zhu, Z., et al. (1998). Monoclonal antibodies targeting the VEGF receptor-2 (Flk1/KDR) as an anti-angiogenic therapeutic strategy. *Cancer Metastasis Rev.* 17(2), 155–161.

Zittermann, S. I., and Issekutz, A. C. (2006). Basic fibroblast growth factor (bFGF, FGF-2) potentiates leukocyte recruitment to inflammation by enhancing endothelial adhesion molecule expression. *Am J Pathol.* 168(3), 835–846.

7

STRUCTURE-BASED DESIGN AND CHARACTERIZATION OF AXITINIB

Robert S. Kania

7.1. INTRODUCTION

Although there have been great advances in the detection and treatment of cancer, it remains one of the greatest medical challenges, with the incidence of some malignancies continuing to increase (Jemal et al., 2007). For many tumor types, established treatments such as cytotoxic chemotherapy and radiotherapy provide only transient therapeutic benefits despite severe side effects (Wilhelm et al., 2006). The need for better treatments has stimulated research into therapies targeting the specific pathways that are dysregulated in human cancer. Among the new therapies now available to cancer patients, those that target the process of angiogenesis (the growth of new blood vessels) are some of the most promising (Ferrara et al., 2004; Wilhelm et al., 2006; Cabebe and Wakelee, 2007; Faivre et al., 2007; George, 2007).

Angiogenesis is a complex, multistage process, normally tightly regulated by endogenous proangiogenic and antiangiogenic factors (Bergers and Benjamin, 2003). It involves the secretion of proteases by endothelial cells lining blood vessels, subsequent degradation of the basement membrane, the migration of circulating endothelial cells through the basement membrane to form new vessel sprouts, proliferation and differentiation of endothelial cells to form sprout extensions (which fuse to form loops), and the secretion of growth factors by endothelial cells to attract supporting cells to form a new basement membrane (Bergers and Benjamin, 2003). In the absence of angiogenesis, solid tumor growth is limited by the extent to which oxygen and

Kinase Inhibitor Drugs. Edited by Rongshi Li and Jeffrey A. Stafford
Copyright © 2009 John Wiley & Sons, Inc.

nutrients can diffuse into the tissue. To grow beyond a few millimeters in diameter, tumors recruit a supporting vasculature by stimulating angiogenesis (Folkman, 1971, 1990), which also increases the risk of metastasis (Folkman, 1990). The complex process of tumor angiogenesis is initiated by a change in the balance of proangiogenic and antiangiogenic factors (the "angiogenic switch"): an increase in expression levels of proangiogenic factors and/or downregulation of antiangiogenic factors (Hanahan and Folkman, 1996).

7.1.1. Vascular Endothelial Growth Factor (VEGF) Role in Angiogenesis

The VEGF family of proangiogenic proteins are key regulators of many of the signaling networks contributing to angiogenesis (Hicklin and Ellis, 2005). The VEGF signaling axis regulates both angiogenic and lymphangiogenic processes that occur in normal physiology, including embryogenesis, skeletal growth, wound healing, and female reproductive functioning (Ferrara, 1999; Ferrara et al., 2003; Hicklin and Ellis, 2005). To initiate angiogenesis, proteins of the VEGF family bind as homodimers to specific high-affinity transmembrane receptor tyrosine kinases (RTKs), expressed primarily on endothelial cells: VEGF receptor 1 (VEGFR1 or fms-like tyrosine kinase [Flt]1); VEGFR2 (or kinase-insert domain-containing receptor [KDR]); and VEGFR3 (or Flt4) (Gille et al., 2001; Ferrara et al., 2003). They also interact with nonsignaling coreceptors (neuropilins) that modulate VEGFR signaling (Ferrara et al., 2003). Binding of a VEGF homodimer to a VEGFR results in receptor dimerization and subsequent activation of the intracellular tyrosine kinase through autophosphorylation of the activation loop. Subsequently, the activated VEGF RTK initiates critical intracellular signaling cascades that ultimately promote the proangiogenic phenotype (Ferrara et al., 2003; Faivre et al., 2007). A correlation between VEGF expression and more aggressive disease and/or poor outcomes has been observed in a range of tumor types (Fontanini et al., 1997; Glade-Bender et al., 2003; Takahashi et al., 2003).

The key role of the VEGF family and VEGFRs in tumor angiogenesis has led to considerable interest in this pathway as an attractive target for the treatment of malignancies. As early as the mid-1990s, anti-VEGF monoclonal antibodies were shown to exhibit antitumor activity in mouse xenografts (Kim et al., 1993; Warren et al., 1995; Borgström et al., 1996), and by 2001 a humanized anti-VEGF monoclonal antibody (mAb) had demonstrated early signs of activity in patients with cancer (Gordon et al., 2001; Margolin et al., 2001). The first-studied member of the VEGF family is VEGF-A, which plays a central role in VEGF signaling through its binding to VEGFR2, the primary mediator of angiogenesis in endothelial cells (it also binds to VEGFR1) (Ferrara et al., 2003; Yamazaki and Morita, 2006). For these reasons, VEGF and VEGF-A have been used interchangeably in much of the early literature (Ferrara et al., 2004), but we now understand that other VEGF family members, including VEGF-B, placenta growth factor (PlGF), VEGF-C, VEGF-D, and the exogenous *parapoxvirus* genome-encoded VEGF (VEGF-E), can also play important roles as ligands in the VEGF signaling network (Ferrara et al.,

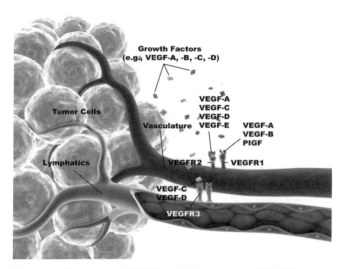

Figure 7.1. Tumor cells express VEGFs, which activate VEGFRs, resulting in the growth of new tumor vasculature and lymphatics. A pan-VEGFR1, 2, and 3 kinase inhibitor approach targets all VEGF signaling in both the vasculature and lymphatics.

2003; Lacal et al., 2005; Yamazaki and Morita, 2006). Unlike VEGF-A, VEGF-B appears to interact only with VEGFR1; signaling through this receptor may play a role in tumor metastasis and has also been shown to support tumor growth in breast cancer cell lines (Ferrara et al., 2003; Kaplan et al., 2005; Wu et al., 2006). PlGF is primarily expressed in the placenta, and also binds only to VEGFR1; it may play a role in pathological angiogenesis (Carmeliet et al., 2001; Yamazaki and Morita, 2006). Both VEGF-B and PlGF have been reported to form heterodimers with VEGF-A (Yamazaki and Morita, 2006). Similarly to VEGF-A, VEGF-C and VEGF-D bind to VEGFR2, but also to VEGFR3, which stimulates lymphangiogenesis and may also contribute to tumor angiogenesis (Mäkinen et al., 2001; Ferrara et al., 2003; Jia et al., 2004; Laakkonen et al., 2007; Tammela et al., 2008). Activation of the VEGF-C/VEGFR3 axis appears to play a role in tumor metastasis, by increasing lymphangiogenesis in and around tumors and enhancing the mobility and invasion capabilities of tumor cells (Su et al., 2007). Blocking the action of VEGF-C has been shown to inhibit the migration of endothelial cells (Jimenez et al., 2005). The binding characteristics and roles of the VEGF family and their receptors are illustrated in Figure 7.1.

7.1.2. Rationale for Targeting VEGFR1, VEGFR2, and VEGFR3 Tyrosine Kinase Activity

Based on the central role of the VEGF signaling axis in the development of malignant disease, we initiated a small-molecule oncology program to target the inhibition of VEGFR1, 2, and 3 kinase activity. This approach to therapeutic intervention, blocking signaling from all three VEGFRs, is expected to have a distinct profile from approaches that aim to neutralize only a subset of VEGFs. The approach targets VEGFRs, which are expressed by normal endothelial cells, whereas, in the disease setting, genetically unstable cancer cells largely control the expression of VEGFs. This difference may have important implications for resistance. The kinase activity of VEGFR1, 2, and 3 can be viewed as the central artery by which multiple growth factors send signals, having the potential consequence for increased scope of effect for blocking kinase activity relative to neutralizing growth factor. The selective blockade of VEGF-A, such as with a mAb (exemplified by the humanized mAb bevacizumab), neutralizes signaling initiated by that growth factor. However, as reviewed earlier, there is a range of identified VEGF growth factor subtypes, all of which play a role in VEGF signaling through the three known VEGFRs. For example, although VEGF-A has been shown to drive much of VEGFR2 signaling, it is clear that it is not the only VEGF ligand for VEGFR2 (Ferrara et al., 2003; Yamazaki and Morita, 2006). Critically, these multiple contributions to VEGF signaling all depend on activation of the tyrosine kinase domain of VEGFRs. Thus regardless of which VEGF or VEGFR is bound, it is this downstream kinase activity that is essential for the initiation of intracellular signaling. As VEGFR1, 2, and 3 have highly conserved ATP-binding catalytic sites in the tyrosine kinase domain (Morabito et al., 2006), a small-molecule inhibitor targeted to this site would likely bind to all three subtypes. Given the central role of VEGFR kinase activity, such a small-molecule pan-VEGFR1, 2, and 3 inhibitor could therefore provide an approach to the complete blockade of VEGF signaling.

In this chapter, we describe the research program, aligned with the above strategy and enabled by structure-based design, that led to the design and characterization of axitinib (AG-013736) (Kania et al., 2001). Axitinib is a potent, selective small-molecule RTK inhibitor of VEGFR1, 2, and 3 that has demonstrated activity against a range of tumor types and shows promise as a novel anticancer agent.

7.2. PROJECT UNDERPINNING

Well-known significant challenges confront research programs targeting kinases for small-molecule drug discovery. The adenine binding portion of the ATP pocket does provide a druggable site for small-molecule inhibitors. However, this site presents obstacles to achieving selectivity, due to the similarity of these binding sites across the kinome (nearly 600 kinases), and to achieving cell potency, due to competitive binding of ATP at high intracellular concentrations. To help rapidly overcome these and other drug discovery challenges, a research program was enabled with structural biology technology to provide atomic-scale insight into inhibitor–protein interactions. The translation of the inhibitor-bound protein structures to meaningful drug optimization was facilitated by drug design strategies that emphasized ligand efficiency and by rigorous assay cascade alignment.

7.2.1. Enabling Structure-Based Design of Novel VEGF RTK Inhibitors

Like other members of the PDGFR family of RTKs, VEGFR2 contains a subdomain, termed the kinase insert domain (KID), that includes docking sites for signal transduction but that is not necessary for catalysis of phosphotransfer from ATP to substrates. As protein constructs containing the large, highly charged KID failed to produce crystals after exhaustive crystallization screening attempts, a construct was designed in which the central 50 residues of the KID were deleted, leaving a loop of 20 residues to mimic the length of the analogous loop in the structure of FGFR1 kinase. The truncated, phosphorylated construct (p-VEGFR2Δ50) crystallized much more readily, producing a structure of the unliganded catalytic domain (McTigue et al., 1999). This structure, which was the first reported structure of VEGFR2 kinase or any member of the PDGFR superfamily, was quickly followed by structures of unphosphorylated kinase (VEGFR2Δ50) complexed with diverse inhibitor leads (Bender et al., 2004). The solved crystal structures of these complexes served to inform and positively influence drug design.

7.2.2. Supporting Assays

A collection of compounds was evaluated in kinase inhibition assays against both full-length protein and the p-VEGFR2Δ50 constructs. The compound structure–activity relationship (SAR) profiles for the two constructs were found to be similar, validating inhibition and structural data arising from p-VEGFR2Δ50. In addition to the phosphorylated kinase p-VEGFR2Δ50, the nonphosphorylated kinase VEGFR2Δ50 was evaluated across compounds. Although SAR was mostly comparable between p-VEGFR2Δ50 and VEGFR2Δ50, for some series, a modest shift to greater potency against VEGFR2Δ50 was observed. However, the shift of SAR was uniform and became understood and predictable based on inhibitor structure type and the corresponding bound protein conformation (see later discussion). Importantly, the SAR generated against the nonphosphorylated form of VEGFR2Δ50 correlated best with IC_{50} results from cellular assays (data not shown). Therefore K_i values were primarily determined using VEGFR2Δ50 and are the reported values throughout this chapter unless otherwise indicated.

A number of readily accessible secondary biochemical assays were utilized to determine selectivity. Early in the drug discovery process, unrelated kinases, such as CHK1 and CDK4, were used to indicate broad-based selectivity. During final optimization, LCK and FGFR1, and finally the closest relatives, PDGFR and cKit, were used to assess selectivity.

In vitro testing in a VEGF-mediated survival assay of human umbilical vein endothelial cells (HUVECs) provided cell-based SAR. Correlation of the

HUVEC IC_{50} values with VEGFR2Δ50 K_i values provided strong validation for the continued use of the VEGFR2Δ50 construct to generate kinase inhibition SAR and the ligand–VEGFR2Δ50 structures to inform the optimization of leads.

7.2.3. Structure-Based Drug Design (SBDD) and Ligand Binding Efficiency

Throughout the program, roughly 50 structures were solved of ligand–protein complexes across three different lead chemical series. A handful of key inhibitor–VEGFR2Δ50 structures proved essential to design highly specific and potent interactions and will be discussed herein. To maximize the chances of delivering compounds that were both potent and likely to exhibit good in vivo performance, ligand binding efficiency was emphasized as a key goal, directing the successful optimization of affinity in a minimalist small-molecule structure. Analysis of SAR, using principles of ligand binding efficiency with respect to molecular weight (MW) and lipophilicity, allowed knowledge to be extracted from inhibitors that were mere fragments of bigger leads, regardless of absolute potency. These principles allowed for optimization of multiple drug properties concurrently. Although the use of simple numerical indices to routinely and quantitatively measure binding efficiency evolved over time, two intuitive and currently used indices are consistently presented throughout this chapter for clarity. A simple index for MW-based ligand efficiency (LE) that approximates free energy of binding per heavy atom (N), based on N ~ MW/14, is presented: LE = $(1.4 \times 14 \times pK_i)$/MW (Andrews et al., 1984; Kuntz et al., 1999; Hopkins et al., 2004). Additionally, the index that reflects lipophilic efficiency (LipE), or the order of magnitude of binding not attributable to nonspecific lipophilic partitioning, is also presented: LipE = pK_i(or pIC_{50}) − log P (Edwards, 2008). A focus on optimization of binding efficiency together with solved structures of ligand–VEGFR2Δ50 complexes and robust SAR resulted in a powerful SBDD approach to discover novel, selective, and potent inhibitors of VEGFR1, 2, and 3 kinases (Bender et al., 2001; Kania et al., 2001).

7.3. LEAD SELECTION: STRUCTURES OF HITS AND OF PROTEINS

Exploratory compound libraries were screened to identify two hit series, the pyrazoles, represented by **1**, and the benzamides, represented by **2** and **3** (Table 7.1). The pyrazole hit **1** is the starting point for drug design efforts that resulted in the discovery of axitinib. The primary reason **1** was selected for optimization was that it had the highest LE compared with other hits. It also presented unique structural features that provided both challenges and opportunities for untapped potential. The core pyrazole ring was presumed, and later confirmed, to bind to the adenine pocket. The two identical styryl substituents produce a long, narrow overall structure made of contiguous sp^2 hybridized carbons, favoring a near-planar geometry, with four rotatable bonds (not counting the

TABLE 7.1. Identified Hit Series from Compound Libraries

Compound	1	2	3 (Optimized)
K_i (μM)	5.1[a]	110[a]	32[a], 4.5
HUVEC IC$_{50}$ (μM)	2.1		0.24
MW	364.4	451.5	378
clog D	4.0	2.1	4.6
LE (K_i/cell)	0.45/0.31	0.30/ND[b]	0.43/0.34
LipE (K_i/cell)	4.3/1.7	4.9/ND	3.7/2.0

[a]Inhibition measured against the phosphorylated construct p-VEGFR2Δ50.
[b]ND, not determined.

terminal methoxy groups). Although the central pyrazole ring can readily tautomerize, equilibrating rapidly to render structural symmetry in solution, it was predicted to make specific H bonds in the adenine pocket to break symmetry. The rotatable bonds can therefore produce up to eight near-planar, low-energy conformations relative to a fixed tautomer, only one of which likely binds the kinase. Structural liabilities, also present in **1**, pointed toward modifications that were needed to make a more drug-like derivative. Specifically, the two phenolic hydroxyls are susceptible to phase II metabolism, the methoxy substituents are liabilities for oxidative demethylation, and electron-rich olefins are potential P450 substrates and possible sites for reactive metabolite formation.

A second series, represented by hit **2** and optimized lead **3**, heavily influenced drug design and is therefore included in this chapter (Bender et al., 2001). The benzamide **2** is a 110 nM inhibitor of p-VEGFR2Δ50 and amenable to rapid synthesis of analogs. Benzamide derivatives, in general, demonstrated high selectivity against a handful of kinases tested (data not shown). Key learning from benzamide derivatives, such as **3**, included the importance of the amide linkage for potency and selectivity, particularly when measured against VEGFR2Δ50 or in the HUVEC. The series also showed a characteristic shift to greater potency when assayed against VEGFR2Δ50 (~8 to 30-fold) relative to p-VEGFR2Δ50. Most importantly, **2** co-crystallized in what was at the time an unprecedented inhibitor-bound kinase conformation. This conformation was immediately recognized as containing an unusual and druggable ligand binding pocket. The literature now documents other kinases (e.g., IGFR, EGFR, cAbl, P38, cKit) that adopt an inactive, auto-inhibited or so-called DFG-out conformation, where the DFG refers to the Asp, Phe, Gly sequence at the beginning of the activation loop (Hubbard et al., 1994; Huse & Kuriyan, 2002; Pargellis et al., 2002; Nagar et al., 2003). Drug successes, such as imatinib and lapatinib, bind to similar inactive conformations (Mol et al., 2004; Wood et al., 2004). However, approximately only 5% of protein kinases have reported DFG-out conformations (Alton and Lunney, 2008).

The two conformations solved for VEGFR2Δ50 are shown in Figure 7.2: ligand-free p-VEGFR2Δ50 in the "open" DFG-in conformation (Figure 7.2A) (McTigue et al., 1999) and the VEGFR2Δ50–**2** complex in the DFG-out conformation (Figure 7.2B) (Bender et al., 2004). Throughout this chapter, graphics of protein–ligand complexes will be provided, viewed from this "standard" frame of reference unless otherwise noted. In Figure 7.2A, the open conformation is labeled to indicate the position of the adenine binding pocket in relation to the commonly known hinge (917–923), catalytic (1024–1030), and activation (1046–1073) loops. For the open conformation in Figure 7.2A, residues 1048–1063 of the activation loop are not modeled due to poorly defined electron density, indicating that this segment is highly dynamic. A small hydrophobic pocket just to the right of the adenine binding pocket is designated with the straightforward label "shallow pocket" to emphasize differentiation from the DFG-out protein conformation. Figure 7.2B shows the

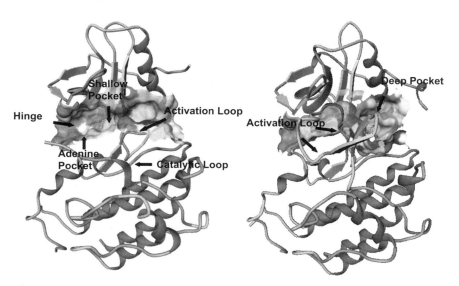

(A) Open Conformation

(B) DFG-Out Conformation

Figure 7.2. Crystal structures of VEGFR2Δ50 are shown in a ribbon diagram of (**A**) unliganded protein in the kinase open conformation, and (**B**) inhibitor **2** bound to the inactive (DFG-out) conformation. The adenine and shallow pockets, labeled in (A), are also present in (B), but covered by the DFG Phe1047 of the rearranged activation loop to form a tunnel in the DFG-out conformation. Protein surface skins are shown to give a sense of shape and size for the two binding sites.

DFG-out conformation where the vast majority of the protein remains in a similar arrangement as is seen in Figure 7.2A. The hinge and catalytic loops remain largely unchanged, as does the position of the adenine binding pocket. However, dramatic rearrangement is seen with the activation loop, for which the entire loop exhibits good electron density in this structure. It has moved over the adenine pocket to occupy the space where the ribose unit and triphosphate chain of ATP would bind, forming a tunnel around **2**. Through its rearrangement, the kinase-conserved DFG motif of the activation loop leaves behind a large "deep pocket" adjacent to, and accessible from, the adenine binding pocket via the tunnel.

The deep pocket that is generated by the DFG-out, autoinhibited conformation has no role to recognize the natural ligand, compared with the "active" conformation ATP site that must recognize a common kinase substrate, ATP, for all kinases. The greater selectivity observed with inhibitors that bind this specific deep pocket, such as the benzamide **2**, is understood in this context since deep pockets across kinases, if they are formed at all, need not function with common molecular recognition.

Phosphorylation of the activation loop is a common regulatory mechanism for destabilizing autoinhibitory conformations (e.g., DGF-out) relative to the active kinase conformations. Deep-pocket inhibitors such as the benzamides (e.g., **3**) must therefore overcome this destabilizing energy barrier to inhibit the phosphorylated kinase, which is consistent with the weaker potency they exhibit against p-VEGFR2Δ50. The potency for DFG-out binders is uniformly greater against VEGFR2Δ50 than against p-VEGFR2Δ50 and is clearly linked to the preferred protein conformation induced by these inhibitors in the bound state.

7.4. DISCOVERY OF THE INDAZOLE SERIES

Two fundamental issues with the pyrazole **1** received priority. The lead exhibited weak potency in HUVEC ($IC_{50} = 2.1\,\mu M$), which may result from lower binding affinity in the cell background and/or low intracellular concentrations due to permeability or efflux issues. The lead also had structural features, if maintained during optimization efforts, which would likely present constant metabolic liability issues. Therefore initial optimization of the pyrazole hit was aimed at three design goals: (1) increase binding affinity to improve cell potency, (2) increase permeability or decrease efflux to improve cell potency, and (3) eliminate several structural features that have inherent metabolic liabilities.

During this initial phase of optimization, co-crystal structures of **1** were not on hand. In the absence of co-crystal structures, models of **1** bound to ligand-free p-VEGFR2Δ50 were used. To optimize for high binding efficiency, two key drug design strategies were pursued that capitalized on the results of these modeling efforts and applied to the permeability and metabolic liability goals as well. The strategy to truncate the lead compound, which systematically removed binding elements from the lead to test for specificity and efficiency of interactions, confirmed structural fragments that exhibited high efficiency and those that did not. The other strategy aimed to introduce conformational constraints to produce rigid analogs of the presumed bound conformations of **1**. Together, these optimization goals and design strategies led to the discovery of indazoles as highly efficient, novel kinase inhibitors (Kania et al., 2001).

7.4.1. Conformational Analysis of Pyrazole 1

One remaining issue figured into the specific design and synthesis of constrained analogs. Tautomerization for **1** results in the facile equilibration of the H-bond donor and acceptor pair, potentially allowing the inhibitor to shift or flip relative to the adenine pocket acceptor–donor–acceptor H-bond triad (Cys919 backbone carbonyl O, NH and Glu917 backbone carbonyl O). Such movement could lead to any of four possible binding modes for new

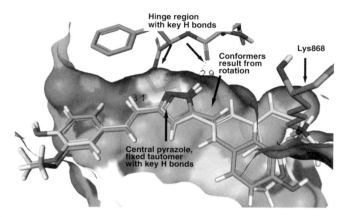

Figure 7.3. Perspective is from the top of the standard viewpoint. Two conformations (one in yellow and one in green) of pyrazole hit **1** are shown modeled into the solved, ligand-free p-VEGFR2Δ50 structure. (See color insert.)

pyrazole derivatives, confounding SAR interpretation. Modeling of **1** into the ligand-free p-VEGFR2Δ50 structure (Figure 7.3) indicated that the preferred tautomer and H bonding was likely to be as shown. However, the styryl substituent could potentially fit into the adenine binding pocket in two conformations (shown), each requiring acceptable side-chain movement of Lys868. To lock the structure into constrained analogs of each of the two putative conformations, a bicyclic indazole core was designed. Utilizing an indazole ring to impose the desired conformational constraint also came with the benefit of a single, energetically preferred tautomer, increasing our confidence that the indazole inhibitor class would exhibit a consistent binding mode orientation.

7.4.2. Indazoles: Constrained and Truncated Pyrazoles

A simplified two-dimensional view of the conformational analysis leading to the constrained indazoles is illustrated in Scheme 7.1. The scheme indicates an equilibrium between solution conformations relative to the rotatable bonds. Rotation about the bond directly attached to the central pyrazole ring gives rise to the two most distinct conformations modeled in Figure 7.3. Both 6- and 7-substituted indazoles **4** and **5** are rigid probe structures that sample the two conformations shown. These probe structures are truncated, partly for synthetic enablement, but they also succeed in removing a significant number of identified metabolic soft spots.

Prepared 7-substituted indazoles and the resulting inhibition data are shown in Table 7.2. Indazole itself has a measurable IC_{50} of ~1 mM. The LE of 0.5 for the stripped-down core served as an early indicator that indazole fits

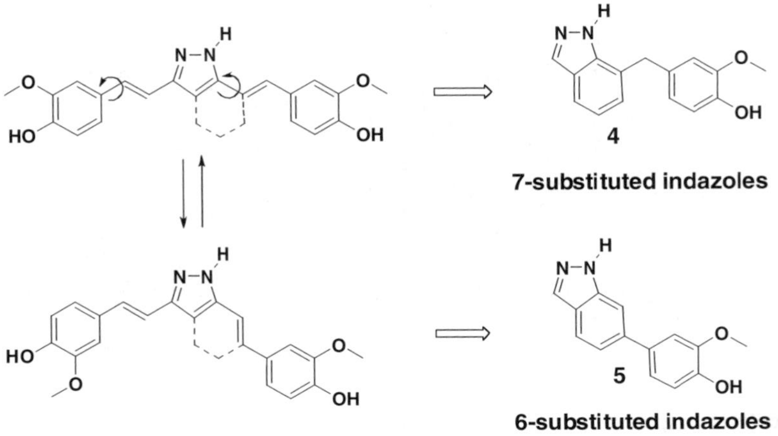

Scheme 7.1. Rationale for 6- and 7-substituted indazoles as probe structures.

TABLE 7.2. 7-Substituted Indazoles Have Poor Efficiencies

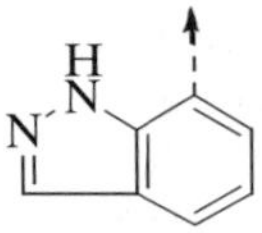	H	I	NO$_2$	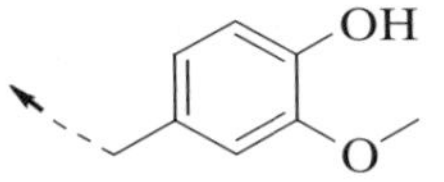	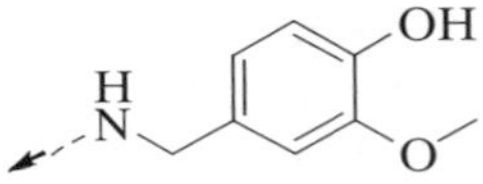
Compound	6	7	8	4	9
VEGFR2Δ50 K_i (μM)	1,000	NI	NI	1,000	476
MW	118			254	269
$c\log D$	1.82			2.78	1.7
LE (K_i)	0.50			0.23	0.24
LipE (K_i)	1.8			0.2	1.6

NI, no inhibition.

well into the binding site and would serve as a good constrained analog of the pyrazole hit **1**. Simple iodo or nitro substitutions in the 7-position result in no measurable inhibition. Analog **4**, which would be expected to mimic the extended styryl conformation shown in Scheme 7.1, resulted in a significant drop in LE relative to **1** and indazole **6**. Taken together, the 7-substituted indazole results did not support the extended bound conformation for **1** and were not attractive leads for further optimization.

In contrast, simple 6-iodo or 6-nitro indazoles demonstrate good LE (Table 7.3). Analog **5**, which simulates the other styryl conformation as depicted in Scheme 7.1, retains high LE comparable to **1**. Additionally, the potency of **12** suggests that the methoxy methyl is not critical, and potentially an area to build selectivity. The phenolic hydroxyl does appear important since capping

TABLE 7.3. 6-Substituted Indazoles Retain High LE Values

Compound	H	I	NO₂	OH/O–	OH/OH	O–/O–
	6	**10**	**11**	**5**	**12**	**13**
VEGFR2Δ50 K_i (µM)	1,000	44	300	2.3	3.0	112
FGF K_i (µM)				16.5		
CHK K_i (µM)				30	7.3	
MW	118	244	163	240	226	254
clog D	1.82	2.85	2.06	2.35	2.18	3.1
LE (K_i)	0.50	0.35	0.42	0.46	0.48	0.30
LipE (K_i)	1.8	1.5	1.5	3.3	3.3	0.9

it as the methyl ether **13** leads to a marked drop in potency. Importantly, the indazole core is shown in its energetically preferred tautomer, fixing the orientation of the H-bond donor and acceptor arrangement relative to the adenine pocket with much greater certainty. The implied orientation explains the importance of the phenol group since these derivatives at the indazole 6-position extend toward the shallow pocket and Lys868, a pocket more demanding of specific interactions than the solvent-exposed region on the other side of the indazole.

Concurrently, 3-substituted indazoles were investigated. Functional groups presumed to be solvent exposed were removed to probe structural feature binding efficiencies. Table 7.4 shows various styryl derivatives in the 3-position of the indazole core. In contrast to the importance of the 4-hydroxyl just discussed for **13** (Table 7.3), neither the 4-hydroxyl nor the 3-methoxy is important to binding for this set of compounds. In fact, the highest LE results from removal of these substituents to give **17**. The conformational constraint and truncation strategies, exemplified by structures in Tables 7.2–7.4, provided important information about the orientation and substitution requirements of the leads while yielding a novel kinase inhibitor core, the indazoles (Kania et al., 2001). Despite the potency findings, none of the truncated indazoles in Tables 7.3 or 7.4 gave measurable inhibition in HUVEC.

Combined learning from compounds **5** and **16** suggested that the composite 3,6-disubstituted indazole, with implicit additivity, would retain high LE and deliver exceptional potency. Accordingly, the full-length indazole **18** was synthesized and shown to be a very potent inhibitor (K_i of 0.3 nM), with high LE and LipE (Table 7.5). Although this also translated well to potent HUVEC activity (IC_{50} = 18 nM), the compound is a nonselective kinase inhibitor. Additionally, this compound demonstrated a poor pharmacokinetic (PK) profile following an oral dose of 50 mg/kg in the mouse (mu), giving an area under the plasma concentration–time curve (AUC mu) of only 0.3 μg·h/mL.

Co-crystallization of **18** with VEGFR2Δ50 allowed the first indazole-bound VEGFR2Δ50 structure to be solved (Figure 7.4). The inhibitor binds to the open conformation of the protein, similar to the ligand-free structure. The orientation and H-bond pattern is as expected, with the Lys868 moving relative to ligand-free structure to accommodate and interact with the phenolic hydroxyl of **18**, which also H-bonds to Glu885. A methoxy group of **18** (R_2 in Table 7.5) points toward the back right of the shallow pocket in Figure 7.4 and only partially fills the hydrophobic shallow pocket. Based on this co-crystal structure, additional 3,6-substituted indazoles (**19–21**) were designed and their inhibition profiles determined. Specifically, structures with modified R_2 ethers that were targeted to fill the lipophilic shallow pocket are reflected in **19** and **21**. Both R_2 substituents were tolerated, with slight drops in LE, and these analogs did lead to improved selectivity against CHK1. Compound **20** represents the first attempt to replace the remaining styryl group with a bicyclic heterocycle, which was tolerated, but demonstrated equal potency against CHK1.

TABLE 7.4. 3-Substituted Indazoles Retain High LE Values

Compound	14	15	16	17
VEGFR2Δ50 K_i (μM)	14	0.4	0.6	0.2
MW	230	266	280	220
clog D	2.6	3.7	4.3	4.4
LE (K_i)	0.41	0.47	0.44	0.60
LipE (K_i)	2.3	2.7	1.9	2.3

TABLE 7.5. 3,6-Disubstituted Indazoles

Compound	18	19	20	21
R$_1$ =				
R$_2$ =	CH$_3$		CH$_3$	Ph
VEGFR2Δ50 K_i (nM)	0.3	1.4	6.6	2.2
FGF K_i (nM)	27	ND[a]	112	ND
CHK K_i (nM) / fold selectivity	5/15x	78/55x	5/1x	1400/600x
HUVEC IC$_{50}$ (nM)	18	>100	93	>100
MW	402	428	356	418
$c\log D$	4.8	5.5	3.2	6.6
LE (K_i/cell)	0.46/0.38	0.41/ND	0.45/0.39	0.41/ND
LipE (K_i/cell)	4.7/2.9	3.4/ND	5.0/3.8	2.1/ND

[a]ND, not determined.

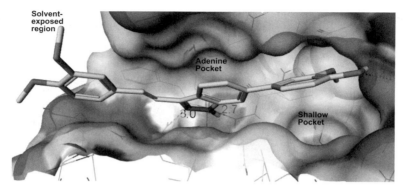

Figure 7.4. The co-crystal structure of the **18**–VEGFR2Δ50 complex reveals that the indazoles bind to the "open" DFG-in conformation of VEGFR2Δ50.

7.5. TARGETING THE DFG-OUT CONFORMATION

Thus far, the two discrete chemical series bind to two distinct protein conformations. The co-crystal structures of indazoles **15** and **18** demonstrated that the indazole series binds to the "open" protein conformation, with molecular recognition of the standard adenine binding pocket. The size and shape of the adenine pockets in the "active" kinase conformations are similar across kinases, providing an explanation for the broad kinase activity observed with these inhibitors. By contrast, compounds such as the benzamide **2**, which has already been discussed to bind the DFG-out conformation, demonstrate inhibition primarily against a subset of DFG-out kinases and are inactive against the majority of kinases. It was concluded that binding the DFG-out conformation, which demonstrated superior kinase selectivity while retaining potent cellular activity in the HUVEC survival assay, would become a target for design within the indazoles chemical class.

7.5.1. Chimera Design to Induce DFG-Out Binding

Toward the design of axitinib, an additional successful strategy to address potency and selectivity goals centered on building structural chimeras from components of separate series. This strategy requires knowledge of the highly efficient ligand–protein interactions across chemical scaffolds. Solved co-crystal structures of ligand–VEGFR2Δ50 complexes revealed the precise relationship of the indazole binding mode to that of the benzamides. This was essential, as structural knowledge was gained from two inhibitor series that bound two significantly different protein conformations to construct a single compound that fully exploits structural features from both series while binding to the favored DFG-out conformation.

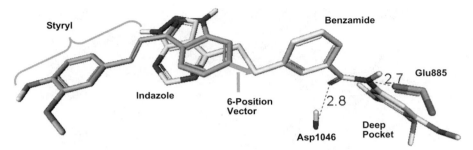

Figure 7.5. From the superimposed co-crystal structures (full protein not shown), indazole **15** (gray) requires a linker atom placed in the 6-position of the indazole to provide the correct extension and bond angle to colocate a ring in the space occupied by the benzamide ring of **2** (white).

Superposition of co-crystal structures of the VEGFR2Δ50–**15** and VEGFR2Δ50–**2** complexes (Figure 7.5) inspired the first application of chimera design to the indazole series, indicating precise three-dimensional placement of key binding elements to induce the DFG-out conformation binding with an indazole.

7.5.2. 6-Linker "Truncated" Indazoles

Each inhibitor has a flat bicyclic heterocycle bound to the adenine pocket that makes two key H bonds to the protein backbone. The styryl group of indazole **15** extends toward solvent on the left of Figure 7.5. However, evaluation of the right side of the inhibitors bound in the crystal structures suggests the benzamide and 6-substituted indazole structural classes, as modified thus far, can only bind their respective protein conformations. The benzamide ring of **2** is the key group that fits to the contours of the DFG-out conformation heading toward the deep pocket. The amide makes two key H bonds in the deep pocket, with Asp1046 backbone NH and Glu885 side chain (only these DFG-out protein atoms are shown for clarity). Conversely, when the full-length indazole **18** is docked to the DFG-out conformation rather than the open conformation, the 6-position aryl group sterically clashes with residues Val848 and Lys868 (not shown). To produce the right pharmacophore to induce and bind the DFG-out conformation from an indazole core, it was hypothesized that an aryl ring from the indazole core must be precisely colocated to overlay with the benzamide ring position observed in the co-crystal structure of **2**–VEGFR2Δ50. Specifically, from the 6-position of the indazole a linker was designed to provide the correct vector, bond angle, and extension, to position an aryl group in the DFG-out-bound benzamide ring space. This design was first tested with highly truncated ligands, which demonstrated comparable LE values to some of the best leads (Table 7.6). The results for

TABLE 7.6. Linkers at 6-Position of Indazoles to Induce DFG-Out

Compound	6	22	23
VEGFR2Δ50 K_i (μM)	1,000	6.6	7.1
MW	118	226	222
$c \log D$	1.82	4.05	2.78
LE	0.50	0.45	0.45
LipE	1.8	1.1	2.4

compounds **22** and **23** supported the hypothesis that indazoles can be designed to induce the DGF-out conformation. Additionally, **22** and **23** were the first examples of high LE compounds that completely lacked phenol and methyl ether functionality, which were viewed as liabilities, as discussed earlier.

7.6. EXTENDED 6-LINKER INDAZOLES: CAPTURING ALL EFFICIENT INTERACTIONS

To capture previously identified inhibitor interactions, styryl substituents were added to the 3-indazole position for both the 6-oxygen linked (**24**) and 6-sulfur linked (**25**) indazoles. The results are shown in Table 7.7. Absolute potency exhibited by **24** and **25** is weaker compared with the full-length indazole **18**, but the biochemical and cellular LE values are similar. In addition to maintaining the high LE, the new compounds delivered on two main design goals. These compounds showed signs of greater kinase selectivity and lacked the metabolically susceptible phenolic hydroxyl and methoxy groups.

Importantly, however, the LipE derived from either the K_i or cell IC_{50} has fallen. The removal of these polar metabolic soft spots came at a price of higher lipophilicity. Despite the low LipE and absolute potencies of **24** and **25**, a key strategic decision was made to focus all further optimization efforts on the new "6-linker" indazole series. This decision followed a key design breakthrough within the indazole series. A solved co-crystal structure of **25**–VEGFR2Δ50 confirmed that the linker strategy succeeded to induce the DFG-out kinase conformation (see Figure 7.6). This achievement allowed for clear and complete structural overlays between the indazoles and the benzamides, paving the way for additional chimera design. The benzamide SAR provided clear evidence that **25** possessed untapped potential in the form of unexploited interactions and pointed the way toward specific binding elements.

TABLE 7.7. Full-Length 6-Linker Indazoles Compared with 18

Compound	18	24	25
VEGFR2Δ50 K_i (nM)	0.3	34	17
FGF K_i (nM)	27	42	ND
CHK K_i (nM)	5	3,200	>10,000
HUVEC IC_{50} (nM)	18	770	280
MW	402	312	328
$c\log D$	4.8	6.4	6.7
LE (K_i/cell)	0.46/0.38	0.47/0.38	0.46/0.39
LipE (K_i/cell)	4.7/2.9	1.1/−0.3	1.1/−0.1

7.7. DEEP-POCKET BINDERS: ADDITION OF AN AMIDE FUNCTIONAL GROUP

The solved structure of **25** bound to VEGFR2Δ50 provides insight into how the indazole series induced the DFG-out conformation with good efficiency. The inhibitor rests in a tunnel that has formed along the adenine binding site, bordered on the front face (from standard perspective shown) by Phe1047 of the DFG motif (Figure 7.6). The indazole H-bond donor makes a strong H bond to the hinge backbone amide oxygen of Glu917 and the indazole H-bond acceptor binds to the backbone amide NH of Cys919. The styryl group of **25** fills the narrow tunnel as it extends out toward solvent, as depicted in Figure 7.6. At this solvent interface, a key crystallographic water (b-factor = 27) is highlighted in close contact with the inhibitor and engaged in an H bond to the backbone carbonyl oxygen of Leu840. At the indazole 6-position, the sulfur-linked phenyl (S-phenyl) occupies an extended shallow pocket, which opens at the far end of the tunnel into the deep pocket. A second key crystallographic water is highlighted just to the right of the inhibitor in close proximity to the S-phenyl group. This water forms a H bond to the backbone NH of Asp1046. These highlighted waters on either side of **25**, and the interactions they make, were useful guides to SBDD.

With a HUVEC IC_{50} = 280 nM, the primary drug design goal for indazole **25** was to increase cell potency. Additionally, the increased lipophilicity of **25**, resulting from removal of offending structural elements, worsened issues such

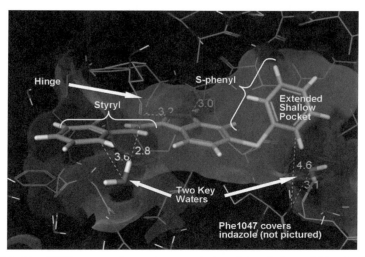

Figure 7.6. The DFG-out conformation was induced by design within the indazole series. The indazole **25** binds tightly in a tunnel. The protein in the foreground has been removed for clarity. To the left is solvent and to the lower right is a deep pocket generated by the rearrangement of the DFG loop. On each side of the ligand is highlighted a key crystallographic water. (See color insert.)

as poor solubility and metabolic stability. The aim was to introduce targeted polar groups into the structure to maintain or enhance binding, but lower lipophilicity. The structure of 25–VEGFR2Δ50 and the highlighted waters in particular pointed toward areas where such polar interactions might be made.

Additional guidance came from an overlay of structures. The inhibitors from the superimposed co-crystal structures of 25 and 2, along with the H-bonding groups from Glu885 and Asp1046 of VEGFR2Δ50, are shown in Figure 7.7. Although there are regions of good inhibitor overlap, there are also significant regions where the two series have unique ligand–protein interactions.

The structure 2 extends further toward the right than does 25, into the deep pocket. The carboxamide oxygen of 2 forms a good H bond with the NH backbone of Asp1046 similar to the H bond formed by water that was highlighted earlier for the 25–VEGFR2Δ50 complex. The amide NH of 2 forms a strong H bond to the side-chain carboxylate oxygen of Glu885. The SAR knowledge generated from the benzamide series (e.g., 2) established that the polar amide functionality was a critical binding element that produced high levels of cell potency and selectivity. The position and vector of this critical amide in 2 suggested modification of 25 with a similar carboxamide attached in the ortho position of the 6-S-phenyl substituent to make these important H-bond contacts and displace the key structural water.

The amide and vector modeled from 25 in this design had close three-dimensional overlap with 2, supporting the expected additivity of the SAR from one series to the other. To select the specific amide substituents to install, the known benzamides SAR was reviewed, which suggested rather large deep-pocket groups would provide inhibitors with high potency. Accordingly, the first two deep-pocket derivatives built into this new design corresponded to the most potent head groups from the benzamides, the methylquinoline in 26 and the 4-(piperazin-1-yl)-3-(trifluoromethyl)-phenyl in 27 (Table 7.8).

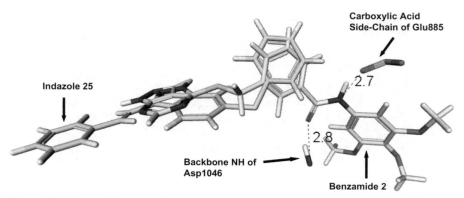

Figure 7.7. From their respective VEGFR2Δ50 bound co-crystal structures, the overlay of benzamide 2 shows clearly that the indazole 25 needs additional functionality (amide) from a specific vector (ortho-position of S-phenyl) to make the two key H bonds to Asp1046 and Glu885.

TABLE 7.8 Deep-Pocket Carboxamides from Chimera Design

Compound	25	26	27
R	H	(2-methylquinolin-6-yl)	(3-CF$_3$-4-piperazinylphenyl)
VEGFR2Δ50 K_i (nM)	17	0.22	72% @ 50 nM
FGF % inhibition at 1 μM	ND	74%	
CHK K_i (nM)	>10,000		
HUVEC IC$_{50}$ (nM)	280	4.5	79
MW	328	512	599
clog P	6.7	7.6	7.5
LE (K_i/cell)	0.46/0.39	0.37/0.32	ND/0.23
LipE (K_i/cell)	1.1/−0.1	2.1/0.7	ND/−0.4

ND, not determined.

Although **26** had impressive absolute biochemical potency (K_i = 0.22 nM) and selectivity, the LE slipped compared with non-amide **25**. It should be noted that accuracy in the standard biochemical assay was limited at these potencies. To support optimization efforts, a shift toward use of HUVEC IC_{50} values was needed. Fortunately, for these deep-pocket inhibitors, the high degree of kinase selectivity gave confidence that HUVEC IC_{50} values were attributable to selective VEGFR kinase inhibition. The cell potencies were confirmed with a number of compounds, including axitinib, in an ELISA-based assay of phospho-VEGFR2 in porcine aorta endothelial (PAE) cells. This validation permitted optimization based on HUVEC data for nanomolar and subnano-molar potencies. In the case of **26** and **27**, the HUVEC IC_{50} supported the conclusions drawn from the biochemical K_i, confirming a drop in efficiencies relative to **25**.

7.8. REFINEMENT AND CHARACTERIZATION OF THE DEEP-POCKET BINDER AXITINIB

To examine the optimization opportunities for the styryl substituent on the solvent-exposed side of the adenine pocket, the co-crystal structure **25**–VEGFR2Δ50 is shown in Figure 7.8A. The inhibitor, residue Phe1047, and the key crystallographic water are displayed in CPK (Corey–Pauling–Koltun) to assess the van der Waals volume. Together, the styryl group and Phe1047 form a hydrophobic pocket that is energetically unfavorable for the water to solvate tightly, as it would require "burying" a H bond. Designs to displace the water or to accommodate the H-bond requirements of the water molecule through appropriate incorporation of an H-bond acceptor on the inhibitor were pursued.

(A) Styryl   **(B) 2-Pyridylvinyl**

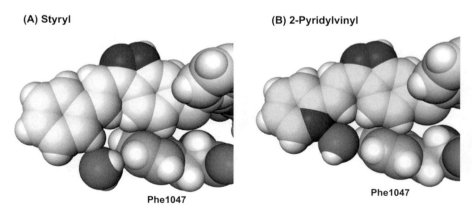

Phe1047   Phe1047

Figure 7.8. Top views of crystal structures compare the (**A**) 3-styryl indazole interactions of **26** with the (**B**) 3-(2-pyridylvinyl) indazole interactions of **28**, demonstrating tighter solvation of the ligand–protein complex for the nitrogen containing analog.

Strategies to displace the water gave compounds with added MW and polar surface area that resulted in undesirable properties. The most elegant design is shown in Figure 7.8B, which replaced the styryl with a 2-pyridylvinyl, featuring a simple N-for-C replacement at the desired location of the inhibitor to give **28**. This design leads to lower $\log P$ and favorable interactions with solvent at the ligand–protein interface. Crystallographically, the water was observed to solvate the **28**–VEGFR2Δ50 composite surface more tightly (Figure 7.8). The benefit to potency for this derivative was readily apparent in HUVEC as a five-fold improvement (IC$_{50}$ = 0.8 nM, Table 7.9). Improvements in both the inhibitor physiochemical and potency attributes contributed to increase the cell-based LE and LipE significantly.

A modeled structure of **26**–VEGFR2Δ50 in the DFG-out conformation in Figure 7.9 illustrates two perspectives into the large, hydrophobic deep pocket. The quinoline ring of **26** fits easily but leaves rather large gaps on the bottom (Figure 7.9A) and the front and back (Figure 7.9B) of the deep pocket. These observations suggested less-than-ideal molecular complementarity of the deep pocket by this rather large and rigid ring system, resulting in poor efficiency. A truncation strategy was targeted for this wide pocket in order to eliminate inefficient binding.

Truncation of the deep-pocket methylquinoline, following the strategy discussed earlier, yielded the phenyl analog **29**, which produced a drop in MW and $c\log P$ while maintaining a similar HUVEC potency (IC$_{50}$ = 0.7 nM) compared with **28**. These improved properties resulted in further increase of cell-based LE and LipE. A more dramatic application of the truncation strategy yielded the methyl analog **30**, axitinib, which resulted from significant truncation of the deep-pocket substituent. Remarkably, this structure also gave an increase in HUVEC potency (IC$_{50}$ = 0.2 nM). The considerable gain in potency and reduction in both MW and $\log P$ produced greatly improved cellular potency efficiencies (LE = 0.49, LipE = 6.4). The outstanding efficiency indices for axitinib are reflected in desirable physiochemical and PK properties. From routine oral PK screening in mice, Table 7.9 reflects the improvements in plasma AUC following a 50 mg/kg dose. Additionally, following 4-hour incubation in rat, dog, and human hepatocytes, the percent axitinib remaining (3%, 43%, and 60%, respectively, average of two runs) indicated species dependence with greatest stability found in human hepatocytes. The in vitro results for axitinib correlated well with in vivo observations, where rat clearance exceeded hepatic blood blow, but dog clearance was moderate to low (15 mL/min/kg), with good bioavailability (71%) and half-life (3.4 h). Additionally, the favorable human in vitro results ultimately translated into a low oral dose in the clinic (5 mg bid starting dose).

Axitinib takes advantage of all the key design elements discussed previously. The core indazole is the constrained analog of the pyrazole in hit **1**, which resulted from efforts to hold the inhibitor rigidly in the bound

TABLE 7.9. Impact of Truncation and Lipophilicity Lowering Strategies

X =	C	N	N	N
Compound	**26**	**28**	**29**	**30 (Axitinib)**
VEGFR2Δ50 K_i (nM)[a]	0.22	0.66	0.28	0.028[b]
Inhibition at 1 μM FGF/LCK	74%/ND[c]	77%/63%	76%/26%	75%/9%
CHK K_i (nM)				>>1,000
HUVEC IC_{50} (nM)[a]	4.5	0.8	0.7[d]	0.2
MW	512	513	448	386
$c \log P$	7.6	6.1	5.1	3.3
LE (K_i/cell)	0.37/0.32	0.35/0.35	0.42/0.40	0.54/0.49
LipE (K_i/cell)	2.1/0.7	3.1/3.0	4.5/4.1	7.3/6.4
AUCmu 50 mg/kg (μg·h/mL)	0.6	4	0.2	19

[a]Due to potency limits in the standard K_i format, HUVEC results are the preferred means of quantifying this level of potency.
[b]Rigorous K_i determination for axitinib (Solowiej et al., 2009).
[c]ND, not determined.
[d]Adjusted from a measured $IC_{50} = 7$ nM in 2.5% BSA conditions to account for protein binding.

(A) Standard View

(B) View from Top

Gap in Back

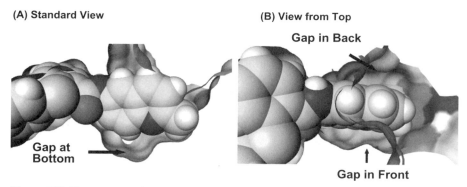

Gap at Bottom

Gap in Front

Figure 7.9. Two perspectives are shown in space-filled CPK models to illustrate how the methylquinoline of **26** does not completely fill the deep pocket.

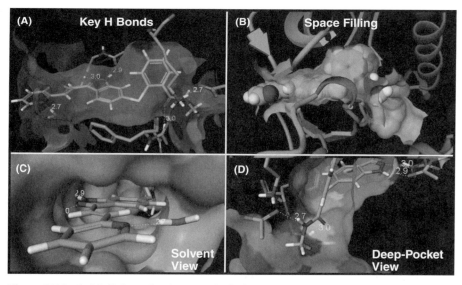

Figure 7.10. Axitinib benefits from each design concept discussed, as can be seen in the four views, to give exceedingly potent inhibition of VEGFR1, 2, and 3 kinases: (**A**) front side view with H bonds highlighted, (**B**) space-filling model demonstrating shape and size complementarity, (**C**) view from left, down the tunnel, and (**D**) view from right, down the tunnel. (See color insert.)

conformation. The indazole core makes two strong H bonds to the hinge region of the protein (Figure 7.10A) and fits the contours of the DFG-out tunnel exquisitely (Figure 7.10B). The vinyl pyridine in axitinib resulted from transformations made to the substituted styryl starting point. The undesired phenolic hydroxyl and methoxy substituents were removed from the terminal phenyl ring, which was then replaced with the more polar

2-pyridyl to allow the ring nitrogen to interact with a crystallographic water (Figure 7.10C). A 6-sulfur-linked phenyl group is incorporated to induce the DFG-out conformation within a series that had not previously bound this important protein conformation. This linker introduction allowed the removal of additional phenolic hydroxyl and methoxy groups found in early lead compounds. Instead, the ortho-substituted carboxamide is installed, following a chimera approach, to make the two key H bonds critical for potency to the DFG-out conformation (Figure 7.10D). And lastly, the highly truncated methyl analog is utilized to leave the oversized deep pocket unfilled, demonstrating the greatest efficiency among amide substituents (Figure 7.10D).

7.9. PRECLINICAL AND CLINICAL DEVELOPMENT OF AXITINIB

Axitinib is a potent and selective inhibitor of all known VEGFRs, critical to the angiogenesis pathway and to tumor growth and development. In preclinical studies, axitinib dose-dependently blocked VEGF-stimulated receptor 1, 2, and 3 autophosphorylation with exceptional kinase-family selectivity measured in cell-based ELISA assays (Table 7.10), leading to the inhibition of endothelial cell proliferation and survival. Evaluation of enzyme inhibition by axitinib across approximately 80 nonfamily protein kinases (Pfizer in-house, Upstate and Dundee panels) showed inhibition ($\geq$60%) of only six protein kinases (Abl, Aurora-2, Arg, AMPK, Axl, and MST2) at $1\,\mu M$ concentration (i.e., approximately 35,000-fold higher concentration than VEGFR2 K_i and 5000-fold higher than PAE ELISA or HUVEC IC_{50} values) and no significant activity in a broad protein kinase screen (Cerep, Seattle, WA). In vivo, axitinib dose-dependently inhibited VEGFR2 phosphorylation in xenograft tumors implanted in mice, as well as VEGF-induced vascular permeability in the skin of mice (Hu-Lowe et al., 2008). The concentration required for the inhibition of in vivo VEGFR2 activity was consistent with that required for in vitro target modulation. Administration of axitinib also resulted in the elimination of endothelial fenestrations and suppression of vascular sprouting in pancreatic islet tumors of RIP-Tag2 transgenic mice (Inai et al., 2004), and led to an overall reduction in tumor vasculature in both RIP-Tag2 tumors and implanted Lewis lung carcinomas (Mancuso et al., 2006).

TABLE 7.10. Cellular Inhibition of Receptor Autophosphorylation by Axitinib

	VEGF			PDGF						
Target	R1	R2	R3	R-α	R-β	KIT	CSF1R	FGFR1	Flt3	RET
IC_{50} (nM)	0.1	0.2	0.1	5.0	1.6	1.7	73	231	>1,000	>1,000

Axitinib has demonstrated antitumor activity in a range of human tumor models, including colon, lung, breast, pancreas, kidney, brain, melanoma, and hematopoietic malignancy (Hu-Lowe et al., 2008). Among other findings, axitinib substantially inhibited spontaneous metastasis of orthotopically implanted human melanoma to the lung and lymph nodes compared with controls in mice (Hu-Lowe et al., 2002). The compound significantly inhibited growth of human breast cancer xenografts in mice and disrupted tumor vasculature, as assessed by dynamic contrast-enhanced (DCE) magnetic resonance imaging (MRI) (Wilmes et al., 2007). In addition to its activity as a single agent, axitinib has also shown antitumor effects when given in combination with other agents in vivo. Combining axitinib with docetaxel in lung and breast cancer models, with carboplatin in an ovarian cancer model, or with gemcitabine in a pancreatic cancer model resulted in enhanced therapeutic benefit compared with the individual agents alone. In a spontaneous metastatic human melanoma model (M24met), coadministration of axitinib and bevacizumab resulted in significantly improved antimetastasis activity compared with either agent alone (Hu-Lowe et al., 2008).

Early clinical studies show that axitinib is absorbed rapidly and demonstrates predictable linear PK, with dose-proportional increases in drug exposure (Rugo et al., 2005). PK/pharmacodynamic analysis indicated that, at clinically relevant levels, the efficacy of axitinib appears to be mainly driven by VEGFR1, 2, and 3 inhibition (Hu-Lowe et al., 2008). In the first study of axitinib in patients with advanced cancer, axitinib showed evidence of clinical activity, with sustained tumor response seen in patients with renal cell cancer as well as adenoid cystic cancer (Rugo et al., 2005). Pharmacodynamic response to axitinib, as measured by DCE MRI, demonstrated a decrease in tumor vascular parameters at this dose (Rugo et al., 2005). Hypertension was the most frequently reported adverse effect; in the majority of cases, this was controlled easily with antihypertensive medication (Rugo et al., 2005). Hypertension has been noted previously with other VEGF-targeted drugs and is expected for this class of agent (Rixe et al., 2007). Further Phase I studies have investigated combining axitinib with paclitaxel and carboplatin in patients with advanced solid tumors (Cohen et al., 2007), or with FOLFOX (oxaliplatin/5-fluorouracil/leucovorin) and bevacizumab in patients with metastatic solid tumors (Abhyankar et al., 2008). Both combinations showed anti-tumor activity and were well tolerated; PK parameters indicated no evidence of an interaction between the constituent agents when administered in combination (Cohen et al., 2007; Abhyankar et al., 2008).

Data from Phase II studies indicates that axitinib, as a single agent, exhibits a broad spectrum of activity against a range of tumor types. Certain tumor types, such as renal cell carcinoma (Rini et al., 2009; Rixe et al., 2007; Dutcher et al., 2008), thyroid cancer (Cohen et al., 2008), and melanoma (Fruehauf et al., 2008), exhibit relatively high objective response rates (ORRs) and prolonged overall survival (OS) with single-agent axitinib; while others, such as non-small-cell lung cancer (Schiller et al., 2009) exhibit a lower ORR but still show evidence of prolonged OS. Continuous dosing with axitinib possesses a safety profile as expected for a VEGFR1, 2, and 3 tyrosine kinase inhibitor that is generally manageable. In patients with cytokine-refractory metastatic renal cell cancer, axitinib showed clinical activity (Rixe et al., 2007). A second Phase II study in patients with metastatic renal cell carcinoma refractory to sorafenib (including subgroups refractory to both sunitinib and sorafenib, or to cytokines and sorafenib) demonstrated that axitinib also has substantial antitumor activity in this population (Rini et al., 2009; Dutcher et al., 2008). In a Phase II study in patients with advanced thyroid cancer refractory to, or unsuitable for, treatment with ^{131}I, axitinib had substantial antitumor effects (Cohen et al., 2008). Pharmacodynamic analysis confirmed its activity as a selective VEGFR inhibitor, with a decrease in levels of soluble VEGFR2 and VEGFR3 from baseline of approximately one-third (Cohen et al., 2008). Encouraging evidence of single-agent antitumor activity has also been observed in a Phase II study of axitinib in patients with advanced non-small-cell lung cancer (Schiller et al., 2009). Axitinib also has single-agent activity in patients with metastatic melanoma, and was shown selectively to decrease blood levels of soluble VEGFR2 and VEGFR3 (compared with soluble KIT) and increase levels of VEGF in this patient population (Fruehauf et al., 2008).

Phase II data have also indicated that axitinib can be safely and effectively combined with other agents in the treatment of cancer. Axitinib combined with docetaxel resulted in a numerical increase in time to progression compared with docetaxel plus placebo in patients with metastatic breast cancer, with a significantly better ORR (Rugo et al., 2007). A significantly longer median time to progression was observed with axitinib plus docetaxel compared with docetaxel plus placebo in patients who had received prior adjuvant chemotherapy (Rugo et al., 2007). The combination regimen had an acceptable safety profile (Rugo et al., 2007). Axitinib was also combined safely with gemcitabine in a Phase II study in patients with advanced pancreatic cancer, and prolonged overall and progression-free survival compared with gemcitabine alone (Spano et al., 2008). The greatest survival benefits were seen in patients with an Eastern Cooperative Oncology Group performance status of 0 or 1, or those with locally advanced disease (Spano et al., 2008). Randomized Phase III clinical studies of axitinib in the treatment of cancer are needed to confirm findings from Phase II studies.

7.10. SUMMARY

A research program was built to design potent, selective, and bioavailable inhibitors of VEGFR1, 2, and 3 kinases. The use of structural biology informed design, which was guided by a strategic focus on maximizing ligand efficiency to achieve drug property goals. A novel VEGFR tyrosine kinase conformation, the DFG-out conformation found with the VEGFR2Δ50 construct, was identified as a key target for small-molecule drug design efforts. To optimize the indazoles, which initially bound only to the open protein conformation, designs deliberately targeted this novel conformation. The approach produced axitinib, a highly efficient ligand that binds the DFG-out conformation, representing the first drug candidate designed to induce such a conformation from a series that had previously bound only the open form. Axitinib is unique among RTK inhibitors in blocking the signaling of VEGFR1, 2, and 3 with exceptionally high potency, subnanomolar HUVEC IC_{50} values, and selectivity. Early clinical data indicate axitinib, as a single agent, exhibits a broad spectrum of activity against a range of tumor types and can be safely and effectively combined with other agents. A Phase III study of axitinib is ongoing in patients with refractory renal cell carcinoma.

ACKNOWLEDGMENTS

The author thanks all the dedicated VEGF project team colleagues: K. Appelt, S. Arthurs, M. Batugo, S. L. Bender, A. Borchardt, J. Braganza, M. Collins, S. Cripps, J. Deal, D. DeLisle, R. Feeley, H. Grettenberger, C. Grove, M. Hallin, D. Hu-Lowe, T. Marrone, M. McTigue, S. Misialek, B. Mroczkowski, B. Murray, M. Niesman, C. Palmer, C. Parast, C. Pinko, D. Rewolinski, D. Romero, S. Sarshar, J. Sarup, D. Shalinsky, G. Stevens, M. Varney, J. Wickersham, E. Wu, H. Zou, and S. Zook. Special thanks to the following for their contributions to the scientific advancements herein and for their help in editing this chapter: S. L. Bender (linker design to induce DFG-out), M. A. McTigue (structural biology), D. Hu-Lowe (nonclinical characterization), and M. P. Edwards (LipE). Editorial assistance was provided by ACUMED® (Tytherington, UK) and funded by Pfizer Inc.

REFERENCES

Abhyankar, V. V., Sharma, S., Trowbridge, R. C., et al. (**2008**). Axitinib (AG-013736) in combination with FOLFOX and bevacizumab in patients with metastatic solid tumors: a Phase I study. *J Clin Oncol.* 26(18S), 206s.

Alton, G. R., and Lunney, E. A. (**2008**). Targeting the unactivated conformations of protein kinases for small molecule drug discovery. *Expert Opin Drug Discov.* 3(6), 595–605.

Andrews, P. R., Craik, D. J., and Martin, J. L. (**1984**). Functional group contributions to drug–receptor interactions. *J Med Chem.* 27(12), 1648–1657.

Bender, S. L., Bhumralkar, D., Collins, M. R., et al. (**2001**). Synthesis of heteroaryl-benzamides and analogs used for inhibiting protein kinases. WO 2001/053274 A1.

Bender, S. L., Kania, R. S., and McTigue, M. A. (**2004**). Crystal structure of human VEGFR2 kinase domain–ligand complexes and use of the atomic coordinates in drug discovery. WO 2004/092217 A1.

Bergers, G., and Benjamin, L. E. (**2003**). Tumorigenesis and the angiogenic switch. *Nat Rev Cancer.* 3(6), 401–410.

Borgström, P., Hillan, K. J., Sriramarao, P., et al. (**1996**). Complete inhibition of angiogenesis and growth of microtumors by anti-vascular endothelial growth factor neutralizing antibody: novel concepts of angiostatic therapy from intravital videomicroscopy. *Cancer Res.* 56(17), 4032–4039.

Cabebe, E., and Wakelee, H. (**2007**). Role of anti-angiogenesis agents in treating NSCLC: focus on bevacizumab and VEGFR tyrosine kinase inhibitors. *Curr Treat Options Oncol.* 8(1), 15–27.

Carmeliet, P., Moons, L., Luttun, A., et al. (**2001**). Synergism between vascular endothelial growth factor and placental growth factor contributes to angiogenesis and plasma extravasation in pathological conditions. *Nat Med.* 7(5), 575–583.

Cohen, E. E., Rosen, L. S., Vokes, E. E., et al. (**2008**). Axitinib is an active treatment for all histologic subtypes of advanced thyroid cancer: results from a Phase II study. *J Clin Oncol.* 26(29), 4708–4713.

Cohen, R. B., Kozloff, M. F., Starr, A., et al. (**2007**). Axitinib (AG-013736; AG) in combination with paclitaxel (P)/carboplatin (C) in patients (pts) with advanced solid tumors. Presented at the *AACR-NCI-EORTC International Conference*, San Francisco, California, October 22–26, Abstract A157.

Dutcher, J. P., Wilding, G., Hudes, G. R., et al. (**2008**). Sequential axitinib (AG-013736) therapy of patients (pts) with metastatic clear cell renal cell cancer (RCC) refractory to sunitinib and sorafenib, cytokines and sorafenib, or sorafenib alone. *J Clin Oncol.* 26(18S), 281s.

Edwards, M. P. (**2008**). Lipophilic efficiency (LipE) as a central concept in optimizing multiple drug properties in parallel. Personal communication.

Faivre, S., Demetri, G., Sargent, W., et al. (**2007**). Molecular basis for sunitinib efficacy and future clinical development. *Nat Rev Drug Discov.* 6(9), 734–745.

Ferrara, N. (**1999**). Role of vascular endothelial growth factor in the regulation of angiogenesis. *Kidney Int.* 56(3), 794–814.

Ferrara, N., Gerber, H. P., and LeCouter, J. (**2003**). The biology of VEGF and its receptors. *Nat Med.* 9(6), 669–676.

Ferrara, N., Hillan, K. J., Gerber, H. P., et al. (**2004**). Discovery and development of bevacizumab, an anti-VEGF antibody for treating cancer. *Nat Rev Drug Discov.* 3(5), 391–400.

Folkman, J. (**1971**). Tumor angiogenesis: therapeutic implications. *N Engl J Med.* 285(21), 1182–1186.

Folkman, J. (**1990**). What is the evidence that tumors are angiogenesis dependent? *J Natl Cancer Inst.* 82(1), 4–6.

Fontanini, G., Vignati, S., Boldrini, L., et al. (**1997**). Vascular endothelial growth factor is associated with neovascularization and influences progression of non-small cell lung carcinoma. *Clin Cancer Res.* 3(6), 861–865.

Fruehauf, J. P., Lutzky, J., McDermott, D. F., et al. (**2008**). Axitinib (AG-013736) in patients with metastatic melanoma: a Phase II study. *J Clin Oncol.* 26(15S), 484s.

George, D. J. (**2007**). Phase 2 studies of sunitinib and AG013736 in patients with cytokine-refractory renal cell carcinoma. *Clin Cancer Res.* 13(2 Pt 2), 753s–757s.

Gille, H., Kowalski, J., Li, B., et al. (**2001**). Analysis of biological effects and signaling properties of Flt-1 (VEGFR-1) and KDR (VEGFR-2). A reassessment using novel receptor-specific vascular endothelial growth factor mutants. *J Biol Chem.* 276(5), 3222–3230.

Glade-Bender, J., Kandel, J. J., and Yamashiro, D. J. (**2003**). VEGF blocking therapy in the treatment of cancer. *Expert Opin Biol Ther.* 3(2), 263–276.

Gordon, M. S., Margolin, K., Talpaz, M., et al. (**2001**). Phase I safety and pharmacokinetic study of recombinant human anti-vascular endothelial growth factor in patients with advanced cancer. *J Clin Oncol.* 19(3), 843–850.

Hanahan, D., and Folkman, J. (**1996**). Patterns and emerging mechanisms of the angiogenic switch during tumorigenesis. *Cell.* 86(3), 353–364.

Hicklin, D. J., and Ellis, L. M. (**2005**). Role of the vascular endothelial growth factor pathway in tumor growth and angiogenesis. *J Clin Oncol.* 23(5), 1011–1027.

Hopkins, A. L., Groom, C. R., and Alex, A. (**2004**). Ligand efficiency: a useful metric for lead selection. *Drug Discov Today.* 9(10), 430–431.

Hubbard, S. R., Wei, L., Ellis, L., and Hendrickson, W. A. (**1994**). Crystal structure of the tyrosine kinase domain of the human insulin receptor. *Nature.* 372, 746–754.

Hu-Lowe, D., Heller, D., Brekken, J., et al. (**2002**). Pharmacological activities of AG013736, a small molecule inhibitor of VEGF/PDGF receptor tyrosine kinases. Presented at the 93rd Annual Meeting of the American Association for Cancer Research, San Francisco, CA, April 6–10, Abstract 5357.

Hu-Lowe, D. D., Zou, H. Y., Grazzini, M. L., et al. (**2008**). Nonclinical anti-angiogenesis and anti-tumor activity of axitinib, an oral, potent, and selective inhibitor of VEGF receptor tyrosine kinases 1, 2, 3. *Clin Cancer Res.* 14(22), 7272–7283.

Huse, M., and Kuriyan, J. (**2002**). The conformational plasticity of protein kinases. *Cell.* 109(3), 275–282.

Inai, T., Mancuso, M., Hashizume, H., et al. (**2004**). Inhibition of vascular endothelial growth factor (VEGF) signaling in cancer causes loss of endothelial fenestrations, regression of tumor vessels, and appearance of basement membrane ghosts. *Am J Pathol.* 165(1), 35–52.

Jemal, A., Siegel, R., Ward, E., et al. (**2007**). Cancer statistics, 2007. *CA Cancer J Clin.* 57(1), 43–66.

Jia, H., Bagherzadeh, A., Bicknell, R., et al. (**2004**). Vascular endothelial growth factor (VEGF)-D and VEGF-A differentially regulate KDR-mediated signaling and biological function in vascular endothelial cells. *J Biol Chem.* 279(34), 36148–36157.

Jimenez, X., Lu, D., Brennan, L., et al. (**2005**). A recombinant, fully human, bispecific antibody neutralizes the biological activities mediated by both vascular endothelial growth factor receptors 2 and 3. *Mol Cancer Ther.* 4(3), 427–434.

Kania, R. S., Bender, S. L., and Borchardt, A. J. (**2001**). Indazole compounds and pharmaceutical compositions for inhibiting protein kinases, and methods for their use. WO 2001/002369 A2.

Kaplan, R. N., Riba, R. D., Zacharoulis, S., et al. (**2005**). VEGFR1-positive haematopoietic bone marrow progenitors initiate the pre-metastatic niche. *Nature.* 438(7069), 820–827.

Kim, K. J., Li, B., Winer, J., et al. (**1993**). Inhibition of vascular endothelial growth factor-induced angiogenesis suppresses tumour growth in vivo. *Nature.* 362(6423), 841–844.

Kuntz, I. D., Chen, K., Sharp, K. A., et al. (**1999**). The maximal affinity of ligands. *Proc Natl Acad Sci USA.* 96(18), 9997–10002.

Laakkonen, P., Waltari, M., Holopainen, T., et al. (**2007**). Vascular endothelial growth factor receptor 3 is involved in tumor angiogenesis and growth. *Cancer Res.* 67(2), 593–599.

Lacal, P. M., Ruffini, F., Pagani, E., et al. (**2005**). An autocrine loop directed by the vascular endothelial growth factor promotes invasiveness of human melanoma cells. *Int J Oncol.* 27(6), 1625–1632.

Mäkinen, T., Jussila, L., Veikkola, T., et al. (**2001**). Inhibition of lymphangiogenesis with resulting lymphedema in transgenic mice expressing soluble VEGF receptor-3. *Nat Med.* 7(2), 199–205.

Mancuso, M. R., Davis, R., Norberg, S. M., et al. (**2006**). Rapid vascular regrowth in tumors after reversal of VEGF inhibition. *J Clin Invest.* 116(10), 2610–2621.

Margolin, K., Gordon, M. S., Holmgren, E., et al. (**2001**). Phase Ib trial of intravenous recombinant humanized monoclonal antibody to vascular endothelial growth factor in combination with chemotherapy in patients with advanced cancer: pharmacologic and long-term safety data. *J Clin Oncol.* 19(3), 851–856.

McTigue, M. A., Wickersham, J. A., Pinko, C., et al. (**1999**). Crystal structure of the kinase domain of human vascular endothelial growth factor receptor 2: a key enzyme in angiogenesis. *Structure.* 7(3), 319–330.

Mol, C. D., Dougan, D. R., Schneider, T. R., et al. (**2004**). Structural basis for the autoinhibition and STI-571 inhibition of c-Kit tyrosine kinase. *J Biol Chem.* 279(30), 31655–31663.

Morabito, A., De, M. E., Di, M. M., et al. (**2006**). Tyrosine kinase inhibitors of vascular endothelial growth factor receptors in clinical trials: current status and future directions. *Oncologist.* 11(7), 753–764.

Nagar, B., Hantschel, O., Young, M. A., et al. (**2003**). Structural basis for the autoinhibition of c-Abl tyrosine kinase. *Cell.* 112(6), 859–871.

Pargellis, C., Tong, L., Churchill, L., et al. (**2002**). Inhibition of p38 MAP kinase by utilizing a novel allosteric binding site. *Nat Struct Biol.* 9(4), 268–272.

Rini, B., Wilding, G., Hudes, G., et al. (**2009**). Phase II study of axitinib in sorafenib-refractory metastatic renal cell carcinoma. *J Clin Oncol.* In press.

Rixe, O., Bukowski, R. M., Michaelson, M. D., et al. (**2007**). Axitinib treatment in patients with cytokine-refractory metastatic renal-cell cancer: a Phase II study. *Lancet Oncol.* 8(11), 975–984.

Rugo, H. S., Herbst, R. S., Liu, G., et al. (**2005**). Phase I trial of the oral antiangiogenesis agent AG-013736 in patients with advanced solid tumors: pharmacokinetic and clinical results. *J Clin Oncol.* 23(24), 5474–5483.

Rugo, H. S., Stopeck, A., Joy, A. A., et al. (**2007**). A randomized, double-blind Phase II study of the oral tyrosine kinase inhibitor (TKI) axitinib (AG-013736) in combination with docetaxel (DOC) compared to DOC plus placebo (PL) in metastatic breast cancer (MBC). *J Clin Oncol.* 25(18S), 32s.

Schiller, J. H., Larson, T., Ou, S. H. I., et al. (**2009**). Efficacy and safety of axitinib in patients with advanced non–small-cell lung cancer: results from a Phase II study. *J Clin Oncol.* In press.

Solowiej, J., Bergqvist, S., McTigue, M. A., et al. (**2009**). Characterizing the effects of the juxtamembrane domain on VEGFR2 enzymatic activity, autophosphorylation, and inhibition by axitinib. *Biochemistry*. In press.

Spano, J.-P., Chodkiewicz, C., Maurel, J., et al. (**2008**). Efficacy of gemcitabine plus axitinib compared with gemcitabine alone in patients with advanced pancreatic cancer: an open-label randomised Phase II study. *Lancet*. 371(9630), 2101–2108.

Su, J. L., Yen, C. J., Chen, P. S., et al. (**2007**). The role of the VEGF-C/VEGFR-3 axis in cancer progression. *Br J Cancer*. 96(4), 541–545.

Takahashi, R., Tanaka, S., Kitadai, Y., et al. (**2003**). Expression of vascular endothelial growth factor and angiogenesis in gastrointestinal stromal tumor of the stomach. *Oncology*. 64(3), 266–274.

Tammela, T., Zarkada, G., Wallgard, E., et al. (**2008**). Blocking VEGFR-3 suppresses angiogenic sprouting and vascular network formation. *Nature*. doi:10.1038/nature07083.

Warren, R. S., Yuan, H., Matli, M. R., et al. (**1995**). Regulation by vascular endothelial growth factor of human colon cancer tumorigenesis in a mouse model of experimental liver metastasis. *J Clin Invest*. 95(4), 1789–1797.

Wilhelm, S., Carter, C., Lynch, M., et al. (**2006**). Discovery and development of sorafenib: a multikinase inhibitor for treating cancer. *Nat Rev Drug Discov*. 5(10), 835–844.

Wilmes, L. J., Pallavicini, M. G., Fleming, L. M., et al. (**2007**). AG-013736, a novel inhibitor of VEGF receptor tyrosine kinases, inhibits breast cancer growth and decreases vascular permeability as detected by dynamic contrast-enhanced magnetic resonance imaging. *Magn Reson Imaging*. 25(3), 319–327.

Wood, E. R., Truesdale, A. T., McDonald, O. B., et al. (**2004**). A unique structure for epidermal growth factor receptor bound to GW572016 (lapatinib): relationships among protein conformation, inhibitor off-rate, and receptor activity in tumor cells. *Cancer Res*. 64(2), 6652–6659.

Wu, Y., Hooper, A. T., Zhong, Z., et al. (**2006**). The vascular endothelial growth factor receptor (VEGFR-1) supports growth and survival of human breast carcinoma. *Int J Cancer*. 119(7), 1519–1529.

Yamazaki, Y., and Morita, T. (**2006**). Molecular and functional diversity of vascular endothelial growth factors. *Mol Divers*. 10(4), 515–527.

PART II

GROWTH FACTOR INHIBITORS: MEK INHIBITORS

8

ROAD TO PD0325901 AND BEYOND: THE MEK INHIBITOR QUEST

JUDITH S. SEBOLT-LEOPOLD AND ALEXANDER J. BRIDGES

8.1. INTRODUCTION

A large proportion of human cancers display dysregulated RAS signaling. It is therefore not surprising that the RAS/RAF/MEK/ERK signaling module (Figure 8.1) continues to be the subject of intense investigation for its amenability to pharmacological intervention. The development of agents targeting this pathway has focused largely on the development of small-molecule inhibitors of enzyme function. The reader is referred elsewhere for comprehensive reviews on the subject of various therapeutic approaches and the complexity of pleiotropic signaling through the RAS–ERK pathway (Downward, 2003; Sebolt-Leopold and Herrera, 2004; Roberts and Der, 2007; Sebolt-Leopold, 2008). This review will chronicle the history of MEK inhibitor research and development that began at Parke–Davis in the 1990s with some updating of other programs to the present. We will discuss the lessons learned from CI-1040, the first MEK inhibitor to undergo clinical evaluation, and how this agent has led to a multitude of structurally related analogs with improved target potency. PD0325901 will be discussed as a prototype member of this new generation of highly selective and highly potent MEK-targeted agents. Looking forward, the easy part is now behind us as there is no longer the need for further improvements in potency. The playing field now shifts to questions on how best to use them. Optimization of clinical activity in light of genetic heterogeneity within patient populations is one of the many current challenges that we now face with PD0325901 and MEK inhibitors in general.

Kinase Inhibitor Drugs. Edited by Rongshi Li and Jeffrey A. Stafford
Copyright © 2009 John Wiley & Sons, Inc.

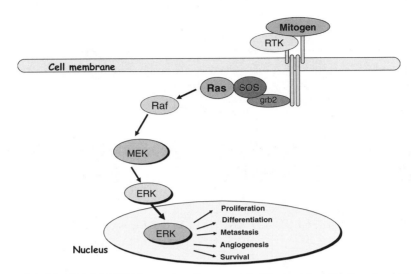

Figure 8.1. The RAS-MAP kinase signaling cascade. Upstream activation through cell surface receptor tyrosine kinases (RTKs) and/or protooncogene products triggers activation of the intracellular MAP kinase signaling cascade. Downstream activation of protein kinases and transcription factors sets the stage for pleiotropic cellular responses including effects on cell growth and survival.

8.2. GENESIS OF THE MEK INHIBITOR PROGRAM AT PARKE–DAVIS

In the early 1990s, three disparate strands came together to forge our MEK inhibitor program. First, the company had a long history of ensuring that it had a complete library of all of its chemical compounds, with the result that by 1992, we had available to us a library of 150,000 individual compounds, the vast majority of which were pure, stable chemical entities in compound space known to be biologically active. Second, Alan Saltiel joined the company to establish a department of signal transduction biology that would be heavily involved in diabetes research. Very soon after the discovery of MAP kinase, his laboratory reported that this kinase was phosphorylated after cells were stimulated with insulin. It soon became obvious that the kinase that activated MAPK, originally MAP kinase kinase (MAPKK), was a very unusual kinase, as it phosphorylated MAPK on both threonine and tyrosine in a unique TEY motif. This was the first example of a true dual specificity kinase, which oddly enough was also the most substrate-specific kinase known. Therefore MAPKK was the subject of considerable intellectual interest and Alan commissioned a postdoctoral scientist, Long Pang, with the assignment of designing a cascade assay involving both MAPKK and MAPK. The assay that he designed utilized phosphorylated myelin basic protein as a readout and could easily be deconvoluted to distinguish MEK from ERK hits. The last thread was the oncology group, which was switching from DNA targeting to signal transduction approaches. With the EGFR program underway, this group had a strong interest in kinase targets. The staurosporins demonstrated that very potent ATP-competitive kinase inhibitors existed for the PKCs. The regular discoveries of new PKC isoforms, as well as unrelated kinases for which staurosporins are very potent inhibitors, reminded one that the selectivity problem would be severe, and probably largely unknowable for the foreseeable future. However, relative ignorance is relative bliss, and at the end of 1992, MAPK appeared to be *the* vital mediator of cellular proliferation, which by unknown effectors was acting downstream of both EGFR and RAS. Over the next few years, the pathway came to be better understood, with MAPK becoming ERK, MAPKK becoming MEK, and additional MAP kinase pathways also emerging. Luckily, when the p38 and jun kinase pathways turned up, the ERK pathway was deemed the critical one with respect to proliferative signaling in tumor cells. By that time, based on mutual interest in ERK by both the oncology and diabetes groups, mass screening for ERK inhibitors, led by the stellar efforts of Jim Fergus and Jim Marks, was now underway. By the very nature of the cascade assay, MEK screening was coming along for the ride.

Initial triaging of screening hits was influenced by our experience in the EGFR program. Anything that contained a thiol (about 30% of the more potent hits) or looked as though it might be an alkylating moiety was immediately discarded. Also discarded were certain classes of compounds that tended to show up in every mass screen, compounds that years later were shown by others to be protein aggregators. Remaining after triage was a pool of roughly two dozen hits, mainly familiar-looking compounds, including several potent staurosporinoids inherited from a prior PKC program carried out at Goedecke. In these early days, we were intrigued by the 100 nM potency of these hits but were faced with the selectivity dilemma. How best to show selectivity was a problem in itself. In the EGFR program, we could get a crude idea of selectivity relative to other receptor tyrosine kinases and their downstream kinases simply by comparing EGF to other different growth factors to stimulate proliferation cascades. With MEK/ERK targeting, no parallel selectivity experiments came to mind at that time and we were at an impasse.

A mixture of careful observation and serendipity came to our rescue before we were lured down the primrose path of the staurosporins. David Dudley determined that the majority of our hits were ERK inhibitors and ATP competitive, a result that was not surprising. However, three hits (Figure 8.2)— PD0098059 (**1**), PD0045443 (**2**), and PD0059563 (**3**)—which were all of the structural outliers in the hit set, were inhibitors of MEK and were not ATP or ERK competitive! With this pivotal discovery, our MEK inhibitor program was born, as we reasoned that we had found an allosteric site on MEK, which had a much larger probability of being unique than did any part of the highly conserved ATP-binding domain. By exploiting such a site, we maximized our

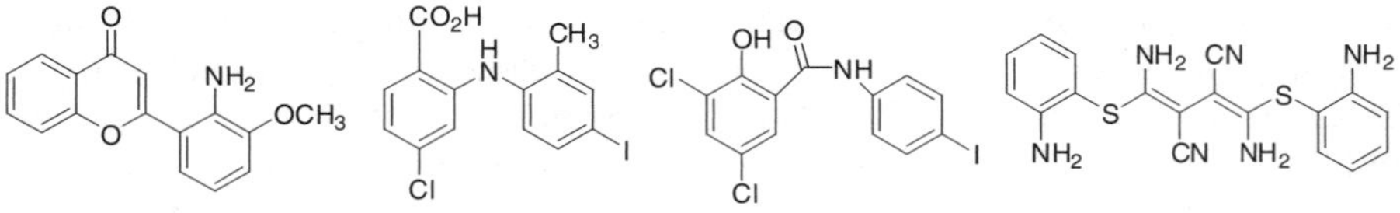

Figure 8.2. Parke–Davis MEK screening hits and U0126.

chances of finding truly selective inhibitors. It was only several years later that we learned that our original MEK screening protein was an intrinsically active truncation mutant rather than a partially phosphorylated form, which, unlike activated phosphoMEK, was susceptible to our original inhibitors. The activity seen in subsequent cellular assays presumably relied on the presence of MEK phosphatases, allowing the enzyme to be trapped by these inhibitors in a dephosphorylated form.

8.3. ROLE OF PD98059 IN TEACHING US THE IMPORTANCE OF THE MAP KINASE PATHWAY

From a chemical viewpoint, none of the leads were anywhere near ideal. PD0098059 is a simple flavone, with a rather weak IC_{50} of 1.3 μM, and has enough known close congeners to preclude there being any likelihood of improving on the potency or of finding patentable space. Furthermore, it is highly insoluble in water and, despite its amine substituent, a solubilizing salt of this compound could not be found. Therefore, although we knew of its remarkable cellular profile with IC_{50} values in the 3–10 μM range, we never bothered to test it in vivo, although others have done so. This compound was rapidly shown to be one of the most selective kinase inhibitors found to date and clearly could be used to explore RAF–MEK–ERK signaling in cells. Publication of the discovery of PD0098059 (Dudley et al., 1995), followed by provision of samples to outside investigators, proved to be greatly beneficial, not only to our development program but also to academia. By the end of 2000, the number of published papers using PD0098059 had exceeded 2000. Consequently, PD0098059 along with SB203580 proved invaluable as tools for mapping the biology around the MAPK cascades. Pivotal studies carried out with PD0098059 showed that MEK inhibition not only impaired prolif-eration but also impacted a diverse array of cellular events, encompassing differentiation, apoptosis, and angiogenesis (Pages et al., 1993; Alessi et al., 1995; Dudley et al., 1995; Pang et al., 1995; Eliceiri et al., 1998; Milanini et al., 1998; Holmstrom et al., 1999; Finlay et al., 2000). Another non-ATP-competitive MEK inhibitor, U0126 (**4**) (Figure 8.2), emerged on the scene shortly after PD0098059 and has also proved to be a useful tool for in vitro studies exploring ERK pathway-mediated signal transduction (Favata et al., 1998).

8.4. STRUCTURE–ACTIVITY RELATIONSHIP (SAR) STUDIES WITH PD0045443

PD0045443 and PD0059563 were clearly structurally related, which suggested that there would be room for SAR development in this area. PD0045443 exhibited a similar IC_{50} to PD0098059, but was only weakly active in cells at $30\,\mu M$. We blamed this lack of potency on permeability barriers, an assumption that was later shown to be correct. PD0059563, however, possessed cellular potency in the submicromolar range. The biologists' hopes were quickly dashed by chemistry colleagues comparing it to powdered obsidian while also pointing to its close relatives in the pesticide patent literature. A depressing in vivo study involving intravenous (IV) administration of a slurry of this compound led to an immediate unanticipated LD_{100} determination and the stark realization that we were down to only one chemical lead, namely, PD0045443. The one piece of encouraging information on this compound was that it belonged to a chemical series that led to Meclomen, an agent that was on the market.

Haile Tecle quickly made an important synthetic breakthrough. He optimized the substrates and conditions for making the chemical core of the molecule with the result that a multiday process with a 30% yield became a single-day process with a 90% yield. For the remainder of the program, formation of the pharmacophore was never problematic, and inhibitors could be assembled at will, even on a multikilogram scale. This breakthrough allowed us to start on a systematic (two-chemist) exploration of the SAR around PD0045443.

One early finding was that the 4-chloro substituent on the anthranilic acid was modestly detrimental to activity. Stephen Barratt then demonstrated that being thorough can be its own reward, because the 4-fluoro analog, PD0169373 (**5**) (Figure 8.3), picked up the vital, but completely unanticipated, H bond at that position, resulting in a 70-fold improvement in potency compared to PD0045443. Soon thereafter, newly synthesized analogs were exhibiting IC_{50} values in the low nanomolar range while retaining their high degree of selectivity. Unfortunately, they also retained a complete lack of cellular activity.

In attempts to mask the acid, carboxylic acid derivatives were explored. These compounds did indeed lead to improvements in cellular potency, but

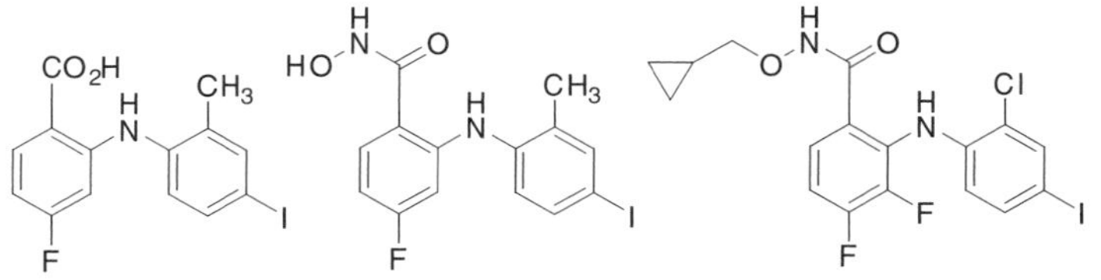

Figure 8.3. Key SAR discoveries leading to CI-1040 (**7**).

unfortunately this came at the expense of reduced enzyme potency. A big SAR breakthrough arrived with the synthesis by Haile Tecle of PD0170611 (**6**) (Figure 8.3), a hydroxamic acid derivative, that exhibited much improved potency compared to PD0169373, as evidenced by an IC_{50} of 7 nM against purified MEK enzyme (2.7-fold improvement) and a cellular IC_{50} of 50 nM when measuring effects on pERK levels (600-fold improvement).

With the emergence of PD0170611, we felt that we now had a MEK inhibitor sufficiently potent to test in vivo and sufficiently soluble to be dosed orally. We turned to the colon 26 (C26) carcinoma model for our early testing. This rapidly growing tumor line, which subsequently became our workhorse in this program, represents a syngeneic model that offers the advantage of revealing potential immunotoxicity. This model was also known to contain a KRAS12V mutation and to constitutively express pERK. The highest dose tested was 200 mg/kg, administered by oral gavage twice a day, with treatment being initiated the day after tumor inoculation. While the outcome revealed modest in vivo activity at the top dose, reflected by tumor growth inhibition of 41% and a growth delay of only 6 days on day 14, we were nonetheless excited with these first hints of in vivo activity from this research program. First, no mice died on treatment, a result that answered one important question; and second, there was a distinct, dose-dependent inhibition of tumor growth. Our validation of MEK as an oncology drug target was moving in the right direction.

Tissue culture studies provided clues on where next to steer the program. While 50 nM PD0170611 elicited a 50% reduction in cellular phosphorylation of ERK after 1 hour, inactivity was observed after 24 h incubation. Cells were not becoming resistant to this compound, as the addition of fresh inhibitor served to depress pERK levels once again. Subsequent time course experiments in cell culture showed that the biological half-life of PD0170611 was approximately 2 h. Up to this time, the project had no input from our PK group. With these data in hand, this group confirmed that rapid metabolism was an issue for PD0170611 by showing that the compound was rapidly converted to a 6:1 mixture of a glucuronide and the parent carboxylic acid. The O-methyl hydroxamate ester was not any better, hinting at N-glucuronidation. Our task was now to find a side chain, which retained potent binding to MEK, while not being a substrate for an unknown UDP-glucuronyl transferase, and at least one unknown hydrolase.

In collaboration with our combinatorial chemistry group, a 5×40 focused array was designed and tested against MEK in the cascade assay. Hits were sequentially triaged after MEK inhibition by testing in KRAS-transformed cells (1 h treatment) followed by cellular testing of active compounds after 24 h treatment. The cyclopropylmethyl hydroxamate esters were the most active compounds in this array and exhibited the best combination of potency and stability. One of them, PD0184352 otherwise referred to as CI-1040 (**7**) (Figure 8.3), would later become the first MEK inhibitor to be tested in humans.

8.5. LESSONS LEARNED FROM CI-1040

From an early stage our oncology programs were strongly dependent on biomarker readouts to give them full intellectual rigor and validation. We were not interested in going down a path that would only add to the literature already replete with studies where one could not distinguish ineffective compounds from inconsequential biological targets. For the MEK program, biomarker assays to measure target modulation were fairly straightforward, as phosphorylated ERK is the product of MEK activity and thus represents a direct measure of MEK inhibition. Therefore, using commercially available antibodies specific for dually phosphorylated ERK1 and ERK2, we reasoned that in vivo evaluation of MEK inhibition could easily be measured in excised samples. Our very first ex vivo study to measure the feasibility of such an approach was also the first in vivo experiment carried out with CI-1040. Specifically, we carried out a pharmacodynamic study aimed at measuring pERK in C26 tumors after oral dosing using relatively high doses of 150 and 300 mg/kg. Tumors were excised at 1 h and 6 h after treatment. Upon learning that ERK phosphorylation was completely inhibited by both doses at both time points, it was hard to distinguish the excitement of the biologists from that of the chemists. We now were in possession of a tool that had the potential to be as useful for in vivo exploration as PD0098059 had been for in vitro studies. The next key question: How would tumors respond to complete pERK suppression?

The scientific leadership of Dick Leopold along with outstanding contributions of Sally Przybranowski taught us the value of having a tumor biology group that viewed mice as miniaturized patients. Before beginning an efficacy study that would answer this question, they carried out an additional pharmacodynamic experiment to address how long pERK was inhibited after a single oral dose of 150 mg/kg. This study taught us that significant activation of the pathway was occurring by 12 h after treatment. By 24 h after dosing, control levels of pERK had been reached. Based on these findings, efficacy studies employed regimens consisting of multiple daily oral doses of CI-1040, generally twice a day (bid). Subsequent efficacy studies carried out with subcutaneous C26 tumors showed that tumor growth was inhibited 53–79% over a wide range of dose levels (48–200 mg/kg per dose). Very importantly, mice did not show any clinical signs of toxicity in these 14 day studies (Sebolt-Leopold et al., 1999).

We went on to more fully characterize CI-1040 by carrying out a number of in vitro and in vivo studies (representative data shown in Figure 8.4). Based on CI-1040's promising preclinical profile that encompassed effects on proliferation, survival, invasion, and angiogenesis, we made the decision to advance this compound into clinical oncology trials.

As CI-1040 represented the first MEK inhibitor to enter the clinic, we approached its development by continuing to fine tune our translational assays. Led by the efforts of Keri Van Becelaere and Roman Herrera, a wide range

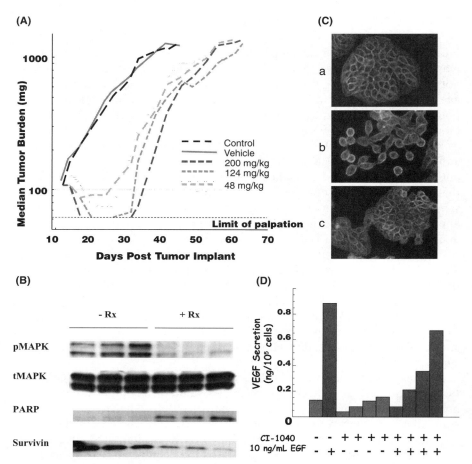

Figure 8.4. Preclinical biological profile of CI-1040. (**A**) Antiproliferative efficacy against BxPC3 human xenografts was measured after oral dosing of CI-1040, administered three times a day at the indicated dose for 14 days. Treatment was initiated on day 13 after tumor implantation. (**B**) Evidence for induction of apoptosis in vivo was obtained in colon 26 tumor-bearing mice that were treated twice daily for 2 days with 150 mg/kg CI-1040. At the end of treatment, ex vivo tumor samples were analyzed by immunoblotting for expression of pMAPK, total MAPK, PARP, and the anti-apoptotic protein survivin. Each lane represents the response of an individual tumor. (**C**) Inhibition of HGF-induced cell scattering in HT-29 cells was measured by F-actin statining (Sebolt-Leopold et al., 1999): (a) control cells, (b) +HGF only, (c) +HGF in addition to 1 μM CI-1040. (**D**) Secretion of VEGF in A431 cells in response to CI-1040 treatment was measured in the presence or absence of EGF stimulation. Concentrations of CI-1040 tested were 5, 0.5, 0.05, and 0.005 μM moving from left to right on the x-axis. (See color insert.)

of assay formats and tissues were studied (Sebolt-Leopold et al., 2003). Several colleagues donated their own skin for punch biopsy analysis of pERK expression, demonstrating their confidence in the project. Our development team, led by Wayne Klohs and Mark Meyer, agreed that we would not recommend continuation of clinical testing if we were unsuccessful in demonstrating translational proof of concept (POC) with this agent. We set the bar for POC rather low at the time and defined it as a result giving $\geq$50% inhibition of pERK in $\geq$25% of evaluable tumor specimens that showed constitutive pERK expression at baseline. In the event that we were unable to secure sufficient biopsy material to make this determination, we developed a surrogate assay that employed PMA-stimulated peripheral blood mononuclear cells (PBMCs).

So what did Phase I clinical trials with CI-1040 teach us? On the positive side, this agent was well tolerated (n = 77 patients) with 98% of the adverse events being of only grade 1 or 2 severity (LoRusso et al., 2005a). The most common toxicities were diarrhea, fatigue, rash, and vomiting. The other encouraging piece of news was the finding that we achieved POC with a mean reduction in pERK levels of 73% observed in ten evaluable biopsies. While we found execution of the PBMC assays to be problematic, including interpatient variation with the degree of ERK activation resulting from PMA stimulation, we learned that plasma levels of CI-1040 > 100 ng/mL generally resulted in >50% reduction of pERK levels in stimulated PBMCs. Importantly, 19 (28%) of the treated patients achieved stable disease of 5.5 months median duration. Most encouraging was a pancreatic cancer patient with a partial response, who remained on therapy for 355 days. The recommended Phase II dose was determined to be 800 mg bid and was more a function of poor absorption at high doses rather than a maximum tolerated dose. Based on these collective findings, we proceeded to Phase II clinical testing in patients with advanced colorectal, breast, non-small-cell lung, or pancreatic cancer. However, clinical activity remained elusive and Phase II trials were terminated, in part because a backup clinical candidate, PD0325901, had entered development, a compound that addressed the pharmaceutical limitations of its predecessor (Rinehart et al., 2004).

8.6. EVOLUTION OF PD0325901

From the time CI-1040 was taken into the clinic, we were looking for a backup compound. We knew that CI-1040 suffered from dose potency issues that stemmed in part from its poor solubility and low bioavailability. What we hadn't anticipated was its exceptionally high propensity for metabolism in patients. Whereas primate testing had shown a threefold higher concentration of the carboxylate metabolite relative to parent compound, the situation was much worse in humans. The high daily dose of 1600 mg administered in Phase II studies was dictated in part by 30-fold higher plasma concentrations of the metabolite compared to parent compound (LoRusso et al., 2005a). Luckily,

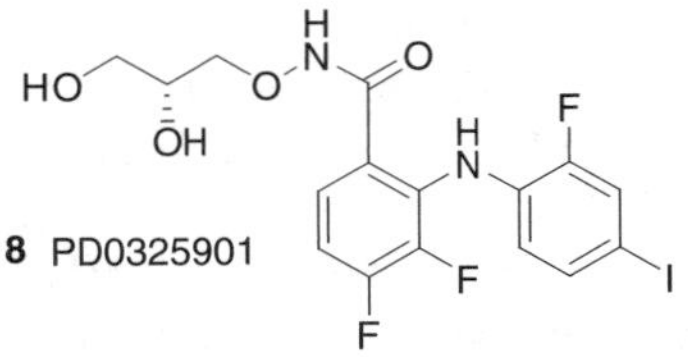

Figure 8.5. Structure of PD0325901.

there were a few clues from our previous SAR studies, which suggested that hydroxyl groups on the side chain might be beneficial. Upon execution of these follow-up studies, conducted by Mike Kaufman, Catie Flamme, and Joe Warmus, we rapidly found ourselves in possession of moderately more potent inhibitors with vastly improved ADME properties. The most potent side chain was shown to be the [R]-2,3-dihydroxypropyl hydroxamate ester. This side chain could be ported with minor modification to the five-membered ring heteroaromatic derivatives (see later section), but found its greatest potency on a minimally modified core structure, thereby giving us PD0325901 (**8**) (Figure 8.5).

Acceleration of our search for a backup compound to CI-1040 was greatly facilitated by our dependence on pharmacodynamic (PD) assays. Using a PD-driven screening approach, we could evaluate a compound within 5 days, whereas the more laborious efficacy-driven approach required 30–60 days per experiment and involved roughly 15–20-fold more mice and compound supply. In addition, without a PD component to the experiment, a negative result is difficult to interpret. Consequently, the MEK program was not comprised of an army of biologists and chemists. It is testimony to the teamwork of lead cellular biologist Heather Valik, pharmacologist Sally Przybranowski, and Haile Tecle's productive group of chemists that we could screen hundreds of newly synthesized compounds in cellular and PD assays in less than a year.

A high point in our program came with the finding that PD0325901 is 100-fold more potent than CI-1040 in whole cells. We then quickly moved to pharmacodynamic and in vivo studies, where we learned that, unlike the case for CI-1040, a maximum tolerated dose (MTD) could be achieved with PD0325901 (25 mg/kg) and that a single oral dose at the MTD inhibited ERK phosphorylation in tumors by >75% as late as 24 h post-treatment. Under the leadership of Ron Merriman, an extensive set of animal studies were then undertaken. Comparative antitumor potency of the two compounds when tested for efficacy in the C26 model revealed a roughly 40-fold difference in doses required to elicit equivalent biological activity. As anticipated, the same broad spectrum activity was observed for PD0325901 as had been observed earlier for CI-1040 when tested against a panel of human tumor xenografts. The comparative biological and biochemical profiles for the two agents are summarized in Table 8.1. Also included here are the comparative pharmaceutical properties of these two compounds. Importantly, the improved target

TABLE 8.1. Comparison of the Biological and Pharmaceutical Properties of PD0325901 and CI-1040

Property	Agent	
	PD0325901	CI-1040
Biochemical activity		
MEK enzyme IC_{50} (nM)[a]	15	18
Cellular IC_{50} (nM)[b]		
Colon 26 (mouse)	0.43	82
Pharmacodynamic activity		
EC_{50} (ng/mL)[c]	16.5	880
EC_{90} (ng/mL)[c]	86	7,900
Ex vivo percentage pERK inhibition[d]	76	14
Antitumor activity[e]		
Total daily dose (mg/kg) producing 70% complete tumor responses	25	900
Tumor growth delay in days at above doses	15.4	12.7
PK profile		
Solubility (μg/mL)	190	<1
Half-life in human liver microsomes (min)	>40	8–15
Oral bioavailability (%) (human)	>30	<5

[a]A cascade assay with raf-1, MEK1, and ERK1 (DELFIA readout) was used to measure enzyme inhibition of MEK1.

[b]Western assays were used to measure MEK inhibition in cultured cells exposed to the indicated compound for 1 hour.

[c]Mice bearing the C26 tumor were treated with various doses of PD0325901 and CI-1040. For the various doses, the plasma concentrations and decreases in tumor pERK levels were determined. From these values, the plasma concentrations required to inhibit ERK phosphorylation by 50% and 90% (EC_{50} and EC_{90}) were calculated.

[d]Tumor-bearing mice were treated orally with PD0325901 at 25 mg/kg and CI-1040 at 300 mg/kg. Twenty-four hours after treatment, tumor levels of pERK were measured by Western blot analysis.

[e]Mice bearing the C26 tumor were treated orally with either PD0325901 or CI-1040 for 14 days. A complete tumor response represents a decrease in tumor mass below the level of detection. The tumor growth delay is the difference in days for the control and treated tumors to reach a specified evaluation size.

potency of PD0325901 was accompanied by improved solubility/bioavailability and metabolic stability. Consequently, the profile of this backup development lead was consistent with its longer-lasting biological effects at significantly reduced doses compared to CI-1040.

However, the development path for PD0325901 incurred bumps along the way, most notably in toxicology. When our toxicologist Alan Brown arrived at a team meeting and announced that we had an interesting compound on our hands, we knew that we were in for a long day. Our 2 week oral dosing studies in rats were showing a severe degree of mineralization of soft tissues and the vasculature at subtherapeutic doses. The findings were consistent with calcium–phosphorus deposition. Over the years we have witnessed lesser toxicities kill many projects. Our team was quite fortunate in having the support of Tim Anderson, who led our Safety Sciences Department, in our desire to pursue additional exploratory toxicology studies in dogs as well as monkeys. We did not observe similar lesions in either of these two species, despite the administration of doses significantly higher than the therapeutic range. Based on further exploratory studies, we concluded that the observed dysregulation of phosphorus and calcium homeostasis was likely due to elevated vitamin D levels in the rat. Consistent with this hypothesis, vitamin D is used as a commercial rodenticide. We then decided to incorporate frequent monitoring of serum calcium and phosphorus in our Phase I trials with the stipulation that we would terminate treatment immediately for any patient showing a perturbation in Ca–P levels. So having gained a better appreciation for the value of toxicology testing in multiple species, our team could now look forward to the initiation of Phase I testing.

Meanwhile, while toxicology studies were underway, we explored the relationship of MEK inhibition to human tumor growth inhibition and plasma drug levels at steady-state conditions in tumor-bearing mice. The models chosen for study are shown in Table 8.2 and had proved to be sensitive in earlier efficacy testing, producing growth delays >10 days in each case. However, the incidence of complete and partial regressions varied substantially, with Colo205 being the most sensitive and HT-29 being the least sensitive. The plasma IC_{50} values of PD0325901 for pERK suppression were measured to serve as pharmacodynamic guide posts in the planned Phase I clinical studies and ranged from approximately 5 to 50 ng/mL. From these studies, it was concluded that maintaining an average steady-state concentration roughly equal to 5 times the IC_{50} would result in near maximal suppression of ERK phosphorylation throughout the dosing interval. Using projected human PK parameter values, a human dose of 1 mg was decided on as the starting dose for

TABLE 8.2. Target Inhibition and In Vivo Antitumor Activity of PD0325901 in Human Tumor Xenografts[a]

Model	Tumor Type	IC_{50} (ng/mL)	Incidence of CR/PR (out of 10)	T-C (days)
MiaPaCa-2	Pancreatic	5.2	1/0	25.5
Colo205	Colon	11.5	4/5	52.8
BxPC3	Pancreatic	40.9	2/8	18.7
HT-29	Colon	53.5	0/0	16.5

[a]The pharmacokinetic–pharmacodynamic relationship of PD0325901 to inhibit pMAPK in the indicated tumor model was evaluated following single oral dosing over a wide dose range. Plasma and tumor samples were collected at varying time points ranging from 1 to 24 hours after treatment. Plasma concentrations of PD0325901 were measured using LC/MS, and tumor pMAPK was determined by immunoblotting. The indicated IC_{50} value corresponds to the plasma concentration required to inhibit tumor pMAPK by 50%.

clinical testing. A dose of roughly 10–15 mg/day was projected to achieve systemic exposure similar to that observed in our preclinical efficacy models. Compared to a dose of 1600 mg/day previously employed for CI-1040, we now had a MEK inhibitor that truly seemed to have the requisite potency and pharmaceutical properties to test the consequences of MEK inhibition in patients.

Throughout the progression of our MEK program, inhibitors were consistently shown to be highly selective for MEK and noncompetitive with respect to ATP as well as ERK. Successful resolution of the crystal structure of MEK1 and MEK2, which had previously remained elusive, was given a boost with the discovery of PD184352 and explained the basis of its specificity. A talented team of crystallographers and molecular biologists led by the efforts of Jeff Ohren, Chris Whitehead, Amy Delaney, and Patrick McConnell, found that truncation of 61 residues at the N terminus of unphosphorylated MEK facilitated its crystallization based on the predictions derived from previous mutagenesis studies (Delaney et al., 2002). As depicted in Figure 8.6, the three-dimensional structure of human MEK1 and MEK2 bound to a variant of PD184352 revealed the existence of a unique inhibitor-binding pocket,

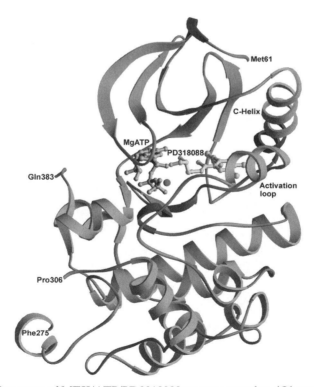

Figure 8.6. Structure of MEK/ATP/PD0318088 ternary complex. (Ohren et al., 2004.) (See color insert.)

rather to our surprise within the catalytic cleft, but adjacent to the MgATP-binding site, thereby explaining how these MEK inhibitors could bind to MEK without preventing the binding of ATP (Ohren et al., 2004). We were just beginning to use the crystal structure for further design work, when, as is the way of our industry, the music stopped.

The crystal structures provided a satisfying explanation for the properties of this family of inhibitors. The first point to note is that the inhibitor-binding site, although also in the interlobal cleft, is adjacent to and does not impinge on the ATP-binding site. Indeed, the best inhibitors, with H-bond donors and acceptors in the amide side chain, may well stabilize the binding of ATP to MEK. Second, this area of the kinase has low sequence homology, with only MEK1 and MEK2 having full sequence identity here, and MKK5, a weakly inhibited kinase, 85% sequence identity. All other kinases have considerably lower homology in this region, explaining the very high selectivity of these inhibitors. The crystal structure shows that the kinase is in a closed form, which is usually associated with catalytic activity, explaining the tight binding. However, several perturbations in the catalytic region, most specifically formation of an α-helix from part of the activation loop, which impinges on the ERK activation loop binding site, and a consequential rotation and displacement of helix C, such that the structurally vital Lys97–Glu114 salt bridge is disrupted, ensure that the conformation is catalytically inactive. Similar activation loop α-helices with displaced C-helices have been seen in a few kinase crystal structures, suggesting that these inhibitors may be stabilizing one of the many natural inactive conformations that these kinases can adopt.

The observed SAR also fits well with the co-complex structure (Figure 8.7). The aniline ring is nearly orthogonal to the anthranilate ring, tightly held in a

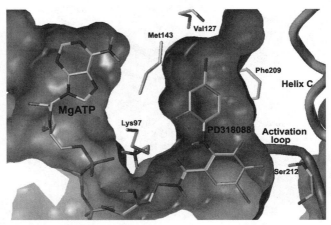

Figure 8.7. Mg-ATP and PD0318088 occupy distinct and adjacent binding sites within the interlobal cleft of MEK kinase. (Ohren et al., 2004.) (See color insert.)

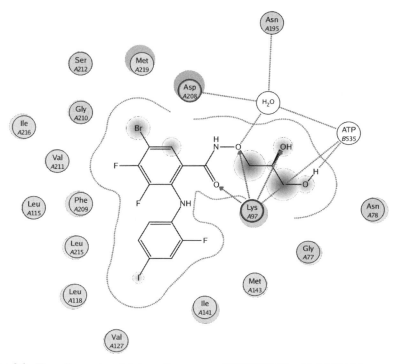

Figure 8.8. Two-dimensional interaction map of PD0318088 with MEK kinase generated from MOE software (Chemical Computing Group, Montreal, QC). Side chain, bound water, and ATP interactions are noted with arrows. Shading represents degree of solvent exposure.

very hydrophobic pocket and making an edge-to-face interaction with Phe209. The iodine atom appears to make a favorable electrostatic interaction with the backbone carbonyl of Val127. The anthranilate phenyl ring is in a somewhat less hydrophobic pocket, and the 4-fluorine atom forms an H bond to the backbone NH of Ser212. The anilide nitrogen and the hydroxamate carbonyl are involved in a six-membered ring H bond and are nearly coplanar. There is some room to build around the 5- and 6-positions of the anthranilate ring, and the hydroxamate does not appear to be involved in any critical interactions, suggesting that it can be replaced with suitably adorned cyclic structures. In addition to its forming multiple polar interactions with Lys97, the hydroxamate side chain hydroxyls come very close to both the magnesium ion and the γ-phosphate of ATP, suggesting that both lone pairs and H-bondable hydrogens may find binding interactions in that very polar region. These interactions are shown schematically in Figure 8.8.

8.7. CLINICAL TRIALS OF PD0325901

Clinical trials with PD0325901 were initiated in 2004. Eligible tumors were restricted to breast, colorectal, and non-small-cell lung cancers, as well as melanomas. It should be pointed out that in the intervening period between clinical testing of CI-1040 and PD0325901, the seminal paper from the Sanger group was published in *Nature*, reporting on the incidence of activating BRAF mutations in human tumors (Davies et al., 2002). Melanomas were reported to show an especially high prevalence of BRAF mutations (nearly 70% in the above publication). Expectations at the time PD0325901 trials were initiated were that a sufficient number of melanoma patients would be accrued to test whether BRAF-mutated tumors would be predisposed toward a better response. Since biopsies were required from all patients, two-thirds of the patients enrolled in this study were in fact melanoma patients, perhaps reflecting the accessibility of tumor tissue in these patients. Early in these clinical trials, we were encouraged by the degree of target inhibition that was consistently being observed in tumor biopsies. Doses as low as 1 mg were resulting in >90% inhibition (LoRusso et al., 2005b). Concentration–time profiles were generated from Phase I testing and were compared to the IC_{50} values previously determined for the tumor xenograft models summarized in Table 8.2. These levels served as minimum threshold targets for PD0325901 plasma concentrations. The first four dose levels tested, 1 mg daily (qd) through 4 mg twice daily (bid), exceeded some or all of the IC_{50} values but only at the C_{max}. The higher dose levels (15, 20, and 30 mg bid) all exceeded the highest of the IC_{50} values, not only at C_{max} but also throughout the 12 hour dosing interval. Importantly, three partial responders (all melanoma patients) provided evidence for the therapeutic potential of PD0325901 (LoRusso et al., 2007).

However, the increased potency of PD0325901 compared to its predecessor CI-1040 was accompanied by increased toxicity concerns. While visual disturbances that took the form of colored spots or halos were observed for both agents, the delayed occurrence of retinal vein occlusions was reported for three patients after 13–38 weeks of therapy (LoRusso et al., 2007). Ocular toxicity of this serious nature was clearly an unwelcome surprise and raised the question of whether this was a target-related adverse event that was a consequence of highly effective ERK pathway suppression.

Alternatively, was this toxicity an off-target effect that would prove to be unique to the PD0325901 chemical template? Would newly emerging MEK inhibitors from other research programs help answer these questions? We will now turn to the chemistry efforts from a multitude of research programs that have continued where PD0325901 left off.

8.8. LEGACY OF PD0325901

Additional SAR development in our program was aimed mainly at protecting the IP around the *N*-arylanthranilate template, with a few representative compounds shown in Figure 8.9. Once we realized that the purpose of the 4-fluorine was to act as a hydrogen-bond acceptor, we were quickly led to the development of several novel series. We learned that almost any way of putting a heteroatom with a lone pair at the 4-position would work. Thus benzimidazoles (**9** and **10**) and pyridones (**11**) formed by the replacement of fluorine with sp^2 hybridized nitrogen and oxygen, respectively, resulted in potent MEK inhibitors. We replaced the hydroxamate with amides (not illustrated), heterocycles as illustrated by oxadiazoles (**10** and **12**), oxysulfonamides (**13**), and cyclized the six-membered ring H bond (**14**). We also replaced the hydroxyl on the side chain with an amine (**12**), and the 4'-iodine atom with propynol, which proved to be the only iodine replacement more potent than bromide, which we found, despite quite extensive searching, largely driven by what proved to be unjustified fears of iodine lability and toxicity.

The rationale that had driven us to adopt MEK as a target proved to be equally persuasive to others, and the clinical data on CI-1040 validated the target, while not exactly providing an intimidating barrier to entry. Lastly, the crystal structure allowed structure-based drug design groups to work out which parts of the molecule could be changed, and by how much, while still retaining the allosteric binding mode of the *N*-arylanthranilamides.

Array BioPharma has provided an exemplary lesson on how ingenious medicinal chemistry can shred the exclusivity dreams of a competitor's patent estate, as laid out in Figure 8.10. They started out with benzimidazoles and heterocyclic replacements for the hydroxamate, very similar to those described previously, of which one, ARRY142886/AZD6244 (**15**), entered clinical trials

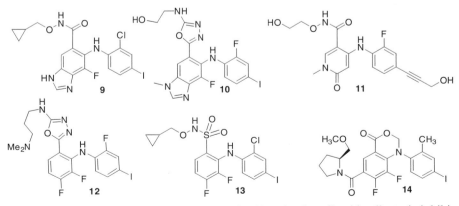

Figure 8.9. Parke–Davis/Pfizer variants on the *N*-arylanthranilamide allosteric inhibitory pharmacophore.

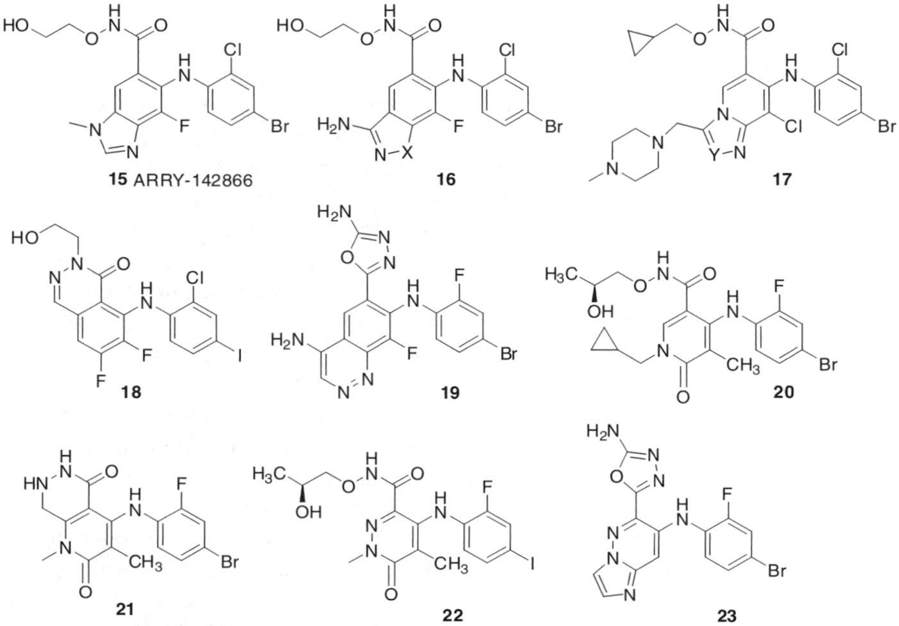

Figure 8.10. Array BioPharma's novel MEK allosteric inhibitor pharmacophores.

in partnership with AstraZeneca (US patent application 2003/0216460). They then went much further and produced many novel variants on the pharmacophore. Substitutions of the benzimidazole by benzisoxazoles (**16**, X=O), pyrazolopyridines (**16**, X=NH), imidazolopyridines (**17**, Y=CH), and triazolopyridines (**17**, Y=N) all appeared in a single patent application (US patent application 2005/0049419). Cyclization of the carboxamide to the 6-position of the anthranilate ring subsequently appeared, with a variety of five- and six-membered ring azaheterocycles involved (US patent application 2005/0130943), exemplified by the phthalazinone (**18**). The 4,5-fused five-membered rings of **15–17** were then expanded to six-membered heteroaromatic rings, containing one or two nitrogen atoms (US patent application 2005/0130976), as exemplified by the cinnoline (**19**). Pyridones, such as **20**, can be used to put in the 4-H-bond acceptor, and this can be combined with the cyclization of the 6-position and carboxamide, to give a variety of 6.6-bicycles containing nitrogen in both rings (US patent application 2005/0250782), exemplified by the pyridopyridazine (**21**). Introduction of a nitrogen atom at the 6-position of the anthranilate ring converted the pyridones (**20**) to pyrazinones (not shown) and pyridazinones, such as **22** (US patent application 2007/0112038), and the benzimidazoles (**15**) to the imidazolopyridazines (**23**) (US patent application 2005/0153942).

As depicted in Figure 8.11, other companies have also expanded the fundamental pharmacophore, in numerous ingenious and patentably distinct

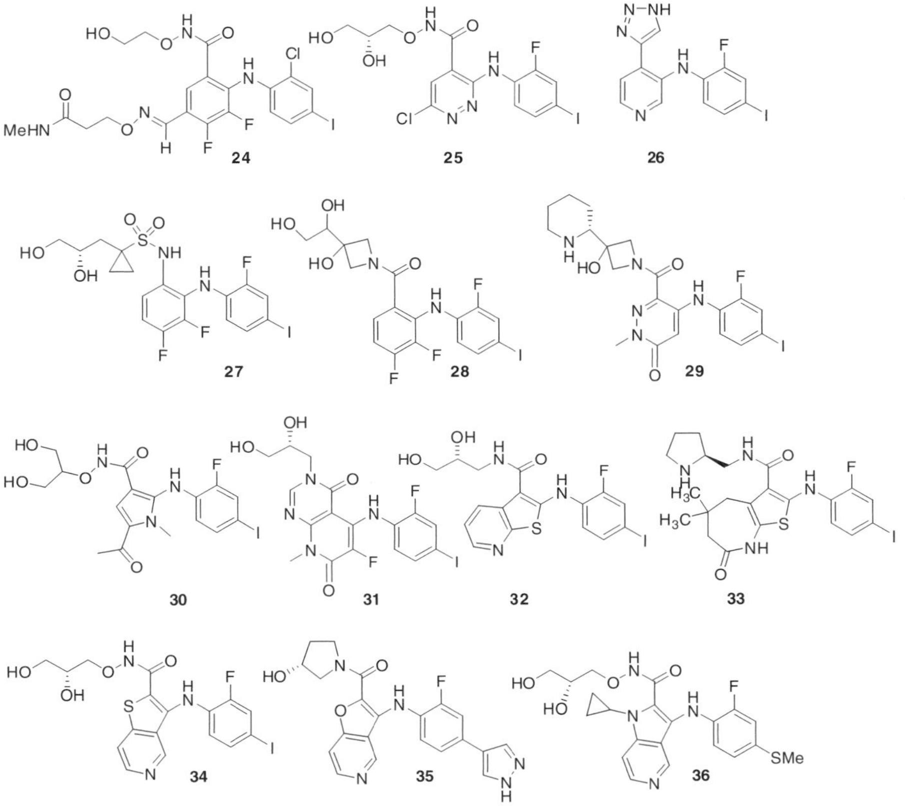

Figure 8.11. Other companies' novel MEK allosteric inhibitor pharmacophores.

ways. Chugai (US patent application 2007/0105859) has introduced novelty
by a 5-aldoxime as illustrated with **24**, whereas Serono (EMD) claimed pyr-
idazines (**25**) (US patent application 2007/0287709) and pyridinyl-1,2,3
-triazoles (**26**) (US patent application 2007/0287737). Another interesting
variant is shown by Ardea (ex-Valeant) exemplified by **27**, an "inverse" sulfonamide (WO2007/014011). Exelixis approached replacement of the hydroxamate with an azetidinyl amide, which is then attached to many of the
aromatics described previously, exemplified by **28** and **29** (WO2007/044515).
Takeda replaced the phenyl ring with either a 5-acetylpyrrole (**30**) or a pyri-
dopyrimidinedione (**31**) in WO2008/055236 and WO2008/079814, respectively.
UCB also replaced the phenyl ring with a five-membered ring heterocycle, a
thiophene, and has described pyridothiophenes (**32**) and many B-ring saturated bicyclic thiophenes, such as the thienoazepinone (**33**) in WO2007/088345
and WO2008/020206, respectively. Genentech has also patented pyridothiophenes (WO2008/024724/5) but managed to reverse the amine and carboxylate functions, as well as placing the pyridyl nitrogen elsewhere (**34**). They
followed on with pyridylfurans and pyrrolopyridines (WO2008/067481),

illustrated by examples where iodine is replaced with a pyrazole (**35**) or a thiomethyl group (**36**).

Some of the compounds encompassed in this condensed review of the patent literature are in active development. The only one with reported clinical trial information is AZD6244, which is reviewed elsewhere in this volume. Returning to the question of whether MEK inhibitors as a class will share the ocular toxicity observed with PD0325901, it is noteworthy that blurred vision was also reported during Phase I evaluation of AZD6244 (Chow et al., 2005; Adjei et al., 2006). However, upon lowering of the dose, this toxicity was not apparent and a maximum tolerated dose of 100 mg administered twice daily was reached. No retinal vein occlusions were reported. However, based on the close structural similarity of this agent to PD0325901 and its reduced potency (nearly one log), it remains difficult to conclude whether the full extent of ocular adverse events have a MEK-related mechanistic basis. The answer to this question may well lie with future clinical evaluation of the new wave of MEK inhibitors that are currently in the development pipeline.

8.9. LOOKING TO THE FUTURE

PD0325901 and the other highly selective and potent MEK inhibitors are now the standard that has come to be expected for agents in this mechanistic class. There does not appear to be any need for further improvement in target potency. We must now shift our attention to ensuring that the potential of these drug candidates in cancer patients is properly evaluated. PD0325901 was the first MEK inhibitor to elicit objective clinical responses in melanoma patients in Phase I evaluation. It is not surprising that all three of these patients harbored either a BRAF or an NRAS mutation (Tan et al., 2007)). The work of Neal Rosen, David Solit, and their team predicted the predisposition of these patients to MEK inhibitor treatment based on their molecularly profiled xenograft studies with PD0325901 (Solit et al., 2006). Despite this, we seem to have entered an era where it is customary to attack the predictive value of preclinical animal models in oncology. In our view, this is either due to a failure to do adequate work to properly understand the animal data in the context of tumor genetics, or a lack of listening to what the science is telling us.

With respect to the failure to trust our preclinical data, a good example is provided by the fact that neither the PD0325901 nor the AZD6244 early trials excluded melanoma patients who were wild type for BRAF and RAS mutational status. Going forward, we must apply the same scientific rigor to selecting our patient population as we generally apply to matching our preclinical models to known target susceptibility. The development of PD0325901 was dealt a serious blow with the observance of ocular toxicities. Many of the newer generation MEK inhibitors hardly penetrate the blood–brain barrier, which may in turn signal decreased retinal penetration. However, a lack of ocular toxicity might also be due to chemotype differences. A completely clean toxicity profile from a signal transduction inhibitor that blocks a pathway as critical as the ERK pathway seems improbable. Rather, anticipation and aggressive management of the observed toxicities will prove critical, both for MEK inhibitors and for all of the other highly potent targeted therapies.

The reader is referred elsewhere for a brief discussion on clinical trial design issues that accompany the development of MEK inhibitors (Sebolt-Leopold, 2008). Clearly, better use of surrogate markers of response, for example, noninvasive PET imaging (Solit et al., 2007), warrants active investigation in future clinical trials, especially in monotherapy settings where cytostasis rather than apoptosis may be detected early in the course of treatment. However, meeting the ultimate challenge of optimizing MEK-targeted therapy against tumors with multiple genetic defects will likely require rational combination strategies. In this regard, the high degree of selectivity shown for PD0325901 and the new generation of MEK inhibitors will be beneficial as we contemplate the design of personalized cocktails carefully tailored to hit choice pathways while minimizing off-target effects. We look forward to watching the clinical science play out, as hopefully, our field starts to practice what is preached when it comes to personalized medicine.

ACKNOWLEDGMENTS

Our attempts to capture the history of the Parke–Davis/Pfizer MEK inhibitor program have focused on key highlights and contributions that we felt to be particularly pertinent to the natural progression of this project. We would like to acknowledge the efforts of the greater MEK team, a truly outstanding group of preclinical and clinical colleagues who enabled the evolution of PD0325901. We especially acknowledge the outstanding contributions of Cho-Ming Loi and Michael Breider.

DEDICATION

This chapter is dedicated to the memory of Han-Mo Koo, a gifted and devoted scientist, whose work will not be forgotten. My life is richer for having known him. [JSL]

REFERENCES

Adjei, A. A., Cohen, R. B., Franklin, W. A., et al. (**2006**). Phase I pharmacokinetic and pharmacodynamic study of the MEK inhibitor AZD6244 (ARRY-142886). Presented at the AACR-NCI-EORTC International Conference on Molecular Targets and Cancer Therapeutics.

Alessi, D. R., Cuenda, A., Cohen, P., et al. (**1995**). PD098059 is a specific inhibitor of the activation of mitogen-activated protein kinase kinase in vitro and in vivo. *J Biol Chem.* 270, 27489–27494.

Chow, L. Q. M., Eckhardt, S. G., Reid, J. M., et al. (**2005**). A first in human dose-range finding study to assess the pharmacokinetics, pharmacodynamics, and toxicities of the MEK inhibitor, ARRY-142886 (AZD6244) in patients with advanced solid malignancies. Presented at the AACR-NCI-EORTC International Conference on Molecular Targets and Cancer Therapeutics.

Davies, H., Bignell, G. R., Cox, C., et al. (**2002**). Mutations of the BRAF gene in human cancer. *Nature* 417, 949–954.

Delaney, A. M., Printen, J. A., Chen, H., et al. (**2002**). Identification of a novel mitogen-activated protein kinase kinase activation domain recognized by the inhibitor PD184352. *Mol Cell Biol.* 22, 7593–7602.

Downward, J. (**2003**). Targeting ras signaling pathways in cancer therapy. *Nat Rev Cancer.* 3, 11–22.

Dudley, D. T., Pang, L., Decker, S. J., et al. (**1995**). A synthetic inhibitor of the mitogen-activated protein kinase cascade. *Proc Natl Acad Sci USA.* 92, 7686–7689.

Eliceiri, B. P., Klemke, R., Stromblad, S., et al. (**1998**). Integrin $\alpha v \beta 3$ requirement for sustained mitogen-activated protein kinase activity during angiogenesis. *J Cell Biol.* 141, 1255–1263.

Favata, M. F., Horiuchi, K. Y., Manos, E. J., et al. (**1998**). Identification of a novel inhibitor of mitogen-activated protein kinase kinase. *J Biol Chem.* 273(9), 18623–18632.

Finlay, D., Healy, V., Furlong, F., et al. (**2000**). MAP kinase pathway signaling is essential for extracellular matrix determined mammary epithelial cell survival. *Cell Death Differ.* 7, 302–313.

Holmstrom, T. H., Tran, S. E., Johnson, V. L., et al. (**1999**). Inhibition of mitogen-activated kinase signaling sensitizes HeLa cells to Fas receptor-mediated apoptosis. *Mol Cell Biol.* 19, 5991–6002.

LoRusso, P., Adjei A., Varterasian, M., et al. (**2005a**). Phase I and pharmacodynamic study of the oral MEK inhibitor CI-1040 in patients with advanced malignancies. *J Clin Oncol.* 23(23), 5281–5293.

LoRusso, P. A., Krishnamurthi, S., Rinehart J. J., et al. (**2005b**). A phase 1–2 clinical study of a second generation oral MEK inhibitor, PD 0325901 in patients with advanced cancer. *J Clin Oncol.* [abstr] 23, 3006.

LoRusso, P. A., Krishnamurthi, S. S., Rinehart, J. J., et al. (**2007**). Clinical aspects of a Phase I study of PD-0325901,a selective oral MEK inhibitor, in patients with advanced cancer. *Mol Cancer Ther.* 6, 3649s [abstr B113].

Milanini, J., Vinals, F., Pouyssegur, J., et al. (**1998**). p42/p44 MAP kinase module plays a key role in the transcriptional regulation of the vascular endothelial growth factor gene in fibroblasts. *J Biol Chem.* 273, 18165–18172.

Ohren, J. F., Chen, H., Pavlovsky, A., et al. (**2004**). Structures of human MAP kinase kinase 1 (MEK1) and MEK2 describe novel noncompetitive kinase inhibition. *Nat Struct Mol Biol.* 11, 1192–1197.

Pages, G., Lenormand, D., L'Allemain, G., et al. (**1993**). Mitogen-activated protein kinases p42mapk and p44mapk are required for fibroblast proliferation. *Proc Natl Acad Sci USA.* 90, 8319–8323.

Pang, L., Sawada, T., Decker, S. J., et al. (**1995**). Inhibition of MAP kinase kinase blocks the differentiation of PC-12 cells induced by nerve growth factor. *J Biol Chem.* 270, 13585–13588.

Rinehart, J., Adjei, A. A., LoRusso, P. M., et al. (**2004**). Multicenter Phase II study of the oral MEK inhibitor, CI-1040, in patients with advanced non-small-cell lung, breast, colon, and pancreatic cancer. *J Clin Oncol.* 22(22), 4456–4462.

Roberts, P. J., and Der, C. J. (**2007**). Targeting the Raf-MEK-ERK mitogen-activated protein kinase cascade for the treatment of cancer. *Oncogene.* 26, 3291–3310.

Sebolt-Leopold, J. S. (**2008**). Advances in the development of therapeutics directed against the RAS-mitogen-activated protein kinase pathway. *Clin Cancer Res.* 14(12), 3651–3656.

Sebolt-Leopold, J. S., and Herrera, R. (**2004**). Targeting the mitogen-activated protein kinase cascade to treat cancer. *Nat Rev Cancer.* 4, 937–947.

Sebolt-Leopold, J. S., Dudley D. T., Herrera, R., et al. (**1999**). Blockade of the MAP kinase pathway suppresses growth of colon tumors in vivo. *Nat Med.* 5, 810–816.

Sebolt-Leopold, J. S., Van Becelaere, K., Hook, K., et al. (**2003**). Biomarker assays for phosphorylated MAP kinase. *Methods Mol Med.* 85, 31–38.

Solit, D. B., Garraway, L. A., Pratilas, C. A., et al. (**2006**). BRAF mutation predicts sensitivity to MEK inhibition. *Nature* 439, 358–362.

Solit, D. B., Santos, E., Pratilas, C. A., et al. (**2007**). 3'-Deoxy-3'-[^{18}F]fluorothymidine positron emission tomography is a sensitive method for imaging the response of BRAF-dependent tumors to MEK inhibition. *Cancer Res.* 67(23), 11463–11469.

Tan, W., DePrimo, S., Krishnamurthi, S. S., et al. (**2007**), Pharmacokinetic (PK) and pharmacodynamic (PD) results of a Phase I study of PD-0325901, a second generation oral MEK inhibitor, in patients with advanced cancer. *Mol Cancer Ther.* 6, 3648s [abstr B109].

9

DISCOVERY OF ALLOSTERIC MEK INHIBITORS

Eli Wallace and James F. Blake

9.1. INTRODUCTION

Cancer is the second leading cause of death in the United States (Minino et al., 2007), with close to 1.5 million new patients diagnosed with some form of cancer every year (Pickle et al., 2007). While the last decade has seen advances in treatment options for patients, there remains a significant need for new therapies for cancer. All forms of cancer are diseases of cellular dysregulation with uncontrolled growth and proliferation, prosurvival, angiogenesis, and differentiation all hallmarks of the disease (Hanahan and Weinberg, 2000). Within this cellular context, more and more molecular signatures of subtypes of cancers are delineated with increasing frequency moving the field of anticancer drug discovery closer to the reality of designing and developing specific, "personalized" anticancer medicines. An attractive molecular target that has both the potential to treat a wide variety of cancers and also to be tailored to patients stricken with cancers harboring specific molecular signatures is the dual specificity protein kinase MEK (mitogen activated protein kinase/extracellular signal-related kinase kinase). MEK plays a pivotal, gatekeeper role in the mitogen-activated protein kinase (MAPK) cascade of growth factor receptor/Ras/Raf/MEK/ERK (Figure 9.1). While there are two MEK and two ERK kinases, MEK1 and MEK2 and ERK1 and ERK2, and studies have delineated some distinct biological roles for the isoforms, both MEK1 and MEK2 have equivalent capability to phosphorylate ERK1 and ERK2 (Giroux et al., 1999; Belanger et al., 2003; Ussar and Voss, 2004; Scholl

Kinase Inhibitor Drugs. Edited by Rongshi Li and Jeffrey A. Stafford
Copyright © 2009 John Wiley & Sons, Inc.

MEK Pathway in Cancer

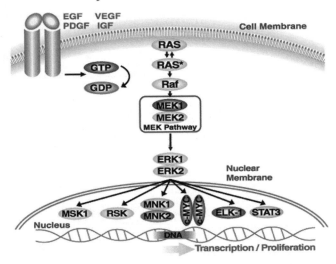

Figure 9.1. Growth factor/Ras/Raf/MEK/ERK pathway.

et al., 2005). Furthermore, a consensus on the distinct roles of the isoforms in the pathophysiology of cancer has not been reached, and the high homology between the isoforms has to date precluded preparation of selective inhibitors. As such, we will refer to MEK1 and MEK2 as MEK and ERK1 and ERK2 as ERK throughout this chapter.

This pathway is inappropriately activated in many human cancers, which results in the activation of ERK via phosphorylation. Once activated, pERK has a plethora of substrates both in the nucleus and the cytosol that control cell proliferation, growth, survival, angiogenesis, and differentiation (Dhillon et al., 2007; Meloche and Pouyssegur, 2007; Turjanski et al., 2007). Constitutive activation of pERK has been found in patient tumor samples in melanoma and cancers of the colon, lung, thyroid, breast, pancreas, and blood (Hoshino et al., 1999; Platanias, 2003; Dhillon et al., 2007). Mechanisms of activation of the pathway include activating mutations in the well-known oncogenes Ras and Raf, as well as overexpression of both growth factors and/or their receptors. Very recently, activating mutations in MEK, which are sensitive to MEK inhibitors, have been found in lung cancer (Marks et al., 2008). Oncogenic Ras has been found in 25% of all human cancers including up to 90% of pancreatic, 50% colorectal, and 30% lung. Point mutations in B-Raf (the Raf isoform most involved in oncogenesis and the one believed to be primarily responsible for activation of MEK) have been identified in a majority of melanomas as well as a significant portion of thyroid and colorectal cancer (Bos, 1989; Davies et al., 2002; Cohen et al., 2003; Xu et al., 2003; Dhillon et al., 2007). Interestingly, oncogenic Ras and B-Raf appear to be mutually exclusive in that tumors may harbor either one or the other, but never both. This evolutionary phenomenon suggests that activation of these oncogenes results in the same downstream consequence. In support of this position is the fact that MEK is the lynchpin protein kinase that links growth factor signaling, and the oncogenic protein kinase B-Raf with ERK. While there is significant redundancy in many of the signaling pathways that are believed to be involved in the development and progression of cancer, the specificity of the MEK–ERK module is noteworthy. The MEK–ERK signaling unit is highly specific, as MEK is the only known activator of ERK, and ERK is the only known substrate for MEK (Roberts and Der, 2007). Thus with the ever-increasing complexity of cellular signaling, the role of MEK in signal transduction is exquisitely selective and, as such, a selective MEK inhibitor will only block the activation of ERK.

While inhibitors of this pathway have the potential to treat a diverse array of cancers, an attractive possibility also exists for treatment of patients found to harbor Ras and B-Raf mutations. As these mutations generally lead to constitutively active pERK via MEK activation, the hypothesis is that these patients will be more likely to respond to MEK inhibitor treatment. Recently, studies in lung and colon cancer have established that patients with activated Ras are resistant to upstream anti-EGFR therapy (Khambata-Ford et al., 2007; Cervantes et al., 2008; Miller et al., 2008; Van Custem et al., 2008). As these patients have limited treatment options, MEK inhibitor therapy in this setting may fill an unmet medical need. Furthermore, selecting B-Raf mutant melanoma patients for treatment regiments that include MEK inhibition may lead to increased efficacy. These intriguing proposals await clinical evaluation where the promise of specific, "personalized" anticancer therapy may be put to the test.

Interestingly, two prototype inhibitors of MEK kinase, PD098059 (**1**) (Alessi et al., 1995; Dudley et al., 1995) and U0126 (**2**) (Duncia et al., 1998; Favata et al., 1998) (Scheme 9.1), have been shown to exhibit kinetics consistent with uncompetitive inhibition with respect to ATP. This kinetic profile of kinase inhibitors is rare and highly desirable, as avoiding the highly conserved ATP binding pocket makes selectivity more readily attainable. Additionally, not having to compete against the millimolar intracellular concentration of ATP, in theory, closes the gap between enzyme and cellular potency. More recently, Parke–Davis (now Pfizer Inc.) discovered and progressed CI-1040 into clinical

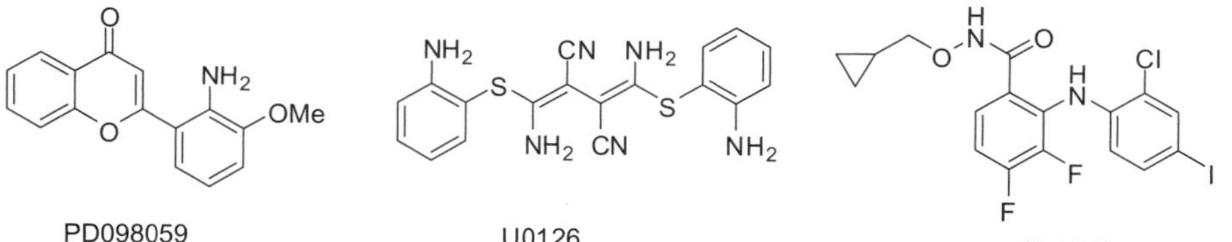

PD098059   U0126

CI-1040

Scheme 9.1. Early MEK inhibitors.

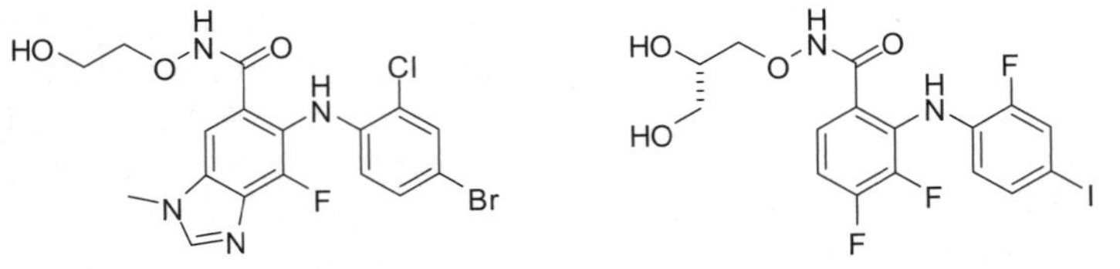

AZD6244 / ARRY-142886   PD0325901

Scheme 9.2. MEK inhibitors.

trials for the treatment of cancer (Scheme 9.1) (Sebolt-Leopold et al., 1999; LoRusso et al., 2005). CI-1040 is a potent and selective MEK inhibitor that was also reported to display ATP noncompetitive kinetics of inhibition.

The combination of its pivotal, specific role in ERK activation, the frequency with which constitutively activated ERK is found in human tumors, the role of the well-known oncogenes Ras and B-Raf in activation of the pathway, and the disclosure of diverse ATP uncompetitive inhibitors of MEK make the dual specificity kinase MEK an attractive target for anticancer drug discovery.

Shortly after the advancement and subsequent clinical failure of CI-1040 (Rinehart et al., 2004), both AZD6244 (ARRY-142886), which was discovered by our group and later licensed to AstraZeneca, and PD0325901 (Pfizer Inc.) (Kaufman et al., 2004) were progressed into clinical development for the treatment of cancer (Scheme 9.2). Preclinical evaluation of these new inhibitors demonstrated they were superior to CI-1040 in nearly every way— potency, hepatic stability, pharmacokinetics, and efficacy (Kaufman et al., 2004; Wallace et al., 2004; Yeh et al., 2007). As with the early MEK inhibitors, AZD6244 and PD0325901 were found to be non-ATP competitive (vide supra). In this chapter, we will describe a pharmacophore model that explains the binding of these inhibitors, show how this model was used to design later generation allosteric MEK inhibitors, summarize the preclinical and clinical activity of AZD6244 including the development and use of a clinical biomarker, and conclude with therapeutic activities of MEK inhibitors outside oncology highlighted by the development of ARRY-438162 for rheumatoid arthritis.

9.2. DEVELOPMENT OF A MEK PHARMACOPHORE MODEL

There was no protein structural information on MEK until late 2004 (Ohren et al., 2004). Accordingly, we sought to build a pharmacophore model that explained the binding of AZD6244, CI-1040, and PD0325901, explained the early reported SAR on anthranilic acid type inhibitors (Tecle, 2002), and allowed the design of new generation analogs (Figure 9.2). From a conformational analysis of the anthranilic acid type inhibitors, we found an internal H

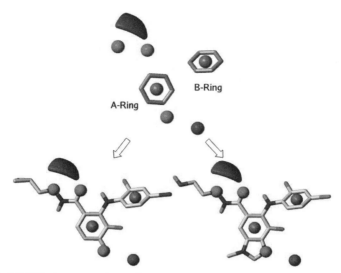

Figure 9.2. MEK1 pharmacophore. Green spheres depict where H-bond acceptors are preferred, with the complementary H-bond donor sites on the protein represented by the red spheres. Hydrophobic centroids are depicted in gold.

bond between the aniline H and the oxygen of the hydroxamate carbonyl defines the positioning of the two aromatic rings (rings A and B in Figure 9.2). We hypothesized that these aniline-linked compounds bound near their energetic minima, with respect to the two aromatic rings. Combination of the conformation analysis with the reported SAR suggested that the potency of these inhibitors was driven primarily via two interactions with the protein through the lipophilic B-ring and hydroxamate contacts. We hypothesized that this latter interaction involved the two oxygens of the hydroxamate acting either as a bifurcated hydrogen-bond acceptor from a charged residue on the protein or coordinated to a bivalent metal cation, similar to the binding mode of hydroxamic acids in metalloproteinases. The activity of these early anthranilic acid analogs was greatly influenced by the nature of the B-ring para substituent as it was reported that *para*-iodo was significantly more potent than bromo, which was more potent than chloro. A subtle and perhaps most intriguing piece of data centered on the potency changes related to substitution at the 4-position of the A-ring. For a series of benzoic acid analogs, substitution of 4-F, relative to hydrogen, resulted in a nearly 30-fold increase in potency. Substitution of 4-Cl was slightly less potent than the unsubstituted compound. This prompted us to speculate that the unusual increase in potency for the 4-F compound was the result of an H bond to the protein, rather than an interaction mediated by hydrophobic contacts, where we would expect more modest potency increases. The ability of aryl fluorides to make H bonds with proteins is controversial (Muller et al., 2007), so including this element in our model was highly speculative. However, we felt this leap was worth exploring as it led us to greatly expand our inhibitor designs and opened us up to analogs with the potential for improved physical properties. The first generation MEK inhibitors, with their apparent reliance on the lipophilic B-ring for potency, often displayed less than optimal drug-like properties— CI-1040 was discontinued from clinical development due to lack of efficacy, which was directly attributed to poor exposure resulting from its physical properties (Kaufman et al., 2004; Rinehart et al., 2004). In order to confidently use the model for the generation of new inhibitors, we felt it imperative that the advanced inhibitors fit our model. As shown in Figure 9.2, both CI-1040 and AZD6244 fit the model with the binding of the Pfizer inhibitor likely relying on the B-ring aryl iodide for potency. Thus we hoped that the design of three-point binding MEK inhibitors resulting from an additional H-bonding element in our pharmacophore model would afford us an opportunity for improving not only the potency but also the drug-like properties of next generation inhibitors.

9.3. PYRIDONE MEK INHIBITORS

Using our pharmacophore model, we designed and prepared several new templates as MEK inhibitors, of which the structure–activity relationships of the pyridones will be highlighted here (Figure 9.3), (Wallace et al., 2005, 2006). Initial results from the pyridones were extremely encouraging as the first analogs exhibited impressive enzymatic and cellular potency (compounds **1** and **2**, Table 9.1). The nature of the 5-substituent modestly influenced enzymatic potency but had a significant effect on cellular activity as the 5-Me analog (**4**) was not significantly more potent against MEK enzyme but was 10–35-fold more active in the mechanistic cell assay (Table 9.1). The importance of the A-ring H-bond acceptor was established with the near complete inactivity of the two pyridine-based inhibitors (**5** and **6**). A brief examination of the carboxylate region SAR showed that a variety of hydroxamates were well tolerated and that a simple primary amide was quite active (Table 9.2). Finally, the role of the B-ring 4-substituent was examined (Table 9.3). Unlike early anthranilic acid type inhibitors (Tecle, 2002), the nature of this moiety did not greatly influence the enzymatic or cellular potency of these inhibitors.

Not only did the activity of the pyridone inhibitors validate our pharmacophore model, but they also supported our three-point binding hypothesis with respect to drug-like properties. As a direct result of strengthening the A-ring H-bond acceptor, potent inhibitors were designed without the B-ring 4-iodide— an unusual moiety for an oral therapeutic. Additionally, replacing the N-O moiety with a simple primary amide was found to be quite potent. In other words, designing MEK inhibitors with three strong protein interactions allowed flexibility in the preparation of potent compounds.

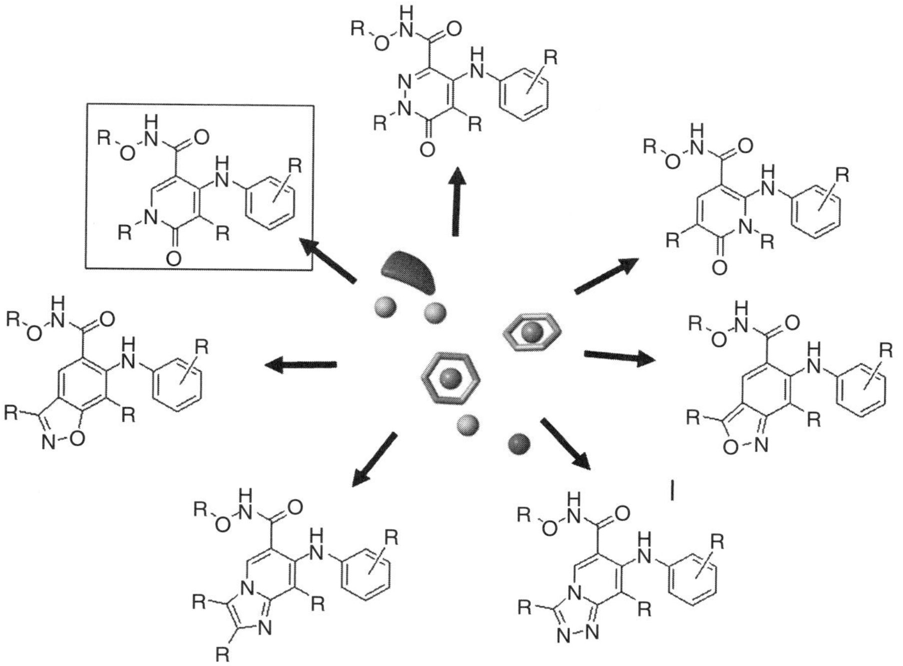

Figure 9.3. Novel MEK inhibitors that can be derived from the pharmacophore model.

A very important aspect of the flexibility garnered from three-point binding was the ability to generate drug-like inhibitors. As evident from all our MEK inhibitors (Figure 9.3), we sought to incorporate more drug-like characteristics by strengthening the A-ring H-bond acceptor, and the pyridones were no exception. As shown in Table 9.4, analogs **11** and **4** (ARRY-509) have low predicted hepatic clearance, good solubility, and excellent rodent pharmacokinetics. Additionally, ARRY-509 demonstrated impressive activity in the HT-29 human colorectal xenograft model and Matrigel model of angiogenesis and greater than 90% bioavailability in dogs (Wallace et al., 2005, 2006).

As mentioned earlier, during the course of our preclinical research, a sizeable number of alternative A-ring templates were investigated. Many of these templates, such as the imidazo[1,2-*a*]pyridine, benzoisoxazole, [1,2,4]triazolo[4,3-*a*]pyridine, and benzimidazole of AZD6244 displayed excellent in vitro, in vivo, and ADME properties, affording us the luxury of choosing among them for further elaboration. Based on a variety of factors, we decided to pursue the benzimidazole ring structure as our platform for further development, leading to the selection of AZD6244 for clinical evaluation in the treatment of cancer (Lee et al., 2004; Wallace et al., 2004; Davies et al., 2007; Yeh et al., 2007). The following section details the preclinical discovery properties of AZD6244 that led to its nomination as a clinical candidate.

TABLE 9.1. MEK Hydroxyethoxy Pyridone C5 SAR

Compound	R	MEK IC$_{50}$ (nM)	pERK^a IC$_{50}$ (nM)
1	H	30	75
2	Cl	45	25
3	F	10	20
4	Me	20	2
5		6,800	>10,000
6		4,500	>10,000

^{a}Malme-3M cells—B-Raf mutant melanoma.

TABLE 9.2. MEK Pyridone SAR

Compound	R	R$_1$	MEK IC$_{50}$ (nM)	pERK^a IC$_{50}$ (nM)
3	HOCH$_2$CH$_2$ONH	F	10	20
7	NH$_2$	F	15	5
8	OH	F	30	>10,000
9	MeNH	F	120	70
10	MeONH	Me	105	40
11	EtONH	Me	80	10

^{a}Malme-3M cells—B-Raf mutant melanoma.

TABLE 9.3. MEK Pyridone B-Ring SAR

Compound	X	MEK IC$_{50}$ (nM)	pERK[a] IC$_{50}$ (nM)
12	Cl	60	15
4	Br	20	2
13	I	5	1
14	SMe	10	3

[a]Malme-3M cells—B-Raf mutant melanoma.

TABLE 9.4. Comparison of Pyridone Inhibitor ADME Properties

Compound	In Vitro Human Hepatic CL[a]	Solubility (pH 6.5)	Rat IV CL[a]/$t_{1/2}$	Rat %F
11	5	60 μg/mL	2/2.5 h	80
4 (ARRY-509)	6	450 μg/mL	8/1.6 h	53

[a]CL units are mL/min/kg.

9.4. PRECLINICAL EVALUATION OF AZD6244

AZD6244 exhibited potent enzymatic and cellular activity with an IC$_{50}$ of 14 nM against constitutively active MEK enzyme and inhibition of ERK phosphorylation in cells with an IC$_{50}$ of 10 nM. AZD6244 did not inhibit any other kinases, receptors, ion channels, or cellular signaling pathways at concentrations up to and exceeding 10 μM. It is interesting that AZD6244 and some of the pyridones (vide infra) were found to be more active in the cell than the enzyme. This cellular phenomenon, along with exquisite selectivity and the fact that the first-generation MEK inhibitors were reported to be noncompetitive with ATP, prompted us to investigate the kinetics of inhibition of AZD6244. Contrary to reports on the early MEK inhibitors, AZD6244 was found to be uncompetitive with ATP. Thus, as shown in Figure 9.4, as the concentration of ATP increases so does the potency of AZD6244. In other words, the mechanism of inhibition requires binding of ATP. Of course, this is distinct from noncompetitive inhibition, where inhibitory potency of the molecules is independent of ATP concentration. This uncompetitive mechanism of inhibition is consistent with the tertiary crystal structure of MEK1/ATP/inhibitor later published (Ohren et al., 2004). It also explains how these

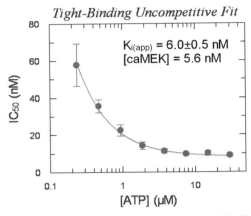

Figure 9.4. Enzymatic kinetic analysis of AZD6244.

and other MEK inhibitors can be more potent in the high ATP concentration found in cellular systems compared to the relatively low levels of ATP in the enzymatic assay.

AZD6244 was found to exhibit moderate plasma protein binding (ca. 3% free in both human and mouse whole blood), high permeability, and low predicted hepatic clearance (CL) across all species evaluated. AZD6244 did not inhibit P450s up to 15 μM free-drug concentration. The pharmacokinetics of AZD6244 were evaluated in mice, rats, monkeys, and dogs. The results are summarized in Table 9.5. Consistent with the in vitro ADME, low CL and moderate half-life were observed in all species after IV administration. Bioavailability in rodents was high (86–98%) and showed dose dependence in monkeys.

Cellular evaluation of AZD6244 demonstrated that it displays antiproliferation and pro-apoptotic activity in a cell-line-specific manner. While inhibition of pERK, whether constitutively active or simulated, was cell-line independent, strong antiproliferation activity of AZD6244 appeared to be correlated with the presence of B-Raf and Ras mutations, with the former most strongly correlated (Table 9.6). The strong correlation with mutant B-Raf is consistent with our current understanding of oncogenic signaling networks as this constitutively active kinase has been shown to signal through MEK and ERK only. On the other hand, Ras mutants may signal through the PI3 kinase–Akt axis, and other pathways, as well as MEK–ERK, and thus some aberrant Ras signaling may not be sensitive to MEK inhibition. Recently, the cellular sensitivity of AZD6244 has been further elaborated and refined by examining activating mutations in B-Raf/Ras and PTEN/PI3K with cell viability as the end point (Dry et al., 2008). The most sensitive cell lines were those containing activating B-Raf/Ras mutations with wild-type PTEN/PI3K. The most resistant were the wild-type B-Raf/Ras cell lines containing activating mutations of PTEN/PI3K. Furthermore, strong synergy was observed combining

TABLE 9.5. Preclinical Pharmacokinetics of AZD6244

Species	Dose (mg/kg)	CL (mL/min/kg)	$t_{1/2}$ (h)	PO AUC ($\mu g\,h/mL$)	PO C_{max} ($\mu g/mL$)	%F
Mouse	IV–2	3.9	3.1			
	PO–10			36.8	12.6	86
Rat	IV–2	0.32	4.8			
	PO–30			1,650	68.4	98
Dog	IV–0.2	3.1	3.4			
	PO–30			34.4	5.1	21
Monkey	IV–3	1.5	10.7			
	PO–1			9.8	0.77	86
	PO–10			18.9	1.5	17

TABLE 9.6. Cellular Evaluation of AZD6244

Cell Line	Type	Ras/Raf Mutation	Cell Viability IC_{50} (nM)	Apoptosis Induction
HT-29	Colon	B-Raf	175	No
HCT-116	Colon	K-Ras	9,500	
Malme-3M	Melanoma	B-Raf	60	Yes
Malme-3	Normal Fibroblast	None	>50,000	
SK-MEL-2	Melanoma	N-Ras	270	Yes
SK-MEL-28	Melanoma	B-Raf	75	No
BxPC3	Pancreatic	None	28,000	
MIA PaCa2	Pancreatic	K-Ras	520	
Zr-75-1	Breast	None	>50,000	
BT474	Breast	None	>50,000	
A549	NSCLC	K-Ras	>50,000	

AZD6244 and an inhibitor of PI3K/mTOR signaling in the A2058 melanoma cell line, which was only moderately sensitive to AZD6244 as a single agent. By examining the influence of these two major oncogenic pathways on the sensitivity of AZD6244, the prediction of potential response is enhanced.

Some oncogenic cell lines undergo apoptosis in addition to growth arrest as a result of MEK inhibition. The molecular determinants of those cells that undergo apoptosis in the presence of AZD6244 have not been elucidated. As shown in Table 9.6, Malme-3M and SK-MEL-2 melanoma cell lines, possessing B-Raf and N-Ras mutations, respectively, undergo apoptosis when treated with AZD6244 (measured by caspase-3/7 activation). However, neither HT-29 nor SK-MEL-28, both B-Raf mutant cell lines, progress to apoptosis even though both were growth inhibited.

AZD6244 demonstrated broad antitumor activity in mouse xenograft models of human cancer including models of melanoma, colorectal, non-small-cell lung, pancreatic, and breast cancer (Table 9.7). For example, the LOX melanoma human xenograft model was extremely sensitive to AZD6244 treatment (Figure 9.5). Treatment with as little as 10 mg/kg/day resulted in 9 of 10 mice experiencing full regression. Interestingly, the mutational status of the tumor line in vivo did not predict response to AZD6244 treatment. Models with B-Raf mutations, Ras mutants, and those with neither deregulated protein

TABLE 9.7. Efficacy of AZD6244 in Tumor Models

Cancer Type	Tumor Model	Ras/Raf Mutation	Potency (mg/kg/d)	Efficacy
Colorectal	Colo205	B-Raf	<25	Regressions
	HCT-116	K-Ras	$EC_{90} < 20$	Cytostatic
	HT-29	B-Raf	EC_{50} 20–40	Cytostatic
	SW620	K-Ras	$EC_{50} < 25$	Cytostatic
NSCLC	A549	K-Ras	$EC_{90} \sim 15$	Cytostatic
	Calu-6	K-Ras	$EC_{90} < 20$	Cytostatic
Pancreatic	BxPC3	None	3–12	Regressions
	PANC-1	K-Ras	EC_{90} 20–40	Cytostatic
	MIA PaCa2	K-Ras	40	Regressions
Breast	Zr-75-1	None	EC_{50} 20	Cytostatic
	MDA-MB-231	K-Ras	$EC_{90} < 20$	Cytostatic
Melanoma	LOX	B-Raf	<20	Regressions

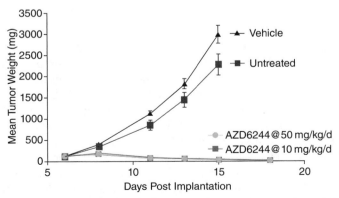

Figure 9.5. Activity of AZD6244 in human melanoma xenograft model (LOX).

responded well to MEK inhibition with AZD6244 (Table 9.7). Extensive research into the in vivo tumor growth inhibition mechanism of action of AZD6244 has recently been published (Davies et al., 2007). The authors found that inhibition of pERK in excised tumors correlated with growth inhibition in vivo and that the IC_{50} for pERK inhibition in these tumors was very similar to the values found in cell culture. They also demonstrated inhibition of proliferation in excised tumors from all models evaluated. Finally, they found that AZD6244 caused tumor cell apoptosis in vivo in two of three models evaluated.

It is clear from the multitude of preclinical studies that the ability of AZD6244 to inhibit cell line growth in vitro does not predict perfectly the in vivo response as BxPC3, HCT-116, A549, and Zr-75-1 models demonstrate (Tables 9.6 and 9.7). In the BxPC3 model, tumor growth was completely inhibited at both doses evaluated and the tumors remained sensitive to AZD6244 even after a dosing holiday that resulted in significant tumor regrowth in the low-dose group (Figure 9.6). The discrepancy between in vitro and in vivo response is not completely understood. One can speculate on any number of factors present in vivo that are not captured in cell culture, including that antiangiogenesis may play a role as inhibition of the MEK–ERK signaling cascade has been shown to inhibit expression of the proangiogenic factor VEGF (Jung et al., 1999; Chang et al., 2006). In support of this hypothesis, we have shown that pyridone MEK inhibitor ARRY-509 inhibited blood vessel formation in an in vivo Matrigel model (Figure 9.7) (Wallace et al., 2005). Finally, AZD6244 has been combined successfully with several other anticancer therapies in vivo, including docetaxel, temozolomide, and radiation, where synergy was observed (Davies et al., 2007; Shannon et al., 2008; Wilkinson et al., 2008).

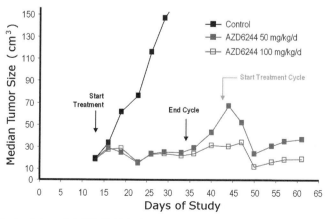

Figure 9.6. Activity of AZD6244 in human pancreatic xenograft model (BxPC3).

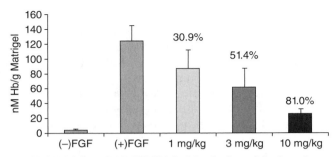

Figure 9.7. Activity of ARRY-509 in Matrigel model of angiogensis.

9.5. CLINICAL EVALUATION OF AZD6244

A two-part Phase I clinical trial of AZD6244 free base (mix and drink formulation) in advanced cancer patients is complete (Adjei et al., 2008). Part A was a dose escalation to determine the maximum tolerated dose (MTD) and pharmacokinetics. AZD6244 was well tolerated in cancer patients, with rash, diarrhea, nausea, and fatigue the most frequent adverse events. The MTD was established as 200 mg bid with rash and diarrhea becoming dose limiting at 300 mg bid. The half-life of AZD6244 was determined to be ca. 8 h and both AUC and C_{max} increased with dose. In order to evaluate the safety and pharmacokinetic data in relation to target inhibition in patients, a whole blood inhibition of ERK phosphorylation mechanistic biomarker assay was developed. As part of the development process, the assay was validated in both ex vivo treated human whole blood and cynomolgus monkeys (Doyle et al., 2005). The assay was found to be robust in both settings and the IC_{50} values from the ex vivo human whole blood and monkey studies were found to be in good agreement, ca. 500 nM and ca. 800 nM, respectively. In cancer patients, rapid (1 h) and strong (up to 100%) inhibition of pERK was observed after oral AZD6244 administration, demonstrating rapid absorption and distribution of the drug. The IC_{50} for pERK in the blood compartment of cancer patients was found to be ca. 340 nM, which agrees well with our preclinical ex vivo results. Furthermore, on repeat dosing an average of 51% inhibition of pERK was observed in trough samples with a maximum of 90% inhibition. The ability to include the mechanistic biomarker data along with the safety and pharmacokinetic data in the evaluation of the first in human studies allowed several important conclusions to be drawn. First, in patients the plasma levels of AZD6244 correlated well with inhibition of the target in this compartment. Second, and importantly, AZD6244 can inhibit MEK at tolerated doses over an extended period in cancer patients. Third, both the half-life and the trough inhibition of ERK phosphorylation data support a twice-daily schedule for this drug in additional clinical studies.

While the Part A clinical results were encouraging, inhibition of ERK phosphorylation in whole blood is only a mechanistic biomarker and not a predictive one. Furthermore, blood is not the target tissue. Thus in Part B of the

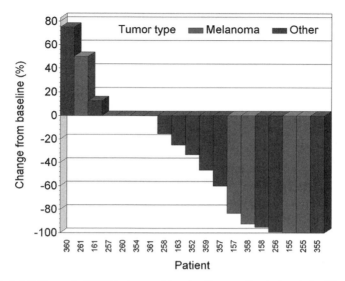

Figure 9.8. Inhibition of pERK in tumor biopsies from patients treated with AZD6244.

Phase I study, in addition to firmly establishing the recommended Phase II dose (examined two doses—200 mg (MTD) and 100 mg (one-half MTD)), tumor biopsies pre- and post-treatment were collected to evaluate pERK and Ki67 (a measure of cellular proliferation) levels. In this expansion phase, it was found that the incidence and severity of rash were unacceptable at 200 mg bid. Thus 100 mg bid was clearly established as the MTD for chronic dosing with this formulation. In the 20 evaluable predose biopsies, all had detectable levels of Ki67 while 19 had significant levels of pERK. Significant and consistent inhibition of ERK phosphorylation was found in the vast majority of post-treatment biopsies with an average of 80% inhibition (Figure 9.8). Inhibition of tumor cell proliferation, as measured by reduced number of Ki67-positive cells, was observed in approximately half of the samples. The differential effect of AZD6244 treatment on tumor ERK phosphorylation and Ki67 levels most likely is an example of the oncogene addiction hypothesis, which relates the reliance of the tumor to a signal transduction pathway or pathways (Weinstein and Joe, 2008). Thus while AZD6244 clearly inhibits its target at the site of action, the functional consequence of MEK inhibition to the fate of the tumor is dependent on the importance of the MEK–ERK pathway to that tumor's progression and survival. The Part B study clearly identified the MTD and the recommended Phase II dose (100 mg/bid) and established that AZD6244 inhibits MEK in tumors, leading to inhibition of tumor cell proliferation in some cases.

As a secondary end point of the Phase I trial, objective clinical response was evaluated by radiological examination after every two cycles (ca. 60 days) on study. A total of 57 patients were dosed with AZD6244 in the study and significant, prolonged stable disease was observed in several patients

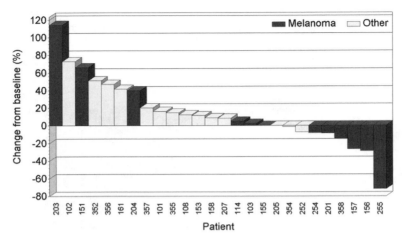

Figure 9.9. Clinical response from Phase I trial of AZD6244 in advanced cancer patients: best percentage change in total lesion length. Lengths are summed across all target lesions per patient.

(Figure 9.9). In one patient diagnosed with malignant melanoma, near complete reduction of levels of ERK phosphorylation and Ki67 was found in the post-treatment biopsy, which correlated with a 70% reduction in the size of the primary tumor. Unfortunately, the patient developed brain metastases that led to disease progression.

AZD6244 has subsequently completed three single-agent Phase II studies as well an additional Phase I study evaluating a new solid oral capsule formulation of the hydrogen-sulfate salt (Agarwal et al., 2008; Dummer et al., 2008; Lang et al., 2008; Tzekova et al., 2008). Objective clinical responses have been observed in several melanoma patients, particularly those with B-Raf positive tumors, and non-small-cell lung cancer patients. In the new formulation Phase I trial, a malignant melanoma patient who had previously failed dacarbazine experienced a compete response lasting 9 months at least; this patient's tumor was found to harbor a B-Raf V600E mutation. As a single agent AZD6244 has a signal for anticancer activity in some patients with advanced solid tumors. Clinical evaluation of AZD6244 continues in oncology with combination studies an important avenue of exploration.

9.6. NEW DIRECTIONS FOR MEK INHIBITIONS

The MEK–ERK signal transduction pathway has been implicated in disease areas outside oncology, including pain and stroke (Ji et al., 2002; Wang et al., 2003; Ma and Quirion, 2005). Besides oncology, the role of MEK inhibitors in inflammation is particularly compelling as we and others have demonstrated

TABLE 9.8. Properties of ARRY-438162

MEK enzyme IC_{50} (nM)	12
pERK IC_{50} (nM)	11
220 Kinase selectivity panel	No activity @ 10 μM
30 Receptor/ion channel panel	No activity @ 10 μM
hERG patch clamp	28% @ 10 μM
Rat, monkey, dog % F	50–75, 30–60, 60

TABLE 9.9. ARRY-438162 Ex Vivo TPA Stimulated Human Whole Blood Cytokine Inhibition

	IL-1b	TNFα	IL-6	pERK
IC_{50} (ng/mL)	9.2 ± 1.8	10.0 ± 0.2	9.3 ± 1.1	123 ± 17

impressive preclinical efficacy in models of rheumatoid arthritis, osteoarthritis, and edema with selective MEK inhibitors (Jaffee et al., 2000; Pelletier et al., 2003; Koch, 2006; Thiel et al., 2007). ARRY-438162 is a potent, selective, uncompetitive inhibitor of MEK with efficacy in several preclinical models of inflammatory disease (Table 9.8) (Koch, 2006). ARRY-438162's anti-inflammatory effects are believed to be a result of its potent anticytokine activity in human cells. In ex vivo human whole blood studies, ARRY-438162 potently inhibited the proinflammatory cytokines IL-1, IL-6, and TNFα at doses that result in only 30% inhibition of pERK (Table 9.9). The demonstration of potent anticytokine inhibition without full inhibition of pERK may lead to significant advances in the treatment of inflammatory diseases. This was confirmed preclinically in the CIA rat model where efficacy was observed at doses that resulted in only 30% inhibition of pERK in inflammatory tissue.

Based on ARRY-438162's efficacy in models of inflammatory disease and drug-like properties, a Phase I clinical trial was recently completed (Carter et al., 2008). In human volunteers, ARRY-438162's exposure was dose proportional with a half-life of ca. 7 hours. In the study, no serious adverse events were reported. Several biomarkers were examined in whole blood of patients treated with ARRY-438162 following ex vivo stimulation with TPA. Consistent with preclinical experiments, potent inhibition of the proinflammatory cytokines IL-1, IL-6, and TNFα was observed in patient samples where pERK inhibition was moderate, demonstrating dissociation of pERK inhibition from anti-inflammatory activity in this ex vivo biomarker setting. In other words, the data generated in the ex vivo setting supports the notion that significant anticytokine activity can be achieved with less than full inhibition of the pathway as measured by inhibition of the formation of pERK. Furthermore, this contrasts the current thinking for MEK inhibition in oncology, where the dogma holds that significant and prolonged inhibition of the pathway is required for anticancer efficacy. Given the tolerability, pharmacokinetics, and ex vivo cytokine inhibition in patients treated with ARRY-438162, a worldwide Phase II trial in rheumatoid arthritis has been initiated.

9.7. MEK PROTEIN–INHIBITOR DOCKING STUDIES

Retrospectively, our pharmacophore model was validated by docking studies with AZD6244 in the published X-ray structure of PD318088, a 4-Br A-ring analog of CI-1040 (Ohren et al., 2004) and later with co-crystal structures with a pyridone analog. Docking studies were performed using the Glide program (Friesner et al., 2004; Halgren et al., 2004) (*Glide V5.0*; Schrodinger, L.L.C.: New York, NY, 2005), using the X-ray crystal structure of MEK1 (PDB code 1SJ9). The results reveal that the B-ring of AZD6244 indeed occupies a hydrophobic pocket formed by Leu118, Ile126, Val127, Phe129, Ile141, Met143, Phe209, and Val211, illustrated in Figure 9.10. Given the hydrophobic nature of this pocket, it is clear that substitution of the B-ring with halogen atoms should lead to increased potency, given their lipophilicity. Interestingly, the 4-Br B-ring group is predicted to sit 3.1 Å from the backbone carbonyl oxygen of Val127, which suggests that it participates in a "halogen bond" (Auffinger et al., 2004), in addition to its numerous hydrophobic contacts. As with the 4-Br substitution on the B-ring, the chloro substituent at the 2-position is accommodated well in this narrow pocket. The 7-fluoro group of the A-ring benzimidazole occupies a small hydrophobic pocket formed by Leu115, Leu118, and Val211. As we hypothesized, a key hydrogen bond is formed between the benzimidazole and the protein. Interestingly, this interaction is even more important than we originally anticipated, as the benzimidazole N1

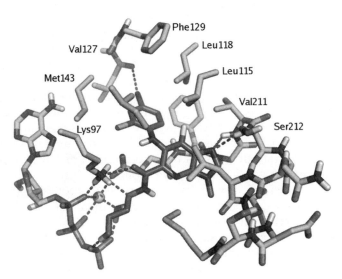

Figure 9.10. Proposed binding mode of AZD6244 to MEK1.

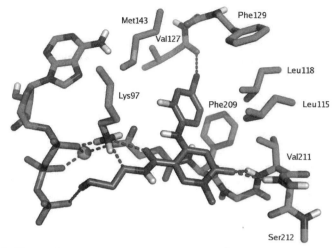

Figure 9.11. X-ray of pyridone bound to MEK1 (3.4 Å resolution). (See color insert.)

makes hydrogen bonds with both backbone amide NHs of Ser212 (N–N distance 3.3 Å) and Val211 (N–N distance 3.5 Å) in a bifurcated manner. The other critical H-bond contacts that we had postulated form between the oxygen atoms of the hydroxamate and the protonated amine portion of Lys97 (catalytic lysine). The hydroxamate oxygen to amine contact is 2.8 Å, while the carbonyl to amine distance is 3.0 Å, which confirms the bidentate nature of this interaction we had postulated from our pharmacophore. The last remaining interaction between AZD6244 and MEK is facilitated by the alcohol of the hydroxamate side chain. In this case, we predict that the hydroxyl group interacts with the terminal phosphate group of ATP, as depicted in Figure 9.10.

In the case of the pyridone series, an X-ray co-crystal of an analog of ARRY-509 verifies our hypothesized binding mode. The primary H-bond contacts occur between the carbonyl oxygen of the pyridone and the backbone NHs of Ser212 and Val211 in a bifurcated manner, analogous to that of AZD6244 (Figure 9.11). The other interactions are identical to those found in the docking studies of AZD6244. The MEK protein–inhibitor structural information clearly demonstrates that our MEK inhibitors utilize the three pharmacophore features we initially proposed, and suggests that additional inhibitors could be designed that utilize these same interactions, limited only by synthetic accessibility.

9.8. SUMMARY

Inhibition of MEK is an attractive target for the treatment of oncology and inflammatory disease as it is the gatekeeper kinase in the activation of the MAP kinase ERK. Activation of ERK leads to activation of a plethora of targets including transcription factors that control cellular proliferation, growth, survival, and angiogenesis as well as the expression of proinflammatory cytokines. We have discovered the potent, selective, ATP uncompetitive MEK inhibitor AZD6244 for the treatment of advanced cancer. AZD6244 has demonstrated anticancer activity in several preclinical models. In Phase I clinical trials in cancer patients, AZD6244 was well tolerated with pharmacokinetics and pharmacodynamics that support twice-daily dosing. In ongoing Phase II studies, several patients with melanoma and lung cancer have experienced objective clinical responses. Single-agent and combination clinical studies continue. Furthermore, ARRY-438162 has shown anticytokine activity in ex vivo samples from Phase I clinical trials, demonstrating the potential utility of MEK inhibition outside oncology. A Phase II trial of ARRY-438162 in rheumatoid arthritis is underway.

REFERENCES

Adjei, A. A., Cohen, R. B., Franklin, W., et al. (**2008**). Phase I pharmacokinetic and pharmacodynamic study of the oral, small-molecule mitogen-activated protein kinase kinase 1/2 inhibitor AZD6244 (ARRY-142886) in patients with advanced cancers. *J Clin Oncol.* 26(13), 2139–2146.

Agarwal, R., Banerji, U., Camidge, D., et al. (**2008**). The first-in-human study of the solid oral dosage form of AZD6244 (ARRY-142886): a Phase I trial in patients (pts) with advanced cancer. *J Clin Oncol.* 26(May 20 Suppl), Abst 3535.

Alessi, D. R., Cuenda, A., Cohen, P., et al. (**1995**). PD098059 is a specific inhibitor of the activation of mitogen-activated protein kinase kinase in vitro and in vivo. *J Biol Chem.* 270(46), 27489–27494.

Auffinger, P., Hays, F. A., Westhof, E., et al. (**2004**). Halogen bonds in biological molecules. *Proc Natl Acad Sci USA.* 101(48), 16789–16794.

Belanger, L. F., Roy, S., Tremblay, M., et al. (**2003**). Mek2 is dispensable for mouse growth and development. *Mol Cell Biol.* 23(14), 4778–4787.

Bos, J. L. (**1989**). ras Oncogenes in human cancer: a review. *Cancer Res.* 49(17), 4682–4689.

Carter, L., Brown, S., Klopfenstein, N., et al. (**2008**). ARRY-162, a novel inhibitor of MEK kinase: Phase 1A–1B pharmacokinetic and pharmacodynamic results. *Ann Rheum Dis.* 67(Suppl II), 87.

Cervantes, A., Macarulla, T., Martinelli, E., et al. (**2008**). Correlation of KRAS status (wild type [wt] vs. mutant [mt]) with efficacy to first-line cetuximab in a study of cetuximab single agent followed by cetuximab + FOLFIRI in patients (pts) with metastatic colorectal cancer (mCRC). *J Clin Oncol.* 26(May 20 suppl; Abst 4129).

Chang, H. J., Park, J. S., Kim, M. H., et al. (**2006**). Extracellular signal-regulated kinases and AP-1 mediate the up-regulation of vascular endothelial growth factor by PDGF in human vascular smooth muscle cells. *Int J Oncol.* 28(1), 135–141.

Cohen, Y., Xing, M., Mambo, E., et al. (**2003**). BRAF mutation in papillary thyroid carcinoma. *J Natl Cancer Inst.* 95(8), 625–627.

Davies, B. R., Logie, A., McKay, J. S., et al. (**2007**). AZD6244 (ARRY-142886), a potent inhibitor of mitogen-activated protein kinase/extracellular signal-regulated kinase kinase 1/2 kinases: mechanism of action in vivo, pharmacokinetic/pharmacodynamic relationship, and potential for combination in preclinical models. *Mol Cancer Ther.* 6(8), 2209–2219.

Davies, H., Bignell, G. R., Cox, C., et al. (**2002**). Mutations of the *BRAF* gene in human cancer. *Nature.* 417(6892), 949–954.

Dhillon, A. S., Hagan, S., Rath, O., et al. (**2007**). MAP kinase signalling pathways in cancer. *Oncogene.* 26(22), 3279–3290.

Doyle, M., Yeh, T., Brown, S., et al. (**2005**). Validation and use of a biomarker for clinical development of the MEK1/2 inhibitor ARRY-142886 (AZD6244). *J Clin Oncol.* 23(16S, Part I of II (June 1 Suppl)), 3075.

Dry, J., Harbron, C., Hickinson, M., et al. (**2008**). Biologically driven interpretation reveals molecular signatures predictive of oncogenic addiction to MEK signaling and cell line response to the MEK1/2 inhibitor AZD6244 (ARRY-142886). *Proc Am Assoc Cancer Res.* 49, Abst 913.

Dudley, D. T., Pang, L., Decker, S. J., et al. (**1995**). A synthetic inhibitor of the mitogen-activated protein kinase cascade. *Proc Natl Acad Sci USA.* 92(17), 7686–7689.

Dummer, R., Robert, C., Chapman, P., et al. (**2008**). AZD6244 (ARRY-142886) vs temozolomide (TMZ) in patients (pts) with advanced melanoma: an open-label, randomized, multicenter, Phase II study. *J Clin Oncol.* 26(May 20 Suppl), Abst 9033.

Duncia, J. V., Santella, J. B. 3rd, Higley, C. A., et al. (**1998**). MEK inhibitors: the chemistry and biological activity of U0126, its analogs, and cyclization products. *Bioorg Med Chem Lett.* 8(20), 2839–2844.

Favata, M. F., Horiuchi, K. Y., Manos, E. J., et al. (**1998**). Identification of a novel inhibitor of mitogen-activated protein kinase kinase. *J Biol Chem.* 273(29), 18623–18632.

Friesner, R. A., Banks, J. L., Murphy, R. B., et al. (**2004**). Glide: a new approach for rapid, accurate docking and scoring. 1. Method and assessment of docking accuracy. *J Med Chem.* 47(7), 1739–1749.

Giroux, S., Tremblay, M., Bernard, D., et al. (**1999**). Embryonic death of Mek1-deficient mice reveals a role for this kinase in angiogenesis in the labyrinthine region of the placenta. *Curr Biol.* 9(7), 369–372.

Halgren, T. A., Murphy, R. B., Friesner, R. A., et al. (**2004**). Glide: a new approach for rapid, accurate docking and scoring. 2. Enrichment factors in database screening. *J Med Chem.* 47(7), 1750–1759.

Hanahan, D., and Weinberg, R. A. (**2000**). The hallmarks of cancer. *Cell.* 100(1), 57–70.

Hoshino, R., Chatani, Y., Yamori, T., et al. (**1999**). Constitutive activation of the 41-/43-kDa mitogen-activated protein kinase signaling pathway in human tumors. *Oncogene.* 18(3), 813–822.

Jaffee, B. D., Manos, E. J., Collins, R. J., et al. (**2000**). Inhibition of MAP kinase kinase (MEK) results in an anti-inflammatory response in vivo. *Biochem Biophys Res Commun.* 268(2), 647–651.

Ji, R. R., Befort, K., Brenner, G. J., et al. (**2002**). ERK MAP kinase activation in superficial spinal cord neurons induces prodynorphin and NK-1 upregulation and contributes to persistent inflammatory pain hypersensitivity. *J Neurosci.* 22(2), 478–485.

Jung, Y. D., Nakano, K., Liu, W., et al. (**1999**). Extracellular signal-regulated kinase activation is required for up-regulation of vascular endothelial growth factor by serum starvation in human colon carcinoma cells. *Cancer Res.* 59(19), 4804–4807.

Kaufman, M. D., Barrett, S. D., Flamme, C. M., et al. (**2004**). Synthesis and SAR development of PD0325901, a potent and highly bioavailable MEK inhibitor. *Proc Am Assoc Cancer Res.* 45, Abst 2477.

Khambata-Ford, S., Garrett, C. R., Meropol, N. J., et al. (**2007**). Expression of epiregulin and amphiregulin and K-ras mutation status predict disease control in metastatic colorectal cancer patients treated with cetuximab. *J Clin Oncol.* 25(22), 3230–3237.

Koch, K. (**2006**). ARRY-438162, a selective, potent inhibitor of MEK 1/2 in clinical development for the treatment of inflammatory disease. Presented at the 14th International Inflammation Research Association Conference, Cambridge, MD.

Lang, I., Adenis, A., Boer, K., et al. (**2008**). AZD6244 (ARRY-142886) versus capecitabine (CAP) in patients (pts) with metastatic colorectal cancer (mCRC) who have failed prior chemotherapy. *J Clin Oncol.* 26(May 20 Suppl), Abst 4114.

Lee, P., Wallace, E., Yeh, T., et al. (**2004**). ARRY-142886, a potent and selective MEK inhibitor: III. Efficacy against human xenograft models correlates with decreased ERK phosphorylaiton. *Proc Am Assoc Cancer Res.* 45, Abst 3890.

LoRusso, P. M., Adjei, A. A., Varterasian, M., et al. (**2005**). Phase I and pharmacodynamic study of the oral MEK inhibitor CI-1040 in patients with advanced malignancies. *J Clin Oncol.* 23(23), 5281–5293.

Ma, W., and Quirion, R. (**2005**). The ERK/MAPK pathway, as a target for the treatment of neuropathic pain. *Expert Opin Ther Targets.* 9(4), 699–713.

Marks, J. L., Gong, Y., Chitale, D., et al. (**2008**). Novel MEK1 mutation identified by mutational analysis of epidermal growth factor receptor signaling pathway genes in lung adenocarcinoma. *Cancer Res.* 68(14), 5524–5528.

Meloche, S., and Pouyssegur, J. (**2007**). The ERK1/2 mitogen-activated protein kinase pathway as a master regulator of the G1- to S-phase transition. *Oncogene.* 26(22), 3227–3239.

Miller, V. A., Riely, G. J., Zakowski, M. F., et al. (**2008**). Molecular characteristics of bronchioloalveolar carcinoma and adenocarcinoma, bronchioloalveolar carcinoma subtype, predict response to erlotinib. *J Clin Oncol.* 26(9), 1472–1478.

Minino, A. M., Heron, M. P., Murphy, S. L., et al. (**2007**). Deaths: final data for 2004. *Natl Vital Stat Rep.* 55(19), 1–119.

Muller, K., Faeh, C., and Diederich, F. (**2007**). Fluorine in pharmaceuticals: looking beyond intuition. *Science.* 317(5846), 1881–1886.

Ohren, J. F., Chen, H., Pavlovsky, A., et al. (**2004**). Structures of human MAP kinase kinase 1 (MEK1) and MEK2 describe novel noncompetitive kinase inhibition. *Nat Struct Mol Biol.* 11(12), 1192–1197.

Pelletier, J. P., Fernandes, J. C., Brunet, J., et al. (**2003**). In vivo selective inhibition of mitogen-activated protein kinase kinase 1/2 in rabbit experimental osteoarthritis is associated with a reduction in the development of structural changes. *Arthritis Rheum.* 48(6), 1582–1593.

Pickle, L. W., Hao, Y., Jemal, A., et al. (**2007**). A new method of estimating United States and state-level cancer incidence counts for the current calendar year. *CA Cancer J Clin.* 57, 30–42.

Platanias, L. C. (**2003**). Map kinase signaling pathways and hematologic malignancies. *Blood.* 101(12), 4667–4679.

Rinehart, J., Adjei, A. A., LoRusso, P. M., et al. (**2004**). Multicenter Phase II study of the oral MEK inhibitor, CI-1040, in patients with advanced non-small-cell lung, breast, colon, and pancreatic cancer. *J Clin Oncol.* 22(22), 4456–4462.

Roberts, P. J., and Der, C. J. (**2007**). Targeting the Raf–MEK–ERK mitogen-activated protein kinase cascade for the treatment of cancer. *Oncogene.* 26(22), 3291–3310.

Scholl, F. A., Dumesic, P. A., and Khavari, P. A. (**2005**). Effects of active MEK1 expression in vivo. *Cancer Lett.* 230(1), 1–5.

Sebolt-Leopold, J. S., Dudley, D. T., Herrera, R., et al. (**1999**). Blockade of the MAP kinase pathway suppresses growth of colon tumors in vivo. *Nat Med.* 5(7), 810–816.

Shannon, A., Telfer, B., Babur, M., et al. (**2008**). Combining the potent MEK1/2 inhibitor AZD6244 (ARRY-142886) with radiotherapy in a lung tumor xenograft model; pharmacodynamic effects, therapeutic benefits and the hypoxia response. *Proc Am Assoc Cancer Res.* 49, Abst 2568.

Tecle, H. (**2002**). *The development of kinase inhibitors with unusual mechanism of action: CI-1040, a selective, non-ATP competitive MEK inhibitor in the clinic.* Presented at the IBC 2nd International Conference on Protein Kinases: Target Validation, Drug Discovery and Clinical Development of Kinase Therapeutics, Boston, MA.

Thiel, M. J., Schaefer, C. J., Lesch, M. E., et al. (**2007**). Central role of the MEK/ERK MAP kinase pathway in a mouse model of rheumatoid arthritis: potential proinflammatory mechanisms. *Arthritis Rheum.* 56(10), 3347–3357.

Turjanski, A. G., Vaque, J. P., and Gutkind, J. S. (**2007**). MAP kinases and the control of nuclear events. *Oncogene.* 26(22), 3240–3253.

Tzekova, V., Cebotaru, C., Ciuleanu, T., et al. (**2008**). Efficacy and safety of AZD6244 (ARRY-142886) as second/third-line treatment of patients (pts) with advanced non-small cell lung cancer (NSCLC). *J Clin Oncol.* 26(May 20 Suppl), Abst 8029.

Ussar, S., and Voss, T. (**2004**). MEK1 and MEK2, different regulators of the G1/S transition. *J Biol Chem.* 279(42), 43861–43869.

Van Custem, E., Lang, I., D'haens, G., et al. (**2008**). KRAS status and efficacy in the first-line treatment of patients with metastatic colorectal cancer (mCRC) treated with FOLFIRI with or without cetuximab: the CRYSTAL experience. *J Clin Oncol.* 26(May 20 Suppl; Abst 2).

Wallace, E., Yeh, T., Lyssikatos, J., et al. (**2004**). Preclinical development of ARRY-142886, a potent and selective MEK inhibitor. *Proc Am Assoc Cancer Res.* 45, Abst 3891.

Wallace, E., Lyssikatos, J., Blake, J., et al. (**2005**). 4-(4-Bromo-2-fluorophenylamino)-1-methyl-pyridin-2(1H)ones: potent and selective MEK 1,2 inhibitors. Presented at the 17th EORTC-NCI-AACR Symposium on Molecular Targets and Cancer Therapeutics, Philadelphia, PA.

Wallace, E. M., Lyssikatos, J., Blake, J. F., et al. (**2006**). Potent and selective mitogen-activated protein kinase kinase (MEK) 1,2 inhibitors. 1. 4-(4-Bromo-2-fluorophenylamino)-1-methylpyridin-2($1H$)-ones. *J Med Chem.* 49(2), 441–444.

Wang, X., Wang, H., Xu, L., et al. (**2003**). Significant neuroprotection against ischemic brain injury by inhibition of the MEK1 protein kinase in mice: exploration of potential mechanism associated with apoptosis. *J Pharmacol Exp Ther.* 304(1), 172–178.

Weinstein, I. B., and Joe, A. (**2008**). Oncogene addiction. *Cancer Res.* 68(9), 3077–3080; discussion 3080.

Wilkinson, R., Logie, A., Haupt, N., et al. (**2008**). Activity of the MEK1/2 inhibitor AZD6244 (ARRY-142886) in combination with standard and approved therapies: impact of in vivo sequencing of drug administration. *Proc Am Assoc Cancer Res.* 49, Abst 4012.

Xu, X., Quiros, R. M., Gattuso, P., et al. (**2003**). High prevalence of BRAF gene mutation in papillary thyroid carcinomas and thyroid tumor cell lines. *Cancer Res.* 63(15), 4561–4567.

Yeh, T. C., Marsh, V., Bernat, B. A., et al. (**2007**). Biological characterization of ARRY-142886 (AZD6244), a potent, highly selective mitogen-activated protein kinase kinase 1/2 inhibitor. *Clin Cancer Res.* 13(5), 1576–1583.

PART III

CELL CYCLE KINASE INHIBITORS: AURORA KINASE AND PLK INHIBITORS

10

DISCOVERY OF MK-0457 (VX-680)

Julian M. C. Golec

10.1. INTRODUCTION

The first Aurora kinase was discovered in 1995 by Glover and colleagues, from a search for mutations that affect the centrosome cycle in *Drosophila* (Glover et al., 1995). The connection between centrosome function and cancer accelerated the discovery of the three human counterparts. Human Aurora-1 (Aurora-B) and Aurora-2 (Aurora-A) were isolated in 1998 in a PCR screen to identify protein kinases that overexpressed in colon carcinomas (Bischoff et al., 1998). Aurora-3 (Aurora-C) came from a human placental cDNA library (Bernard et al., 1998). From 1998 onwards the interest in the Aurora kinases exploded, both from the perspective as targets for drugs against cancer and for the sake of better understanding the processes involved in the cell cycle. The interest continues unabated as judged by the number of recent reviews (Carvajal et al., 2006; Gautschi et al., 2006; Matthews et al., 2006; Naruganahalli et al., 2006; Fu et al., 2007).

Vertex became interested in the Aurora kinases as targets for new cancer drugs toward the end of the year 2000. The available knowledge at that time was well summarized in reviews by Bischoff and Plowman (1999) and Giet and Prigent (1999). The three Auroras were known to share high sequence identity (67–76%) in their catalytic domains (Bischoff and Plowman, 1999). Both *Aurora-A* and *Aurora-B* transcripts were found to be expressed at low levels in most tissues yet were abundant in mitotically active cells such as thymus. Both transcripts were highly expressed in a majority of human cell lines representing diverse tumor types. The kinase activity associated with Aurora-A was found to peak prior to the activation of Aurora-B, being maximal

Kinase Inhibitor Drugs. Edited by Rongshi Li and Jeffrey A. Stafford
Copyright © 2009 John Wiley & Sons, Inc.

in late G2 and prophase (Bischoff et al., 1998) (see Figure 10.1 for a schematic representation of the cell cycle and explanation of terms). Aurora-A-deficient cells were found to arrest in mitosis. They were able to form a bipolar mitotic spindle, but the chromosomes failed to align on the metaphase plate, suggesting that the arrest point is in prophase (Bischoff and Plowman, 1999). The cellular localization and kinase activity of Aurora-B pointed to a role in the later stages of mitosis, namely, the anaphase and telophase. Experiments using the rat ortholog AIM1 of Aurora-B and a catalytically inactive form led to greater insight of the function of Aurora-B and what a small-molecule kinase inhibitor might do. In mink lung epithelial cells, induction of catalytically inactive AIM1 led to cells that had more than two nuclei. Similar results were seen in NRK-49F and KD cells. These multinucleated cells had normal spindle functions, normal condensation, and segregation of chromosomes and had no defect in nuclear division. Instead, expression of the AIM1 mutant appeared to disrupt formation of the cleavage furrow and prevents the ultimate separation of the two daughter cells at the final step of cytokinesis (Terada et al., 1998). Far less was known about Aurora-C. Its expression is limited to the testis, though levels were shown to be elevated in several cancer cell lines, highest during G2/M, localizing to the centrosome during mitosis from anaphase to cytokinesis and reducing after mitosis (Kimura et al., 1999).

Both Bischoff (Bischoff and Plowman, 1999) and Giet (Giet and Prigent, 1999) made a strong case for Aurora-A as the cancer target of choice. Aurora-B and Aurora-C were hardly mentioned in this context. Whereas the *Aurora-B* gene maps to chromosome 17p13 that is often deleted in a variety of human cancers, the *Aurora-A* gene maps to human chromosome 20q13, whose amplification is common to a variety of human malignancies and correlates with poor prognosis for patients with node-negative breast cancer. The fact that *Aurora-A* can act as an oncogene and is able to transform both Rat1 fibroblasts and mouse NIH3T3 cells added further weight to the argument (Bischoff et al., 1998). Therefore, in accordance with the wisdom of the day, we decided that our crystallography and screening campaigns would be directed toward Aurora-A. This decision was taken with some trepidation since cell death, the ultimate aim of any antimitotic drug, had only been mentioned in the context of Aurora-B kinase disruption (Terada et al., 1998). We took some comfort from the view that the kinase active sites were likely to be so similar that it would be some time before we were able to prepare compounds that demonstrated good selectivity between the two kinases. Aurora-C was barely considered.

Despite the fact that all three Aurora kinases share similar sequences, especially in their catalytic domains, their localization and functions are quite different. All three Aurora enzymes reach peak expression at the G2/M point of the cell cycle. Aurora-A is primarily associated with the centrosomes and regions of microtubules that are proximal to them. Aurora-B is a chromosomal passenger protein that is nuclear in the prophase, found in the inner centromere in the metaphase, on the spindle midzone at anaphase and finally concentrates in the midbody at the point of cytokinesis. The two kinases, Aurora-A

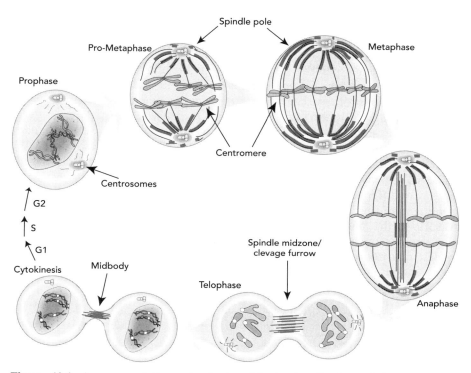

Figure 10.1. A representation of mitosis with the localization of Aurora-A and Aurora-B kinases highlighted in blue and orange, respectively. The mitotic phase of the cell cycle is characterized by six phases. *Prophase*: loosely coiled duplicated genetic material (chromatin) in the nucleus is condensed into the ordered chromosomes (comprising two sister chromatids). The centrosomes, which were duplicated earlier in the cell cycle, begin to segregate and nucleate microtubule material that will form the spindle pole. *Pro-metaphase*: the centrosomes migrate to opposite ends of the cell, the nuclear envelope breaks down, and the microtubule network of the spindle is extended. Microtubules begin to attach to the middle of the chromosome (kinetochore) and tension within the spindle begins to exert a force on the microtubule-kinetochore, pulling it toward the centrosome. *Metaphase*: the spindle checkpoint machinery is activated to ensure microtobules from opposing centrosomes successfully capture kinetochores from each of the two sister chromatids in the chromosome. Opposing tension in the spindle leads to alignment of the chromosomes at the metaphase plate in the middle of the cell. Progression beyond this phase of the cell cycle requires that all chromosomes are correctly captured and aligned. This is policed by the spindle checkpoint. *Anaphase*: the two sister chromatids are separated by the anaphase promoting complex. Each chromatid is pulled toward the opposing pole and the microtubule network begins to extend, elongating the cell. *Telophase*: the two identical copies of genetic material accumulate at opposite ends of the elongated cell and unfold back to form the chromatin. A new nuclear envelope is formed around each set of genetic information forming two nuclei. The extended microtubule network pinches at the middle of the cell between the two nuclei where the metaphase plate used to be, forming a cleavage furrow. *Cytokinesis*: a contractile ring is formed at the cleavage furrow that pinches off the two separate nuclei into two identical daughter cells.

and Aurora-B, require different proteins for their regulation and activation. The most studied protein associated with Aurora-A is TPX2. This activates the enzyme and targets it to the microtubules proximal to the centrosome. Aurora-B becomes part of a complex with the inner centromere protein (INCENP) and survivin. Complex formation activates Aurora-B and INCENP targets the complex to the centromeres, the spindle midzone, and the cleavage furrow, dependent on the stage of mitosis. Of course, all this is a great over-simplification and more detailed information can be found in several excellent reviews (Carmena and Earnshaw, 2003; Warner et al., 2006; Agnese et al., 2007; Ruchaud et al., 2007). It is now clear that small-molecule kinase inhibitors with different selectivity profiles between the Aurora kinases can be expected to have very different effects on cells and consequently different utilities in the treatment of cancer. Since taking the decision to focus our attention on Aurora-A, the understanding of the function of the three Aurora kinase enzymes has improved dramatically. This increasing knowledge has helped to explain many of the strange structure–activity relationships we saw in the lead optimization phase of the program.

10.2. EARLY MEDICINAL CHEMISTRY

A screen against full-length Aurora-A (1–403) yielded several reversible inhib-itors that were shown to be competitive with ATP. We chose to work on the most potent, a pyridine (compound **1**; Table 10.1) that had a $K_i = 62$ nM. For a preliminary view on selectivity, compounds were also tested for inhibition of full-length GSK-3β, the kinase that was regarded as the most similar in sequence to the Auroras, and full-length Src kinase as a guide to general kinase inhibition. Owing to problems in protein production, we were unable to measure Aurora-B inhibition in the early stages of the project. Cell potency was checked against inhibition of the proliferation of Colo205 cells as mea-sured by thymidine uptake and general cytotoxicity was checked for in periph-eral blood mononuclear cells (PBMCs) that were not cycling. In order to check that Colo205 cells were not giving misleading results, the lead compound was tested against ten different cell lines and activated lymphocytes. Results were consistent.

Prior to obtaining the first crystal structure of Aurora-A, medicinal chem-istry exploration revealed quite a lot about the lead molecule. It was quickly established that a whole host of substitutions at the 2-position of the quinazo-line core could yield active molecules and gains in potency. A series of quin-azolines carrying substituted phenyl groups at the 2-position were prepared, as epitomized by compound **3** (Table 10.1). Although only small gains in potency against Aurora-A were observed, selectivity against GSK-3β was enhanced in some examples. Changes to the 3-aminopryrazole portion of the molecule clearly showed that this group provided the key hydrogen-bonding interaction with the hinge region of Aurora-A and that the function could be

TABLE 10.1.

Compound	Structure	Aurora-A K_i (nM)	GSK-3β K_i (nM)	Colo205 IC$_{50}$ (nM)
1		62	76	2,500
2		58	30	1,300
3		11	70	1,500
4		7	20	700
5		20	170	3,000

TABLE 10.1. *Continued*

Compound	Structure	Aurora-A K_i (nM)	GSK-3β K_i (nM)	Colo205 IC$_{50}$ (nM)
6		1	253	700
7		1	>15,000	>12,000
8		12	200	>12,000

replicated by alternative heterocycles. The system proved very sensitive to substitution at the 4- and 5-posions of the pyrazole. The majority of lager substitutions diminished Aurora-A inhibition, though smaller substitutions (e.g., compound **4**; Table 10.1) enhanced activity at the expense of selectivity. A linking heteroatom, either nitrogen or sulfur at the 2-position of the quinazoline, was found to enhance potency without detriment to selectivity (e.g., compound **5**). The use of an oxygen linker was not as successful. With a combination of heteroatom-linked aryls at the 2-postion of the quinoline and small substitutions at the 5-position on the pyrazole, compounds with K_i values of around 1 nM and 100-fold selectivity against GSK-3β were prepared (e.g., compounds **6** and **7**).

While this short medicinal chemistry campaign had given many insights, many problems remained. Most obviously, no real gains in cell potency had been achieved and selectivity against Src kinase, our indicator for general kinase selectivity, did not follow our successes in the area of selectivity against GSK-3β. Several explanations for the poor cell potency were put forward. A trend connecting lower lipophilicity to increased cell potency was observed, but the fact that the most potent compounds had poor overall kinase selectivity and in some cases were generally cytotoxic clouded the issue. Inhibition of GSK-3β was also blamed since it had been shown that inhibition of this enzyme might inhibit apoptosis (Pap and Cooper, 1998; Bijur et al., 2000). The thought that the compounds may have been selective between the Aurora kinases themselves and that this might influence the observed cell potency was never raised.

10.3. FIRST CRYSTAL STRUCTURES

The first Aurora-A crystal structure to be solved was of a complex between compound **4** (Table 10.1) (Aurora-A $K_i = 7$ nM) and a truncated version of the enzyme (residues 107–403) (Figure 10.2). Co-complex structures of Aurora-A with adenosine (Cheetham et al., 2002) and GSK-3β with compound **1** (Table 10.1) were also solved. Although Aurora-A was shown to have an overall structure and topology that is closely related to both the Src and the AGC family of kinases, the structure did reveal how selectivity for Aurora-A over Src kinase and kinases with a similar active site sequence such as GSK-3β and CDK-2 might be attained. For instance, the 6-amino group of adenosine points toward a deep hydrophobic pocket formed by the flexible glycine-rich loop and the hinge region. This pocket contains several residues that are not conserved in Src kinase, GSK-3β, or CDK-2. In addition, when compared with GSK-3β and CDK-2, the hinge regions of Aurora-A and Src kinase contain a single glycine insertion that reduces the size and changes the conformation of the adenosine-binding pocket. The prospects for gaining selectivity between the Aurora kinases themselves were regarded as poor. In the sphere of protein

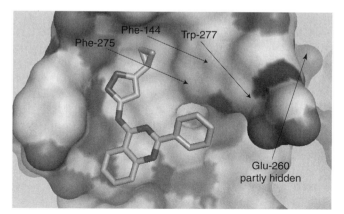

Figure 10.2. The first Aurora-A co-complex crystal structure (compound **4**) identified the binding orientation of the *N*-(1*H*-pyrazol-3-yl)quinazolin-4-amine inhibitors in the ATP-binding site.

residues surrounding the bound adenosine, only residue 217, which is threonine in Aurora-A and glutamic acid in both Aurora-B and Aurora-C, is not conserved. In Aurora-A, the side chain of Thr217 made a hydrogen bond with the main chain of residue Glu260 and appeared to play an important role in stabilizing the tertiary structure of the C-terminal kinase lobe. This residue difference was regarded as poorly accessible to a small-molecule inhibitor.

10.4. FIRST IN VIVO EXPERIMENTS

Despite the availability of this crystallography data, an explanation for the exquisite selectivity of the naphthalene compound **7** (Table 10.1) was not forthcoming. Owing to the compound's poor solubility, we were unable to obtain a co-crystal structure or more detailed biological data. One of the first attempts to produce a more polar mimic of the naphthalene led to the acetamide **9** (Table 10.2). This compound retained the potency and selectivity of the naphthalene and was found to be the most potent inhibitor of cell proliferation that we had seen so far. Compound **9** turned out to be a potent inhibitor of all three Aurora kinases—A, B, and C—giving K_i values of 4, 27, and 9 nM, respectively. When tested against 49 other kinases, it only showed a significant effect against Fyn kinase ($K_i = 280$ nM) and Tie-2 ($K_i = 230$ nM). IC_{50} values for inhibition of proliferation in a 96 hour [^{3}H]thymidine uptake assay involving a wide variety of normal and transformed mammalian cell types ranged from 100 to 1400 nM. No effects were seen on noncycling cells. Compound **9** caused the accumulation of cells in the G2/M phase of the cell cycle. As expected, the compound appeared to block cytokinesis and the percentage of cells with >4N DNA increased. These cells did not remain viable in prolonged culture; this was the first indication that a "selective" pan-Aurora inhibitor would cause the death of cycling cells. Although the compound had poor pharmacokinetic properties (bioavailability ≈ 40% and half-life ≈ 1.5 h in rats), it was tested in several xenograft models of cancer. Results were consistent: oral doses of 300 mg/kg twice daily (bid) were required to reduce tumor growth by around 50% in three xenografts. The body weights of the animals were largely unaffected, although the total white blood cell count in a rat model was reduced. Compound **9** had provided hope that a pan-Aurora inhibitor could provide a viable cancer therapy. However, the doses required for effect in the xenograft models showed that significant improvements in cell potency and ADME properties were essential.

10.5. THE DISCOVERY OF MK-0457 (VX-680)

Although no crystal structures of compounds analogous to **9** (Table 10.2) that incorporated a thioether at the 2-position of the quinazoline were available, co-complex structures of a couple of compounds carrying a nitrogen atom at

TABLE 10.2.

Compound	Structure	Aurora-A K_i (nM)	GSK-3β K_i (nM)	SRC K_i (nM)	Colo205 IC_{50} (nM)
9		4	>1,000	>1,000	300
10		<1	>1,215	965	900
11		3	1,700	1,600	500
12		2.5	>4,000	225	350

the same place gave direction for the next steps. The crystal structures led us to believe that further potency could be extracted by slightly increasing the size of the amide moiety on compound **9**. This proved to be the case. Too big an amide moiety caused loss of potency and a derivative of cyclopropane carboxylic acid (compound **10**; Table 10.2) proved optimal. Unfortunately, cell potency was diminished. High lipophilicity and low solubility were regarded as detrimental to cell potency and ADME properties. The crystal structures suggested that polar groups might be added to either the acetate carbon of compound **9** or to positions 7 or 8 of the quinazoline system. Most groups added to the acetate portion resulted in a loss of potency. However, the addition of a dimethylamino group resulted in compound **11** that was less lipohilic, more soluble, and with unchanged enzyme potency. Unfortunately, cell potency was essentially unchanged also and the compound was rapidly metabolized by rat liver microsomes. Substitutions in the 8-position of the quinazoline generally resulted in a drop in potency. Substitution at the 7-position gave better results as illustrated by compound **12**. A crystal structure of compound **12** in complex with Aurora-A showed why substitution at the 7-position was preferable. The compound itself offered no advantage over the original quinazoline **9**.

Despite having prepared many compounds with Aurora-A K_i values of around 1 nM and having decreased lipophilicity and improved solubility over compound **9**, no real progress had been made in improving cell potency. It was clear that a change in approach was called for. It had already been noted (compound **8**; Table 10.1) that the quinazoline scaffold was not essential for good inhibition of Aurora-A and that the smaller pyrimidine scaffold may provide greater potential for advantageous modification. As expected, a 6-phenylpyrimidine analog **13** (Table 10.3) of quinazoline **9** proved to be potent against Aurora-A, and gratifyingly, it had good ADME properties with bio-availability of nearly 60% and half-life of 3–4 h in rats. Unfortunately, there was no sign of improved cell potency. Despite this, compound **13** opened up the prospect of altering polarity and solubility without significantly increasing molecular weight. Compounds **14–17** (Table 10.3) provide examples of how this was done. Since a tenfold increase in cell potency had been obtained with essentially no change in potency against Aurora-A, the view that compound polarity and cell penetration was the key to good cell potency continued to hold sway. The discovery of compound **18**, that is, MK-0457, and compounds like its *t*-butylpiperazine analog **19**, where cell potency had increased from tenfold to several hundredfold over compounds with similar or "better" calculated log *P* and superior potency against Aurora-A, caused us to take serious issue with this view.

For reasons associated with physical and pharmacokinetic properties, MK-0457 was chosen as the compound to be examined more deeply (Harrington et al., 2004). It proved to be remarkably selective for the Aurora kinase family. K_i values were 0.6, 18, and 4.6 nM against Auroras-A, -B, and -C, respectively, and it showed over 100-fold selectivity for the Aurora-A against 55 out of 56 other kinase enzymes tested. The exception was the Fms-related tyrosine kinase (FLT3), where MK-0457 inhibited with a K_i value of 30 nM. MK-0457 potently inhibited proliferation of a wide variety of tumor cell types with IC_{50} values ranging from 15 to 113 nM and caused the accumulation of cells with 4N DNA content (polyploidy). Kawasaki et al. (2001) had shown that TPA-induced polyploidization of K562 cells was canceled by Aurora-B but not Aurora-A expression and that the downregulation of Aurora-B but not of Aurora-A was effective in inducing polyploidization. Therefore cells treated

TABLE 10.3.

Compound	Structure	Clog P	Auror-A K_i (nM)	Aurora-B K_i (nM)	Aurora-C K_i (nM)	GSK-3β K_i (nM)	SRC K_i (nM)	Colo205 IC$_{50}$ (nM)
13		5.6	<1	140	20	1,000	>2,000	1,000
14		4.2	<3	50	50	1,000	750	385
15		5.1	1	8	150	3,300	940	770

TABLE 10.3. *Continued*

Compound	Structure	Clog P	Auror-A K_i (nM)	Aurora-B K_i (nM)	Aurora-C K_i (nM)	GSK-3β K_i (nM)	SRC K_i (nM)	Colo205 IC$_{50}$ (nM)
16		3.7	1	15	130	>3,000	400	108
17		3.7	3.5	18	70	>7,500	550	680

Compound	Structure	$C\log P$	Auror-A K_i (nM)	Aurora-B K_i (nM)	Aurora-C K_i (nM)	GSK-3β K_i (nM)	SRC K_i (nM)	Colo205 IC$_{50}$ (nM)
18		4.3	0.6	18	4.6	>10,000	300	30
19		5.4	1	11	15	>10,000	280	1.5
20		5.0	1.3	10	12	1,000	>3,000	250

with MK-0457 showed a phenotype more consistent with what one might expect for Aurora-B inhibition rather than Aurora-A inhibition. Although the quinazoline **9** (Table 10.1) had given us faith that an Aurora inhibitor would cause the death of cycling cells, the potential was probed more deeply with MK-0457. MK-0457 induced cell death through apoptosis in a wide panel of tumor cell lines. Leukemia, lymphoma, and colorectal cancer cell lines were particularly sensitive. In addition to killing immortalized tumor cell lines, MK-0457 completely ablated colony formation of primary leukemic cells from patients with acute myeloid leukemia (AML) (CFU-L) who were refractory to standard therapies and primary leukemic cells possessing FLT3 ITD mutations. Activating mutations of FLT3 confer a poor prognosis (Sawyers, 2002; Gale et al., 2008) in AML cases and the fact that MK-0457 had been found to be a good inhibitor of FLT3 was seen as an advantage for the compound. As expected, MK-0457 was found to inhibit the proliferation of PHA-stimulated primary human lymphocytes (IC_{50} = 79 nM) but had no effect on the viability of noncycling peripheral blood mononuclear cells at concentrations as high as 10 μM. The lack of toxicity on resting cells increased our expectation that Aurora inhibition is a viable target for intervention in oncology.

To evaluate its potential in vivo, MK-0457 was tested in four xenograft types. In three of them, MK-0457 caused tumor regression to a greater or lesser degree. For instance, in a human AML (HL-60) xenograft model, MK-0457 dosed intraperitoneally at 75 mg/kg bid for 13 days reduced mean tumor volumes by 98% in comparison to the control group. In 4 out of 10 animals, the final tumor volume was lower than the initial volume prior to dosing. MK-0457 was well tolerated with a 5% decrease in body weight observed only at the highest dose. By comparison, treatment with a previously determined maximum tolerated dose (MTD) schedule of cisplatin gave only a 27% inhibition of tumor growth. Similar results were seen in a model of pancreatic cancer (MIA PaCa-2), where MK-0457 dosed intraperitoneally at 50 mg/kg bid induced regression in 7 out of 10 tumors with a 22% decrease in mean tumor volume relative to initial tumor size prior to dosing. In comparison, 5-fluorouracil, administered intravenously on every fourth day at a maximum tolerated dose of 50 mg/kg, gave a 77% inhibition of tumor growth versus control. For an orthotopic cancer model we used the human breast tumor line MDA-MB-231. In vitro studies indicated that this cell line was one of the most resistant to the cytotoxic effects of MK-0457. The fact that MK-0457 and taxol gave similar results of 35% inhibition of tumor growth versus control at their respective maximum tolerated doses was regarded as encouraging.

In order to obtain information regarding the likely therapeutic index of the molecule, we developed a human colon xenograft model in nude rats. This allowed us to more easily look at white blood cell counts and administer the compound by intravenous infusions. Using the interperitoneal route of administration, a 3 day/week dosing cycle was found to give maximal efficacy and allow control over the myelotoxicity. Two doses per day of 50 mg/kg resulted in a 93% decrease in tumor growth and a body weight loss of 15%

that recovered during the dosing holiday. This almost total inhibition of tumor growth was obtained with a well-tolerated drop of 27% in the neutrophil counts. Inhibition of tumor growth was paralleled by a reduction of histone H3 phosphorylation and a significant increase in apoptosis as measured by TUNEL staining within the tumor tissue. In the infusion experiment, MK-0457 was administered at 0.5, 1, and 2 mg/kg/h continuously for 3 days via an indwelling femoral catheter. This was followed by a saline infusion for 4 days before repeating the dose cycle. Tumor growth was halted in the 1 mg/kg/h group with 4 out of 7 tumors showing regression. This was achieved with no loss of body weight, and only transient effects on white blood cell counts. No signs of mechanism-independent toxicity of the compound were observed. In normal, as opposed to nude rats, MK-0457 was administered at 1 mg/kg/h for 5 days and caused no outward signs of toxicity, no clinical chemistry changes, and only a 50% reduction of white blood cell count. These data indicated that MK-0457 had a chance of providing a high enough therapeutic index for use as chemotherapy.

10.6. INSIGHTS INTO MECHANISM AND STRUCTURE–ACTIVITY RELATIONSHIPS

Studies with MK-0457 had provided further good evidence that inhibition of Aurora kinases would provide a new approach to cancer therapy. The compound's overall properties, biological and physical, recommended it as suitable for clinical development. However, the path to the discovery of MK-0457 had thrown up many questions, the answers to which would help in the design of backup and improved follow-up molecules: (1) Is there an explanation for the selectivity profile? (ii) What causes the anomalies in the structure–activity relationships; (iii) What are the causes of the cell phenotype that gives the appearance that Aurora-B inhibition overrides Aurora-A?

In our first Aurora-A crystal structure (Cheetham et al., 2002) and 16 further co-complexes prior to the discovery of MK-0457, residues 273–278, located at the N-terminal end of the activation loop were clearly visible and appeared to adopt a unique conformation. Other kinase crystal structures published up to this point were similar to each other but different from the Aurora-A structure. In these structures the activation loop adopts an extended conformation irrespective of whether an activated or dephosphorylated kinase was used for crystallization. Crystal structures of cAMP-dependent protein kinases complexed with ATP or adenosine and a peptide substrate were thought to represent the bioactive conformations of protein kinases (Bossemeyer et al., 1993; Narayana et al., 1997). In contrast, the activation loop residues of Aurora-A—Asp274, Phe275, Gly276, and Trp277—adopted a closed conformation where Trp277 folds into the active site and where the expected salt bridge interaction between the catalytic residues Asp274 and Lys162, seen in most other kinase structures, was not observed. Although these observations may have been a crystallization artifact, they prompted us to ask if they might explain some of the structure–activity relationship anomalies and possibly the selectivity profile. Interestingly, the methodology used for the procurement of co-complex crystals had to be varied considerably from compound to compound. The MK-0457–Aurora-A co-complex crystals were the most difficult to obtain and we suspected that compounds were causing enough changes to the protein conformation to disrupt crystallization.

It was originally believed that one of the reasons that Aurora-A formed a closed conformation in the co-complex crystal structures is its ability to form an interaction between Trp277 and Phe275 of the activation loop with Phe144 in the flexible glycine-rich loop (see Figure 10.2 for positions in early structures). Although similarly placed combinations of aromatic residues are found in many other kinases, including FLT (Griffith et al., 2004) and BCR-ABL (Schindler et al., 2000), such interactions between the activation loop and glycine-rich loop had not been reported. Since Trp277 is conserved in all three human Aurora kinases and there appeared to be no other kinase with a tryptophan located at this position, this conformational behavior was considered to be unique to the Aurora family and dependent on the tryptophan. In our extended checks on MK-0457 selectivity, four kinases were inhibited with $IC_{50} < 1\,\mu M$: Lck (leukocyte-specific protein tyrosine kinase) (estimated $K_i = 75\,nM$), Src ($K_i = 300\,nM$), FLT3 ($K_i = 30\,nM$), and BCR-ABL ($K_i = 30\,nM$). It was therefore clear that our original ideas concerning selectivity predictions needed to be revised. Based on pure sequence analysis, we had thought that obtaining selectivity against GSK-3β would be the most difficult, yet MK-0457 gave a K_i value against this enzyme of $>10\,\mu M$. Lck, Src, FLT3, and BCR-ABL all turned out to be kinases that have combinations of aromatic residues in similar places to residues Trp277, Phe275, and Phe144 in Aurora-A. It seemed that Trp277 on its own was not so important and that selectivity could be better explained by the propensity for certain kinases to adopt a particular conformation.

The ability of MK-0457 to inhibit FLT3 was seen as a potential advantage since mutations in this receptor tyrosine kinase are present in approximately 30% of patients with newly diagnosed AML. These mutations come in two forms; their relationship to other genetic lesions and clinical outcome is complex and has been much studied. Clinical investigations by Gale et al. (2008) and Bacher et al. (2008), together with references therein, provide much insight. The potency of MK-0457 against ABL was regarded as more exciting. During the 1970s it was reported that most patients with chronic myeloid leukemia (CML) carried the Philadelphia chromosome abnormality that had originally been described 13 years earlier. The Philadelphia chromosome causes a gene fusion between *BCR* and *ABL* that transforms the native ABL tyrosine kinase into one that is constitutively activated and enhances proliferation and viability of myeloid lineage cells. By 1990, the oncogenic capabilities of BCR-ABL were demonstrated in mouse models, where expression was shown to be sufficient to cause leukemia, and in 1996 scientists from

Ciba-Geigy had shown that a molecule designed to inhibit ABL was able to kill cell lines expressing the fusion protein but did not kill the cell lines from which they were derived. This compound, imatinib, went on to become the benchmark for targeted cancer therapies and a highly successful drug. Most chronic phase CML patients respond well to imatinib treatment although some relapsed and/or progressed to an accelerated phase or blast crisis. For patients with advanced phases of CML, imatinib treatment gives an early response in most instances, followed by relapse. Relapse is generally associated with reactivation of BCR-ABL signaling. The most common mechanisms by which this occurs are through point mutations of the kinase domain that either decreased sensitivity to imatinib by mutation of the binding residues (e.g., T315I, F317L, and F359V) or mutation of residues that cause overall conformational changes that also decrease imatinib binding. This subject has been reviewed extensively; for a recent synopsis see Sherbenou and Druker (2007). In 2002 Shah et al. (2002) conducted a BCR-ABL kinase domain sequencing analysis of 45 CML patients that had shown resistance to imatinib. They found that mutations in the BCR-ABL kinase domain occurred in over 90% of patients that relapsed after an initial response. They provided definitive evidence that at least eight mutants, the most common, play a causal role in imatinib resistance. Three mutations (T315I, E255K, and M351T) were found to account for more than 60% of the resistance cases in the study. MK-0457 turned out to have a K_i value of 42 nM against the T315I mutant, similar to that against the wild-type ABL kinase. In a more detailed study by Carter et al. (2005), binding constants for MK-0457 against eight imatinib-resistant ABL mutants were measured. Although MK-0457 was found to bind to wild-type ABL with an order of magnitude less potency than imatinib, its ability to bind the three most common resistant mutations was remarkably unchanged. In fact, where imatinib had K_d values of 2 nM and 6000 nM against wild-type ABL and T315, respectively, MK-0457 showed K_d values of 20 nM and 5 nM.

Crystallography was to provide some insight into the selectivity profile of MK-0457 and its ability to inhibit imatinib-resistant ABL mutants. Following the determination of binding constants for MK-0457 against resistant mutants, Young and colleagues attempted to provide a crystal structure of a co-complex between MK-0457 bound to Abl with a mutation at the gatekeeper position (e.g., T315I) (Young et al., 2006). Although they were not successful in doing this, they were able to provide a structure of the inhibitor bound to another imatinib-resistant mutant, ABL H396P, for which MK-0457 has K_d = 7 nM. The structure of this mutant form of the Abl kinase domain was seen to be in an active form, which closely mimics the structure of activated and phosphorylated Lck. Comparisons were made between this structure and the structure of what was regarded as an active form of Aurora-A (Nowakowski et al., 2002). Eight of the 14 contact side chains were found to be identical between ABL and Aurora, and four of the remaining six sites involved conservative substitutions. One of the nonconservative substitutions is at the periphery of the inhibitor-binding site and was not predicted to make close contact with the

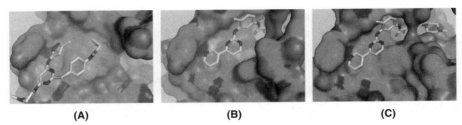

(A)   **(B)**   **(C)**

Figure 10.3. The crystal structures of MK-0457 bound to Aurora-A (**A**), imatinib bound to cKit kinase (**B**), and imatinib bound to ABL kinase (**C**). All three kinases have similar conformation in which the DFG activation loop presents a hydrophobic cap to the ATP-binding site. Although imatinib cannot easily be fitted into the inactive conformation of Aurora-A, MK-0457 can easily be modeled into the inactive conformations of ABL and Kit kinases (MK-0457 K_i(cKit) = 150 nM; K_i(ABL) = 30 nM).

inhibitor. The other nonconservative substitution is found at the gatekeeper position, where Thr315 in ABL is replaced by Leu210 in Aurora-A. By aligning the structures of ABL and Aurora-A on the hinge regions of the two kinases, it was shown that MK-0457 can be accommodated into Aurora-A with a small adjustment in side-chain conformation that should be readily accessible to the protein. Taking this model further and by considering hydrogen-bond interactions, MK-0457 was predicted to bind the ABL (T315I) mutant, where imatinib is ineffective. Thus an explanation for the MK-0457 selectivity profile was provided.

The crystal structure of MK-0457 in complex with the unphosphorylated catalytic domain of Aurora-A (Cheetham et al., 2007) (Figure 10.3) suggested a different approach to understanding the ability of MK-0457 to inhibit imatinib-resistant mutations of ABL might be taken. Further to the original crystal structure of Aurora-A where the enzyme can be considered closed and inactive (Cheetham et al., 2002), two more important crystal structures were published that provided insight into Aurora-A activation. The Nowakowski structure (Nowakowski et al., 2002) used in the comparison with the MK-0457–ABL(H396P) complex, was different and regarded as showing an open and active confirmation. Aurora-A is activated by phosphorylation and association with the protein TPX2 that also localizes it to spindle microtubules. Bayliss et al. (2003) provided great insight into the mechanisms involved in Aurora-A activation by solving a crystal structure of a phosphorylated form of Aurora-A in complex with a 43 residue long domain of TPX2. This structure was different from the previous two and can probably be regarded as a good representation of the fully functional activated kinase. The MK-0457 –Aurora-A co-complex showed Aurora-A in a different conformation to either the Nowakowski or the Bayliss structure. Although several residues in the activation loop were only partially ordered, residues Asp274, Phe275, and Trp277 were clearly visible and formed a cap to the active site that would have obstructed the binding of ATP. These residues created a hydrophobic

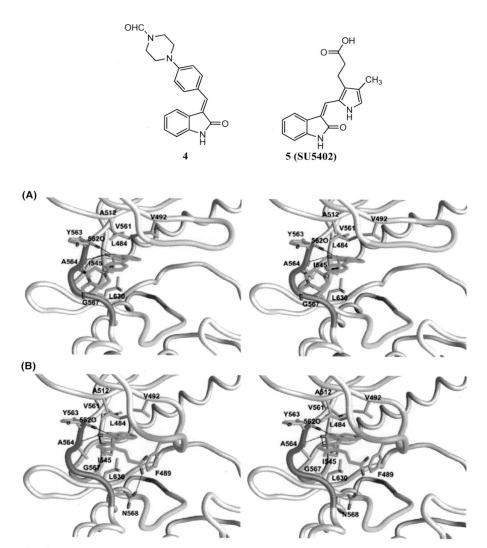

Figure 1.2. Co-crystal structure of SU5402 and compound 4 in FGFR1 kinase domain (Mohammadi et al., (1997). Stereoviews of the inhibitor binding sites. The side chains of residues that interact with the inhibitors are shown. Carbon atoms of the inhibitor and FGFR1K are green and orange, respectively; oxygen atoms are red and nitrogen atoms are blue. Selected hydrogen bonds are shown as black lines. (**A**) FGFR1K-4. (**B**) FGFR1K-SU5402.

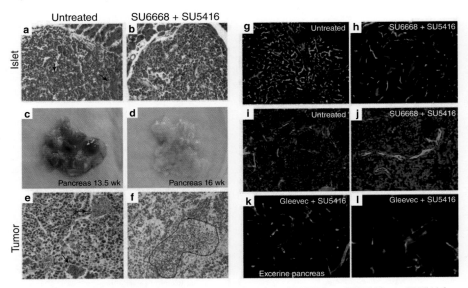

Figure 1.9. Effects of the combined therapy using SU5416 + SU6668 or SU5416 + imatinib. (See text for full caption.)

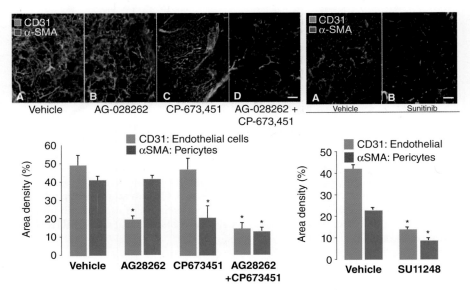

Figure 1.12. Effects of SU11248, a selective VEGFR inhibitor, or a selective PDGFR inhibitor on density of CD31 positive microvessels or α-SMA positive perivascular endothelia in RIP1-Tag2 islet cell tumors (Yao et al. 2006). (See text for full caption.)

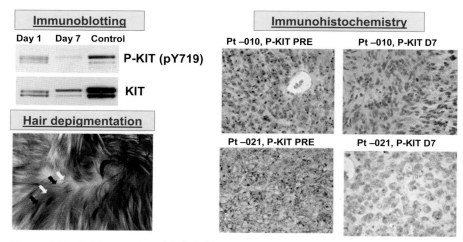

Figure 1.16. Evidence of sunitinib inhibition of KIT in repeat GIST tumor biopsies and KIT-dependent hair pigmentation (Moss et al., 2003; Demetri et al., 2004; Davis et al., 2005). (*Upper left panel*) Repeated resected biopsies (baseline and day 7 post–treatment) were obtained from a GIST patient, frozen, protein lysates were created and resolved by SDS-PAGE, transferred and immunoblots were performed utilizing total KIT and phosphorylated KIT (phosphotyrosine 719) antibodies. Results indicated a qualitative reduction in the levels of phosphorylated KIT following 7 days of sunitinib administration at 50 mg/day. (*Right panel*) Repeated biopsies (baseline and day 7 post– treatment) were obtained from 2 GIST patients (patients 010 and 021), were formalin-fixed and paraffin-embedded, and immunohistochemistry was performed utilizing a phosphorylated KIT (phosphotyrosine 719) antibody. Results indicated a qualitative reduction in the levels of phosphorylated KIT following 7 days of sunitinib administration at 50 mg/day. (*Lower left panel*) Images of study subject with metastatic synovial sarcoma undergoing treatment with SU11248. This subject received multiple 6 week cycles of treatment over a 4 week period receiving 50 mg SU11248 daily and a 2 week break from treatment. Cyclical hair depigmentation is evident that was concordant with the treatment regimen. Depigmented bands of hair grown during periods when the patient was receiving SU11248 (*white arrows*) are distinct from pigmented bands of hair grown during drug-free breaks (*black arrows*).

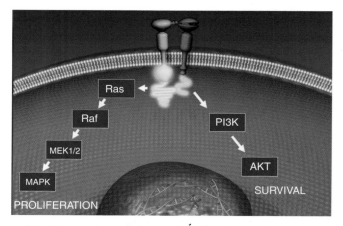

Figure 2.2. Schematic rendition of the erbB family signaling pathway.

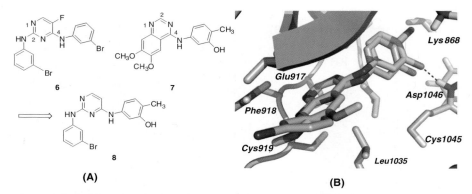

Figure 3.3. (**A**) The binding modes of screening hits **6** and **7** suggested the synthesis of pyrimidine **8** (**B**) Pyrimidine **8** is overlaid with quinazoline **7**, revealing an identical interaction to the Asp1046 NH by both hydroxyaniline OH groups.

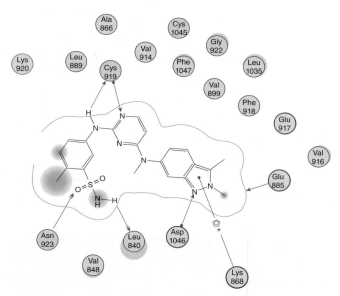

Figure 3.13. Two-dimensional interaction map of pazopanib with VEGFR2 kinase generated from MOE software (Chemical Computing Group, Montreal, QC). Amino acids with polar side chains are depicted as lavender and nonpolar side chains as light green. Side chain interactions are noted with green arrows and backbone interactions are noted with blue arrows. Shading represents degree of solvent exposure.

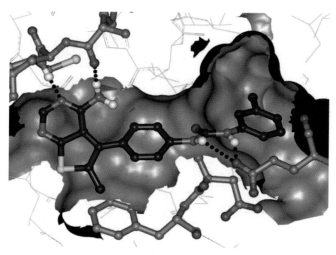

Figure 4.6. Model of **6b** bound to KDR kinase. Hydrogen bonds in black are shown between the urea NHs and Glu885 carboxylate, between the exocyclic amine and Glu917 backbone carbonyl, and between the ring nitrogen and Cys919 N-H. Also in thick bond are residues Asp1046-Phe1047 of the "DFG" motif in the "inactive" conformation ("DFG-out"). Reprinted with permission from *J Med Chem*. 2005, 48, 6066–6083. Copyright © 2005 American Chemical Society.

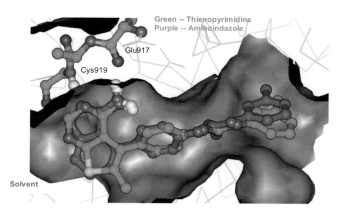

Figure 4.10. Overlap of thienopyrimidine **6b** (green) and aminoindazole **9b** (purple) bound to KDR kinase.

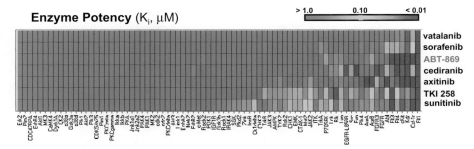

Figure 4.14. Kinase inhibition profile.

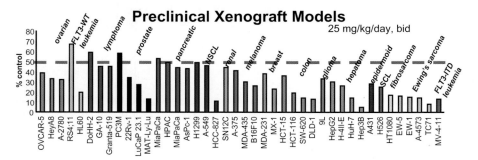

Figure 4.20. Summary of the effects of ABT-869 in preclinical xenograft models.

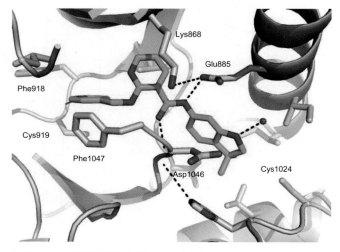

Figure 5.6. Active site of VEGFR2 kinase with bound motesanib. The red sphere is a tightly bound water molecule (PDB code 3EFL). Construct: E815 through D1171 with a C-terminal His-tag. Mutations: C817A; E990V; kinase insert domain (T940-E989) deleted. Resolution: 2.2 Å.

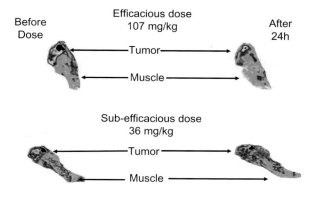

Higher contrast uptake, i.e., higher blood flow   Lower contrast uptake, i.e., lower blood flow

Figure 6.9. DCE-MRI analysis of coronal single slice images through the tumor and the muscle of the hind limb area before and 24 hours after administration of brivanib in the L2987 lung xenograft mouse model showing a markedly reduced uptake of contrast agent with brivanib 107 mg/kg compared with the 36 mg/kg dose, indicating lower blood flow to the tumor.

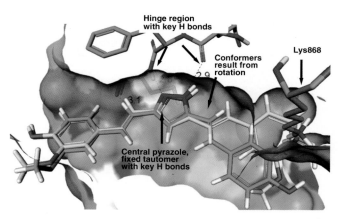

Figure 7.3. Perspective is from the top of the standard viewpoint. Two conformations (one in yellow and one in green) of pyrazole hit **1** are shown modeled into the solved, ligand-free p-VEGFR2Δ50 structure.

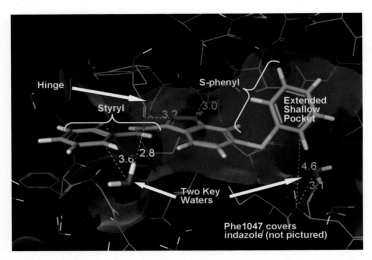

Figure 7.6. The DFG-out conformation was induced by design within the indazole series. The indazole **25** binds tightly in a tunnel. The protein in the foreground has been removed for clarity. To the left is solvent and to the lower right is a deep pocket generated by the rearrangement of the DFG loop. On each side of the ligand is highlighted a key crystallographic water.

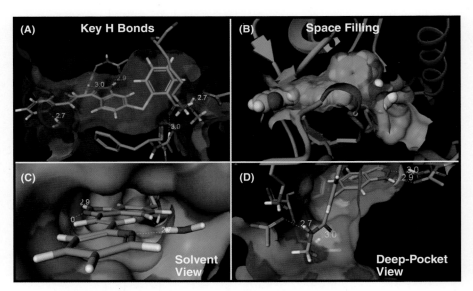

Figure 7.10. Axitinib benefits from each design concept discussed, as can be seen in the four views, to give exceedingly potent inhibition of VEGFR1, 2, and 3 kinases: (**A**) front side view with H bonds highlighted, (**B**) space-filling model demonstrating shape and size complementarity, (**C**) view from left, down the tunnel, and (**D**) view from right, down the tunnel.

(C)

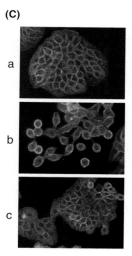

Figure 8.4. Preclinical biological profile of CI-1040. (**C**) Inhibition of HGF-induced cell scattering in HT-29 cells was measured by F-actin statining (Sebolt-Leopold et al., 1999): (a) control cells, (b) +HGF only, (c) +HGF in addition to 1 μM CI-1040. (See text for full caption.)

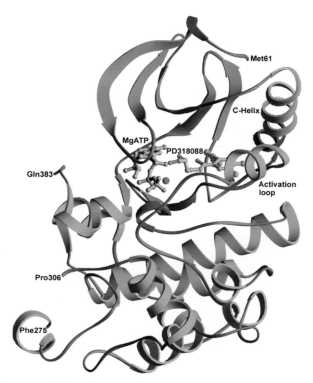

Figure 8.6. Structure of MEK/ATP/PD0318088 ternary complex. (Ohren et al., 2004.)

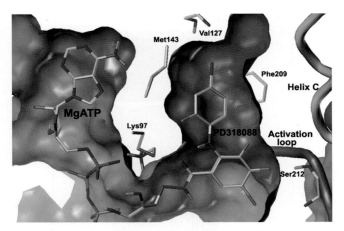

Figure 8.7. Mg-ATP and PD0318088 occupy distinct and adjacent binding sites within the interlobal cleft of MEK kinase. (Ohren et al., 2004.)

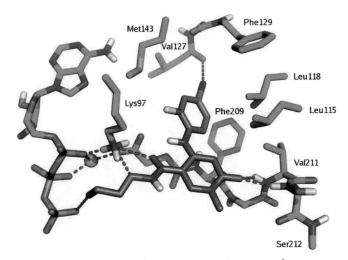

Figure 9.11. X-ray of pyridone bound to MEK1 (3.4 Å resolution).

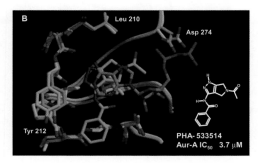

Figure 11.4. (**B**) Superposition of the Aurora-A complex with PHA-533514 (green carbon atoms for the protein, cyan for the compound) on that of the structure of Aurora-A complexed with ADP.

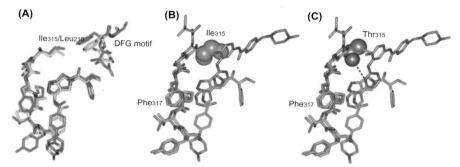

Figure 11.7. (**A**) Details of the binding of PHA-739358 to Abl (green carbon atoms) and to Aurora-A (yellow carbon atoms). (**B, C**) PHA-739358 complex (green carbon atoms) superimposed with the structure of imatinib (magenta carbon atoms). The gatekeeper residues Ile315 of PHA-739358 complex (A) and Thr315 of the imatinib complex (B) are shown with van der Waals spheres. In the T315I mutant, the isoleucine side chain causes a steric clash with imatinib; in addition, the hydrogen bond between imatinib and the side chain oxygen of threonine is lost. Adapted from *Cancer Res.* **2007**, 67, 7987– 7990.

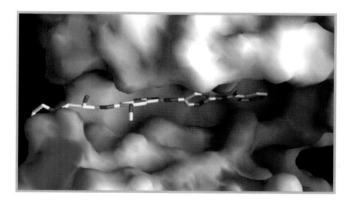

18

Figure 12.2. X-ray crystal structure (2.1 Å) of GSMH-[T287D]Aurora-A (122–400) and compound **18**.

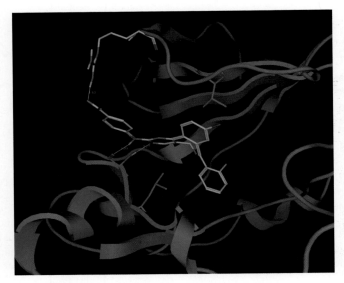

Figure 13.6. ML2 docked in Aurora-A active site.

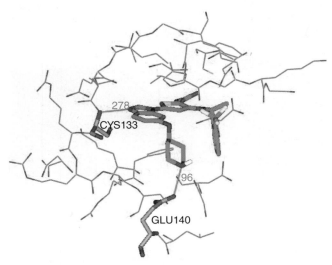

Figure 14.3. Homology model of compound **91** docked into Plk1.

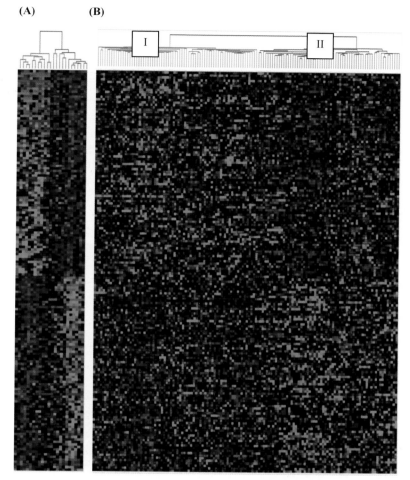

Figure 15.2. Hierarchical clustering analysis depicting the expression patterns of "dasatinib sensitivity gene signature." This figure is adopted from Huang et al. 2007. Each column represents a cell line or tumor and each row represents a gene. The matrix represents normalized expression patterns for each gene. Red indicates relatively high expression and green indicates relatively low expression. (**A**) The relative expression levels of 161 genes ("dasatinib sensitivity gene signature") that are highly correlated with dasatinib sensitivity/resistance classification in 23 breast cell lines. The sensitive cell lines are labeled in blue and resistant cell lines are labeled in red. (**B**) The expression patterns of "dasatinib sensitivity gene signature" in 134 breast tumors. Cluster I is the potential dasatinib nonresponder population labeled in red and cluster II is the potential dasatinib responder population labeled in blue.

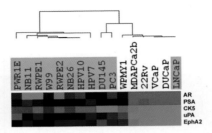

Figure 15.3. (D) Expression pattern of a five-gene set (AR, PSA, CK5, uPA, and EphA2) in prostate cell lines. Hierarchical clustering analysis of 16 cell lines using the five gene set with expression level highly correlated with dasatinib sensitivity/resistance classification. The sensitive cell lines are highlighted. This figure, courtesy of Dr. Xi-De Wang, is adapted from Wang et al. (2007).

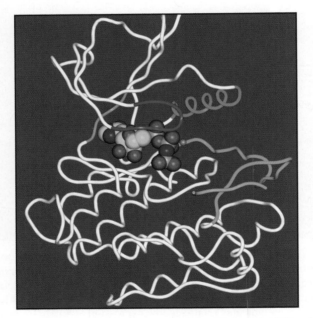

Figure 16.1. Representative protein kinase structure (Hubbard, 1997; pdb code 1IR3). ATP (nonhydrolyzable analog in this structure) binds into a cleft formed between the primary N (top) and C (bottom) terminal domains and engages in hydrogen bonding with the flexible hinge region (orange) that links the two domains. Key regulatory regions are the glycine-rich loop colored in magenta and draping over the phosphate-binding site; the activation loop colored in cyan; and the C-helix colored in green. A subset of kinase inhibitors target variations in conformation of these regulatory regions. Peptide inhibitor is shown is light green.

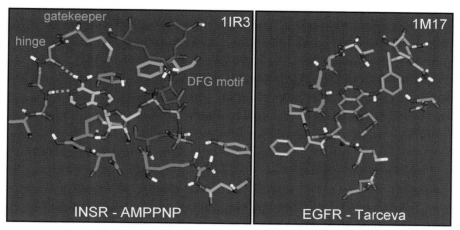

Figure 16.2. (*Left*) Close-up view of the insulin receptor ATP-binding site as determined by X-ray (Hubbard, 1997; pdb code 1IR3). Backbone atoms of the hinge region (orange) engage in hydrogen bonds with adenine N1 and exocylic amine N6 while the adenine ring system lies sandwiched between hydrophobic residues. Conserved catalytic residues are shown in magenta. The phenylalanine of the DFG motif is highlighted in cyan and the conformation is DFG in. On bottom left a portion of an inhibitor peptide (light green) is shown with tyrosine hydroxyl group proximal to gamma phosphate of AMPPNP analog. (*Right*) EGFR–Tarceva active sight as determined by X-ray (Stamos et al., 2002; pdb code 1M17). The anilino group projects into a back hydrophobic pocket made accessible by a small gatekeeper residue (Thr790). The catechol ether moiety of Tarceva also projects into a hydrophobic space, and then to solvent, at the front of the binding site. Both of these regions are unoccupied by ATP.

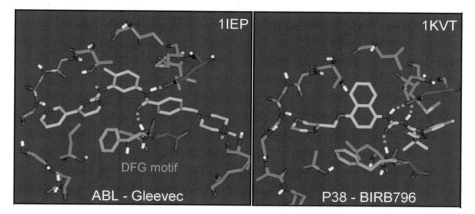

Figure 16.3. (*Left*) ABL–Gleevec structure as determined by X-ray crystallography (Schindler et al., 2000; pdb code 1IEP). The structure exemplifies the DFG-out kinase motif in which the phenylalanine is relocated from its position in a catalytically active kinase to, in this case, a position roughly adjacent to where the ATP ribose would be. The phenyl amide moiety occupies the region where the phenylalanine normally resides and makes hydrogen bonds to both the backbone NH of the DFG aspartate and carboxyl group of the catalytic glutamate from the C-helix. The piperazine group reaches solvent on the backside of the protein. (*Right*) P38– BIRB796 structure as a second example of the DFG-out binding motif (Pargellis et al., 2002; pdb code 1KVT). A *tert*-butyl-pyrazole-urea functionality provides pharmacophore elements analogous to the phenyl-amide group of Gleevec. Because of the strong interactions with the allosteric binding region, the ligand has a diminished need for strong interactions in the adenine-binding region, which is occupied by the morpholino group.

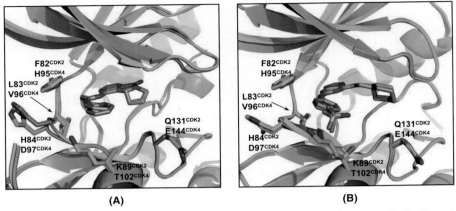

Figure 17.4. Overlays of CDK2 and CDK2/CDK4 chimeras. For both panels, the ligand and residues that impact residue specificity are shown in stick representations. (**A**) The crystal structures from Ikuta et al. (2001) of CDK2 (PDB code: 1GII, blue) and a CDK2/CDK4 chimera (PDB code: 1GIJ, green). Residues His84 and Gln131, which can impact specificity but aren't mutated, are colored orange. (**B**) The crystal structures from Pratt et al. 2006 of two different CDK2/CDK4 chimeras (PDB codes: 2IW9, blue and 2IW8, green). Residue Gln131, which can impact specificity but isn't mutated in either of the chimeras, is colored orange.

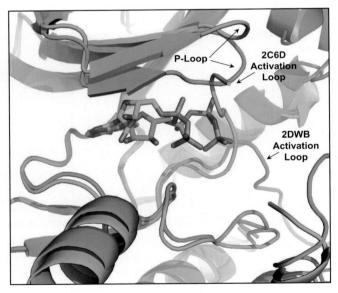

Figure 17.7. Two different crystal structures of Aurora-A bound to AMPPNP. The structure of the T287D construct (PDB code: 2C6D; Heron et al., 2006) is shown in blue. The wild-type construct is shown in green (PDB code: 2DWB). There is a significant amount of structural divergence between the two structures—mainly in the regions of the activation loop and P-loop. This is likely arising due to a combination of the T287D mutation and crystallization conditions. Note that for the sake of clarity, only one of the two conformations of the 2C6D AMPPNP molecule is shown. Also, the γ-phosphate of the 2CSD AMPPNP is disordered.

pocket that appeared to facilitate MK-0457 binding. The catalytic residues Asp275, Lys162, and Glu181 were disrupted such that Asp275 is rotated by approximately 180° from the normal (a 7 Å shift), thus converting a hydrophilic pocket that provides the enzyme's metal binding capability into a hydrophobic pocket. The cyclopropyl group of MK-0457 made a series of hydrophobic interactions that would not have been possible if the enzyme were in an open conformation. This Aurora-A conformation turned out to be remarkably similar to the conformation adopted by ABL when bound to imatinib (Nagar et al., 2002) and an analog (Schindler et al., 2000) (Figure 10.3). Both ABL and Aurora-A exhibited closed inactive conformations that appeared to be stabilized by inhibitor interactions. The propensity for MK-0457 to bind to an inactive Aurora conformation provides an explanation for its high degree of selectivity; most kinases are either unable to adopt a comparable closed conformation or lack key residues that form the critical hydrophobic pocket. Those that can adopt such a conformation include FLT3 and ABL kinases. Comparison between the Aurora-A/MK-0457 structure and the ABL/imatinib structures shows that these inhibitors exploit a different set of interactions with their respective kinases. Imatinib appears to derive most of its binding affinity through extensive interactions with a hydrophobic pocket present only in the inactive conformation of ABL kinase, whereas MK-0457 forms a greater number of hydrogen bonds with the hinge region and exploits a lipophilic pocket that, although unused by imatinib, is present in both enzymes and imatinib-resistant mutants. Modeling the ABL-resistant mutants in the context of the closed ABL/imatinib conformation predicts results that are consistent with experimental observation (Carter et al., 2005).

Crystal structures had gone some way to explaining the selectivity profile of MK-0457 but had not explained the anomalies in the structure–activity relationships or the observed cellular phenotypes. The most obvious anomaly in structure–activity relationships was the disconnection between enzyme and cell potency. This is clearly illustrated in comparing compounds **18**, **19**, and **20** (Table 10.3). The three compounds have similar K_i values against the three Aurora enzymes but widely differing IC_{50} values against Colo205 cell proliferation. This could not be explained by differing cell penetration capabilities since each compound was found to be an equally potent inhibitor of Aurora-A within cells, as measured by inhibition of Aurora-A autophosphorylation. The crystallographic studies invoked the idea of a two-step binding mechanism for the inhibition of the Auroras by MK-0457. In the first step, the enzyme might behave toward the inhibitor as if it were in the open active form where hydrogen-bonding interactions provide the main binding energy. In the second step, further binding energy is derived by a conformational change toward a more closed ATP binding site, the extent and nature of which is determined by the inhibitor. All three compounds—**18**, **19**, and **20**—showed normal first-order kinetics in Aurora-A inhibition. So although crystal structures of inhibitors in complex with Aurora-A had invoked the notion of a two-step inhibition process, it did not apply to inhibition of this enzyme. The situation with regard to Aurora-B was different. For compound **20**, first-order kinetics was maintained, whereas compound **18** (MK-0457) and compound **19** were slow to establish steady-state kinetics and deeper examination showed that their inhibition kinetics were most compatible with the predicted two-step mechanism. This manifested itself in compound **20** having a very short residency time on Aurora-B (half-life < 0.01 h) while MK-0457 and compound **19** had longer residency times, with half-lives of 0.6 and 8 h, respectively. The K_i values for these compounds had been calculated on the assumption that first-order kinetics are maintained and potencies against Aurora-B appear to be the same as each other. However, if off-rates are used as a measure of absolute potency, then compounds **18** and **19** are at least 60- and 800-fold more potent, respectively, than compound **20** against Aurora-B. The structure–activity relationship anomalies and cell phenotype observations had now been explained at a stroke: cell potency correlated with residency time on Aurora-B, standard Aurora-A K_i measurements were clearly giving misleading results, the most cell potent compounds were the most potent inhibitors of Aurora-B, and selectivity against kinases such as Src and GSK-3β could be better explained in the context of the notion of a two-step binding mechanism and closed Aurora conformation. These correlations were applicable to a wide range of compounds and were used, together with crystallographic data, to design further compounds with selectivity within the Aurora enzyme family. Interestingly, Tyler and colleagues were able to show that MK-0457 blocks the phosphorylation and activation of both Aurora-A and Aurora-B, suppresses the phosphorylation of specific substrates of each enzyme, and induces cell phenotypes associated with the inhibition of either enzyme (Tyler et al., 2007).

10.7. MK-0457 (VX-680) AND ABL

While some imatinib-resistant forms of CML had succumbed to new ABL inhibitors such as nilotinib and dasatinib, the T315I mutant remained stubborn to treatment. The fact that MK-0457 appeared to be a potent inhibitor of this mutation and several other resistant ABL mutations made it a very exciting prospect for the treatment of CML. Tetzuso Tauchi and co-workers showed what might be done with MK-0457 at a 2006 meeting of the American Society of Hematology. They found that VE-465, a very close analog of MK-0457, inhibited the proliferation of K562 cells and BaF3 cells expressing p185 BCR-ABL or T315I BCR-ABL with IC_{50} values <500 nM. Treatment with VE-465 also prolonged the survival in mice injected with BaF3 cells expressing wild-type or T315I mutant form of BCR-ABL. Shah and colleagues showed that MK-0457 is also effective against the other commonly encountered dasatinib-resistant mutation, V299L (Shah et al., 2007). Most importantly, Giles and colleagues used MK-0457 to provide the first observed clinical activity of a kinase inhibitor against the T315I phenotype (Giles et al., 2007). In a Phase I/II study, three patients—two with chronic myeloid leukemia (CML) and one with Philadelphia (Ph) chromosome-positive acute lymphocytic leukemia (ALL)—carried the T315I ABL mutant. All had been refractory to various treatments including imatinib, dasatinib, and nilotinib, yet all achieved a hematological response. A drop in T315I mutant to undetectable levels was seen in the CML patients after two cycles of MK-0457.

10.8. OTHER AURORA INHIBITORS

Besides MK-0457, there are now several Aurora inhibitors in clinical trials. The Millennium compounds, MLN-8327 and MLN-8054 (Hoar et al., 2007; Manfredi et al., 2007), are noteworthy for their selectivity for Aurora-A over Aurora-B. The AstraZeneca compound AZD-1152, on the other hand, has exquisite selectivity for Aurora-B (Mortlock et al., 2007). Glaxo's GSK1070916 is also selective for Aurora-B (Aur-B/INCENP $K_i^* = 0.4$ nM ; Aur-C/INCENP $K_i^* = 1.5$ nM ; Aur-A/TPX2 $K_i^* = 500$ nM). Like MK-0457, GSK1070916 inhibits Aurora-B in a time-dependent fashion. The enzyme–inhibitor dissociation half-life is more than 40 hours. As well as being selective for Aurora-B, Nerviano's PHA-739358 is a potent inhibitor of ABL and its resistant T315I mutant and is in a Phase II trial that includes CML patients with this mutation (Gontarewicz et al., 2008). A crystal structure (Modugno et al., 2007) of a complex between PHA-739358 and the ABL T315I mutant had an open active conformation similar to the conformation found for the MK-0457/WT ABL complex (Young et al., 2006). Other Aurora inhibitors in early clinical trials include CYC-116 (Cyclacel), AT-9283 (Astex), PF-3814735 (Pfizer), and R-763 (Merck-Serono).

10.9. SUMMARY

Nearly 10 years have elapsed between Parry's discovery of the Aurora kinases in *Drosophila* and the first Aurora kinase inhibitor to enter clinical trials. During that time, enormous strides have been made in understanding the mechanisms of these enzymes' actions and their importance in the normal cell cycle and the pathogenesis of cancer. At the beginning of the Vertex Aurora project, we were pessimistic about the possibility of achieving selectivity between the three Aurora kinases. Early crystal structures, structure–activity relationships, and the notion of a two-step binding mechanism showed how selectivity might be achieved. MK-0457 itself is probably best classified as tending toward an Aurora-B selective agent, but the compounds from Millennium, AstraZeneca, and Glaxo appear to take such selectivity to a new level. It is likely that these compounds will prove to be exceptional tools to further elucidate the mechanism involved in the cell cycle. In addition, they are likely to find various utilities in cancer therapy dependent on their selectivity profile. Little has been published on the utility of Aurora inhibitors in combination with other drugs, but encouragingly, AZD1152, the Aurora-B selective agent, was found to enhance the antiproliferative effect of vincristine, a tubulin depolymerizing agent, in vitro as well as in vivo (Yang et al., 2007). Aurora inhibitors have also been found to sensitize cells to ionizing radiation. AZD1152 was found to be an effective radiosensitizer of p53-deficient cells both in vitro and in vivo (Tao et al., 2008). The effect was mimicked by knockdown of Aurora-B or by inhibition of Aurora-B by transfection with an inducible kinase-dead Aurora-B. On the other hand, Guan and colleagues found that inhibition of Aurora kinase by MK-0457 upregulated p53 levels and sensitized cells to radiotherapy (Guan et al., 2007). Although it is clear that we have much to learn about these fascinating enzymes and their inhibitors, it is also clear that they are providing a rich seam for drug discovery. Combinations of selectivity within the Aurora family and outside it, for instance, MK-0457, and its ability to inhibit resistant ABL mutants, should provide drugs for various oncology settings. The discovery of MK-0457 can be regarded as one of the first steps into a new era of antimitotic cancer drugs that do not rely on tubulin interference.

ACKNOWLEDGMENT

My thanks to the numerous scientists at Vertex Pharmaceuticals and at Merck and Co. who contributed to the MK-0457 project.

REFERENCES

Agnese, V., Bazan, V., Fiorentino, F. P., et al. (**2007**). The role of Aurora-A inhibitors in cancer therapy. *Ann Oncol.* 18(Suppl 6), 47–52.

Bacher, U., Haferlach, C., Kern, W., et al. (**2008**). Prognostic relevance of FLT3-TKD mutations in AML: the combination matters—an analysis of 3082 patients. *Blood.* 111(5), 2527–2537.

Bayliss, R., Sardon, T., Vernos, I., et al. (**2003**). Structural basis of Aurora-A activation by TPX2 at the mitotic spindle. *Mol Cell.* 12(4), 851–862.

Bernard, M., Sanseau, P., Henry, C., et al. (**1998**). Cloning of STK13, a third human protein kinase related to *Drosophila* Aurora and budding yeast Ipl1 that maps on chromosome 19q13.3-ter. *Genomics.* 53(3), 406–409.

Bijur, G. N., De Sarno, P., and Jope, R. S. (**2000**). Glycogen synthase kinase-3β facilitates staurosporine- and heat shock-induced apoptosis. *J Biol Chem.* 275(11), 7583–7590.

Bischoff, J. R., and Plowman, G. D. (**1999**). The Aurora/Ipl1p kinase family: regulators of chromosome segregation and cytokinesis. *Trends Cell Biol.* 9(11), 454–459.

Bischoff, J. R., Anderson, L., Zhu, Y., et al. (**1998**). A homologue of *Drosophila aurora* kinase is oncogenic and amplified in human colorectal cancers. *EMBO J.* 17(11), 3052–3065.

Bossemeyer, D., Engh, R. A., Kinzel, V., et al. (**1993**). Phosphotransferase and substrate binding mechanism of the cAMP-dependent protein kinase catalytic subunit from porcine heart as deduced from the 2.0 Å structure of the complex with Mn^{2+} adenylyl imidodiphosphate and inhibitor peptide PKI(5-24). *EMBO J.* 12(3), 849–859.

Carmena, M., and Earnshaw, W. C. (**2003**). The cellular geography of aurora kinases. *Nat Rev Mol Cell Biol.* 4(11), 842–854.

Carter, T. A., Wodicka, L. M., Shah, N. P., et al. (**2005**). Inhibition of drug-resistant mutants of ABL, KIT, and EGF receptor kinases. *PNAS.* 102(31), 11011–11016.

Carvajal, R. D., Tse, A., and Schwarz, G. K. (**2006**). Aurora kinases: new targets for cancer therapy. *Clin Cancer Res.* 12(23), 6869–6875.

Cheetham, G. M. T., Knegtel, R. M. A., Colle, J. T., et al. (**2002**). Crystal structure of Aurora-2, an oncogenic serine/threonine kinase. *J Biol Chem.* 277(45), 42419–42422.

Cheetham, G. M. T., Charlton, P. A., Golec, J. M. C., et al. (**2007**). Structural basis for potent inhibition of the Aurora kinases and a T315I multi-drug resistant mutant form of Abl kinase by VX-680. *Cancer Lett.* 251(2), 323–329.

Fu, J., Bian, M., Jiang, Q., et al. (**2007**). Roles of aurora kinases in mitosis and tumorigenesis. *Mol Cancer Res.* 5(1), 1–10.

Gale, R. E., Green, C., Allen, C., et al. (**2008**). The impact of FLT3 internal tandem duplication mutant level, number, size, and interaction with NPM1 mutations in a large cohort of young adult patients with acute myeloid leukaemia. *Blood.* 111(5), 2776–2784.

Gautschi, O., Mack, P. C., Davies, A. M., et al. (**2006**). Aurora kinase inhibitors: a new class of targeted drugs in cancer. *Clin Lung Cancer.* 8(2), 93–98.

Giet, R., and Prigent, C. (**1999**). Aurora/Ipl1p-related kinases, a new oncogenic family of mitotic serine–threonine kinases. *J Cell Sci.* 112(21), 3591–3601.

Giles, F. J., Cortes, J., Jones, D., et al. (**2007**). MK-0457, a novel kinase inhibitor, is active in patients with chronic myeloid leukemia or acute lymphocytic leukemia with the T315I BCR-ABL mutation. *Blood.* 109(2), 500–502.

Glover, D. M., Leibowitz, M. H., McLean, D. A., et al. (**1995**). Mutations in *aurora* prevent centrosome separation leading to the formation of monopolar spindles. *Cell.* 81(1), 95–105.

Gontarewicz, A., Balabanov, S., Keller, G., et al. (**2008**). Simultaneous targeting of Aurora kinases and Bcr-Abl kinase by the small molecule inhibitor PHA-739358 is effective against imatinib-resistant BCR-ABL mutations including T315I. *Blood.* 111(8), 4355–4364.

Griffith, J., Black, J., Faerman, C., et al. (**2004**). The structural basis for autoinhibition of FLT3 by the juxtamembrane domain. *Mol Cell.* 13(2), 169–178.

Guan, Z., Wang, X., Zhu, X., et al. (**2007**). Aurora-A, a negative prognostic marker, increases migration and decreases radiosensitivity in cancer cells. *Cancer Res.* 67(21), 10436–10444.

Harrington, E. A., Bebbington, D., Moore, J., et al. (**2004**). VX-680, a potent and selective small-molecule inhibitor of the Aurora kinases, suppresses tumor growth in vivo. *Nat Med.* 10(3), 262–267.

Hoar, K., Chakravarty, A., Rabino, C., et al. (**2007**). MLN8054, a small-molecule inhibitor of Aurora A, causes spindle pole and chromosome congression defects leading to aneuploidy. *Mol Cell Biol.* 27(12), 4513–4525.

Kawasaki, A., Matsumura, I., Miyagawa, J., et al. (**2001**). Downregulation of an AIM-1 kinase couples with megakaryocytic polyploidization of human hematopoietic cells. *J Cell Biol.* 152(2), 275–287.

Kimura, M., Matsuda, Y., Yoshioka, T., et al. (**1999**). Cell cycle-dependent expression and centrosome localization of a third human Aurora/Ipl1-related protein kinase, AIK3. *J Biol Chem.* 274(11), 7334–7340.

Manfredi, M. G., Ecsedy, J. A., Meetze, K. A., et al. (**2007**). Antitumor activity of MLN8054, an orally active small-molecule inhibitor of Aurora A kinase. *Proc Natl Acad Sci USA.* 104(10), 4106–4111.

Matthews, N., Visintin, C., Hartzoulakis, B., et al. (**2006**). Aurora A and B kinases as targets for cancer: will they be selective for tumors? *Expert Rev Anticancer Ther.* 6(1), 109–120.

Modugno, M., Casale, E., Soncini, C., et al. (**2007**). Crystal structure of the T315I Abl mutant in complex with the Aurora kinases inhibitor PHA-739358. *Cancer Res.* 67(7), 7987–7990.

Mortlock, A. A., Foote, K. M., Heron, N. M., et al. (**2007**). Discovery, synthesis, and in vivo activity of a new class of pyrazoloquinazolines as selective inhibitors of Aurora B kinase. *J Med Chem.* 50(9), 2213–2224.

Nagar, B., Bornmann, W. G., Pellicena, P., et al. (**2002**). Crystal structures of the kinase domain of c-Abl in complex with the small molecule inhibitors PD173955 and imatinib (STI-571). *Cancer Res.* 62(15), 4236–4243.

Narayana, N., Cox, S., Shaltiel, S., et al. (**1997**). Crystal structure of a polyhistidine-tagged recombinant catalytic subunit of cAMP-dependent protein kinase complexed with the peptide inhibitor PKI(5–24) and adenosine. *Biochemistry.* 36(15), 4438–4448.

Naruganahalli, K. S., Lakshmanan, M., Dastidar, S. G., et al. (**2006**). Therapeutic potential of aurora kinase inhibitors in cancer. *Curr Opin Invest Drugs.* 7(12), 1044–1051.

Nowakowski, J., Cronin, C. N., McRee, D. E., et al. (**2002**). Structures of the cancer-related Aurora-A, Fak and Epha2 protein kinases from nanovolume crystallography. *Structure.* 10(12), 1659–1667.

Pap, M., and Cooper, G. M. (**1998**). Role of glycogen synthase kinase-3 in the phosphatidylinositol 3-Kinase/Akt cell survival pathway. *J Biol Chem.* 273(32), 19929–19932.

Ruchaud, S., Carmena, M., and Earnshaw, W. C. (**2007**). Chromosomal passengers: conducting cell division. *Nat Rev Mol Cell Biol.* 8(10), 798–812.

Sawyers, C. L. (**2002**). Finding the next Gleevec: FLT3 targeted kinase inhibitor therapy for acute myeloid leukemia. *Cancer Cell.* 1(5), 413–415.

Schindler, T., Bornmann, W., Pellicena, P., et al. (**2000**). Structural mechanism for STI-571 inhibition of Abelson tyrosine kinase. *Science.* 289(5486), 1938–1942.

Shah, N. P., Nicoll, J. M., Nagar, B., et al. (**2002**). Multiple *BCR-ABL* kinase domain mutations confer polyclonal resistance to the tyrosine kinase inhibitor imatinib (STI571) in chronic phase and blast crisis chronic myeloid leukemia. *Cancer Cell.* 2(2), 117–125.

Shah, N. P., Skaggs, B. J., Branford, S., et al. (**2007**). Sequential ABL kinase inhibitor therapy selects for compound drug-resistant BCR-ABL mutations with altered oncogenic potency. *J Clin Invest.* 117(9), 2562–2569.

Sherbenou, D. W., and Druker, B. J. (**2007**). Applying the discovery of the Philidelphia chromosome. *J Clin Invest.* 117(8), 2067–2074.

Tao, Y., Zhang, P., Girdler, F., et al. (**2008**). Enhancement of radiation response in p53-deficient cancer cells by the Aurora-B kinase inhibitor AZD1152. *Oncogene.* 27(23), 3244–3255.

Terada, Y., Tatsuka, M., Suzuki, F., et al. (**1998**). AIM-1: a mammalian midbody-associated protein required for cytokinesis. *EMBO J.* 17(3), 667–676.

Tyler, R. K., Shpiro, N., Marquez, R., et al. (**2007**). VX-680 inhibits Aurora A and Aurora B kinase activity in human cells. *Cell Cycle.* 6(22), 2846–2854.

Warner, S. L., Gray, P. J., and Von Hoff, D. D. (**2006**). Tubulin-associated drug targets: Aurora kinases, Polo-like kinases, and others. *Semin Oncol.* 33(4), 436–448.

Yang, J., Ikezoe, T., Nishioka, C., et al. (**2007**). AZD1152, a novel and selective Aurora B kinase inhibitor, induces growth arrest, apoptosis, and sensitization for tubulin depolymerizing agent or topoisomerase II inhibitor in human acute leukemia cells in vitro and in vivo. *Blood.* 110(6), 2034–2040.

Young, M. A., Shah, N. P., Chao, L. H., et al. (**2006**). Structure of the kinase domain of an imatinib-resistant Abl mutant in complex with the Aurora kinase inhibitor VX-680. *Cancer Res.* 66(2), 1007–1014.

11

DISCOVERY OF PHA-739358

Daniele Fancelli and Jürgen Moll

11.1. INTRODUCTION

Vinca alkaloids and taxanes remain some of the most relevant drugs of anti-cancer therapy, validating the approach of antimitotic drugs in the treatment of cancer (Jordan, 2002; Jordan and Wilson, 2004). These drugs target microtubules, which are necessary for mitosis, during which duplicated chromosomes are separated and distributed into two daughter cells. Based on their mechanism of action, drugs targeting microtubules have side effects, such as neurotoxicity, which are related to the physiological roles of microtubules in essential processes other than mitosis. To specifically target mitosis, keeping the anticancer activity of microtubule-targeting drugs while avoiding their undesired side effects is the aim of several molecular-targeted drug development programs in the preclinical or clinical phase of development. The molecular targets of these programs include ATPases, such as kinesins, and protein kinases, such as Polo-like kinases and Aurora kinases. Cyclin-dependent kinases (CDKs) are also targeted to some extent, although most CDK family members have no role in mitosis and the most advanced inhibitors target multiple CDKs (de Carcer et al., 2007; Sharma et al., 2008). With respect to kinesins, ispinesib is currently the most advanced kinesin inhibitor with others following close behind (Bergnes et al., 2005). The commercial success of kinase inhibitors and the strong growth of the global cancer drug market have attracted a lot of new players in the field of oncology. Therefore it is not surprising that for some of the most attractive targets, which include Aurora kinases, there are numerous preclinical and clinical programs ongoing (Carpinelli and Moll, 2008; Gautschi et al., 2008). Based on the published

Kinase Inhibitor Drugs. Edited by Rongshi Li and Jeffrey A. Stafford
Copyright © 2009 John Wiley & Sons, Inc.

Phase I results of the first-generation Aurora kinase inhibitors, some patients experience stable disease while others show objective responses following administration of PHA-739358 (Cohen et al., 2008). With improved dosing schedules and dose level selection, increasing clinical experience, and better patient stratification, there is hope that these new drugs will be added to the arsenal against cancer in the near future.

The first Aurora kinase was identified by a screen for mitotic spindle pole mutants in *Drosophila* (Glover et al., 1995). Soon after, additional Aurora kinase family members were characterized. At present, three closely related Aurora kinases (A, B, and C) are known in vertebrates, with all of them orchestrating critical events during mitosis. However, some functions outside mitosis have been postulated, in particular, for Aurora-A, in mRNA stabilization, cilia formation, and NFκB signaling (Sasayama et al., 2005; Pugacheva and Golemis, 2006; Briassouli et al., 2007). Aurora-B and Aurora-C seem to have overlapping functions in mitosis, whereas Aurora-A shows diverse functions. This is reflected in different subcellular localization and timing of expression for Aurora-A. For simplicity, only the vertebrate Aurora kinase members are considered for further review, keeping in mind that lower eukaryotic cells such as yeast possess only one Aurora kinase (Ipl1) with essential functions during mitosis overlapping with different Aurora members in higher organisms (Ke et al., 2003).

Aurora-A is localized at centrosomes and is associated with the spindle poles in early mitosis. The maturation of centrosomes into a mature mitotic spindle is one of the major tasks of Aurora-A and inhibition of its kinase activity results in spindle defects. Interacting proteins such as TPX-2 or Ajuba modulate the kinase activity of Aurora-A by facilitating autophosphorylation and by protecting Aurora-A from inactivation by phosphatases (Kufer et al., 2002; Hirota et al., 2003). Aurora-A also seems to regulate p53 stability and transcriptional activity by directly phosphorylating p53 in position Ser315 and Ser215, respectively (Katayama et al., 2004; Liu et al., 2004). Of all the Aurora kinase family members, Aurora-A shows the strongest link to cancer. First, overexpression is oncogenic (Bischoff et al., 1998; Zhou et al., 1998); second, the gene is located on chromosome 20q13, which is frequently amplified in multiple cancers and this is usually accompanied by overexpression of Aurora-A; and third, a polymorphic allele is known as low penetrance tumor susceptibility gene in different tumors including breast cancer (Ewart-Toland et al., 2005). Together with its easy druggability, these properties make Aurora-A highly attractive as an anticancer target.

Aurora-B is known to regulate multiple events during different stages of mitosis. In prophase, it is responsible for the phosphorylation of histone H3, which might contribute to chromosome condensation. In addition, phosphorylation of histone H3 is supposed to be a label, which marks the successful execution of cellular events in metaphase and enables cells to enter anaphase, the subsequent step in mitosis (Hans and Dimitrov, 2001). During metaphase, Aurora-B acts on the kinetochores, where it is located outside the chromosomal passenger complex. A function as a mitotic checkpoint kinase has been proposed by acting as a sensor of microtubule attachment and force (Murata-Hori and Wang, 2002; Dewar et al., 2004). When cells enter anaphase, Aurora-B can be activated by a subpopulation of microtubules to create a spatial phosphorylation gradient in anaphase, where it is centered at the spindle midzone, and from its location gives positional information for the cell division plane (Fuller et al., 2008). An additional function in anaphase might be to increase chromosome condensation by axial shortening of chromosomes (Mora-Bermúdez et al., 2007). Finally, proper execution of cytokinesis seems to depend on Aurora-B, where it phosphorylates critical substrates including desmin, vimentin, MKLP1, TACC, and MgcRacGAP (Fu et al., 2007). In summary, Aurora-B is a master regulator of mitosis. It is an absolutely essential kinase for proper execution of mitosis by acting on chromosome condensation; it is a mitotic spindle checkpoint controlling microtubule attachments of kinetochores; it also orchestrates cytokinesis. The link of Aurora-B to disease is less strong as compared to that of Aurora-A, although overexpression of Aurora-B in multiple tumors has been observed (Katayama et al., 2003). When Aurora-B is inhibited by specific small molecules or the protein is downregulated by RNA interference, most cells enter endoreduplication cycles, which can lead to polyploidy and potentially cell death.

Aurora-C is functionally more closely related to Aurora-B than Aurora-A but has additional roles in meiosis, for example, during spermatogenesis. Additional Aurora-C-specific functions have been proposed such as the modification of telomere-associated protein, TRF2, which is specifically phosphorylated in position Thr358 by Aurora-C (Spengler, 2007). Ectopic expression of a hyperactive mutant of Aurora-C indicates a role as a regulator of cell morphology and cell growth, an action different from those of Aurora-A or Aurora-B.

In summary, both Aurora-A and Aurora-B are independently promising targets for anticancer therapy and selective inhibitors of each have shown good preclinical activity. Interestingly, inhibitors of Aurora-A and Aurora-B show a dominant Aurora-B-related phenotype, which can be explained by the mitotic checkpoint functions of Aurora-B (Yang et al., 2005). This chapter will focus on the discovery and development of PHA-739358 (Figure 11.1), a

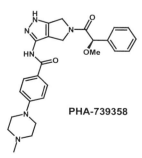

PHA-739358

Figure 11.1. Chemical structure of PHA-739358.

potent pan-inhibitor of Aurora kinases that also shows low nanomolar potency against additional anticancer kinase targets such as Abl, including the T315I mutant, Ret, Trk-A, and FGFR1.

PHA-739358, which in 2004 was the first Aurora kinase inhibitor to enter clinical trials, is currently being evaluated in various Phase I and II studies in solid and hematological tumors. The results from the most advanced of these trials will be discussed. Finally, an attempt is made to predict the future prospects of the compound based on the initial results of clinical studies, including the relevant responses of patients with chronic myeloid leukemia (CML) relapsing on imatinib and second-generation Abl inhibitors.

11.2. DISCOVERY OF PHA-739358

11.2.1. Lead Identification

11.2.1.1. Chemical Libraries Targeting Kinase Inhibition. The identification and development of the chemical series that eventually produced PHA-739358 were strictly linked to an initiative carried out during the years 2000–2004 in the Nerviano site of Pharmacia, aimed to build a proprietary collection of chemical libraries that inhibit protein kinases.

These "kinase-targeted libraries" (KTLs) were designed around novel, proprietary ATP-mimetic scaffolds and expanded by combinatorial chemistry methods. The final goal was to accelerate new kinase projects by rapidly screening a small (approximately 5×10^4 compounds) subset of our Research Chemical Collection that would provide a significantly enhanced hit rate and lead to the identification of high-quality active compounds. These compounds would ideally be proprietary, drug-like, and easily expandable by previously established combinatorial methods.

KTL scaffolds were designed by exploiting both structural similarities and differences across the ATP binding sites of the kinase family (Vulpetti and Bosotti, 2004). Typically, these scaffolds are recognized by different kinases through a pattern of hydrogen bonds mimicking those between the ATP adenine and the highly conserved hinge region located in the ATP binding site of kinases, while their diversity elements, which point more toward variable pockets of the ATP binding site, can be used to modulate potency and selectivity (Figure 11.2).

Following this strategy, a number of novel series of kinase inhibitors (Figure 11.3) were produced, providing an important source of lead compounds (Berta et al., 2002; Fancelli et al., 2002, 2005b; Tonani et al., 2004a,b; Traquandi et al., 2004; Vanotti et al., 2004). In several kinase-targeted projects, these leads have evolved into clinical candidates.

11.2.1.2. Screens for Aurora-A Inhibitors. The kinase-targeted subset of the collection, still under construction at the time of the screens for Aurora-A

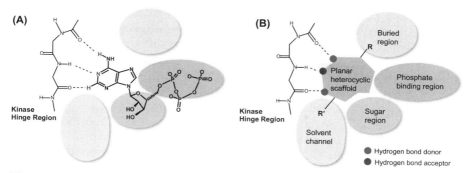

Figure 11.2. (**A**) Schematic representation of ATP in the kinase-binding site, with the H-bond pattern (acceptor–donor–acceptor) between adenine and the kinase hinge region. (**B**) Schematic representation of a generic adenino-mimetic scaffold. Typically, it is a heterocycle able to reproduce one or more of the three H bonds with the hinge region and endowed with variable elements (e.g., R and R′) that can explore different regions of the binding site.

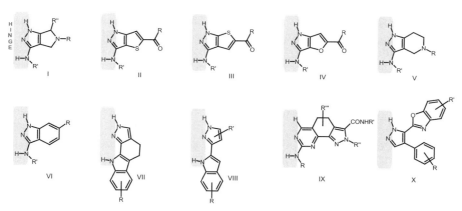

Figure 11.3. Examples of scaffolds of Kinase Targeted Libraries. Atoms in blue color represent the primary recognition element for the kinase hinge region (experimentally confirmed by X-ray crystallography). R and R′ groups can be varied using combinatorial chemistry methodologies. Only one of the different possible binding modes of scaffold X is shown.

inhibition, was screened in different runs as soon as the new libraries became available. For this purpose, a biochemical assay was established that measures the kinase activity of recombinant Aurora-A (Carpinelli et al., 2007). Overall, about 20,000 compounds were tested, allowing the identification of a remarkable number of active compounds ($IC_{50} < 10 \mu M$), corresponding to a hit rate of about 0.9%. In comparison, the hit rate for the remaining part of the Pharmacia corporate chemical collection at the time, which was composed of approximately half a million compounds, was 0.06%.

Aurora-A inhibitors were identified in almost all the KTL sublibraries screened, but priority was initially given to the expansion of the tetrahydropyrrolopyrazole series (Figure 11.2, scaffold I). The main factors that guided this decision were the high hit rate of the class, the immediate identification of some SAR trends, and the particularly high synthetic versatility of this series. In fact, the methods set up for the production of the combinatorial libraries could easily be transferred to the production of smaller libraries by parallel syntheses routinely carried out in our medicinal chemistry laboratories. This allowed us to move from the synthesis of the very first tetrahydropyrrolopyrazole derivative to the clinical candidate PHA-739358 (corresponding to the "lead finding" and "lead optimization" stages of the conventional drug discovery project outline) in only 18 months, a time frame that is well aligned with the best standards in the drug development industry.

11.2.1.3. Pyrrolopyrazole Aurora Kinase Inhibitors. The design of the pyrrolopyrazole series was originally derived from an elaboration of the 3-aminopyrazole moiety, a well-known adenine mimetic pharmacophore present in several classes of kinase inhibitors. The NH_2–C–N–NH pattern of the 3-aminopyrazole moiety, which is stereochemically well suited to form hydrogen bonding interactions with the kinase hinge region of the ATP pocket, was embedded within the 1,4,5,6-tetrahydropyrrolo[3,4-c]pyrazole to give an original scaffold endowed with additional anchoring points for combinatorial expansion (Figure 11.4A) (Fancelli et al., 2005a). In particular, the nitrogen atom at position 5 can be regarded as a handle for a great variety of synthetic manipulations, which can allow extensive exploration of the phosphate binding region of the ATP pocket.

The expected binding mode was initially confirmed by the X-ray structure of PHA-533514, a simple prototype element of the series that was crystallized as a complex with the kinase domain of Aurora-A (Figure 11.4B). The

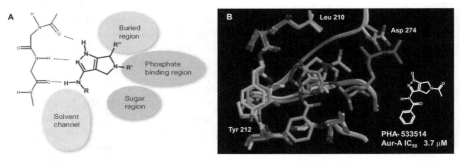

Figure 11.4. (**A**) Schematic representation of the tetrahydropyrrolopyrazoles scaffold in the ATP binding site. (**B**) Superposition of the Aurora-A complex with PHA-533514 (green carbon atoms for the protein, cyan for the compound) on that of the structure of Aurora-A complexed with ADP. (See color insert.)

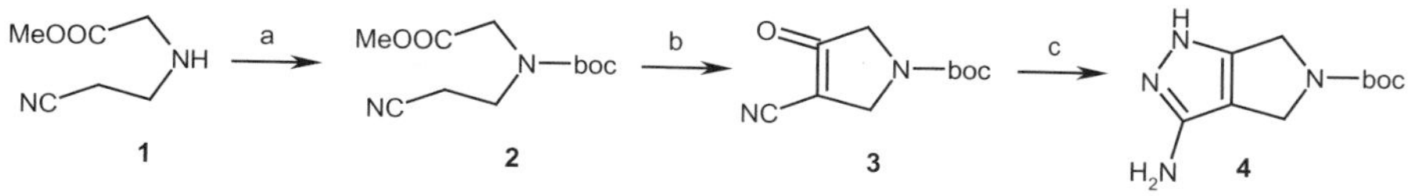

Scheme 11.1. Reagents and conditions: (a) di-*tert*-butyl dicarbonate, DCM/aq NaHCO$_3$ (1:1), 24 h, 22 °C; (b) MeONa, toluene, 3 h, 80 °C, then 2 N HCl; (c) hydrazine hydrochloride, EtOH, 3 h, 60 °C, then aq NaHCO$_3$.

3-amino-tetrahydropyrrolo[3,4-*c*]pyrazole scaffold, protected as the *N*-*tert*-butyloxycarbonyl derivative at position 5, is obtained in three synthetic steps from the commercially available *N*-(2-cyanoethyl)glycine methyl ester through a high yielding and easily scalable process (Scheme 11.1).

The key step of the following expansion is the acylation of the 3-aminopyrazole moiety. This reaction is known to be subject to kinetic or thermodynamic control. The 1(2)-acylation on ring nitrogen is the faster reaction, followed by a second acylation on the exocyclic nitrogen. Both the 1(2)-acylderivative and the 1,3-bis-acylderivative give the thermodynamically stable 3-monoacylderivative under equilibrating conditions. Thus, using a solid-supported acylating agent, the kinetic product distribution can be frozen and the bis-acylation avoided. Following this strategy a novel and simple method to load pyrazoles onto solid support was developed, by treating tetrahydropyrrolopyrazole **4** with polystyrene isocyanate resin. The resulting urea linker between one of the ring nitrogens and the resin is stable to the acidic conditions employed in the synthesis and sufficiently labile to allow a clean cleavage of the final compounds by alkaline hydrolysis. The complete process is outlined in Scheme 11.2.

A related solution-phase process, based on protection of the pyrazole ring nitrogen as an ethyl carbamate (Scheme 11.3), is used for large-scale syntheses, including the preparation of PHA-739358.

According to Scheme 11.2, 22 acyl chlorides were used in step b and 46 acylating agents in step d to produce an initial set of about 1000 pyrrolopyrazoles. This kinase-targeted library was routinely used in screens against different kinase targets. This set was designed to integrate a diversity-oriented approach with medicinal chemistry experience. Thus building block selection was carried out by first filtering the combined sets of commercial and proprietary reagents according to synthetic constraints and medicinal chemistry criteria and then by clustering the resulting lists by structural similarity (a set of two-dimensional molecular descriptors, mainly based on the MDL® ISIS keys, was used in this step). One representative reagent per cluster was finally selected, strictly based on medicinal chemistry criteria.

11.2.1.4. Initial Hits for Aurora-A Inhibition.

In a screen against Aurora-A, this library gave a hit rate (IC$_{50}$ < 10 μM) exceeding 10%, with 7% exhibiting submicromolar activity. Even though understanding of SAR was not a primary objective of the screen of this diversity set, it became apparent that the most

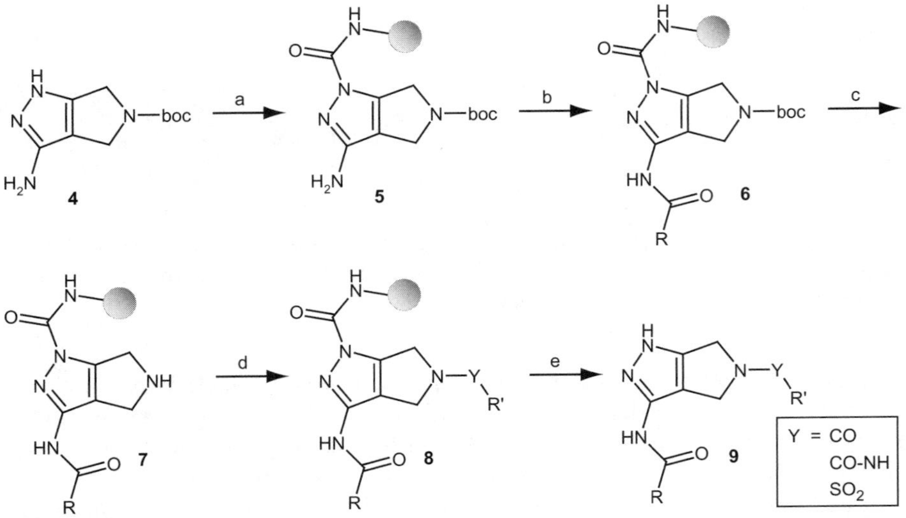

Scheme 11.2. Reagents and conditions: (a) PS-NCO, DCM, 20 h, 22 °C; (b) RCOCl, DIEA, DCM, 16 h, 22 °C; (c) TFA/DCM (1:1), 3 h, 22 °C; (d) R′NCO or R′SO₂Cl or R′COOH, TBTU, NMM, DCM or DMF, 24 h, 22 °C; (e) NaOH aq, MeOH, 72 h, 40 °C, then HCl 35%.

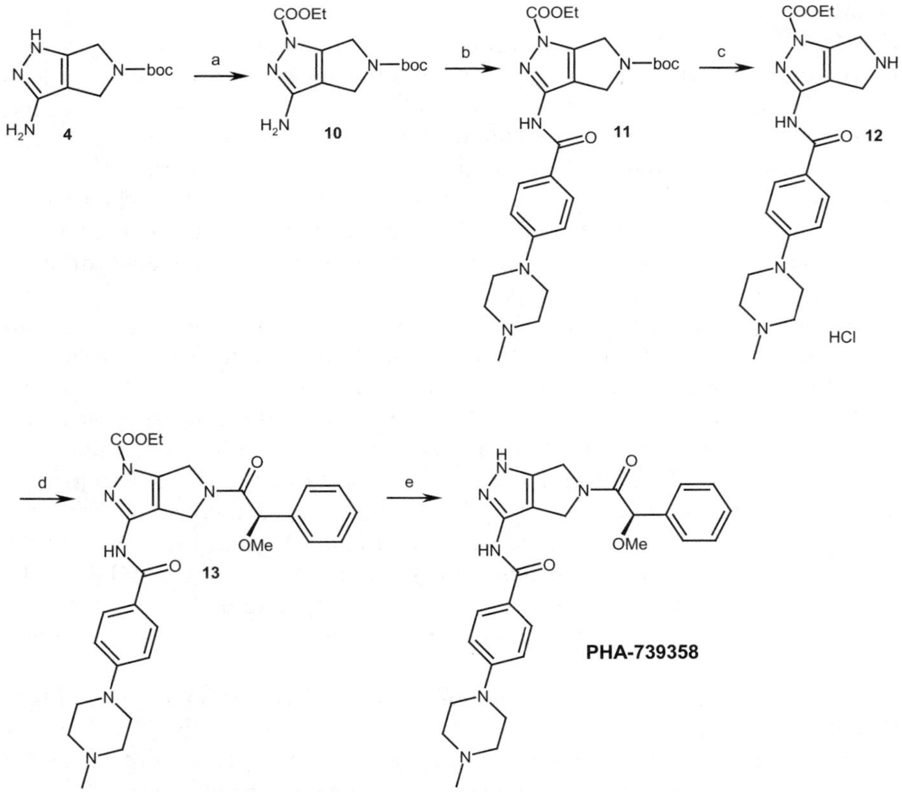

Scheme 11.3. Reagents and conditions: (a) EtCOOCl, THF, 20 h, 22 °C; (b) *p*-piperazinylbenzoyl chloride, DIEA, THF, 16 h, 22 °C; (c) HCl (12 equiv, 4N in dioxane), DCM, 24 h, 22 °C; (d) acylchloride, DIEA, DCM 6–8 h, 22 °C; (e) Et₃N 10% in MeOH, 3–6 h, 22 °C.

potent Aurora inhibitors in this set were characterized by para-substituted benzamido groups at position 3. In particular, the array of 4-*tert*-butylbenzamide derivatives provided several compounds endowed with high inhibitory activities on Aurora-A and promising antiproliferative effects on the human colon carcinoma cell line HCT-116 (Table 11.1). By contrast, a relatively wider range of substituents was tolerated at position 5, and relatively potent inhibitors emerged from both the 5-urea and 5-amino series (Table 11.1).

By combining the data in Table 11.1 with preliminary assessments of selectivity and mechanism of action (as measured by the ability of the compound

TABLE 11.1. Structure and Aurora-A Inhibition of Representative *N*-(tetrahydropyrrolo[3,4-*c*]pyrazol-3-yl)-4-*tert*-butyl-benzamides

Entry	R'	Aur-A[a]	HCT-116[b]
14	H	>10	Not tested
15	—Me	0.85	Not tested
16		0.041	2.1
17		0.005	2.0
18		0.13	3.0
19		0.016	1.6
20		0.10	2.2

[a]Enzyme inhibition IC_{50} (µM).
[b]Antiproliferation IC_{50} (µM).

to arrest cells in the G2/M cell cycle phase and inducing accumulation of cells with ≥4 N DNA content), compounds **17**, **18**, and **19** were chosen as the parent compounds for the development of 5-amido and 5-ureido pyrrolopyrazole Aurora inhibitors.

11.2.2. Lead Optimization

Despite their promising activity, these initial hits also showed important drawbacks that hampered their assessment in in vivo tumor models and precluded any further development. In particular, they turned out to be poorly soluble compounds (<15 μM in pH 7 buffer) with very short in vivo half-lives (<15 minutes following intravenous administration in mice). These short half-lives were due to metabolic oxidation of the *tert*-butyl moiety. Thus the subsequent lead optimization was directed primarily to the preparation of soluble, metabolically stable analogs. Based on the hypothesis that the *tert*-butyl is directed toward the outside of the enzyme (Figure 11.3), and having in mind that substituents placed in that region have often been used for optimization of physicochemical properties in other kinase inhibitor series, we planned the parallel synthesis of several arrays of analogs of the initial hits bearing different hydrophilic moieties at position 4'.

Indeed, simple replacement of *tert*-butyl with the 4-methylpiperazin-1-yl moiety led to analogs with high potency and greatly increased aqueous solubility (>200 μM in buffer pH 7, Table 11.2).

In particular, the ureido derivative **23** (PHA-680632), which showed higher potency in both enzymatic and antiproliferative assays, was selected for more extensive characterization (Fancelli et al., 2005a; Soncini et al., 2006). The overall profile of **23** was sufficiently interesting to warrant further investigation. In fact, this compound was considered the endpoint of the expansion of the urea class and progressed to preclinical development.

To highlight areas for further optimization of the inhibitory activity of the amido series, the crystal structure of compound **21** was solved as a complex with Aurora-A kinase and refined at a resolution of 2.0 Å (Figure 11.5).

By comparing the binding modes of compound **21** with PHA-680632, it was envisaged that a substituent at the pro-R position of the benzylic methylene could adopt a position similar to the diethyl benzene of PHA-680632 under the glycine-rich loop and near the amino nitrogen of Lys162. By contrast, substitutions at the pro-S position were thought to be less favorable due to the proximity of Val147. Following this hypothesis, and assuming that the phenyl group of compound **2** would adopt the same position as the thiophene of compound **21**, we carried out the synthesis of a small series of pyrrolopyrazoles branched at the CH₂ of the phenylacetyl moiety in position 5, mainly with H-bond acceptor groups targeting a possible interaction with the Lys162 hydrogens.

Results shown in Table 11.3 indicate that benzylic substitution at the pro-R position effectively led to compounds endowed with significantly increased

TABLE 11.2. Structure and Aurora-A Inhibition of Representative *N*-(tetrahydropyrrolo[3,4-*c*]pyrazol-3-yl)- 4-(4-methyl-piperazin-1-yl)benzamides

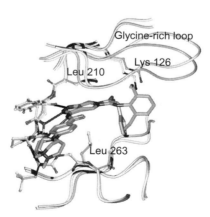

Entry	R′	Aur-A[a]	HCT-116[b]
21	O S (2-thienyl acetyl)	0.065	0.57
22	O (phenyl acetyl)	0.14	0.22
23	H–N, Et / O, Et (2,6-diethylphenyl)	0.027	0.045

[a]Enzyme inhibition IC_{50} (μM).
[b]Antiproliferation IC_{50} (μM).

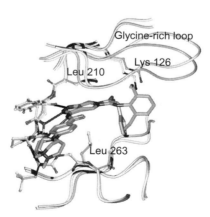

Figure 11.5. Structure of Aurora-A in complex with compound **21** (yellow, tan carbon atoms) superposed on the structure with PHA-680632 (light green carbon atoms). Reproduced with permission from *J Med Chem.* **2006**, 49(24), 7247–7251. Copyright © 2006 American Chemical Society.

TABLE 11.3. Structure and Aurora-A Inhibition of 5-α-Substituted-(Phenylacetyl)pyrrolopyrazoles

Entry	R	R′	Aur-A[a]	HCT-116[b]
24	H	H	130	220
25	F	H	9	50
26	OH	H	6	97
27	Me	H	24	21
28	OMe	H	13	31
29	H	Me	452	Not tested
30	H	OMe	354	Not tested

[a]Enzyme inhibition IC_{50} (μM).
[b]Antiproliferation IC_{50} (μM).

inhibitory and antiproliferative potency. Among them, compound **28** (PHA-739358) emerged as the molecule with the best balance in terms of kinase inhibition profile, pharmaceutical properties, efficacy, and safety profile in animal models (Fancelli et al., 2006; Carpinelli et al., 2007).

11.3. PROFILE OF PHA-739358

11.3.1. Kinase Inhibition Profile

PHA-739358 inhibits Aurora kinases in a biochemical assay with IC_{50} values of 13, 79, and 61 nM for Aurora-A, -B, and -C, respectively. Its selectivity was assessed on a panel of more than 200 kinases, chosen to represent diverse families of Tyr and Ser–Thr kinases. For a smaller array of 25 kinases, the K_m values for ATP and the specific substrate were initially determined, and each assay was then run at optimized ATP ($2 \times K_m$) and substrate ($5 \times K_m$) concentrations. This setting enabled direct comparison of IC_{50} values of PHA-739358 across the screening panel (Pevarello et al., 2004).

As reported in Table 11.3, besides inhibiting the three Aurora kinases, PHA-739358 also inhibits with high potency an additional set of tyrosine kinases, in particular, Abl, including the T315I mutant, Ret, Trk-A, and FGFR1 (and other family members). These kinases are involved in a number of malignancies that include chronic myelogenous leukemia (CML), acute lymphoblastic leukemia (ALL), and thyroid, prostate, and breast carcinomas (Soncini et al., 2006; Modugno et al., 2007).

Based on these data, PHA-739358 can be defined as a spectrum-selective kinase inhibitor for cancer-related kinases.

11.3.2. Inhibition of Wild-Type and Mutated Forms of Abl Protein Kinase

Although the treatment of chronic myelogenous leukemia (CML) has been revolutionized by the introduction of the Bcr-Abl kinase inhibitor imatinib, the drug resistance derived by reactivation of Abl signaling via several different point mutations remains a critical unmet medical need. In fact, none of the second-generation Bcr-Abl inhibitors in clinical development, which are active on the majority of imatinib-resistant mutants, is able to target the mutation of threonine315 to isoleucine (T315I), which confers resistance to all existing therapies.

Thus the significant cross-reactivity with the wild-type Abl kinase by PHA-739358 in the biochemical assay (Table 11.4) prompted us to immediately investigate whether our compound was capable of inhibiting the tyrosine kinase activity of the imatinib-resistant Abl mutants.

A biochemical kinase assay was initially carried out using WT Abl kinase domain in parallel with three of the most frequent imatinib-resistant mutants: T315I, E255V, and M351T. As shown in Figure 11.5, PHA-739358 efficiently inhibits substrate phosphorylation by WT and mutant proteins, being even more active against the T315I mutant (Figure 11.6).

To confirm the in vitro kinase assay data, an ATP-binding site-dependent displacement assay, which uses an indolinone ligand as the probe, was used for quantitative affinity evaluation for recombinant WT and Abl kinase domain mutants (Modugno et al., 2007). Inhibitor affinities for different Abl forms measured using this assay are shown in Table 11.5. Imatinib showed a higher affinity for the dephosphorylated compared with the phosphorylated form of Abl (0.021 and 0.23 µM, respectively), whereas no displacement was observed on the T315I mutant, in agreement with published data. Lower affinity was observed for the E255V and M351T mutants. On the contrary, PHA-739358 binds all of the Abl forms, showing a highest affinity for the T315I mutant (0.005 µM) in agreement with the initial biochemical assay.

TABLE 11.4. Kinase Inhibition Profile of Compound PHA-739358

Kinase	Aur-A	Aur-B	Aur-C	Abl	Trk-A	Ret	FGFR1
IC_{50} (nM)	13	79	61	25	30	31	47

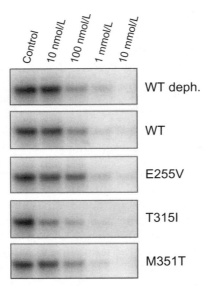

Figure 11.6. Inhibitory activity of PHA-739358 on a panel of imatinib-resistant mutants representative of the most frequent mutations observed in imatinib-resistant patients. Adapted from *Cancer Res.* **2007**, 67, 7987–7990.

TABLE 11.5. PHA-739358 Affinities for Wild-Type and Mutated Abl

	Displacement K_d (µM)				
	WT no P	WT	E255W	T315I	M315T
Imatinib	0.021	0.230	0.610	No displacement	0.100
PHA-739358	0.014	0.021	0.014	0.005	0.015

From a structural viewpoint, the mutation T315I occurs at the "gatekeeper" position, the residue that flanks the variable hydrophobic pocket at the rear of the ATP-binding site. The increased steric hindrance imposed by the substitution of threonine by isoleucine would interfere with the binding of inhibitors, such as imatinib, which make use of that pocket.

In the case of PHA-739358, the crystal structure of the inhibitor–protein complex demonstrates that the binding mode of PHA-739358 is very similar to that of the complex of the same compound with Aurora-A (Figure 11.7A), although the conformations of the proteins around the ATP-binding site show some differences. In the Aurora-A structure, the DFG motif is more similar to the "out" conformation, while the mutated Abl protein is in the typical conformation of active kinases, with the activation loop in the extended DFG "in" conformation.

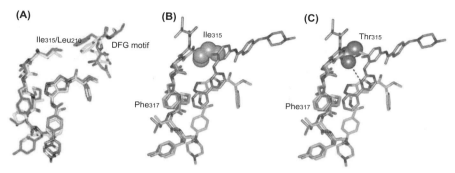

Figure 11.7. (**A**) Details of the binding of PHA-739358 to Abl (green carbon atoms) and to Aurora-A (yellow carbon atoms). (**B**, **C**) PHA-739358 complex (green carbon atoms) superimposed with the structure of imatinib (magenta carbon atoms). The gatekeeper residues Ile315 of PHA-739358 complex (A) and Thr315 of the imatinib complex (B) are shown with van der Waals spheres. In the T315I mutant, the isoleucine side chain causes a steric clash with imatinib; in addition, the hydrogen bond between imatinib and the side chain oxygen of threonine is lost. Adapted from *Cancer Res.* **2007**, 67, 7987–7990. (See color insert.)

In particular, PHA-739358 binds in the ATP-binding pocket of the two kinases without occupying the hydrophobic pocket, and without any steric hindrance from the gatekeeper residue. The gatekeeper for the Aurora kinases is Leu210, a large and hydrophobic residue very similar to the isoleucine of mutated Abl. Consistently, the T315I mutation has no impact on the binding potency of PHA-739358.

As has been also observed for other kinases, the gatekeeper residue is a key determinant of the binding potency of many ATP-competitive kinase inhibitors and drug resistance is frequently attributed to mutations at this position.

Therefore the approach of developing inhibitors that do not require occupancy of the hydrophobic pocket for reaching adequate potency and selectivity is a viable strategy to address the issue of emerging resistance to drugs targeting other kinases known to escape through gatekeeper substitutions, such as PDGFR, KIT, and EGFR (Böhmer et al., 2003; Kobayashi et al., 2005; Tamborini et al., 2006).

11.3.3. Effect on Tumor Cell Proliferation and Mechanism of Action

The kinase inhibitory activity showed by PHA-738358 in the biochemical assays was fully confirmed in cellular assays: the compound has strong activity on Aurora-A, as determined by inhibition of autophosphorylation in position Thr288 and also on Aurora-B as determined by inhibition of phosphorylation of its substrate, histone H3, in position Ser10. In HeLa cells, inhibition for both Aurora kinases starts to be seen from about 0.1 µM concentrations upward.

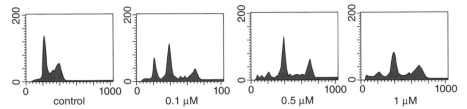

Figure 11.8. Flow cytometric analysis of DNA content in human colon carcinoma cells (HCT-116) treated for 24 hours with increasing concentrations of PHA-739358. Reproduced with permission from *J Med Chem.* **2006**, 49(24), 7247–7251. Copyright © 2006 American Chemical Society.

Inhibition of Abl, Ret, and Trk-A by PHA-739358 was assessed using cell lines where these proteins are relevant for growth or survival. The Ret and Trk-A kinase-inhibitory activities of PHA-739358 were evaluated for dose-related inhibition of receptor autophosphorylation in appropriate cell-based assays using TT and PC-12 cells, respectively. TT cells were derived from a tumor of a patient with sporadic medullary thyroid carcinoma. These cells contain a Ret allele with a constitutively activating mutation (C634W) in the extracellular domain. Inhibition of ligand-induced Trk-A phosphorylation by PHA-739358 was examined in PC-12 cells, a NGF-responsive cell line established from a rat pheochromocytoma. Both Ret and Trk-A kinases were inhibited at low micromolar concentrations of PHA-739358 in agreement with the inhibitory activity observed in the biochemical assay. The compound also inhibits Abl autophosphorylation and its downstream pathway, as well as histone H3 phosphorylation as a read-out for inhibition of Aurora-B. Consistent with the typical phenotype induced by Aurora-A and Aurora-B dual inhibitors, the incubation of different tumor cell lines with PHA-739358 results in a substantial increase in 4N DNA and polyploidy (>8N DNA) populations, with a variable extent of polyploidy induction depending on the genetic background of the tested cell line (Figure 11.8).

Finally, the antiproliferative effects of the compound were assessed on a panel of exponentially growing cell lines from different tumor types, which were treated for 72 hours with different concentrations of PHA-739358. All cell lines examined were highly sensitive to the compound (Figure 11.9), with the antiproliferation IC_{50} values ranging between 28 and 300 nM (A2780 and U2OS, respectively).

11.3.4. Pharmacokinetic and Antitumor Activity in Animal Models

The pharmacokinetic profiles of PH-739358A were investigated in the mouse, rat, dog, and monkey. In all species, the compound showed moderate–high systemic clearance and a high volume of distribution, suggesting extensive tissue distribution. Pharmacokinetic parameters estimated in CD-1 mouse are

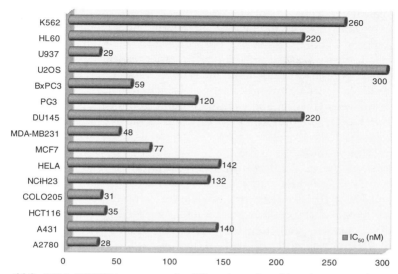

Figure 11.9. PHA-739358 treatment of cell lines in antiproliferation assays (IC$_{50}$ values at 72 hours).

TABLE 11.6. Average Pharmacokinetic Parameters Estimated in Male CD-1 Mice (Three Animals) Following a Single Intravenous Bolus at the Dose of 10 mg/kg

C_{max}	(μM)	9.6
$T_{1/2}$	(h)	1.4
AUC	(μM·h)	6.5
CL	(L/h/kg)	3.6
V_{ss}	(L/kg)	3.7

reported in Table 11.6. Negligible exposure is observed when the compound is administered orally.

In vitro studies in liver slices with PHA-739358 showed that the major route of metabolism involves the formation of the N-oxide of the N-alkyl piperazine moiety and a minor route involving dealkylation of the same moiety. In vivo metabolism results for PHA-739358 from mouse, rat, dog, and monkey urine and/or plasma confirmed the in vitro findings.

To understand the relationship between the time–concentration profiles of PHA-739358 and the tumor growth curves in different xenograft models, a pharmacokinetic/pharmacodynamic model (PK/PD) was applied (Simeoni et al., 2004). In this model, it is assumed that the cells, after being exposed to the drugs, are irreversibly damaged and subsequently enter an irreversible death process. The severity of the damage is defined as the potency and the rate at which the cells go to death (cell death distribution). These parameters can be calculated using the model after appropriate fitting of the experimental data. Quantitatively, the potency of the compound is related to two model parameters: K_2 and C_t. K_2 is the proportionality factor linking the plasma concentration to the effect and can be regarded as a drug-specific measurement of the potency of the compound. The C_t value provides an estimate of the steady-state drug concentration in plasma that must be maintained to observe tumor regression and eventually tumor eradication ($C_{ss} > C_t$). In the case of PHA-739358, the estimated C_t value in the A2780 model was about 1.5 µM, and the potency factor K_2 was between 0.0055 and 0.0096 h/µM independent of the tumor size at the start of treatment. For comparison, the same values for paclitaxel are 0.545 µM and 0.022 h/µM (C_t and K_2, respectively). No dependency of dose and schedule was observed, and the activity was maintained with the same potency as when the compound was given to tumors in more advanced stages. These parameters were helpful to guide schedules in clinical trials and predictions of active doses and target plasma levels.

PHA-739358 was tested in several animal models for efficacy and safety. Results obtained in these preclinical experiments demonstrate a broad spectrum of activity against a number of cell lines in vivo. Tumor growth inhibition and regression have been noted at exposures with acceptable toxicity, defining an overall pharmacology profile that is highly promising for further development.

A summary of the results of in vivo efficacy experiments is reported in Figure 11.10 and Table 11.7.

11.4. DEVELOPMENT OF PHA-739358

11.4.1. Aurora Kinase Inhibitors in Clinical Development

Numerous Aurora kinase inhibitors have begun clinical phase testing. The various clinical candidates differ in their selectivity profiles for both Aurora kinase family members and other kinases, and in their pharmaceutical properties, in particular, bioavailability. There are several recent reviews, which touch on the advantages and disadvantages of more or less selective inhibitors (Carpinelli and Moll, 2008; Gautschi et al., 2008). The next section summarizes the properties of some of the current Aurora kinase inhibitors in clinical development.

AstraZeneca is developing AZD1152, a quinazoline prodrug that shows some degree of selectivity for Aurora-B (Wilkinson et al., 2007). The compound is in Phase I trials for the treatment of advanced solid tumors given as a weekly 2 hour infusion. Also, alternative schedules are currently being tested, including a biweekly and continuous infusion. In the initial study, the dose-limiting toxicity (DLT) has been neutropenia and at present no objective responses are reported, although some patients experienced stable disease.

Merck and Vertex are codeveloping a series of pyrimidine derivatives, for which VX-680/MK-0457 is the most advanced (Harrington et al., 2004). The compound inhibits all Aurora kinases and was reported to have

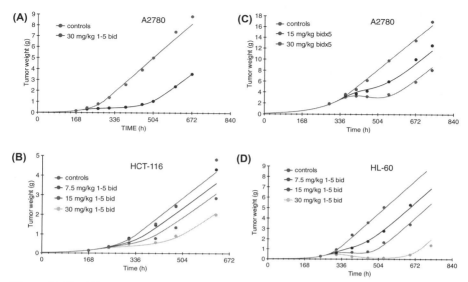

Figure 11.10. (**A**) A2780 xenograft tumors were treated intravenously with the vehicle or PHA-739358 at 30 mg/kg bid for 5 days from day 8. (**B**) As in A) with the exception that large tumors were treated intravenously with the vehicle or PHA-739358 at 15 and 30 mg/kg bid for 5 days from day 13. Mice bearing HCT-116 (**C**) or HL-60 (**D**) xenograft tumors were treated intravenously with the vehicle or PHA-739358 at 7.5, 15, and 30 mg/kg bid for 5 days from day 8. Adapted from *Mol Cancer Ther.* **2007**, 6(12), 3158–3168.

cross-reactivities with Flt3 and Abl, including the Abl T315I mutant (Cheetham et al., 2007). It has been examined in Phase I clinical trials in patients with advanced solid tumors and in those with chronic myelogenous leukemia expressing mutant Abl (T315I). For the latter indication, some promising responses were described (Giles et al., 2007). After observation of a QTc prolongation in a patient, development of the compound was halted, and a backup compound is in development.

MLN8054 is an orally available inhibitor developed by Millennium Pharmaceuticals (now Takeda) with activity mainly on Aurora-A (Manfredi et al., 2007). The compound entered clinical trials in 2005 and was investigated in solid tumors. Due to nonmechanism of action related sideeffects, a second-generation compound (MLN8327) subsequently entered clinical trials. There are several other compounds in late preclinical development or early clinical trials (AT-9283, R763/AS-703569, Cyc-116, PF-03814735, GSK1070916, ENMD-981693), which have been described in some recent reviews (Gautschi et al., 2008).

The reasons for the attractiveness of Aurora kinases as anticancer targets are related to their convincing preclinical target validation, the unique mechanism of action upon inhibition, the strong link to disease, and the ease of finding small-molecule inhibitors.

TABLE 11.7. In Vivo Activity of PHA-739358

Model[a]	Dose (mg/kg)	Schedule	Maximal TGI % (day)	Maximum Weight Loss (%)
Xenograft models in nude mice				
A2780, human ovarian carcinoma	30	IV qd D1–10	80 (19)	18
HCT-116, human colon carcinoma	30	IV bid D1–5	66 (17)	22
HL-60, human acute myelog-enous leukemia	30	IV bid D1–5	98 (22)[b]	16
Transgenic models in mice				
MMTV-RAS, mammary carcinoma	25	IV bid D1–3 q wk × 2	75 (10)	10
TRAMP, prostate carcinoma	30	IV bid D1–3 q wk × 2	68 (23)	15
Rat model				
DMBA-induced mammary carcinoma	25	IV bid D1–3 q wk × 2	75 (10)[c]	10

[a]n = 8–10 animals/study.
[b]Two out of eight animals showed complete regression.
[c]One out of ten animals showed complete regression; one out of ten, death at day 5.
Abbreviations: IV = intravenous, qd = daily, bid = twice per day, TGI = tumor growth inhibition, PR = partial response, SD = stable disease.

11.4.2. PHA-739358 Clinical Trials

11.4.2.1. Solid Tumors. There are two major directions for the development of PHA-739358 in the clinic: first, as an inhibitor of Aurora kinases having a primary effect at mitosis; and second, as an inhibitor of additional cancer-relevant kinases such as BCR-ABL (T315I) in chronic myelogenous leukemia or FGFR-3 in multiple myeloma. In these settings, inhibition of Aurora kinases is expected to contribute to the antitumor effects observed.

PHA-739358 was the first Aurora kinase inhibitor to enter clinical trials in the middle of 2004. The initial Phase I trials had classical primary endpoints of pharmacokinetics and toxicity with secondary endpoints being responses or effects on survival and biomarker modulation. Two Phase I trials in solid tumors were initiated simultaneously applying different schedules. In the first trial the compound was given in cycles of 24 hour infusions every 2 weeks and

40 patients were treated at seven dose levels (Cohen et al., 2008). The compound was escalated up to $650 \, mg/m^2$, with $500 \, mg/m^2$ being the recommended Phase II dose. PK parameters showed low interpatient variability and dose-proportionate increases in AUC and C_{max}, and plasma levels predicted to be efficacious from preclinical models were exceeded at $500 \, mg/m^2$. The half-life of the drug was in the range of 18–26 hours.

Biomarker modulation was followed by measuring phosphorylation of histone H3, a direct substrate of Aurora-B kinase, in skin biopsies before and at the end of infusion. The modulation of this biomarker was observed at the recommended Phase II dose as assessed by immunohistochemistry and Western blot.

Dose-limiting toxicities were neutropenia and lymphocytopenia observed in 72% and 55% of patients, respectively. These side effects were expected based on the mechanism of action and the preclinical assessment of the compound. Forty-six percent of evaluable patients showed stable disease (SD) as best response, with 28% having SD for more than 3 months and with one ovarian patient having a regression of 27% in tumor size accompanied by a reduction of plasma tumor marker (CA125). Since neutropenia was the major dose-limiting toxicity, the original protocol was amended to allow growth factor support. An increase of the MTD of 50% ($750 \, mg/m^2$) was achieved and 43% of evaluable patients showed stable disease. Also, a partial response in a small-cell lung cancer patient was reported, lasting for half a year.

In the second study, a 6 hour weekly infusion was administered to patients for 3 weeks in a 4 week cycle (De Jonge et al., 2008). The maximum tolerated dose was $330 \, mg/m^2$ and, in this case, the dose-limiting toxicity was neutropenia as in the study mentioned previously. Of 30 evaluable patients, 7 (23%) experienced stable diseases with 4 of these responses lasting more than 6 months. A non-small-cell lung cancer patient was treated for more than 31 months (still on treatment). Also, in this case, the phosphorylation of histone H3 in skin was determined and inhibition was observed starting at $190 \, mg/m^2$.

In summary, both Phase I studies showed similar results. PHA-739358 shows excellent PK properties, a MOA related DLT, exposures expected to be efficacious based on preclinical data, pharmacodynamic biomarker modulation at the recommended Phase II doses, and clinically relevant stable diseases with one partial response in heavily pretreated patients.

Further Phase I and II studies of PHA-739358 as monotherapy or in combination are underway to better judge the value of this compound for the treatment of cancer.

11.4.2.2. Clinical Opportunities in CML. Since PHA-739358 shows cross-reactivity with BCR-ABL and, in particular, with one of the most common and currently untreatable mutants T315I, a clinical study was performed to test activity in CML patients. Although treatment of CML patients with imatinib is a very effective option for patients in the chronic phase of the disease, this treatment is only marginally effective in patients in the accelerated phase of CML or in a blast crisis. In addition, once treatment in responsive CML patients is stopped, relapse is observed (Jabbour et al., 2008).

One of the reasons for resistance to imatinib is the appearance of point mutations that either interfere directly with binding of the drug or prevent the adoption of the inactive conformation required for binding. One of the most commonly identified mutations occurs in the gatekeeper residue Thr315 of Abl. Even the second-generation BCR-ABL inhibitors such as dasatinib, nilotinib, or bosutinib are inactive against this mutation. The reasons for the good activity of PHA-739358 are due to its unique binding mode, as seen when the compound was crystallized in complex with the T315I Abl mutant (Modugno et al., 2007).

PHA-738358 was tested preclinically for its ability to inhibit proliferation of cell lines expressing wild-type or imatinib-resistant BCR-ABL mutants including the T315I mutant. In these cells, the activity of both Abl and Aurora kinases was inhibited and PHA-739358 showed pharmacological synergy with imatinib in cell lines with a partial resistance to imatinib. Strong antiproliferative activity is also seen in $CD34^+$ cells from CML patients in chronic phase or blast crisis, including those bearing the T315I mutation (Gontarewicz et al., 2008). Based on this strong preclinical data, a clinical development plan was established to evaluate the potential of the compound in CML and, in particular, in the T315I-positive subpopulation of patients.

In a first study (see www.clinicaltrials.gov, NCT00335868), the drug was administered for 3 hours at $250\,mg/m^2$ and, although effects were seen on the number of blasts in bone marrow and blood in many patients, a fast rebound was observed after treatment. This led to the application of more aggressive regimens, such as increasing the dose to $400\,mg/m^2$ and/or giving the dose over a shorter time frame. Highly relevant clinical responses were seen in patients bearing the T315I mutation. This might be due to the high affinity of the compound for this mutant, as mentioned previously (Modugno et al., 2007). The crystal structure of PHA-739358 bound to the T315I Abl kinase domain has been solved and the binding mode explains why the compound is able to inhibit this mutant more effectively than other known inhibitors of ABL. It is worth noting that at least two other Aurora kinase inhibitors are active on ABL T315I: VX-680/MK-0457 and AT-9283. The CML trial is still ongoing but a few long-term responses were observed in T315I-bearing patients for more than a year.

Although PHA-739358 shows a clear dominant cellular phenotype related to inhibition of Aurora-B, some of the other cross-reactivities, identified upon screening of more than 200 kinases, could open additional venues for development or might contribute to the compound's antitumor activity. As mentioned previously, kinases in this group include FGFRs, VEGFRs, Ret, and Trk-A.

FGFR family members are key players in cancer development and progression (Jeffers et al., 2002). In particular, a role for FGFR3 in bladder cancer has been defined and in urothelial cancer a high percentage of cases show mutations (Tomlinson et al., 2007). In approximately 15% of multiple myeloma patients, a translocation of FGFR3 is found and inhibitors of FGFR3 are currently in development for this group of patients (Onwuazor et al., 2003). PHA-739358 has been shown to inhibit FGFR3 signaling at submicromolar doses in cells and this concept is currently being tested in clinical trials. Other interesting cross-reactivities, which could be targeted for an anticancer treatment, are the inhibition of Ret and Trk-A. Both are oncogenes known to be mutated and activated in thyroid carcinoma (Kodama et al., 2005). Since Aurora-B levels also are correlated with thyroid carcinoma phenotype and its inhibition has antiproliferative activity, the combined inhibition of RET, TRK-A, and Aurora-B could be a promising approach in this indication.

11.5. SUMMARY

Looking back at the discovery of PHA-739358, it is interesting to reevaluate some of the crucial decisions we needed to make at the time and the lessons learned. First, concerning the use of the combinatorial techniques, we decided to use them mainly as a tool for expanding the capability of classical medicinal chemistry. Following this approach, the size of combinatorial libraries was limited well below the capacity of the available process. The library design was based on a compromise favoring medicinal chemistry experience over diversity maximization, and a low automation process was developed for library production. At least in the present case, this strategy turned out to be extremely time and cost effective. This conclusion is in line with recent discussions about the pitfalls of some of the original combinatorial chemistry approaches, which were based on exploring chemical space with huge, diversity-driven compound libraries.

A second crucial decision to be made was on the selectivity profile of the candidate. We decided to pursue the development of a pan-Aurora kinase inhibitor, which also is extremely active against additional anticancer kinase targets. In this, we were guided by a pragmatic approach, which favored the overall in vivo safety–efficacy profile over the paradigm of highly selective molecular-targeted anticancer therapeutics. As of today, the additional activities of PHA-739358 have not resulted in any unexpected toxicity. By contrast, they are offering promising therapeutic opportunities and interesting elements for differentiation in the crowded field of Aurora kinase inhibitors. Indeed, the approach of developing multikinase inhibitors has rapidly become a widely accepted strategy.

Being the first Aurora kinase inhibitor in clinical trials, PHA-739358 was and is still a compound that may provide the first clinical proof-of-concept for Aurora inhibition. In clinical trials, the compound shows good tolerability and promising anticancer activities in both solid and nonsolid tumors. The most promising indications are currently being investigated using optimized schedules. The study of combinations could offer further opportunities to increase the efficacy of the compound. It is hoped that PHA-739358 will become a new weapon against cancer for the benefit of many patients.

REFERENCES

Bergnes, G., Brejc, K., and Belmont, L. (2005). Mitotic kinesins: prospects for antimitotic drug discovery. *Curr Top Med Chem.* 5(2), 127–145.

Berta, D., Felder, E. R., Villa, M., et al. (2002). WO 02/62804.

Bischoff, J. R., Anderson, L., Zhu, Y., et al. (1998). A homologue of *Drosophila* aurora kinase is oncogenic and amplified in human colorectal cancers. *EMBO J.* 17(11), 3052–3065.

Böhmer, F. D., Karagyozov, L., Uecker, A., et al. (2003). A single amino acid exchange inverts susceptibility of related receptor tyrosine kinases for the ATP site inhibitor STI-571. *J Biol Chem.* 278(7), 5148–5155.

Briassouli, P., Chan, F., Savage, K., et al. (2007). Aurora-A regulation of nuclear factor-kappaB signaling by phosphorylation of IkappaBalpha. *Cancer Res.* 67(4), 1689–1695.

Carpinelli, P., and Moll, J. (2008). Aurora kinase inhibitors: identification and preclinical validation of their biomarkers. *Expert Opin Ther Targets.* 12(1), 69–80.

Carpinelli, P., Ceruti, R., Giorgini, M. L., et al. (2007). PHA-739358, a potent inhibitor of Aurora kinases with a selective target inhibition profile relevant to cancer. *Mol Cancer Ther.* 6(12 Pt 1), 3158–3168.

Cheetham, G. M., Charlton, P. A., Golec, J. M., et al. (2007). Structural basis for potent inhibition of the Aurora kinases and a T315I multi-drug resistant mutant form of Abl kinase by VX-680. *Cancer Lett.* 251(2), 323–329.

Cohen, R. B., Jones, S. F., von Mehren, M., et al. (2008). Phase I study of the pan aurora kinases (AKs) inhibitor PHA-739358 administered as a 24 h infusion without/with G-CSF in a 14-day cycle in patients with advanced solid tumors. *J Clin Oncol.* 26(Suppl), Abst 2520.

de Carcer, G., Perez de Castro, I., and Malumbres, M. (2007). Targeting cell cycle kinases for cancer therapy. *Curr Med Chem.* 14(9), 969–985.

De Jonge, M., Steeghs, N., Verweij, J., et al. (2008). Phase I study of the Aurora kinases (AKs) inhibitor PHA-739358 administered as a 6 and 3-h IV infusion on days 1, 8, 15 every 4 wks in patients with advanced solid tumors. *J Clin Oncol.* 26(Suppl), Abst 3507.

Dewar, H., Tanaka, K., Nasmyth, K., et al. (2004). Tension between two kinetochores suffices for their bi-orientation on the mitotic spindle. *Nature.* 428(6978), 93–97.

Ewart-Toland, A., Dai, Q., Gao, Y. T., et al. (2005). Aurora-A/STK15 T+91A is a general low penetrance cancer susceptibility gene: a meta-analysis of multiple cancer types. *Carcinogenesis.* 26(8), 1368–1373.

Fancelli, D., Pittala, V., and Varasi, M. (2002). WO 02/012242.

Fancelli, D., Berta, D., Bindi, S., et al. (2005a). Potent and selective Aurora inhibitors identified by the expansion of a novel scaffold for protein kinase inhibition. *J Med Chem.* 48(8), 3080–3084.

Fancelli, D., Forte, B., Moll, J., et al. (2005b). WO 05/005427.

Fancelli, D., Moll, J., Varasi, M., et al. (2006). 1,4,5,6-Tetrahydropyrrolo[3,4-c]pyrazoles: identification of a potent Aurora kinase inhibitor with a favorable antitumor kinase inhibition profile. *J Med Chem.* 49(24), 7247–7251.

Fu, J., Bian, M., Jiang, Q., et al. (**2007**). Roles of Aurora kinases in mitosis and tumorigenesis. *Mol Cancer Res.* 5(1), 1–10.

Fuller, B. G., Lampson, M. A., Foley, E. A., et al. (**2008**). Midzone activation of Aurora B in anaphase produces an intracellular phosphorylation gradient. *Nature.* 453(7198), 1132–1136.

Gautschi, O., Heighway, J., Mack, P. C., et al. (**2008**). Aurora kinases as anticancer drug targets. *Clin Cancer Res.* 14(6), 1639–1648.

Giles, F. J., Cortes, J., Jones, D., et al. (**2007**). MK-0457, a novel kinase inhibitor, is active in patients with chronic myeloid leukemia or acute lymphocytic leukemia with the T315I BCR-ABL mutation. *Blood.* 109(2), 500–502.

Glover, D. M., Leibowitz, M. H., McLean, D. A., et al. (**1995**). Mutations in Aurora prevent centrosome separation leading to the formation of monopolar spindles. *Cell.* 81(1), 95–105.

Gontarewicz, A., Balabanov, S., Keller, G., et al. (**2008**). Simultaneous targeting of Aurora kinases and Bcr-Abl kinase by the small molecule inhibitor PHA-739358 is effective against imatinib-resistant BCR-ABL mutations including T315I. *Blood.* 111(8), 4355–4364.

Hans, F., and Dimitrov, S. (**2001**). Histone H3 phosphorylation and cell division. *Oncogene.* 20(24), 3021–3027.

Harrington, E. A., Bebbington, D., Moore, J., et al. (**2004**). VX-680, a potent and selective small-molecule inhibitor of the Aurora kinases, suppresses tumor growth in vivo. *Nat Med.* 10(3), 262–267.

Hirota, T., Kunitoku, N., Sasayama, T., et al. (**2003**). Aurora-A and an interacting activator, the LIM protein Ajuba, are required for mitotic commitment in human cells. *Cell.* 114(5), 585–598.

Jabbour, E., Cortes, J. E., Ghanem, H., O'Brien, S., and Kantarjian, H. M. (**2008**). Targeted therapy in chronic myeloid leukemia. *Expert Rev Anticancer Ther.* 8(1), 99–110.

Jeffers, M., LaRochelle, W. J., and Lichenstein, H. S. (**2002**). Fibroblast growth factors in cancer: therapeutic possibilities. *Expert Opin Ther Targets.* 6(4), 469–482.

Jordan, M. A. (**2002**). Mechanism of action of antitumor drugs that interact with microtubules and tubulin. *Curr Med Chem Anticancer Agents.* 2(1), 1–17.

Jordan, M. A., and Wilson, L. (**2004**). Microtubules as a target for anticancer drugs. *Nat Rev Cancer.* 4(4), 253–265.

Katayama, H., Brinkley, W. R., and Sen, S. (**2003**). The Aurora kinases: role in cell transformation and tumorigenesis. *Cancer Metastasis Rev.* 22(4), 451–464.

Katayama, H., Sasai, K., Kawai, H., et al. (**2004**). Phosphorylation by Aurora kinase A induces Mdm2-mediated destabilization and inhibition of p53. *Nat Genet.* 36(1), 55–62.

Ke, Y. W., Dou, Z., Zhang, J., and Yao, X. B. (**2003**). Function and regulation of Aurora/Ipl1p kinase family in cell division. *Cell Res.* 13(2), 69–81.

Kobayashi, S., Boggon, T. J., Dayaram, T., et al. (**2005**). EGFR mutation and resistance of non-small-cell lung cancer to gefitinib. *N Engl J Med.* 352(8), 786–792.

Kodama, Y., Asai, N., Kawai, K., et al. (**2005**). The RET proto-oncogene: a molecular therapeutic target in thyroid cancer. *Cancer Sci.* 96(3), 143–148.

Kufer, T. A., Sillje, H. H., Korner, R., et al. (**2002**). Human TPX2 is required for targeting Aurora-A kinase to the spindle. *J Cell Biol.* 158(4), 617–623.

Liu, Q., Kaneko, S., Yang, L., et al. (**2004**). Aurora-A abrogation of p53 DNA binding and transactivation activity by phosphorylation of serine 215. *J Biol Chem.* 279(50), 52175–52182.

Manfredi, M. G., Ecsedy, J. A., Meetze, K. A., et al. (**2007**). Antitumor activity of MLN8054, an orally active small-molecule inhibitor of Aurora A kinase. *Proc Natl Acad Sci USA.* 104(10), 4106–4111.

Modugno, M., Casale, E., Soncini, C., et al. (**2007**). Crystal structure of the T315I Abl mutant in complex with the Aurora kinases inhibitor PHA-739358. *Cancer Res.* 67(17), 7987–7990.

Mora-Bermúdez, F., Gerlich, D., and Ellenberg, J. (**2007**). Maximal chromosome compaction occurs by axial shortening in anaphase and depends on Aurora kinase. *Nat Cell Biol.* 9(7), 822–831.

Murata-Hori, M., and Wang, Y. L. (**2002**). The kinase activity of Aurora B is required for kinetochore–microtubule interactions during mitosis. *Curr Biol.* 12(11), 894–899.

Onwuazor, O. N., Wen, X. Y., Wang, D. Y., et al. (**2003**). Mutation, SNP, and isoform analysis of fibroblast growth factor receptor 3 (FGFR3) in 150 newly diagnosed multiple myeloma patients. *Blood.* 102(2), 772–773.

Pevarello, P., Brasca, M. G., Amici, R., et al. (**2004**). 3-Aminopyrazole inhibitors of CDK2/cyclin A as antitumor agents. 1. Lead finding. *J Med Chem.* 47(13), 3367–3380.

Pugacheva, E. N., and Golemis, E. A. (**2006**). HEF1–Aurora A interactions: points of dialog between the cell cycle and cell attachment signaling networks. *Cell Cycle.* 5(4), 384–391.

Sasayama, T., Marumoto, T., Kunitoku, N., et al. (**2005**). Over-expression of Aurora-A targets cytoplasmic polyadenylation element binding protein and promotes mRNA polyadenylation of Cdk1 and cyclin B1. *Genes Cells.* 10(7), 627–638.

Sharma, P. S., Sharma, R., and Tyagi, R. (**2008**). Inhibitors of cyclin dependent kinases: useful targets for cancer treatment. *Curr Cancer Drug Targets.* 8(1), 53–75.

Simeoni, M., Magni, P., Cammia, C., et al. (**2004**). Predictive pharmacokinetic–pharmacodynamic modeling of tumor growth kinetics in xenograft models after administration of anticancer agents. *Cancer Res.* 64(3), 1094–1101.

Soncini, C., Carpinelli, P., Gianellini, L., et al. (**2006**). PHA-680632, a novel Aurora kinase inhibitor with potent antitumoral activity. *Clin Cancer Res.* 12(13), 4080–4089.

Spengler, D. (**2007**). Aurora-C-T191D is a hyperactive Aurora-C mutant. *Cell Cycle.* 6(14), 1803–1804.

Tamborini, E., Pricl, S., Negri, T., et al. (**2006**). Functional analyses and molecular modeling of two c-Kit mutations responsible for imatinib secondary resistance in GIST patients. *Oncogene.* 25(45), 6140–6146.

Tomlinson, D. C., Baldo, O., Harnden, P., et al. (**2007**). FGFR3 protein expression and its relationship to mutation status and prognostic variables in bladder cancer. *J Pathol.* 213(1), 91–98.

Tonani, R., Bindi, S., Fancelli, D., et al. (**2004a**). WO 04/007504.

Tonani, R., Bindi, S., Fancelli, D., et al. (**2004b**). WO 04/013146.

Traquandi, G., Brasca, M. G., D'Alessio, R., et al. (**2004**). WO 04/104007.

Vanotti, E., Cervi, G., Pulici, M., et al. (**2004**). WO 04/071507.

Vulpetti, A., and Bosotti, R. (**2004**). Sequence and structural analysis of kinase ATP pocket residues. *Farmaco*. 59(10), 759–765.

Wilkinson, R. W., Odedra, R., Heaton, S. P., et al. (**2007**). AZD1152, a selective inhibitor of Aurora B kinase, inhibits human tumor xenograft growth by inducing apoptosis. *Clin Cancer Res*. 13(12), 3682–3688.

Yang, H., Burke, T., Dempsey, J., et al. (**2005**). Mitotic requirement for Aurora A kinase is bypassed in the absence of Aurora B kinase. *FEBS Lett*. 579(16), 3385–3391.

Zhou, H., Kuang, J., Zhong, L., et al. (**1998**). Tumour amplified kinase STK15/BTAK induces centrosome amplification, aneuploidy and transformation. *Nat Genet*. 20(2), 189–193.

12

DISCOVERY OF AZD1152: A SELECTIVE INHIBITOR OF AURORA-B KINASE WITH POTENT ANTITUMOR ACTIVITY

KEVIN M. FOOTE AND ANDREW A. MORTLOCK

12.1. INTRODUCTION

The Aurora proteins are a small family of serine/threonine kinases that are expressed during mitosis and have been suggested to be attractive drug targets (Keen and Taylor, 2004). They have roles in chromosome segregation and cytokinesis and ensure that a complete copy of the duplicated genome is precisely partitioned into the two daughter cells. There are three human Aurora kinase paralogues, Aurora-A, -B and -C, two of which (Aurora-A and -B) are commonly overexpressed in human tumors (Bischoff et al., 1998). With their key role in mitosis and their being aberrantly overexpressed in tumor cells, there has been considerable interest in developing specific Aurora kinase inhibitors and in understanding the therapeutic value of selectively inhibiting Aurora-A and -B.

While there are now considerable data supporting a link between Aurora-A and -B kinase expression and cancer, it is still unclear whether inhibition of Aurora-A and/or Aurora-B could be advantageous in terms of providing therapeutic benefit in oncology. Studies using both pharmacological and genetic disruption of Aurora kinases in cells have shown that the mitotic defects described following exposure of cells to Aurora kinase inhibitors seem largely due to inhibition of Aurora-B (Ditchfield et al., 2003; Hauf et al., 2003;

Kinase Inhibitor Drugs. Edited by Rongshi Li and Jeffrey A. Stafford
Copyright © 2009 John Wiley & Sons, Inc.

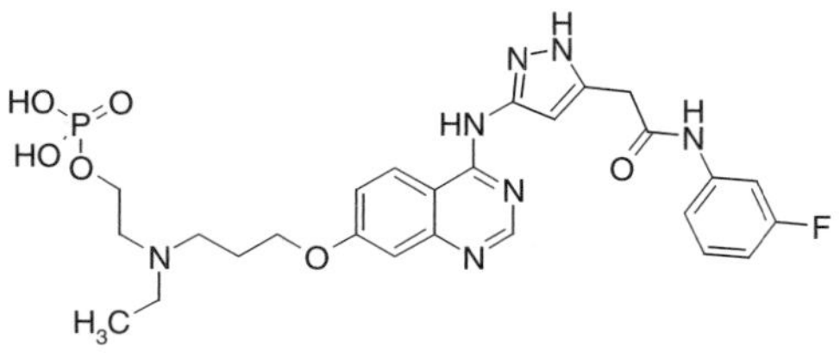

Figure 12.1. Structure of AZD1152.

Yang et al., 2005; Girdler et al., 2006, 2008). When Aurora-B is inhibited in tumor cells, the cells are forced through a catastrophic mitotic exit leading to polyploid cells that rapidly lose viability. In contrast, selective inhibition of Aurora-A kinase activity causes a mitotic delay and abnormalities in centrosome separation leading to the formation of a monopolar spindle (Girdler et al., 2006).

Several potent and structurally diverse small-molecule inhibitors of the Aurora kinases have demonstrated antitumor activity and have subsequently entered clinical evaluation. Some of these compounds inhibit both Aurora-A and Aurora-B (Harrington et al., 2004; Fancelli et al., 2006; Carpinelli et al., 2007); others produce cellular phenotypes indicative of selective Aurora-A kinase inhibition (Hoar et al., 2007; Manfredi et al., 2007) and we have described the preclinical activity of the first Aurora-B selective inhibitor, AZD1152, to enter clinical evaluation (Mortlock et al., 2007; Wilkinson et al., 2007).

AZD1152 (Figure 12.1) was developed following optimization, in multiple iterations, of a series of aryl-substituted quinazolines. AZD1152 is selective for Aurora-B over Aurora-A and is a readily activated phosphate prodrug with high solubility in simple pH-adjusted aqueous vehicles, making it suitable for parenteral delivery using a range of dosing schedules. AZD1152 possesses robust antitumor activity in preclinical xenograft models and has the potential for activity in multiple tumor types.

12.2. ANILINOQUINAZOLINES AND CORRESPONDING PYRIMIDINE AND PYRIDINE ANALOGS

Screening of the AstraZeneca compound collection, with an assay measuring in vitro kinase activity using truncated Aurora-A protein, was used to establish a range of starting points for medicinal chemistry. At the time of screening, Aurora-A, in particular, had been identified as a drug target given the observation that it can act as an oncogene and transform cells when ectopically expressed (Bischoff et al., 1998). Attractive chemical hits were found from a number of well-known kinase inhibitor series (as well as many more novel small clusters), but a subseries of anilinoquinazolines, exemplified by compound **1** (Table 12.1), stood out in terms of both potency and selectivity

TABLE 12.1. In Vitro SAR of Quinazoline Leads

Compound	X	Aurora-A IC$_{50}$ (μM)	MCF7 Cell IC$_{50}$ (μM)	Log $D_{7.4}$
1		0.393	1.25	3.7
2		0.11	0.198	3.5
3		0.003	0.21	2.7
4		0.629		

for Aurora-A over other serine/threonine and tyrosine kinases. Clear structure–activity relationship (SAR) was evident from the primary screening data and suggested that compounds where the aniline group contained an extended *para*-substituent showed good potency toward the kinase. Knowledge from other quinazoline-based kinase inhibitors, such as Iressa™, suggested that the quinazoline should bind into the adenine site (with N-1 making a critical interaction with the protein backbone) and indicated that the extended benzamido group should occupy the selectivity pocket.

Based on this simple hypothesis of the binding mode of compound **1**, a number of compounds were made with more elaborate groups at the C-6 and C-7 positions of the quinazoline core, both to introduce polar groups to improve compound solubility and to pick up additional binding in the channel between the adenine binding site and the solvent-accessible region. From this preliminary work, compound **2** (ZM447439) was prepared, which showed much improved cellular potency (MCF7 antiproliferation assay), making it an attractive tool to probe further the mechanism and cellular phenotype of an Aurora kinase inhibitor. Evaluation of compound **2** in a panel of in vitro kinase inhibition assays demonstrated good activity against Aurora-A kinase (IC$_{50}$ = 0.11 μM) with good selectivity across a limited kinase panel. Published studies with compound **2** later showed equivalent potency against Aurora-B kinase (IC_{50} = 0.13 µM) and in cell studies was shown to cause a dose-dependent increase in 4N DNA, due to a failure of cytokinesis, that is consistent with the proposed mechanism of action (Ditchfield et al., 2003). Furthermore, compound **2** selectively induced apoptosis in cycling cells but had relatively little effect on G1-arrested MCF7 cells when profiled in in vitro clonigenicity assays, again consistent with the proposed mechanism of action.

Despite the utility of compounds such as **1** and **2** as tools for exploring Aurora kinase function, both compounds have relatively low aqueous solubility and are also highly protein bound (compound **2** rat plasma protein binding = 99.7%), probably due to high lipophilicity. In an effort to improve these physical properties, a number of strategies to lower the $\log D$ of the core structure were followed. Greatest success was achieved when the phenyl ring of the aniline substituent was replaced with a pyrimidine group. The enzyme potency was highly sensitive to the specific pyrimidine isomer that was employed. The 5-pyrimidinyl isomer (compound **3**) showed increased potency in the enzyme assay compared with the phenyl analog (compound **2**). In contrast, the 2-pyrimidyl isomer (compound **4**) was over 100 times less potent against Aurora-A than compound **3**. The reduced $\log D$ for compound **3** resulted in a significant reduction in plasma protein binding (compound **3** rat plasma protein binding = 95.5%), although the compound's aqueous solubility remained poor. Selectivity over other kinases was also improved with many other kinases being intolerant of the heterocyclic ring.

While the improved physicochemical properties of compounds such as **3** are readily attributed to a reduction in lipophilicity, the increase in potency is more difficult to rationalize, even when the X-ray structural data is used (see Section 12.3). There is no obvious eclipsing interaction between the meta hydrogens in compound **3** and the protein, nor is it obvious the compounds can populate significantly different conformation space.

Further improvements in Aurora-A enzyme potency were achieved by introduction of small lipophilic substituents, especially in the meta and/or para positions, on the phenyl ring of the benzamido group. Substituents such as 3-chloro or 3-chloro-4-fluoro (compounds **5** and **6**, Table 12.2) gave excellent enzyme potency and also resulted in a significant improvement in the cell activities (80 and 20 nM, respectively). The introduction of larger groups (compounds **7** and **8**) had a detrimental effect on potency while introduction of a very large sulfonamido group (compound **9**) resulted in a 1000-fold drop in activity when compared with compound **3**. Replacement of the phenyl ring with either a heterocyclic group (e.g., 4-pyridyl, compound **10**) or an alkyl substituent (e.g., n-butyl, compound **11**) gave compounds with much improved aqueous solubility but the drop in potency against both enzyme and cell assays was unacceptable.

Although beneficial for potency, the introduction of the halogens on the pendant phenyl ring, and the associated increase in lipophilicity, negated some

TABLE 12.2. Benzamide In Vitro SAR

5–11

Compound	X	Aurora-A IC$_{50}$ (μM)
5		<0.001
6		<0.001
7		0.070
8		0.085
9		3.9
10		0.69
11	n-Bu	0.017

of the improvement in physical properties resulting from the introduction of the pyrimidine ring. With the inhibitor now refined with respect to the adenine and selectivity pocket binding groups, attention returned to the C-7 side chain as the key substituent to ameliorate physical properties. While substitution was not tolerated on the methylene unit nearest to the quinazoline, there was considerable scope for introduction of one or more solubilizing groups on the second or third methylene units in the chain. The level of aqueous solubility can be increased dramatically by increasing the basicity of the nitrogen such that it is effectively completely protonated at physiological pH, for example,

TABLE 12.3. C-7 In Vitro SAR in Pyrimidine–Quinazoline Series

12–17

Compound	R_1R_2N	X	Y	Aurora-A IC_{50} (µM)	Aqueous Solubility (µM)	pK_a[a]
12		H	H	0.0008	3,600	9.3
13		OH	H	0.0006	600	8.7
14		OH	H	0.002	0.1	7.0
15		H	F	0.015	3,300	9.7
16		H	F	0.0007	1,400	8.4
17		H	F	0.007	2,440	9.0

[a]Estimated from ACD pK_a suite of software.

compound **12** (Table 12.3), and/or by introduction of polar substituents, for example, compound **13**. Furthermore, it was clear that neither the Aurora-A enzyme potency nor the activity of these compounds in the MCF7 antiproliferative assay was adversely affected by these modifications (Mortlock et al., 2005). The strong correlation between the basicity of the nitrogen and the aqueous solubility can clearly be seen with compounds **14–17**, which demonstrate the dramatic change (10^3–10^4) in solubility resulting from modulating pK_a.

12.3. CRYSTALLOGRAPHIC STUDIES

Following crystallization of a fragment of the Aurora-A protein, the determination of the structure of a protein–inhibitor complex was achieved using compound **18** (Figure 12.2), the direct analog of compound **13** with an unsubstituted benzamido phenyl group. The docking mode of compound **18** into the active site of Aurora-A is illuminating and provided additional powerful evidence to support the SAR models that were being developed from the biochemical data (Heron et al., 2006).

The structures show the bilobal shape characteristic of protein kinases with the inhibitor binding site situated in the cleft between the two lobes (Figure 12.2). Compound **18** adopts a near-planar, extended, conformation in complex with Aurora-A, demonstrating the extent of the available binding pocket. A classical (adenine mimetic) kinase–inhibitor hydrogen bond interaction with the main chain peptide is made between the N-1 of the quinazoline ring and the amide of Ala212, while the piperidine moiety at the end of the quinazoline C-7 side chain extends into solvent.

The protein–inhibitor structure adopts a conformation typical of catalytically inactive kinases. The benzoyl moiety in compound **18** fits into a hydrophobic pocket occupied by Phe274 in the conserved DFG motif in the absence of the inhibitor. The inhibitor stabilizes a "DFG-out" conformation, which

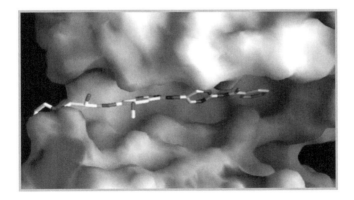

Figure 12.2. X-ray crystal structure (2.1 Å) of GSMH-[T287D]Aurora-A (122–400) and compound **18**. (See color insert.)

typically prevents the activation loop from adopting a productive conformation for activation by phosphorylation and may contribute to the inhibitory mechanism (Heron et al., 2006).

12.4. QUINAZOLINES SUBSTITUTED WITH AMINOTHIAZOLES OR AMINOTHIOPHENES

The observation that certain six-membered ring heterocycles could be substituted for the aniline group in compound **2** stimulated a parallel line of work to explore the corresponding five-membered ring compounds. A number of quinazolines with five-membered rings of various structure with directly linked amide groups (compounds **19–22**, Table 12.4) were evaluated, with the 2-thiazole (**19**) and 5-thiophene (**20**) analogs being of greatest interest (Mortlock et al., 2005; Jung et al., 2006).

Modeling studies suggested that compounds **19–22** were characterized by a different conformational relationship between the quinazoline system (notably the key N-1 hydrogen bond acceptor) and the benzamido group when compared to earlier pyrimidinoquinazolines, such as compound **18**. This observation suggested the kinase enjoys significant conformational flexibility and that different inhibitors could potentially bind to different kinase conformations. Such a hypothesis suggested that further improvements in selectivity and potency might be achievable by further optimizing the heterocycle–benzamide moiety.

TABLE 12.4. In Vitro SAR Across a Range of Five-Membered Ring Heterocycles

19–23

Compound	X	Y	Z	n	Aurora-A IC$_{50}$ (μM)	MCF7 Cell IC$_{50}$ (μM)
19	S	N	CH	0	0.004	0.19
20	S	CH	CH	0	0.10	
21	NH	CH	CH	0	0.37	
22	NH	N	CH	0	4.9	
23	S	N	CH	1	<0.001	0.008

Of the many compounds prepared in this area, one series where an extra methylene unit had been inserted between the amide carbonyl and the five-membered heterocyclic ring stood out in terms of enzyme and cell potency (compound **23**). When compounds containing this novel linking group were tested in the MCF7 cellular proliferation assay, a considerable increase in cellular potency over compounds that do not possess this group was seen. While no crystal structure has been reported with a compound of this type, molecular modeling studies indicate that the thiazole and benzamido phenyl rings are no longer able to adopt the relatively planar conformation observed in the structure of compound **18** bound into Aurora-A (Jung et al., 2006).

Numerous analogs, focused principally on thiazole derivatives, were made with the broad SAR paralleling that seen with the earlier series. Thus introduction of small lipophilic groups (such as 3-chloro) into the terminal phenyl group was advantageous in terms of potency, while at the other end of the molecule, hydrophilic groups on the end of the propoxy side chain allowed the retention of excellent cellular potency but kept aqueous solubility and plasma protein binding in the desired range. Compounds **24–30** (Table 12.5) are representative of the many compounds made in this series and were used as probe compounds in further studies (Mortlock et al., 2005; Jung et al., 2006).

12.5. THE SCREENING CASCADE UPDATED

The project had identified compounds with good potency in cell proliferation assays together with acceptable general kinase specificity and PK properties to warrant exploration of their in vivo activity. At this stage two particular facets of the program came into sharp focus which would set the scene for the eventual discovery of AZD1152. First, we hypothesized that continued exposure of an Aurora kinase inhibitor may maximize the chance of delivering tolerated pharmacological effects in vivo. To provide tools to explore the effects of longer-term exposure of an Aurora kinase inhibitor, it was necessary to obtain compounds with high aqueous solubility (>10 mg/mL) that could be infused via subcutaneous minipumps. Second, the maturing of the Aurora kinase biology field resulted in a shift in focus away solely from Aurora-A kinase. The first generation compound, ZM447439, together with the chemically unrelated inhibitor, Hesperadin (Hauf et al., 2003), were pivotal to this understanding of Aurora kinase function in cells and indicated a much greater role for Aurora-B kinase in the observed cellular phenotype than had at first been realized.

12.5.1. Phosphate Derivatives

The use of subcutaneous minipumps to administer inhibitors over a number of days was seen as an attractive way to explore the relationship between blood level, duration of exposure, and pharmacodynamic effect. Use of such infusion pumps requires compounds with very high solubility (given the small

TABLE 12.5. C-7 In Vitro SAR in the Thiazole–Quinazoline Series

24–30

Compound	R	X	Aurora-A IC$_{50}$ (µM)	MCF7 Cell IC$_{50}$ (µM)
24	HO—piperidine	Cl	0.0003	0.0056
25	N-methylpiperazine	Cl	0.0005	0.006
26	HO—pyrrolidine	Cl	0.0003	0.012
27	HO—N(CH)—	Cl	0.0003	0.029
28	morpholine	Cl	0.0004	0.039
29	N,N-dimethylaminoethylamine	Cl	0.0017	0.059
30	HO—piperidine	F	<0.001	0.004

volumes involved) and synthesis of prodrugs was attempted in parallel with model development.

As many compounds of interest included an aliphatic hydroxy group in the C-7 side chain, the preparation of prodrugs based on introduction of a covalently bound solubilizing group onto this hydroxy group was explored. Preliminary in-house evaluation identified phosphate as offering the potential for high solubility and rapid in vivo cleavage by alkaline phosphatases (for an overview see Sherwood, 1996). Phosphate analogs of compounds such as **30** were prepared from the corresponding hydroxy compounds according to the general scheme shown in Figure 12.3. These phosphate derivatives are typically highly soluble in pH-adjusted saline (10–25 mg/mL at pH 9) and undergo rapid conversion to the corresponding drug in plasma. The great versatility of dosing possible with these phosphate derivatives allowed exploration of both short-term (bolus) and longer-term exposure and contributed significantly

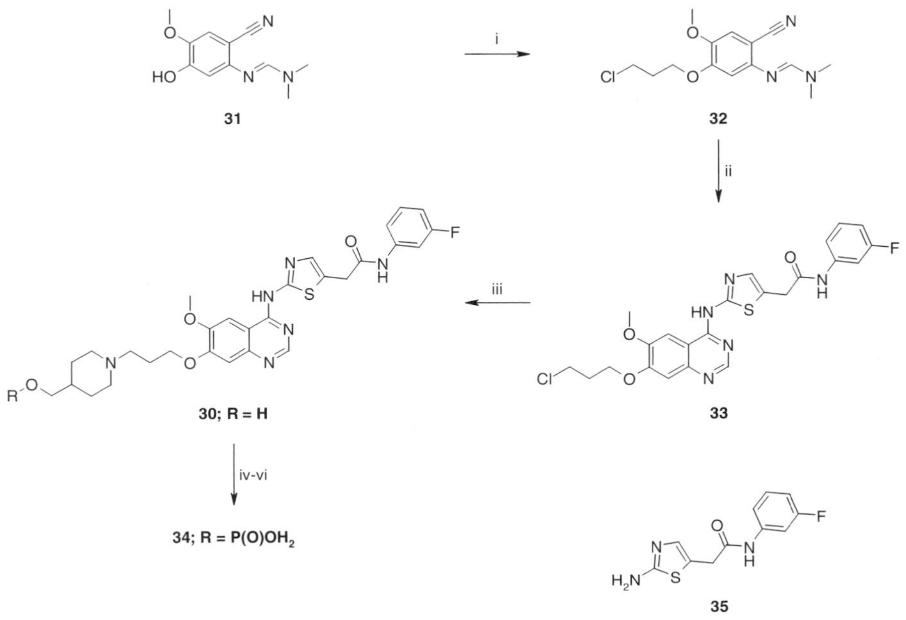

Figure 12.3. Synthetic route to **30** and the phosphate derivative **34**. Reagents: (i) 1-chloro-3-bromopropane, Cs_2CO_3, MeCN, 80 °C; (ii) **35**, AcOH, Δ; (iii) 4-hydroxy-methylpiperidine, NMP, KI, 60 °C; (iv) $Et_2NP(Ot\text{-}Bu)_2$, DMA, r.t.; (v) H_2O_2, −10 °C; (vi) HCl, dioxane, r.t.

to the understanding of the complex balance between concentration and duration of exposure on efficacy and tolerability.

When compound **30** was administered as its dihydrogen phosphate derivative **34** (as an infusion over a period of 48 hours using a minipump), a significant inhibition of histone-H3 phosphorylation in human SW620 colorectal adenocarcinoma tumors could be demonstrated (Mortlock et al., 2005; Jung et al., 2006). Histone-H3 is a cellular substrate of Aurora kinase and is therefore a useful marker of Aurora kinase inhibition in vivo. While the identification of a compound with in vivo activity against a relevant biomarker represented significant progress, this activity was somewhat variable and antitumor studies with this compound were ultimately inconclusive. As the focus of the medicinal chemistry effort shifted away from thiazoles onto alternative core structures, synthesis of prodrugs to allow use of the minipump assay became an increasingly important part of the overall strategy.

12.5.2. Aurora Kinase Inhibition Profile

A detailed analysis of the cellular phenotype of ZM447439 was carried out in Stephen Taylor's laboratory at the University of Manchester. This work showed that the phenotype observed for ZM447439 closely resembled that described for inhibition of Aurora-B, rather than Aurora-A, despite possessing equal potency against both kinases in recombinant enzyme assays (Ditchfield et al., 2003). ZM447439 caused inhibition of both phosphorylation of histone H3 on serine 10 and cytokinesis. However, cells treated with ZM447439 did not undergo a simple mitotic arrest; rather, the cell cycle proceeded with normal timing with entry/exit from mitosis being unaffected. Treated cells either continued to cycle (without cytokinesis), becoming highly polyploid (and ultimately died), or alternatively underwent a G1-like cell cycle arrest (Ditchfield et al., 2003).

The growing interest in Aurora-B kinase led to the introduction of an Aurora-B inhibition assay and the acquisition of data for both Aurora-A and Aurora-B on all newly prepared compounds. Clearly at this point in the project we had yet to identify compounds with high selectivity between Aurora-A and Aurora-B; with a screening cascade collecting data for both kinases, there was an opportunity to identify more selective compounds and probe further the precise roles of these two closely linked kinases.

12.6. QUINAZOLINES SUBSTITUTED WITH AMINOPYRAZOLES

In parallel to the thiazole series, we continued to evaluate a range of other chemical options based around the quinazoline core. The major focus was to fully explore the various heterocyclic replacements for the phenyl ring in compound 1, with the aim of achieving the optimum balance between potency and physical properties. As experience with the thiazole series had demonstrated that the conformation of the kinase must be fairly dynamic, the full range of five-membered ring heterocycles was explored. From this extensive set of compounds, the three series based on the possible isomers of the pyrazole were particularly interesting as they all boasted significant improvements in physicochemical properties. While the series where the terminal aryl group was attached through nitrogen (the "4-pyrazole series" in our nomenclature) contained compounds of exceptional potency (Foote et al., 2008), the series selected for most detailed study was based on 5-acetanilide substituted 3-aminopyrazoles ("3-pyrazole series"), which ultimately led to the discovery of AZD1152 (Mortlock et al., 2007).

The 3-pyrazole series delivers high Aurora-B kinase inhibitory potency but shows less activity against Aurora-A kinase (Mortlock et al., 2007). The SAR followed the same broad trends as described in the earlier series with fluoro groups being particularly favored in the terminal lipophilic binding pocket, especially in the ortho and meta positions. Larger and more polar functional groups are also tolerated but are less preferred, especially in terms of cellular potency. These data suggest the binding conformations of the thiazole and pyrazole series are likely to be comparable although the presence of a further hydrogen bond donor in the pyrazole ring (compared to the thiazole ring) could, in theory, allow additional binding to the protein backbone although analysis is difficult due to the two tautomeric forms of the pyrazole, which can place the proton on either one of the two ring nitrogens.

The pyrazole compounds are generally less lipophilic than the corresponding thiazole analogs, for example, $\log D_{7.4} = 3.2$ versus 2.1 for compounds **30** and **36** (Table 12.6), respectively, resulting in an improvement in general

TABLE 12.6. Pyrazole C-7 and Acetanilide In Vitro SAR

36–43

Compound	R	X	Aurora-A K_i (µM)	Aurora-B –INCENP K_i (µM)	SW620 Cell IC$_{50}$ (µM)
36	3-F		0.45	0.002	0.68
37	3-F		0.11	0.001	0.33
38	2,3-di-F		0.094	0.001	0.042
39	3-F		0.69	0.001	0.63
40	3-F		0.19	0.001	0.27
41	2,3-di-F		0.36	<0.001	0.045
42	2,3-di-F		0.087	<0.001	0.018
43	2,3-di-F		0.018	<0.001	<0.001

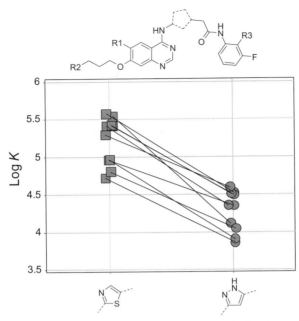

Figure 12.4. Log K values measured in rat plasma for matched-pair analogs in the thiazole (■) and 3-pyrazole (●) series. Each marker represents an individual compound matching the substructure shown. Lines connect exact (R^1, R^2, R^3) matches. Average log K values for thiazole and 3-pyrazole compound sets in the study are 5.2 and 4.3, respectively.

physicochemical related properties such as plasma protein binding (Figure 12.4).

Optimization of the quinazoline C-7 side chain resulted in an enhancement of cellular potency. The presence of an amino functional group increased potency while its basicity helps to reduce the compound's binding to plasma albumin. With a strategy requiring synthesis of in vivo hydrolyzable phosphate esters, the C-7 side chain was also required to contain a pendant hydroxyl functional group. This hydroxyl group plays a second critical role in the drug as, depending on its proximity to the basic nitrogen, it exerts a powerful role in moderating the basicity of the latter group. Both cyclic and noncyclic amine side chains are tolerated by the Aurora kinases, giving rise to excellent levels of cellular potency (measured by the inhibition of histone-H3 phosphorylation in SW620 human tumor cells), in most cases, without a significant increase in lipophilicity (Table 12.6). In the cyclic amine series, the prolinol group was found to have the greatest cellular activity with little noticeable difference in terms of potency, between the two enantiomers. Six-membered cyclic amines were found to be marginally less active in cells (Mortlock et al., 2007). In the acyclic series, *N*-substituted ethanolamines were found to be optimal with a clear relationship between the lipophilicity of the N-substituent and cellular potency (compounds **39–43** in Table 12.6) with the N-isobutyl-substituted compound **43** having an IC_{50} in SW620 cells of less than 1 nM. However, as lipophilicity and cellular potency increased, protein binding increased concomitantly. In addition, compounds with high lipophilicity were found to be more likely to inhibit the major cytochrome P450 isoforms, especially against 3A4, for example, compare compound **43** (log $D_{7.4}$ = 3.6; 3A4 IC_{50} = 0.4 μM) versus compound **41** (log $D_{7.4}$ = 1.9; 3A4 IC_{50} > 10 μM). Within this set of compounds the 2,3-difluorophenyl group gave greater cellular potency compared with the 3-fluorophenyl group. The 2,3-difluorophenyl group also resulted in lower protein binding (compare compounds **38** vs. **37** and **41** vs. **40**: 85% vs. 95% bound and 83% vs. 95% bound in rat plasma, respectively). By appropriate combination of the quinazoline C-7 side chain and anilide groups, as described, it is possible to balance attractive physicochemical-based properties (high free-drug levels and no cytochrome P450 inhibition) with high potency in cell assays.

Important roles for the quinazoline C-7 side chain and the lipophilic pocket binding group had been established in the earlier series and these roles and the associated SAR also broadly applied to the new pyrazole series, albeit with some detailed differences. In contrast, the role of the substituent at the C-6 position on the quinazoline ring was less well understood. It was hypothesized that this group was not involved in direct binding to the protein (although it did have the potential to influence the hydrogen bond acceptor properties of the quinazoline ring in its key interaction with the hinge) and that its removal would allow a reduction in molecular weight and remove any risk of reactive metabolites being formed resulting from oxidative metabolism of the methyl group. Surprisingly, it was found that replacing the C-6 methoxy group with a proton generally reduced potency versus Aurora-A kinase but maintained very high potency versus Aurora-B kinase; improved potency was also observed in the SW620 cell assay (compounds **44–49** in Table 12.7). The cellular phenotype observed for these Aurora-B selective compounds is identical to that described previously for ZM447439. The Aurora-B selective inhibitors inhibit phosphorylation of histone-H3 on serine 10, resulting in a failure of cell division and polyploidy without affecting the core cell cycle timing through mitosis (Girdler et al., 2006). The selectivity for Aurora-B kinase over Aurora-A shown by these pyrazole compounds is unprecedented among Aurora kinase inhibitors described in the literature. This feature together with general high kinase specificity shown by the 3-pyrazole series may be important in future human studies. Compounds such as these should allow the role and clinical utility of Aurora-B inhibition compared with Aurora-A inhibition to be explored while at the same time limiting non-Aurora kinase related toxicities.

The 3-pyrazole compounds possess a particularly good balance of properties. Compounds in this class are selective for Aurora-B kinase over Aurora-A, have high kinase specificity, and have highly potent cellular activities. The reduced lipophilicity of the pyrazole subclass allows potency to be balanced

TABLE 12.7. Quinazoline C-6 H In Vitro SAR

44–49

Compound	R	X	Aurora-A K_i (µM)	Aurora-B –INCENP K_i (µM)	SW620 Cell IC$_{50}$ (µM)
44	2,3-di-F	HO~~N]	0.16	<0.001	0.007
45	2,3-di-F	HO~~N]	0.35	<0.001	0.002
46	2,3-di-F	HO (pyrrolidine)	0.95	<0.001	0.005
47	3-F	HO~~N]	1.4	<0.001	0.017
48	3-F	HO~~N]	0.98	<0.001	0.007
49	3-F	HO (pyrrolidine)	1.4	<0.001	0.024

with attractive physicochemical and pharmacokinetic properties and led to the identification of compounds with striking in vivo activity.

12.7. AZD1152

AZD1152 is the dihydrogen phosphate prodrug of the pyrazoloquinazoline inhibitor **47** (AZD1152-HQPA [hydroxyquinazoline pyrazol anilide]). A synthesis of AZD1152 is shown in Figure 12.5 (Mortlock et al., 2007).

AZD1152-HQPA shows 1000-fold greater potency for Aurora-B than for Aurora-A in recombinant enzyme assays. At the same time it retains the high

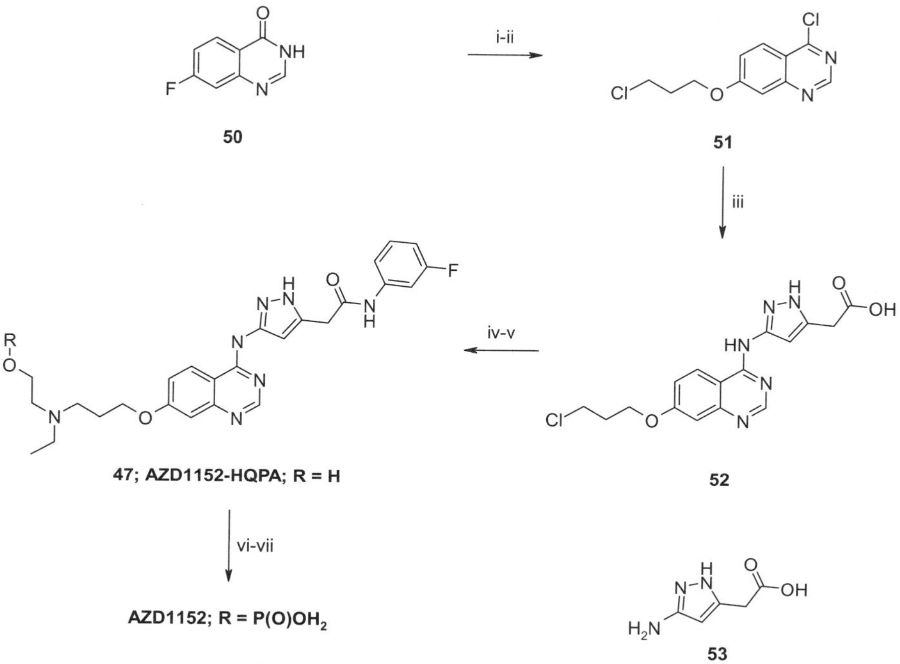

Figure 12.5. Synthetic route to AZD1152-HQPA and AZD1152. Reagents: (i) NaH, 1,3-propanediol, DMF, 60 → 110 °C; (ii) SOCl₂, DMF, 85 °C; (iii) **53**, DMF, HCl (dioxane), 90 °C; (iv) pentafluorophenyl trifluoroacetate, pyridine, DMF; 3-fluoroaniline 0 °C → r.t.; (v) *N*-(ethylamino)ethanol, KI, DMA, 90 °C; (vi) di-*tert*-butyldiethylphosphoramidite, tetrazole, DMF, r.t.; H₂O₂, −10 °C → r.t.; (vii) HCl, dioxane, r.t.

TABLE 12.8. Selectivity Profile of AZD1152-HQPA in a Panel of Kinases

Kinase	IC$_{50}$ (µM)	Kinase	IC$_{50}$ (µM)
Aurora-A	1.4	KDR	1.8
Aurora-B–INCENP	<0.001	PHK	1.8
Aurora-C–INCENP	0.017	ZAP70	8.2
LCK	0.17	Others[a]	>10

[a]JAK3, vABL, CSK, FAK, SRC, IGFR, EGFR, FGFR, P38A, PAK1, CDK2, JNK1A, PKA, MEK, CHK1, PLK1.

specificity for Aurora kinases demonstrated in the earlier series; in a panel of other serine/threonine and tyrosine kinases, AZD1152-HQPA showed very little other kinase activity (Table 12.8) with the exception of Aurora-C–INCENP. Consistent with inhibition of Aurora-B kinase, addition of AZD1152-HQPA to tumor cells in vitro induces chromosome misalignment, prevents cell division, and consequently reduces cell viability and induces apoptosis (Wilkinson et al., 2007).

AZD1152-HQPA has moderate lipophilicity and excellent free-drug exposure and shows no significant safety pharmacological liabilities (Mortlock et al., 2007). Selected properties of AZD1152-HQPA and AZD1152 are summarized in Table 12.9. Despite the presence of a basic side chain ($pK_a = 8.8$), AZD1152-HQPA does not significantly inhibit the hERG ion channel at concentrations up to 30 μM when measured in a whole cell assay. AZD1152-HQPA also has attractive pharmacokinetic properties, displaying no significant inhibition of the major cytochrome P450 isoforms and low to moderate clearance following intravenous bolus injections in rats leading to high systemic exposure in vivo when dosed parenterally. The phosphate derivative (AZD1152) is freely soluble in 0.3 M Tris buffer at pH 9 at a concentration of 25 mg/mL.

AZD1152 is converted to the parent AZD1152-HQPA following parenteral administration (Mortlock et al., 2007). The mean plasma concentration of AZD1152 and AZD1152-HQPA following a single intravenous infusion of 68 μmol/kg of AZD1152 is shown in Figure 12.6. The peak mean plasma concentrations (C_{max}) of both AZD1152 and AZD1152-HQPA occurred at 2 minutes post-dose (t_{max}), indicating that AZD1152 was rapidly converted into the active drug AZD1152-HQPA. These data demonstrate that conversion of the phosphate prodrug to the corresponding active drug compound is both rapid and complete following intravenous (IV) administration in rats. The noncleavable phosphonate analog of AZD1152-HQPA does not have significant activity in cell-based assays ($IC_{50} > 1$ μM). As expected, the highly charged nature of the phosphonate moiety at physiological pH results in low cell permeability and demonstrates, by analogy, that conversion of AZD1152 into AZD1152-HQPA is essential for activity in vivo.

Administration of AZD1152 by subcutaneous infusion (osmotic minipump) over 48 hours leads to inhibition of Aurora-B kinase activity in human tumor xenografts established in nude mice (Wilkinson et al., 2007). Flow cytometric analysis of disaggregated SW620 colon tumor xenografts showed that the proportion of phosphohistone-H3 (PhH3) positive cells within the G2-M phase of the cell cycle declined in a dose-dependent fashion in AZD1152-treated animals compared with vehicle-treated controls (Figure 12.7). Significant inhibition of histone-H3 phosphorylation was observed at doses as low as 0.5 mg/kg/day. Inhibition of histone-H3 phosphorylation correlated with an increased proportion of cells with a 4N and >4N DNA content. Moreover, histological analysis of tumor sections showed an increase in large multinucleated cells in AZD1152-treated tumors. Together these data demonstrate that AZD1152 leads to pharmacodynamic changes in tumors characteristic of Aurora-B kinase inhibition.

The robust pharmacodynamic activity of AZD1152 led to potent and dose-dependent inhibition of growth in human tumors (Wilkinson et al., 2007). At doses between 10 and 150 mg/kg/day for 48 hours (subcutaneous minipump infusion), AZD1152 inhibits tumor growth in multiple xenograft models

TABLE 12.9. Physicochemical, Pharmacokinetic, and Safety Pharmacology Properties of AZD1152-HQPA and AZD1152

Compound	Log $D_{7.4}$	pK_a	Solubility (mg/mL)[a]	Percentage Bound[b]	Rat Cl (mL/min/kg)[c]	3A4 Inhibition IC$_{50}$ (μM)[d]	hErg IC$_{50}$ (μM)[e]
AZD1152-HQPA	2.3	8.8, 5.0		96	14	>10	>30
AZD1152			25				

[a]Tris buffer pH 9.
[b]Rat serum albumin.
[c]Compounds were dosed to male Han Wistar rats at 5 mg/kg formulated in a mixture of 10% DMSO in water.
[d]The activity of human CYP3A4 determined by inhibiting the biotransformation of 7-benzyloxy-4-(trifluoromethyl)-coumarin to the fluorescent metabolite 7-hydroxy-4-trifluoromethyl-coumarin.
[e]Activity against the human ether-a-go-go-related gene (hERG)-encoded potassium channel was determined using automated whole-cell electrophysiology.

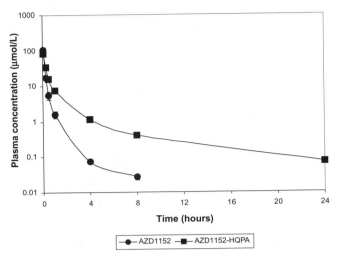

Figure 12.6. Group mean plasma concentrations (±SE) of AZD1152 and AZD1152-HQPA in male and female Wistar Hannover rats ($n = 3$ for each sex) following single intravenous bolus dosing of AZD1152 at 68 µmol/kg.

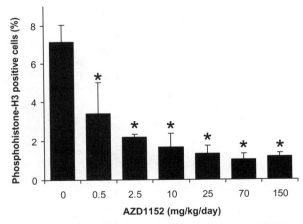

Figure 12.7. AZD1152 dose–response showing percentage PhH3-positive cells in SW620 tumors analyzed by flow cytometry. *Columns*, PhH3-positive cells (%); *bars*, SE; $P < 0.05$ (Wilkinson et al., 2007).

(colorectal: SW620, HCT-116, Colo205; lung: A549, Calu-6; and hematological: HL-60). The inhibition of tumor growth in individual models ranged from 55% to ≥100% (summarized in Table 12.10) and in a dose-dependent manner (Figure 12.8). Significant antitumor activity was also observed when AZD1152 was dosed episodically to mice using other parenteral routes (i.e., intravenous

TABLE 12.10. In Vivo Activity of AZD1152 Against a Range of Human Tumor Xenograft Models

Tumor Model	Dose (mg/kg/d)	Route (duration)	Inhibition of Tumor Volume (%)	
			Maximum	End of Study
SW620	150	Subcutaneous minipump (48h, days 7–9)	87 (day 23)	87 (day 23)
	25	Subcutaneous minipump (48h, days 7–9)	65 (day 14)	49 (day 23)
	10	Subcutaneous minipump (48h, days 7–9)	55 (day 10)	28 (day 23)
	25	Intraperitoneal bolus daily (4d, days 6–9)	65 (day 13)	54 (day 24)
	25	Intravenous bolus daily (3d, days 6–8)	91 (day 13)	47 (day 24)
Colo205	150	Subcutaneous minipump (48h, days 5–7)	>100 (day 18)	94 (day 21)
HCT-116	150	Subcutaneous minipump (48h, days 11–13)	93 (day 18)	74 (day 25)
A549	150	Subcutaneous minipump (48h, days 13–15)	79 (day 26)	69 (day 29)
	25	Subcutaneous minipump (48h, days 13–15)	74 (day 15)	36 (day 29)
Calu-6	150	Subcutaneous minipump (48h, days 20–22)	67 (day 29)	55 (day 41)
HL-60	150	Subcutaneous minipump (48h, days 16–18)	>100 (day 18)	>100 (day 35)

Source: Wilkinson et al. (2007).

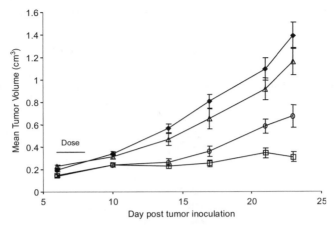

Figure 12.8. Inhibition of tumor growth by AZD1152 at doses of 10 ($\triangle$), 25 ($\bigcirc$), and 150 ($\square$) mg/kg/d (subcutaneous infusion) compared with control treated ($\blacklozenge$) in SW620 human tumor xenografts established in nude mice. Mean tumor volume (cm^3) of 8 to 10 mice; *vertical bars*, SE; *horizontal bar*, duration of dosing (Wilkinson et al., 2007).

or intraperitoneal bolus injections). For example, three consecutive daily bolus intravenous injections of AZD1152 (25 mg/kg/day) in SW620-bearing mice led to a maximal tumor volume inhibition of 91% (Table 12.10). AZD1152 was generally well tolerated at doses where antitumor efficacy was observed with transient myelosuppression being the only toxicity evident in these studies (Wilkinson et al., 2007).

12.8. SUMMARY

The Aurora kinases continue to generate significant interest as attractive drug targets in oncology. Through the work carried out at AstraZeneca, selective inhibitors of Aurora-B kinase have been profiled and have allowed a novel mechanism of action (failure of cell division) to be determined which is distinct from the classical antimitotic agents.

The quinazoline core has shown itself to be an excellent template in which to develop potent Aurora kinase inhibitors while an understanding of the binding mode (supported by X-ray crystallography) has allowed rapid optimization of the series with respect to potency and selectivity for the Aurora kinases. Pyrazolo-substituted quinazolines have been especially interesting in that they combine potent inhibition of Aurora kinase activity with excellent physicochemical properties and safety profile. The elucidation of detailed SAR has led to the development of compounds with high selectivity for Aurora-B kinase (over Aurora-A) and improved cellular activity such as AZD1152.

When prepared as in vivo hydrolyzable phosphate esters, the compounds possess high solubility in simple pH-adjusted aqueous vehicles, allowing flexibility in dosing route and schedule. AZD1152 has been demonstrated to undergo rapid systemic conversion to the active drug, AZD1152-HQPA, which has pharmacokinetic properties that cause dose-dependent plasma exposure. When AZD1152 is dosed to nude mice, pharmacodynamic effects in the tumor are evident, consistent with the inhibition of Aurora-B kinase (reduction of histone-H3 phosphorylation followed by a failure of tumor cell division and apoptosis). Parenteral administration of AZD1152 caused profound and durable antitumor effects in a range of human tumor xenograft models at well-tolerated doses (transient myelosuppression was the only observed toxicity at doses required to elicit potent antitumor activity). AZD1152 has the potential for efficacy in multiple tumor types and is currently undergoing clinical evaluation.

ACKNOWLEDGMENT

We would like to acknowledge the excellent contributions made by all scientists at AstraZeneca and elsewhere who worked or collaborated on the Aurora kinase program, in particular, Madeleine C. Brady, Claire Crafter (neé Ditchfield), Nicola M. Heron, Nicholas J. Keen, Stephen Green, Frédéric H. Jung, Rajesh Odedra, Stephen R. Wedge, and Robert W. Wilkinson.

REFERENCES

Bischoff, J. R., Anderson, L., Zhu, Y., et al. (**1998**). A homologue of *Drosophila* Aurora kinase is oncogenic and amplified in human colorectal cancers. *EMBO J.* 17(11), 3052–3065.

Carpinelli, P., Ceruti, R., Giorgini, M. L., et al. (**2007**). PHA-739358, a potent inhibitor of Aurora kinases with a selective target inhibition profile relevant to cancer. *Mol Cancer Ther.* 6(12, Pt 1), 3158–3168.

Ditchfield, C., Johnson, V. L., Tighe, A., et al. (**2003**). Aurora B couples chromosome alignment with anaphase by targeting BubR1, Mad2, and Cenp-E to kinetochores. *J Cell Biol.* 161, 267–280.

Fancelli, D., Moll, J., Varasi, M., et al. (**2006**). 1,4,5,6-Tetrahydropyrrolo[3,4-c]pyrazoles: identification of a potent Aurora kinase inhibitor with a favorable antitumour kinase inhibition profile. *J Med Chem.* 49, 7247–7251.

Foote, K. M., Mortlock, A. A., Heron, N. M., et al. (**2008**). Synthesis and SAR of 1-acetanilide-4-aminopyrazole-substituted quinazolines: selective inhibitors of Aurora B kinase with potent anti-tumor activity. *Bioorg Med Chem Lett.* 18(6), 1904–1909.

Girdler, F., Gascoigne, K. E., Eyers, P. A., et al. (**2006**). Validating Aurora B as an anti-cancer drug target. *J Cell Sci.* 119, 3664–3675.

Girdler, F., Sessa, F., Patercoli, S., et al. (**2008**). Molecular basis of drug resistance in Aurora kinases. *Chem Biol.* 15(6), 552–562.

Harrington, E. A., Bebbington, D., Moore, J., et al. (**2004**). VX-680, a potent and selective small-molecule inhibitor of the Aurora kinases, suppresses tumour growth in vivo. *Nat Med.* 10, 262–267.

Hauf, S., Cole, R. W., LaTerra, S., et al. (**2003**). The small molecule Hesperadin reveals a role for Aurora B in correcting kinetochore–microtubule attachment and in maintaining the spindle assembly checkpoint. *J Cell Biol.* 161(2), 281–294.

Heron, N. M., Anderson, M., Blowers, D. P., et al. (**2006**). SAR and inhibitor complex structure determination of a novel class of potent and specific Aurora kinase inhibitors. *Bioorg Med Chem Lett.* 16(5), 1320–1323.

Hoar, K., Chakravarty, A., Rabino, C., et al. (**2007**). MLN8054, a small-molecule inhibitor of Aurora A, causes spindle pole and chromosome congression defects leading to aneuploidy. *Mol Cell Biol.* 27(12), 4513–4525.

Jung, F. H., Pasquet, G., Lambert-van der Brempt, C., et al. (**2006**). Discovery of novel and potent thiazoloquinazolines as selective Aurora A and B kinase inhibitors. *J Med Chem.* 49, 955–970.

Keen, N., and Taylor, S. (**2004**). Aurora-kinase inhibitors as anticancer agents. *Nat Rev Cancer.* 4(12), 927–936.

Manfredi, M. G., Ecsedy, J. A., and Meetze, K. A., et al. (**2007**). Antitumor activity of MLN8054, an orally active small-molecule inhibitor of Aurora A kinase. *Proc Natl Acad Sci USA.* 104(10), 4106–4111.

Mortlock, A. A., Keen, N. J., Jung, F. H., et al. (**2005**). Progress in the development of selective inhibitors of Aurora kinases. *Curr Top Med Chem.* 5(8), 807–821.

Mortlock, A. A., Foote, K. M., Heron, N., et al. (**2007**). Discovery, synthesis, and in vivo activity of a new class of pyrazolylamino quinazolines as selective inhibitors of Aurora B kinase. *J Med Chem.* 50(9), 2213–2224.

Sherwood, R. F. (**1996**). Advanced drug delivery reviews: enzyme pro-drug therapy. *Adv Drug Deliv Rev.* 22(3), 269–288.

Wilkinson, R. W., Odedra, R., Heaton, S., et al. (**2007**). AZD1152, a selective inhibitor of Aurora B kinase, inhibits human tumor xenograft growth by inducing apoptosis. *Clin Cancer Res.* 13(12), 3682–3688.

Yang, H., Burke, T., and Ye, X., et al. (**2005**). Mitotic requirement for Aurora A kinase is bypassed in the absence of Aurora B kinase. *FEBS Lett.* 579, 3385–3391.

13

CASE STUDY OF AURORA-A INHIBITOR MLN8054

CHRISTOPHER F. CLAIBORNE AND MARK G. MANFREDI

13.1. INTRODUCTION

One of the hallmarks of cancer is the ability for unregulated proliferation under conditions where normal cells would not survive. Cancer cells divide by progressing through phases of the cell cycle (G1, S, G2, and M) unsupervised due to defects in checkpoints that normally monitor DNA and environmental status. Several US Food and Drug Administration (FDA) approved chemotherapies perturb cancer cell division through inhibition at various phases of the cell cycle (Blagosklonny, 2004). Agents that are particularly effective are those that interfere with mitosis (antimitotics). Mitosis is a well orchestrated process by which cells segregate their duplicated chromosome to prepare for cell division (cytokinesis). All approved antimitotic agents act by binding tubulin and changing the dynamics of the structural microtubule network. The vinca alkaloids (vincristine, vinblastine, and vinorelbine) promote microtubule disassembly, while the taxanes (paclitaxel, docetaxel) and epothilones promote mictrotubule assembly (Bhalla, 2003; Rowinsky and Calvo, 2006). Other agents that antagonize microtubules, such as the combretastatins, are in various stages of clinical development (Lawrence et al., 2001; Hande et al., 2006; Simoni et al., 2006; Meng et al., 2008). Toxicities associated with antimitotics include bone marrow suppression and peripheral neuropathy (Kohler and Goldspiel, 1994; Marupudi et al., 2007). The latter effect is due to the function of microtubules in postmitotic neurons and is not associated with cell division.

Kinase Inhibitor Drugs. Edited by Rongshi Li and Jeffrey A. Stafford
Copyright © 2009 John Wiley & Sons, Inc.

Over the last decade, several kinases and kinesins have been identified to play critical roles in mitosis (Miglarese and Carlson, 2006; de Carcer et al., 2007; Schmidt and Bastians, 2007). Based on the success of the classic antimitotic agents exemplified by the taxanes, newer mitotic mediators have been pursued as therapeutic targets in oncology. These include polo-like kinases, Eg5, CENP-E, Nek family, and Aurora kinases. However, mechanistically it is clear that inhibition of these newer mitotic enzymes has consequences to cells that do not completely overlap with classic antimitotics (Ditchfield et al., 2003; Hoar et al., 2007; Lenart et al., 2007; Manfredi et al., 2007). Individually, therefore, each target holds the potential to add clinical value to the existing antimitotic therapies.

The Aurora serine/threonine kinase family consists of three members: A, B, and C (Andrews, 2005; Marumoto et al., 2005). The expressions of all members are highly regulated within mitosis, and their function and localization are divergent. Aurora-A expression is upregulated in late G2 and degraded by the proteasome in an anaphase promoting complex (APC) dependent fashion (Honda et al., 2000). Aurora-A localizes to centrosomes and proximal mitotic spindles and plays a role in centrosome maturation and separation. This kinase has also been shown to phosphorylate target proteins that have additional roles in mitosis. Aurora-A has been identified as an oncogene, based on the finding that ectopic overexpression results in tumorigenesis of normal cells that are injected in nude mice (Dutertre et al., 2002). The Aurora-A gene is amplified and the protein is overexpressed in many different malignancies (Bischoff et al., 1998; Zhou et al., 1998; Li et al., 2003). Moreover, overexpression of Aurora-A has been associated with poor prognosis in several cancer types (Landen et al., 2007). Aurora-B is expressed in prophase and is degraded in late mitosis (Nguyen et al., 2005). Aurora-B localizes to the kinetochores during metaphase and the midbridge during telephase, where it plays a role in chromosome segregation and cytokinesis. Aurora-C has overlapping functions with Aurora-B; however, due to infrequent expression in tumors, its relevance in oncology is likely limited (Sasai et al., 2004). Targeting Aurora-A and Aurora-B for the treatment of cancer has been an area of intense focus over the last several years.

13.2. MLN8054 CASE STUDY

During the 2001–2003 period, the emerging literature on Aurora-A and Aurora-B supported both kinases as attractive oncology targets. However, there was no clear evidence to suggest that selective inhibition of either kinase afforded a higher probability for success as an anticancer target. The few industry publications available suggested a focus on Aurora-B for small-molecule discovery efforts (Ditchfield et al., 2003; Hauf et al., 2003). As a research organization, we had a particular interest in the discovery of first-in-class molecules. Since no selective inhibitors of Aurora-A had been reported, this kinase represented an attractive opportunity. Furthermore, we were intrigued by the reports of Aurora-A amplification as a distinguishing feature that deserved more attention. We therefore set out to assess the possibility of developing a selective Aurora-A inhibitor. Since the two kinases are structurally related with 86% similarity in the ATP binding pocket, we expected challenges in achieving the desired selectivity. We anticipated that success depended, in part, on developing reliable whole cell assays that would provide direct readouts of Aurora-A and Aurora-B function to guide compound selection and design. We proceeded to establish four in vitro systems to steer our efforts: (1) routine enzymatic screens, (2) whole cell systems reporting Aurora kinase activity, (3) phenotypic evaluation (cellular morphology), and (4) BrdU-based viability readouts.

In cells, Aurora-A and Aurora-B coordinate with partner proteins that have been shown to modulate their kinase activity (Bolton et al., 2002; Kufer et al., 2002; Honda et al., 2003; Anderson et al., 2007). In particular, Aurora-B exists as a complex with INCENP and survivin, both of which are required for full Aurora-B enzymatic activity. TPX2 binds Aurora-A in cells and is involved in localization and activation of Aurora-A (Kufer et al., 2002; Eyers et al., 2003). We developed DELFIA-based assays for both Aurora-A and Aurora-B that did not attempt to reconstitute the relevant protein complexes. Instead, we emphasized the whole cell readouts for target/countertarget evaluation, since these intact systems provided the pertinent milieu.

Toward the task of setting up cell-based assays for Aurora-A and Aurora-B that were suitable for evaluating 10–15 compounds per week, we employed high-content automated immunofluorescent microscopy. Aurora-A was activated through autophosphorylation on threonine 288 (pT288). Since pT288 immunostaining localized to centrosomes, quantification of the signal proved to be difficult. This was overcome through immunodetection optimization (signal amplification) and by increasing the number of regions on the 96-well plates that were imaged. In the case of Aurora-B, it was well established that this kinase phosphorylates histone H3 on serine 10 (pHisH3). The immunofluorescence detection of pHisH3 in cells was robust, and therefore developing this cell-based assay for Aurora-B was fairly straightforward. In order to establish preliminary validation for Aurora-A, Aurora-B, and dual inhibition in these assays, we employed RNAi and cell cycle flow cytometry to determine distinguishing phenotypes. Aurora-A inhibition led to mitotic spindle abnormalities and a delay in mitosis. Spindle defects were identified by immunofluorescence staining of alpha tubulin, and mitotic accumulation was determined by fluorescence activated cell sorting (FACS). These same two methods were also employed to evaluate Aurora-B inhibition. Aurora-B inhibition resulted in chromosome congression and cytokinesis defects that result in multinucleation. Multinucleation was then quantified by looking for the presence of 8N DNA cells (FACS analysis). It was determined through RNAi knockdown of both kinases that the multinucleation phenotype was dominant. This was described later in the literature (Yang et al., 2005). When Aurora-A-selective

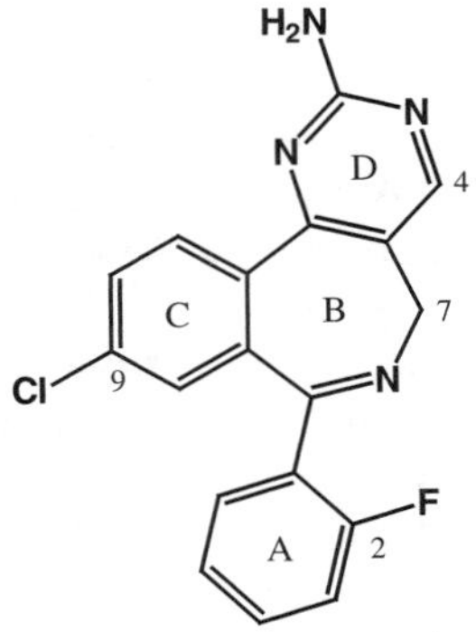

Figure 13.1. Chemical structure of the anti-mitotic agent BBL22 (Bessor and Bessor Labs).

compounds were ultimately identified, a good correlation developed between the pT288 assay and BrdU-based cell viability. Furthermore, at concentrations where compounds inhibited pT288 staining, cells exhibited the expected phenotype associated with Aurora-A inhibition (Marumoto et al., 2002, 2003). This combination of corroborating data (phenotype, dose response, and viability) along with excellent reproducibility garnered our confidence in employing this assay as a primary driver for compound selection.

Concurrent with the development of the necessary assays, a high-throughput (HTS) Aurora-A enzymatic assay was carried out to identify chemical matter. Several suitable (MW < 400) series were identified for initiating medicinal chemistry (data not included). While the project team had commenced the early discovery efforts with the small-molecule hits from this HTS, we came across an interesting article by Xia et al. (2000) on an unadorned benzazepine, BBL22 (Figure 13.1), that produced G2/M arrest and apoptosis in cancer cells. This report did not identify a mechanism of action other than to rule out a likely suspect, the peripheral benzodiazepine receptor (PBR). As part of our oncology research focus on agents that trigger mitotic arrest, we decided to evaluate cells treated with BBL22. Through the use of immunofluorescence imaging, it was discovered that BBL22 produced increased mitotic index, abnormalities in the mitotic spindle, and chromosome segregation errors. This phenotype was reminiscent of the effects caused by our early stage Aurora inhibitors and RNAi, which led us to inquire if Aurora was playing a role in the biology.

We evaluated BBL22 in the Aurora-A DELFIA assay and found it to have micromolar activity. The prospect that this compound could be optimized for Aurora-A and serve as a point of departure for medicinal chemistry was intriguing. A scan of the literature for the structural family represented by BBL22 indicated that a majority of the publications arose from work performed more than 15 years ago. The benzodiazepines and, to a lesser extent,

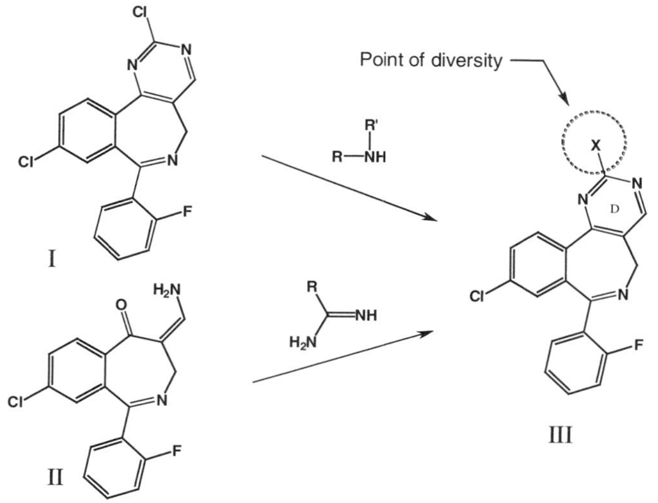

Figure 13.2. Synthetic route to 2-substituted pyrimidine analogs of BBL22.

the benzazepine heterocyclic systems had been intensely investigated in the central nervous system (CNS) field as modulators of $GABA_A$. The $GABA_A$ receptor is a ligand-gated ion channel involved in mediating the effects of GABA (γ-aminobutyric acid), the major inhibitory neurotransmitter in the brain. The $GABA_A$ receptor complex is also the molecular target of the benzodiazepine class of sedative/hypnotic drugs, and is commonly referred to as the benzodiazepine receptor. Given the well-established history of the benzodiazepine structural class, the observation that BBL22 was a potential kinase inhibitor was unexpected.

The team suggested a small exploratory chemistry effort to evaluate substitution effects on Aurora-A activity. To limit the impact on resources and scope of this proposal, an empirical approach emphasizing substitutions introduced late in the synthetic sequence was undertaken (Figure 13.2).

Building on established methods for the synthesis of BBL22, slight sequence modifications were made to facilitate the desired derivatizations on the 2-position of the pyrimidine (ring D). It was envisaged that approximately 20–30 analogs would be prepared and evaluated for Aurora-A activity. The selection of this probe set of compounds was guided primarily by a desire to maintain molecular weight low and to examine substitutions that would sample a range of physical properties. This first round of Aurora-A data revealed an informative structure–activity relationship (SAR) on the narrow molecular space examined (data not shown). The "analoging" effort exposed noteworthy potency enhancements over BBL22, as exemplified by the catechol dimethyl ether derivative, ML1, which was a 610 nM (IC_{50}) inhibitor in the T288 assay. Furthermore, ML1 demonstrated the potential for Aurora-A selectivity with

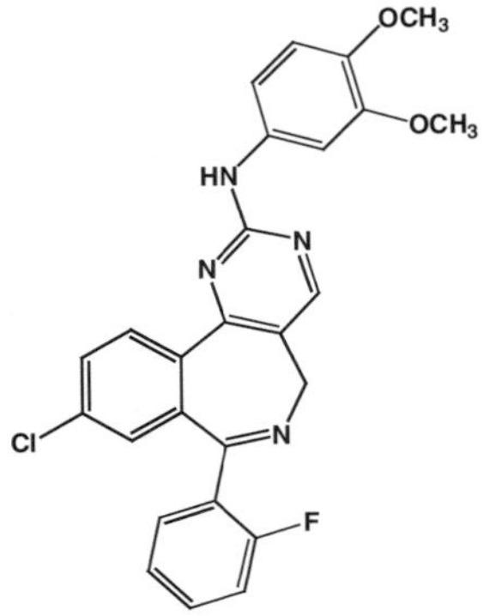

	ML1
Aur-A Enzyme	360
T288 (nM)	610
Aur-B Enzyme	2,000
pHisH3 (nM)	>10,000

Figure 13.3. Chemical structure of ML1, a compound with poor physical properties that nevertheless captured our interest in expanded optimization efforts.

the pHisH3 IC_{50} above 10 μM. Although the other HTS-derived screening leads that were available to the team were significantly more potent, the team was attracted to the novel kinase inhibitor scaffold represented by ML1 (Figure 13.3) and consequently shifted its focus to this series.

Encouraged by this result, a more comprehensive plan for analog synthesis was devised. Computational chemistry, structural biology, and biochemistry were engaged to start investigating the binding interactions. It was determined that ML1 was ATP competitive, and logic dictated that the pyrimidine in ML1 was binding to the adenosine recognition site (hinge region). The strategy for fleshing out the SAR for the scaffold involved modification of all available sites and included ring deletions and/or replacement (Figure 13.4). A number of distinct synthetic routes were developed to gain access to each of the proposed analogs (US patent application 2005256102 A1).

While pursuing the more synthetically complex derivatives, further modification of the pyrimidine amino group afforded a critical discovery. The efforts focused on improving solubility by adding ionizable functionality on the E aryl ring, resulting in identification of the benzoic acid compound ML2, a nanomolar inhibitor of Aurora-A (Figure 13.5). Further characterization demonstrated that ML2 was also functionally selective for Aurora-A, soluble, and orally bioavailable. In the pT288 and HCT-116–BrdU viability assays, ML2 showed IC_{50} values of 170 nM and 900 nM, respectively. Computational analysis indicated that the increased Aurora-A inhibitory activity might be derived from an interaction between the benzoic acid carbonyl on ML2 and Arg137 (Figure 13.6). Since this amino acid residue was conserved in Aurora-B, the carboxylic acid was anticipated to confer a proportional increase in Aurora-B inhibitory activity. Indeed, this proved to be the case in the biochemical assay. On the other hand, the whole cell results continued to show no measurable Aurora-B activity at the upper limit of the assay (10 μM). We maintained our focus on the cellular readouts for compound design decisions and ascribed the apparent

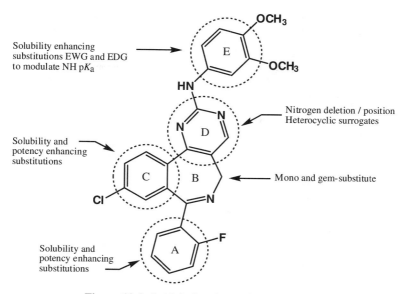

Figure 13.4. Initial plan for optimizing ML1.

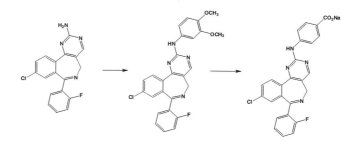

	BBL22	**ML1**	**ML2**
Aur-A Enzyme **T288 (nM)**	1,700 6,000	360 610	33 170
Aur-B Enzyme **pHisH3 (nM)**	ND >10,000	2,000 >10,000	160 >10,000
HTC-116 (nM)	11,000	1,900	950
Bioavailability	ND	0%	80%

Figure 13.5. ML2 data summary vs. BBL22 and ML1.

assay discordance to the aforementioned Aurora-B complexing proteins, INCENP and survivin.

The discovery of ML2 provided an attractive opportunity to initiate in vivo studies. Although overexpression and amplification (Aurora-A) could

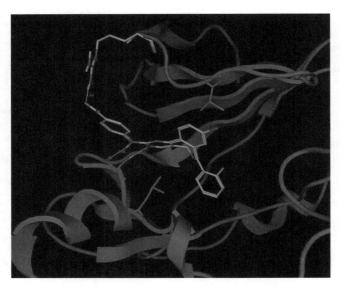

Figure 13.6. ML2 docked in Aurora-A active site. (See color insert.)

provide a rationale for selection of a specific xenograft model, theoretically, inhibitors of Aurora-A should be effective in most if not all cells passing through mitosis. We therefore selected one of our workhorse models, HCT-116, to initiate in vivo studies while we characterized cell lines for an abnormal Aurora-A profile (overexpression and/or amplification). The HCT-116 colon xenograft tumor model was chosen for pharmacodynamic and efficacy screening based on reproducible growth kinetics, duration of study (approximately 3 weeks), and the expression of the indirect pathway pharmacodynamic (PD) marker pHisH3 (phosphohistone H3 Ser10), a readout for mitotic index. Because HisH3 was a direct substrate of Aurora-B and phosphorylation would be inhibited upon Aurora-B inhibition, we used MPM2 as a second marker of mitosis. MPM2 staining would not be expected to change upon short-term Aurora-B inhibition. As determined from cell-based assays, mitotic accumulation was a phenotype of Aurora-A inhibition. To understand the kinetics of mitotic accumulation in the HCT-116 xenograft, the antimitotic paclitaxel was used at a high dose of 50 mg/kg. Following treatment with paclitaxel, cells accumulated in mitosis within 2 hours (5.8-fold above baseline) and continued for more than 9 hours. Using this data as guidance for evaluating the Aurora inhibitors, we assessed mitotic index at 4, 6, and 8 hours (post-administration of compound) for the initial pharmacodynamic screening paradigm.

In order to maintain close control of exposures, ML2 was dosed intravenously to support the development of the in vivo markers. We initiated studies at 15 mg/kg, which resulted in a transient but significant increase in the mitotic

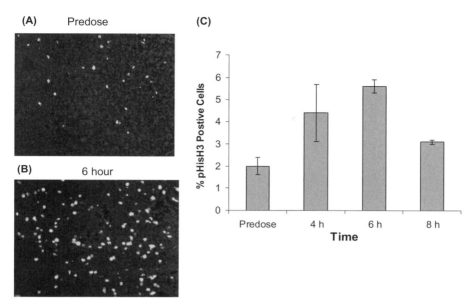

Figure 13.7. Detection of mitotic cells in HCT-116 xenograft tissue through immuno-fluorescence staining for pHisH3. (**A, B**) Pre-dosing and 6 hour post-dosing (ML2) tissue sections stained with DAPI (blue) to detect all cells and with an antibody to pHisH3 to detect mitotic cells (green). (**C**) Percentage of mitotic cells was calculated at each time point ($N = 3$ mice/time point) using automated microscopy (Metamorph software) by dividing the pHisH3 cell counts by the total cell counts.

index (Figure 13.7). The mitotic index increased by 2.2-fold at 4 hours post-dosing and peaked at 2.8-fold at 6 hours (Figure 13.7C). The mitotic index fell significantly by the 8 hour time point.

ML2 had a less significant effect on mitotic index than paclitaxel. At the time, we attributed this difference to incomplete inhibition of Aurora-A or the difference in mechanism between the two agents (mitotic arrest for paclitaxel and mitotic delay for Aurora-A inhibition). To determine if the duration and magnitude of the PD (mitotic index) response observed for ML2 was sufficient for tumor growth inhibition, we conducted an efficacy study in the HCT-116 tumor model at 5, 15, and 25-mg/kg IV. Cell washout experiments with ML2 suggested that we needed a minimum of 72–96 hours of Aurora-A inhibition to produce optimal antiproliferative effects. We therefore designed a schedule of five contiguous days of dosing followed by 2 days off (Figure 13.8). Tumor growth inhibition (TGI) was apparent within 1 week of dosing and reached a maximum after 2 weeks. All doses were well tolerated and demonstrated a dose–response trend. These results represented the first proof of concept, to our knowledge, for Aurora-A-mediated tumor growth inhibition in a mouse xenograft model.

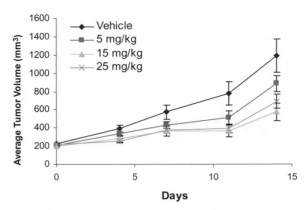

Figure 13.8. Anti-tumor activity of ML2 administered i.v. in the HCT-116 colon tumor xenograft grown subcutaneously.

The PD data demonstrated that the mitotic index increased only transiently, suggesting that Aurora-A was not inhibited beyond 6–8 hours per day. To extend the duration of Aurora-A inhibition, other routes of administration were explored. When ML2 was dosed orally, the plasma exposure saturated at a relatively low dose (5–10 mg/kg). We reasoned that absorption was the limiting factor in achieving higher exposures. Indeed, when the gastrointestinal tract of the mouse was examined, unabsorbed, precipitated compound was identified. Although the dosing solutions were homogeneous, we proposed taking a new look at formulation. We approached the problem as a simple acid–base mediated event and developed a highly base-buffered dosing solution to ensure that the test article would remain ionized upon introduction to the acidic stomach environment. The new dosing solutions significantly enhanced oral exposures and provided an avenue to run studies at higher doses. This result ultimately played an important role in how we formulated all future carboxylic acid containing derivatives. ML2 represented a milestone contribution to the Aurora-A program by establishing that this molecular series could lead to orally bioavailable, selective inhibitors of Aurora-A.

Concurrent with the characterization activities for ML2 and still relatively early in the medicinal chemistry efforts, the SAR was emerging from modifications on distinct regions of the scaffold. A number of highly cell active compounds were identified, but one stood out as particularly interesting. The addition of an second *ortho*-fluorine on the A-aryl ring yielded a 34 nM compound, ML3, in the pT288 assay, uniquely distinguished in the whole cell assay, while the enzymatic data was relatively unremarkable (Figure 13.9). ML3 was also more potent on Aurora-B but retained >200-fold cellular selectivity for Aurora-A versus Aurora-B.

Motivated by the noteworthy improvements in the in vitro data, we initiated in vivo characterization. The team designed a study to look at mitotic

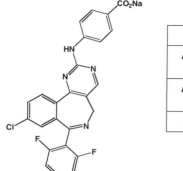

	ML3
Aur-A Enzyme T288 (nM)	31 34
Aur-B Enzyme pHisH3 (nM)	37 5,200
HTC-116 (nM)	220

Figure 13.9. Structure and primary data for ML3.

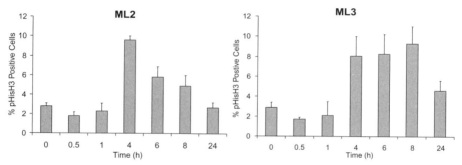

Figure 13.10. Detection of mitotic cells in ML2 or ML3 treated HCT-116 xenograft tissue. Immunofluorescent detection and quantification done as described in figure 13.7.

accumulation in HCT-116 tumor model over 24 hours following a single oral 30 mg/kg dose. As a point of comparison, ML2 was added to the study. Interestingly, the peak mitotic index value for the two compounds was similar and only the duration of the pharmacodynamics changed (Figure 13.10). This suggested that we saturated the pharmacodynamics produced by inhibition of Aurora-A. ML3 demonstrated a significantly more durable PD effect, which was likely a consequence of its greater Aurora-A potency. To understand how this observation would translate to antitumor activity, we proceeded to carry out a head-to-head study in the HCT-116 xenograft efficacy model.

The efficacy study was conducted at daily (qd) doses of 3, 10, and 30 mg/kg for 21 days (Figure 13.11). ML3 resulted in dose-dependent efficacy with tumor stasis at the top dose. These results suggested that the duration of pharmacodynamics and not magnitude, led to superior tumor growth inhibition. The data was also consistent with the cell viability washout studies, which suggested longer duration of inhibition was important for antiproliferation activity.

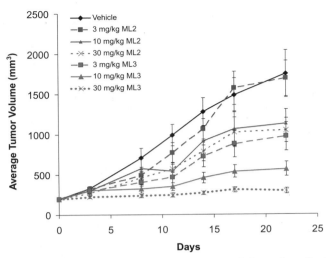

Figure 13.11. Anti-tumor activity of ML2 and ML3 administered orally in the HCT-116 colon tumor xenograft grown subcutaneously.

The convincing ML3 activity in the HCT-116 xenograft tumor model warranted further evaluation of this compound in additional models. ML3 was profiled in eight additional subcutaneous xenograft models and one disseminated non-Hodgkin's lymphoma model (Figure 13.12). ML3 demonstrated robust efficacy at 30 mg/kg dosed either daily or twice daily in the majority of models. With the exception of the MDA-MB-231 breast and Calu-6 lung tumor models, other models examined showed similar efficacy when ML3 was dosed at 30 mg/kg daily (qd) or twice daily (bid).

To develop a more comprehensive understanding of the pharmacodynamics–efficacy relationship, we sought to evaluate intermittent dosing schedules. In the event that continuous inhibition of the target was required for efficacy, an oral drug may be essential for clinical development. However, if shorter durations of target inhibition prove to be equally therapeutic, intravenous dosing strategies could be considered. Dose scheduling studies were performed in the HCT-116, Calu-6 (lung), and H460 (lung) tumor models. The maximum tolerated dose (MTD) on a continuous schedule was 30 mg/kg bid. Higher doses were tolerated only with the introduction of dose holidays. An efficacy study in the HCT-116 was conducted with MTD dosing on a continuous (30 mg/kg bid), 5 days per week (60 mg/kg bid), 3 days per week (90 mg/kg bid), and 2 days per week (120 mg/kg bid) schedule. While all doses were efficacious, continuous dosing resulted in the greatest and most durable tumor growth inhibition.

Since extended duration of Aurora-A inhibition correlated with improved efficacy, we reasoned that durable exposures (high AUC or sustained C_{min}), as opposed to high transient exposures (C_{max}), were central to optimal antitumor

Histology	Model	30 mg/kg qd	30 mg/kg bid
Breast	MDA-MB-231	0	46%
Colon	HCT-116	84%	96%
	DLD-1	ND[2]	47%
	SW480	81%	83%
Lung	Calu-6	0	84%
	H460	72%	81%
Lymphoma	Ly3	99%	ND
Ovarian	SKOV3	54%	65%
Pancreatic	HPAC	ND	54%
Prostate	PC3	85%	94%
	CWR22	ND	95%

Figure 13.12. Percent tumor growth inhibition of preclinical tumor xenografts treated with various doses of MLN8054 once (qd) or twice (bid) per day. (Percent tumor growth inhibition is calculated as $[100 - (d\text{Treated}_{vol}/d\text{Control}_{vol}) * 100]$.

activity. We next set out to determine the plasma concentrations associated with target inhibition. This data would later be used for the efficacious human dose estimation. Alzet osmotic minipumps were used to deliver steady-state plasma levels of ML3. Solutions containing 1, 5, 10, and 25 mg/mL of ML3 were used in pumps that delivered 0.5 μL/h over 48 hours (Figure 13.13). Plasma levels achieved steady-state concentrations within 8 hours following implantation. The increased mitotic index was apparent at the 8 hour time point and was maintained for 24 hours. By 48 hours, the mitotic index decreased. This effect was most apparent in the 25 mg/mL group. We reasoned that this was due to cells undergoing apoptosis, which was corroborated by an increase in cleaved caspase 3 positive cells (data not shown) at the 48 hour time point.

The 25 mg/mL continuous delivery provided sustained elevation in mitotic index comparable to those observed transiently using a 30 mg/kg oral dose. This suggested that the high C_{max} achieved using oral dosing was not necessary for maximal Aurora-A inhibition. We next conducted an efficacy study in the HCT-116 xenograft model to compare tumor growth inhibition when ML3 is delivered over 12 days by osmotic pump and through oral dosing where higher C_{max} levels (approximately 30 μM) are achieved. For this study 7 day pumps were used with a pump replacement needed on day 6. A concentration-dependent effect was observed in the minipump study with near complete tumor growth inhibition seen at 25 mg/mL (Figure 13.14). Moreover, a similar degree and duration of tumor growth inhibition was seen between 30 mg/kg qd dosing and

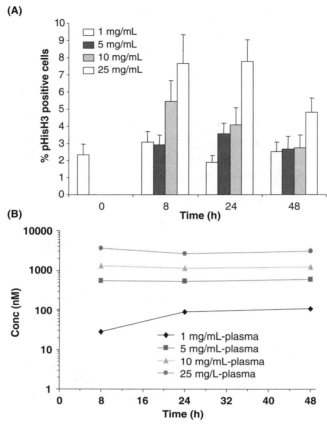

Figure 13.13. Steady-state plasma concentration of ML3 results in increased mitotic index as determined by pHisH3 staining. Various concentrations of ML3 in 7 day Alzet minipumps were implanted subcutaneously in the flanks of HCT-116 tumor-bearing nude mice. (**A**) Mitotic index was determined at each time point as described above. (**B**) Plasma samples were analyzed for ML3 concentration at 8, 24, and 48 hours after implantation of primed pumps.

25 mg/mL osmotic minipumps (data not shown). Pharmacodynamics and efficacy were plotted versus plasma concentration using an E_{max} model. This data suggests that both PD and efficacy responses saturated at a plasma concentration of approximately 2 μM (Figure 13.14). The coincident saturation of pharmacodynamics and efficacy supported the concept that the antitumor effects were Aurora-A mediated. We conceptualized that the 2 μM concentration would be an appropriate target for efficacious human exposure.

While ML3 was highly selective in a broad kinase panel (>180 targets: in house and published), we did not free ourselves from the GABA$_A$ binding liability that we suspected this chemical series to carry. The GABA$_A$ binding

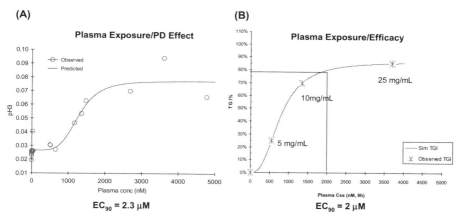

Figure 13.14. Relationship of ML3 plasma concentration with pharmacodynamic effect and efficacy in HCT-116 osmotic minipump study. (**A**) Individual animals were plotted for plasma concentration and mitotic index, which was calculated 8 hours post-implantation. Pumps delivered 1, 5, 10, or 25 mg/mL ML3. (**B**) Tumor growth inhibition of cohorts ($N = 10$/cohort) of mice with pumps was plotted against plasma steady-state concentrations at 8 hours post-implantation. Pumps delivered 5, 10, and 25 mg/ML ML3. TGI was calculated on day 12.

value provided by NovaScreen was 90 nM. Since these binding data were of limited value in predicting GABAA pharmacology, we asserted that rat behavioral studies should be utilized to differentiate lead compounds. Function observational battery (FOB) analysis in rats showed cognitive deficits at high doses (twofold over projected therapeutic levels), providing evidence that ML3 was most likely a competent $GABA_A$ agonist. The broad array of $GABA_A$ agonists on the market had an excellent safety record despite the reported potential for dependency. In an oncology setting, it could easily be rationalized that, if efficacious, limited sedative liabilities could be managed. By all other assessments of safety, ML3 yielded a profile consistent with the mechanism of action (prometaphase arrested cells in all proliferating tissue). From an overall drug discovery perspective, objectives for development had been met. We made a recommendation for initiation of investigatory new drug enabling studies that acknowledged the possibility of sedating side effects but provided a path forward for establishing rapid proof of concept with an Aurora-A inhibitor. The goal of reducing $GABA_A$ mediated effects, if proved to be a substantive clinical issue, could be relegated as an objective for a backup program.

ML3, also known as MLN8054, commenced Phase I clinical trials at three US and two Spanish sites in late 2005 to assess safety and pharmacokinetics. In addition, the team had developed protocols that afforded the opportunity to biopsy skin and tumor pre- and post-treatment with MLN8054 to look for Aurora-A mediated pharmacodynamic effects (preliminary details and results shown at ASCO 2007). We were able to observe phenotypic changes in harvested tissue that were consistent with Aurora-A inhibition, thus providing valuable human pharmacodynamic data. This included mitotic spindle abnormalities and an increased proportion of abnormal mitotic cells that were delayed in prometaphase. Sedative effects, presumably $GABA_A$ mediated, did arise as an adverse event during the dose escalation process, confounding our ability to rapidly progress toward the projected efficacious concentrations. Successful strategies were developed to mitigate the sedative potential of MLN8054 through more frequent dosing to reduce peak concentrations, and coadministration of methylphenidate (stimulant). The discovery team, nevertheless, worked toward identifying a new molecule with a superior separation between Aurora-A and $GABA_A$ activity. Approximately 1 year after learning of the MLN8054 mediated sedating effects in humans, the team was able to identify, develop, and initiate clinical trails with a backup molecule, MLN8237, to address this deficit.

We remain highly sanguine about the therapeutic potential of Aurora-A. The debate continues regarding which Aurora kinase (A or B) is more likely to demonstrate clinical proof of concept and ultimately enter the realm of therapeutic options available to patients with cancer.

REFERENCES

Anderson, K., Yang, J., Koretke, K., et al. (**2007**). Binding of TPX2 to Aurora A alters substrate and inhibitor interactions. *Biochemistry*. 46(36), 10287–10295.

Andrews, P. D. (**2005**). Aurora kinases: shining lights on the therapeutic horizon? *Oncogene*. 24(32), 5005–5015.

Bhalla, K. N. (**2003**). Microtubule-targeted anticancer agents and apoptosis. *Oncogene*. 22(56), 9075–9086.

Bischoff, J. R., Anderson, L., Zhu, Y., et al. (**1998**). A homologue of *Drosophila* Aurora kinase is oncogenic and amplified in human colorectal cancers. *EMBO J*. 17(11), 3052–3065.

Blagosklonny, M. V. (**2004**). Analysis of FDA approved anticancer drugs reveals the future of cancer therapy. *Cell Cycle*. 3(8), 1035–1042.

Bolton, M. A., Lan, W., Powers, S. E., et al. (**2002**). Aurora B kinase exists in a complex with survivin and INCENP and its kinase activity is stimulated by survivin binding and phosphorylation. *Mol Biol Cell*. 13(9), 3064–3077.

de Carcer, G., de Castro, I. P., and Malumbres, M. (**2007**). Targeting cell cycle kinases for cancer therapy. *Curr Med Chem*. 14(9), 969–985.

Ditchfield, C., Johnson, V. L., Tighe, A., et al. (**2003**). Aurora B couples chromosome alignment with anaphase by targeting BubR1, Mad2, and Cenp-E to kinetochores. *J Cell Biol*. 161(2), 267–280.

Dutertre, S., Descamps, S., and Prigent, C. (**2002**). On the role of Aurora-A in centrosome function. *Oncogene*. 21(40), 6175–6183.

Eyers, P. A., Erikson, E., Chen, L. G., et al. (**2003**). A novel mechanism for activation of the protein kinase Aurora A. *Curr Biol*. 13(8), 691–697.

Hande, K. R., Hagey, A., Berlin, J., et al. (**2006**). The pharmacokinetics and safety of ABT-751, a novel, orally bioavailable sulfonamide antimitotic agent: results of a Phase I study. *Clin Cancer Res.* 12(9), 2834–2840.

Hauf, S., Cole, R. W., LaTerra, S., et al. (**2003**). The small molecule Hesperadin reveals a role for Aurora B in correcting kinetochore–microtubule attachment and in maintaining the spindle assembly checkpoint. *J Cell Biol.* 161(2), 281–294.

Hoar, K., Chakravarty, A., Rabino, C., et al. (**2007**). MLN8054, a small-molecule inhibitor of Aurora A, causes spindle pole and chromosome congression defects leading to aneuploidy. *Mol Cell Biol.* 27(12), 4513–4525.

Honda, K., Mihara, H., Kato, Y., et al. (**2000**). Degradation of human Aurora2 protein kinase by the anaphase-promoting complex–ubiquitin–proteasome pathway. *Oncogene.* 19(24), 2812–2819.

Honda, R., Korner, R., and Nigg, E. A. (**2003**). Exploring the functional interactions between Aurora B, INCENP, and survivin in mitosis. *Mol Biol Cell.* 14(8), 3325–3341.

Kohler, D. R., and Goldspiel, B. R. (**1994**). Paclitaxel (taxol). *Pharmacotherapy.* 14(1), 3–34.

Kufer, T. A., Sillje, H. H., Korner, R., et al. (**2002**). Human TPX2 is required for targeting Aurora-A kinase to the spindle. *J Cell Biol.* 158(4), 617–623.

Landen, C. N. Jr., Lin, Y. G., Immaneni, A., et al. (**2007**). Overexpression of the centrosomal protein Aurora-A kinase is associated with poor prognosis in epithelial ovarian cancer patients. *Clin Cancer Res.* 13(14), 4098–4104.

Lawrence, N. J., Rennison, D., Woo, M., et al. (**2001**). Antimitotic and cell growth inhibitory properties of combretastatin A-4-like ethers. *Bioorg Med Chem Lett.* 11(1), 51–54.

Lenart, P., Petronczki, M., Steegmaier, M., et al. (**2007**). The small-molecule inhibitor BI 2536 reveals novel insights into mitotic roles of polo-like kinase 1. *Curr Biol.* 17(4), 304–315.

Li, D., Zhu, J., Firozi, P. F., et al. (**2003**). Overexpression of oncogenic STK15/BTAK/ Aurora A kinase in human pancreatic cancer. *Clin Cancer Res.* 9(3), 991–997.

Manfredi, M. G., Ecsedy, J. A., Meetze, K. A., et al. (**2007**). Antitumor activity of MLN8054, an orally active small-molecule inhibitor of Aurora A kinase. *Proc Natl Acad Sci USA.* 104(10), 4106–4111.

Marumoto, T., Hirota, T., Morisaki, T., et al. (**2002**). Roles of Aurora-A kinase in mitotic entry and G2 checkpoint in mammalian cells. *Genes Cells.* 7(11), 1173–1182.

Marumoto, T., Honda, S., Hara, T., et al. (**2003**). Aurora-A kinase maintains the fidelity of early and late mitotic events in HeLa cells. *J Biol Chem.* 278(51), 51786–51795.

Marumoto, T., Zhang, D., and Saya, H. (**2005**). Aurora-A—a guardian of poles. *Nat Rev Cancer.* 5(1), 42–50.

Marupudi, N. I., Han, J. E., Li, K. W., et al. (**2007**). Paclitaxel: a review of adverse toxicities and novel delivery strategies. *Expert Opin Drug Safety* 6(5), 609–621.

Meng, F., Cai, X., Duan, J., et al. (**2008**). A novel class of tubulin inhibitors that exhibit potent antiproliferation and in vitro vessel-disrupting activity. *Cancer Chemother Pharmacol.* 61(6), 953–963.

Miglarese, M. R., and Carlson, R. O. (**2006**). Development of new cancer therapeutic agents targeting mitosis. *Expert Opin Invest Drugs.* 15(11), 1411–1425.

Nguyen, H. G., Chinnappan, D., Urano, T., et al. (**2005**). Mechanism of Aurora-B degradation and its dependency on intact KEN and A-boxes: identification of an aneuploidy-promoting property. *Mol Cell Biol.* 25(12), 4977–4992.

Rowinsky, E. K., and Calvo, E. (**2006**). Novel agents that target tublin and related elements. *Semin Oncol.* 33(4), 421–435.

Sasai, K., Katayama, H., Stenoien, D. L., et al. (**2004**). Aurora-C kinase is a novel chromosomal passenger protein that can complement Aurora-B kinase function in mitotic cells. *Cell Motil Cytoskeleton.* 59(4), 249–263.

Schmidt, M., and Bastians, H. (**2007**). Mitotic drug targets and the development of novel anti-mitotic anticancer drugs. *Drug Resistance Update.* 10(4–5), 162–181.

Simoni, D., Romagnoli, R., Baruchello, R., et al. (**2006**). Novel combretastatin analogues endowed with antitumor activity. *J Med Chem.* 49(11), 3143–3152.

Xia, W., Spector, S., Hardy, L., et al. (**2000**). Tumor selective G2/M cell cycle arrest and apoptosis of epithelial and hematological malignancies by BBL22, a benzazepine. *Proc Natl Acad Sci USA.* 97(13), 7494–7499.

Yang, H., Burke, T., Dempsey, J., et al. (**2005**). Mitotic requirement for Aurora A kinase is bypassed in the absence of Aurora B kinase. *FEBS Lett.* 579(16), 3385–3391.

Zhou, H., Kuang, J., Zhong, L., et al. (**1998**). Tumour amplified kinase STK15/BTAK induces centrosome amplification, aneuploidy and transformation. *Nat Genet.* 20(2), 189–193.

14

DISCOVERY OF GSK461364: A POLO-LIKE KINASE 1 INHIBITOR FOR THE TREATMENT OF CANCER

KEVIN W. KUNTZ AND KYLE A. EMMITTE

14.1. INTRODUCTION

The journey to the discovery of GSK461364 began many years ago. The first publication in 1994 about a human homolog to the *drosophila polo* with expression that varied with the cell cycle led to interest in inhibiting the kinase to disrupt mitosis (Golsteyn et al., 1994; Holtrich et al., 1994). Since the effort to discover an inhibitor was initiated, hundreds of papers have appeared, further increasing our knowledge about the polo-like kinases (Strebhardt and Ullrich, 2006). The polo-like kinase family is made up of four evolutionarily conserved serine/threonine kinases characterized by a carboxy-terminal polo-box domain. Plk1 is the most studied of the family and a critical regulator of mitosis (Yap et al., 2007). Plk2 (Snk) is believed to have a critical role in synaptic plasticity (Seeburg et al., 2008). Plk3 (Prk/Fnk) is also involved in mitosis and may have a role as a tumor suppressor (Yang et al., 2008). Plk4 (Sak) has only one polo-box domain (the others have two) and is the most dissimilar from the other family members (Bettencourt-Dias et al., 2005). From the onset of this effort, the focus of our work was the inhibition of Plk1 activity, as there was clear evidence for the role of Plk1 in mitosis.

The lack of proper cell cycle control and regulation is a hallmark of cancer cells. Inhibition of the cell cycle through the use of antimitotics has been established as an effective approach to cancer therapy (Wood et al., 2001). Plk1 plays important roles throughout mitosis and is involved in the regulation

Kinase Inhibitor Drugs. Edited by Rongshi Li and Jeffrey A. Stafford
Copyright © 2009 John Wiley & Sons, Inc.

of mitotic progression, including mitotic entry, spindle formation, chromosome segregation, and cytokinesis (Barr et al., 2004; Lowery et al., 2005). Inhibition of Plk1 in vitro has been shown to induce mitotic arrest and can lead to apoptosis (Goh et al., 2004). In addition, the inhibition of Plk1 using antisense oligonucleotides has shown activity in mouse tumor xenograft models (McInnes et al., 2005). Plk1 expression is elevated in numerous cancer types and has been correlated with poor clinical prognosis (Takai et al., 2005).

14.2. BACKGROUND

GlaxoSmithKline's interest in Plk dates back to the former organizations where both GlaxoWellcome and SmithKline Beecham had independently developed Plk1 enzyme assays and run high-throughput screens (HTS) on their respective compound collections. After the corporate merger and sharing of best practices, a Plk1 construct from GlaxoWellcome was used with the peptide substrate from SmithKline Beecham for further screening. To obtain a robust signal, a kinase domain-only construct was used for routine screening. (Lansing et al., 2007). A select few of the lead compounds were also screened in a full-length enzyme assay for Plk1, which confirmed the validity of using only the kinase domain for screening purposes (Erskine et al., 2007).

It was felt that an intracellular mechanistic assay for inhibition of Plk1 activity would help guide the design of cell-permeable Plk1 inhibitors. While there are numerous published substrates of Plk1, many problems exist for using the natural substrates as markers of Plk1 activity. For some substrates, no tools existed for detecting specific phosphorylations. Many of the substrates appear and disappear as the cell progresses through mitosis, leading to the unusual problem of having low basal level of the substrate in the absence of an inhibitor. However, because Plk1 inhibitors cause an accumulation of cells in mitosis, substrate levels increase dramatically in the presence of the inhibitor. It is possible to measure the ratio of phosphorylated to unphosphorylated substrate, but this assay lacked the robustness needed for routine screening. Instead, what was developed was a tet-inducible p53–Plk1 fusion construct (Lansing et al., 2007) where a nonnatural substrate can be added, since there was no good natural substrate. Full-length p53 was tethered to the kinase domain of Plk1 with the T210D mutation to increase its kinase activity. When the cells were treated with doxycycline, they would express this fusion protein, and the p53 portion would be phosphorylated by the Plk1 portion. In the presence of an inhibitor, the phosphorylation would be blocked, and this activity correlated well with the cell proliferation data (for a graph of the correlation see Lansing et al., 2007), giving us confidence that the antiproliferation activity was due to Plk1 inhibition.

A cell proliferation assay was used to determine the cell activity of the compounds. The routine assay involved treatment for 72 h with compound and comparing the number of cells in treated wells to untreated wells at the end of the 72 h treatment period. The number of cells was determined either by staining with methylene blue to determine protein content or by cell-titer glo to determine ATP content. A few cell lines were used for routine screening, but there were no significant differences in the SAR between the cell lines, so for simplicity sake, only data from HCT-116 cells will be cited in this chapter when discussing cell-based structure–activity relationships (SARs).

14.3. Plk1 STRUCTURE–ACTIVITY RELATIONSHIPS

The high-throughput screen for Plk1 identified several potential series. Analogs were made in a few of these series, and they were useful in confirming the phenotype of a Plk inhibitor. However, a very selective chemotype was discovered from the kinase cross-screening effort and soon all effort was placed in optimizing this series.

Novel thiophene benzimidazole (**1**) was identified as a promising lead with good enzyme potency and selectivity (Figure 14.1). The synthesis of this class of compounds begins with known compound methyl 2-chloro-3-oxo-2,3-dihydro-2-thiophenecarboxylate (**3**) (Scheme 14.1). Conjugate addition of a benzimidazole to **3** led to *N*-aryl benzimidazole derivative **4**. In the case of 5-substituted benzimidazoles, this reaction produced a regioisomeric mixture of products. Appendage of the benzyl ether moiety was accomplished through alkylation of a benzyl bromide or Mitsunobu coupling of the corresponding benzyl alcohol to provide **5**. Treatment of **5** with methanolic ammonia in a sealed tube at elevated temperatures afforded the final amide product **6**.

An initial survey of the benzyl ether portion of the inhibitor was conducted using an unsubstituted benzimidazole. Highlights of these results are summarized in Table 14.1. Analysis of the data revealed a slight preference for substitution at the ortho position. Substitution at the meta position showed modest potency improvements while substitution at the 4-position was generally neutral.

Docking of compound **1** into a Plk1 homology model built from the active confirmation of the protein PKA C-α (Figure 14.2) showed that the benzimidazole portion of the molecule offered an area for exploration due to the space

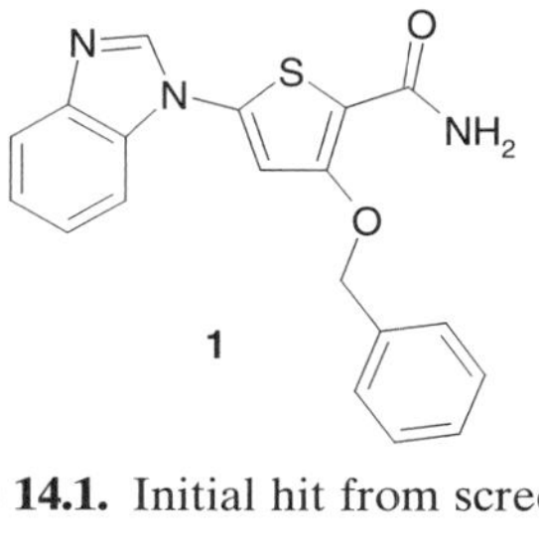

Figure 14.1. Initial hit from screening.

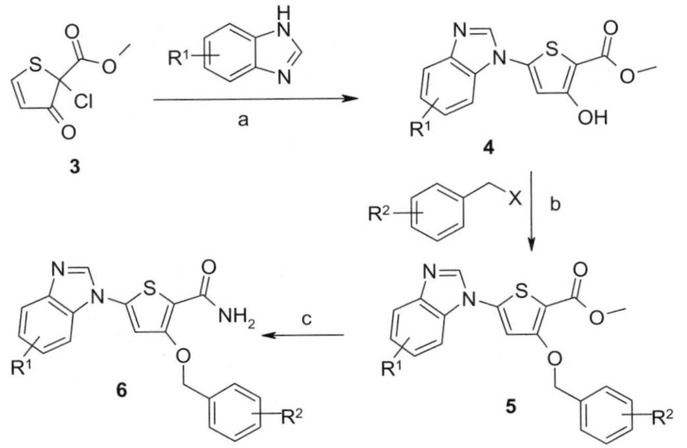

Scheme 14.1. Reagents and conditions: (a) CHCl₃, *N*-methylimidazole; (b) K₂CO₃, DMF (X = Br) or PPh₃, DIAD, CH₂Cl₂ (X = OH); (c) 7 N NH₃ in methanol, 80 °C, sealed tube.

TABLE 14.1. Benzyl Ether Substitutions

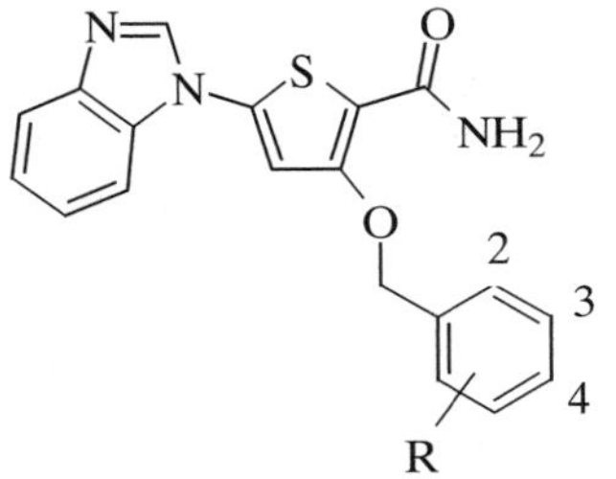

Compound	R	Plk1 IC$_{50}$ (nM)
1	H	61
7	2-Me	12
8	3-Me	12
9	4-Me	70
10	2-OMe	12
11	3-OMe	28
12	4-OMe	35
13	2-Cl	12
14	3-Cl	22
15	4-Cl	100
16	2-CF$_3$	15
17	2-Br	11
18	2-F	14

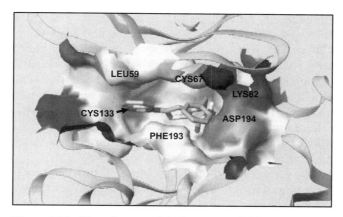

Figure 14.2. Homology model of compound **1** bound to Plk1.

TABLE 14.2. Benzimidazole Substitution SAR

Compound	R1	R2	Plk1 IC$_{50}$ (nM)	HCT-116 IC$_{50}$ (µM)
19	5-Cl	2-Me	21	29.3
20	6-Cl	2-Me	4	1.69
21	6-Br	2-CF$_3$	3	0.781
22	5-CONH$_2$	2-CF$_3$	8	5.16
23	6-CONH$_2$	2-CF$_3$	32	14.3
24	5-CF$_3$	2-Br	300	>30
25	6-CF$_3$	2-Br	9	3.59
26	5-SO$_2$Me	2-CF$_3$	250	>30
27	6-SO$_2$Me	2-CF$_3$	12	2.96
28	5-OMe	2-CF$_3$	8	2.70
29	6-OMe	2-CF$_3$	2	1.23
2	5,6-di-OMe	2-CF$_3$	2	0.699

at the solvent front. In search of a more significant potency boost, we turned our attention to modification of this area. These new analogs were prepared using some of the optimal benzyl ethers previously identified. The data from this set of analogs appear in Table 14.2. Benzimidazoles substituted at the C6 position were generally more potent than the corresponding C5-substituted analogs, with compounds **22** and **23** representing the exception. Comparing compounds **20** and **29**, which were both quite potent, may indicate that the electronic nature of the substituent may not be of primary importance. Overall, the dimethoxy analog **2** (GW843682) proved to be the most potent compound from this set with respect to both the enzyme and cellular assay. In addition, the symmetrical benzimidazole was desirable from a synthetic standpoint since it did not produce regioisomers in the previously described conjugate addition reaction. With these facts in mind, the 5,6-dimethoxybenzimidazole became the preferred template for further SAR exploration.

At this point, we returned to the benzyl ether in order to more thoroughly evaluate this portion of the molecule. Table 14.3 summarizes the key data from this effort. As was the case with the unsubstituted benzimidazole, small lipophilic groups at the 2-position were generally potent (compounds **2**, **31**, and **32**). In addition, some difluorinated benzyl ethers were potent (compounds **43**

TABLE 14.3. Benzyl Ether SAR with the 5,6-Dimethoxybenzimidazole

Compound	R	Plk1 IC$_{50}$ (nM)	HCT-116 IC$_{50}$ (μM)
2	2-CF$_3$	2	0.699
30	H	13	1.09
31	2-Br	3	0.926
32	2-Cl	2	0.999
33	2-CN	6	2.63
34	2-SO$_2$Me	32	5.43
35	2-COMe	20	2.64
36	2-OCF$_3$	5	1.15
37	2-OMe	8	2.11
38	3-NMe$_2$	32	3.47
39	3-NH$_2$	20	2.27
40	3-CN	100	>30
41	4-OMe	13	12.1
42	4-SO$_2$Me	79	>30
43	2,6-di-F	3	0.751
44	2,5-di-F	3	1.09

and **44**). Larger groups at the 2-position (compounds **34** and **35**) were approximately tenfold less potent than small lipophilic groups (compounds **2**, **31**, and **32**). Substitution at either the 3- or 4-position also resulted in a drop in potency regardless of the size of the substituent (compounds **38–42**).

In order to expand the SAR of this template, a series of analogs was prepared in which the benzyl ether moiety was replaced with other ethers. This series included saturated alkyl, aryl, and heteroaryl containing ethers. The results of this exercise are summarized in Table 14.4. Although saturated alkyl ethers **52** and **53** maintained similar enzyme potency to benzyl ether **30**, there was a noticeable drop in the cellular potency. Extending the length of the alkyl chain between oxygen and the aryl ring was not effective (compounds **45** and **46**). Heterocycles linked by a methylene unit were reasonably effective replacements, especially the thienylmethyl analogs **47–49**. Halogenated pyridinyl replacements for the benzyl ether maintained good levels of potency (compounds **55** and **56**).

In order to determine if the primary amide was the optimal group for the 2-position of the thiophene, we took a further look at this area. The synthesis

TABLE 14.4. Potency of Benzyl Ether Replacements

Compound	R	Plk1 IC$_{50}$ (nM)	HCT-116 IC$_{50}$ (μM)
2	2-CF$_3$benzyl	2	0.699
30	benzyl	13	1.09
45	CH$_2$CH$_2$Ph	130	24.1
46	CH$_2$CH$_2$CH$_2$Ph	63	7.75
47	2-thienylmethyl	10	1.54
48	3-thienylmethyl	16	1.52
49	(3-Cl-2-thienyl) methyl	2	1.48
50	2-furylmethyl	25	27.6
51	3-furylmethyl	200	19.0
52	cyclopentylmethyl	32	3.38
53	cyclohexylmethyl	16	3.09
54	4-pyridinylmethyl	130	21.0
55	(2-Br-4-pyridinyl) methyl	13	1.77
56	(2-F-3-pyridinyl) methyl	10	1.73

TABLE 14.5. Primary Amide Replacements

Compound	R	Plk1 IC$_{50}$ (nM)	HCT-116 IC$_{50}$ (μM)
2	CONH$_2$	2	0.699
57	CO$_2$Me	5,000	—
58	CO$_2$H	2	7.66
59	CN	630	—
60	1H-tetrazol-5-yl	79	>30
61	CSNH$_2$	6	>30
62	CONHMe	2,000	—
63	CONMe$_2$	10,000	—
64	COMe	79	—

of these analogs and a summary of their data are contained in Table 14.5. Only the acid **58** and the thioamide **61** maintained acceptable enzyme potency; however, both molecules suffered from poor cellular potency. It may be that these compounds lack the necessary properties to penetrate the cell. It is clear that the primary amide is uniquely effective, and that there is little room for substitution (compounds **62** and **63**).

While compound **2** is a useful tool compound for in vitro models (Lansing et al., 2007), it was necessary to improve the potency and pharmacokinetics to develop a compound for in vivo models. One of the breakthroughs for addressing these properties came from the addition of a methyl group to the benzyl carbon of the benzyl ether. The substitution to give the R enantiomer was significantly more potent than the S enantiomer. While small substitutions on the chiral methyl group were tolerated, the simple, unsubstituted methyl proved most potent (Table 14.6). Additionally, alcohols (**74**) and fluoroalkyls (**75**) provided substantial potency, but for various other reasons, these compounds were not further pursued.

Many reasons have been hypothesized for the significant increase in cell potency from addition of the methyl group, but none is fully satisfying. For this reason the group became known as the "magic methyl." One possible explanation is that these methyl-bearing compounds were reaching the limit of detection in our enzyme assay (2 nM nominal enzyme concentration) and could actually be more potent against the kinase enzyme than measured. Another hypothesis is that the methyl increases the solubility of the compounds and decreases the nonspecific binding to the plastic of the test wells,

TABLE 14.6. Substitution at Benzyl Position

Compound	R1	Configuration	R2	Plk1 IC_{50} (nM)	HCT-116 (nM)
2	H		CF_3	1.6	699
65	Me	R	CF_3	1	76
66	H		Cl	1.6	999
67	Me	S	Cl	25	4,020
68	Me	R	Cl	0.63	33
69	Et	S	Cl	40	3,110
70	Et	R	Cl	0.63	120
71	*n*-Pr	R	Cl	1.6	165
72	*i*-Pr	R	Cl	1.6	145
73	*c*-Pentyl	Rac	Cl	13	1,310
74	CF_3	Rac	Cl	0.79	97
75	CH_2OH	S	Cl	2	96
76	CH_2NH_2	Rac	Cl	63	1,400

thereby increasing the available compound inside the cell. As compounds both with and without the methyl showed high permeability, it is unlikely that permeability is the issue. Whatever the reason, this "magic methyl" gave us the potency needed to see activity in our in vivo models and thus was included in all subsequent derivatives.

The exploration of SAR around the phenyl ring is provided in Table 14.7. It was shown clearly that while potent inhibitors of Plk1 enzyme could be found, ortho substitution, especially with electron-withdrawing groups, led to extremely potent compounds in both enzyme and cell assays.

At this time in the development of the Plk1 inhibitor, a decision was made to focus on intravenous (IV) delivery for the initial drug candidate. An internal goal of achieving 10 mg/mL solubility in an acceptable IV formulation led to the incorporation of solubility-enhancing substituents on the benzimidazole. Substitution from the 6-position (Table 14.8) not only improved solubility but also increased cell potency and provided selectivity over Plk3. The carbon-linked piperazine provided the best balance of potency, pharmacokinetics, and developability properties (Table 14.9).

Further characterization of the lead compounds in a variety of assays led to the selection of GSK461364 (**96**) as the clinical candidate (Kuntz et al., 2007). GSK461364 is a very selective Plk1 inhibitor. In an external kinase panel screened against 260 protein kinases, GSK461364 demonstrated an IC_{50}

TABLE 14.7. Substitution on the Chiral Benzyl Ether

Compound	R	Plk1 IC$_{50}$ (nM)	HCT-116 IC$_{50}$ (nM)
77	H	5	487
78	2-F	0.63	71
68	2-Cl	0.63	33
79	2-Br	1	48
80	2-Me	2.5	461
81	2-OCF$_3$	1	44
82	3-F	7.9	463
83	3-Br	10	1,320
84	3-Me	5	502
85	3-CF$_3$	63	7,250
86	3-OMe	50	6,100
87	3-NH$_2$	20	1,670
88	3-NO$_2$	16	1,340
89	4-F	6.3	806
90	4-Cl	63	6,630

TABLE 14.8. Adding Solubility-Enhancing Groups

Compound	X	Y	R	Plk1 IC$_{50}$ (nM)	HCT-116 IC$_{50}$ (nM)
91	O	C	H	3.2	20
92	O	C	Me	2.5	15
93	NH	C	H	3.2	111
94	NH	C	Me	2	20
95	CH$_2$	N	H	6.3	51
96	CH$_2$	N	Me	1.6	14
97	CO	N	H	160	8,370

TABLE 14.9. Adjusting the Basicity of the Piperazine Nitrogen

Compound	R	Plk1 IC$_{50}$ (nM)	HCT-116 IC$_{50}$ (nM)
96	Me	1.6	14
98	COMe	5	365
99	CH$_2$CH$_2$F	4	224
100	CH$_2$CH$_2$SO$_2$Me	7.9	8,556
101	SO$_2$Me	6.3	870
102	CH$_2$CN	7.9	118

TABLE 14.10. Enzyme Inhibition Profile of GSK461364 (96)

Kinase	IC50 (nM)
Plk1*	2
Plk2*	860
Plk3*	1,000
Lok	126
Nek2	264
CaMKIIδ	727
Flt4	996
Mlk1	803
Pim-1	343
Prk2	566
Rsk2	255
Rsk3	432
Rsk4	219

*in house data.

value < 1 μM against only 10 other kinases (Table 14.10). The nearest kinase inhibitory activity of GSK461364 was detected against Lok (>50-fold selective), which may be the kinase that activates Plk1 (Walter et al., 2003). Recently, however, it has been suggested that Aurora-A serves that role (Macurek et al., 2008).

Interestingly, GSK461364 was very selective against other members of the Plk family. While the importance of this selectivity is as yet unknown, this

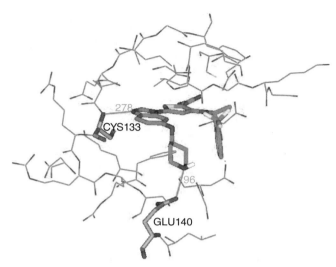

Figure 14.3. Homology model of compound **91** docked into Plk1. (See color insert.)

TABLE 14.11. Cellular Proliferation Inhibition Activity for GSK461364 (96)

Cell Line	Tumor Type	IC_{50} (nM)
A549	Lung adenocarcinoma	9.7
COLO205	Colorectal carcinoma	4.3
HCT116	Colorectal carcinoma	6.6
HT29	Colon adenocarcinoma	2.4
MX-1	Breast carcinoma	8.1
P388	Leukemia	28
SKOV-3	Ovarian carcinoma	14

Plk-family selectivity was obtained when large groups were attached to the 6-position of the benzimidazole. Docking studies to a Plk1 homology model suggest that compounds with basic nitrogens pointing to the solvent-exposed region of the site may be interacting with Glu140 (Figure 14.3). It is not understood whether this interaction is important in delivering kinase selectivity, but in Plk2 and Plk3 this Glu140 residue is a histidine, therefore incapable of making the same favorable, salt-bridge interaction.

GSK461364 is broadly active against several hundred tumor cell lines with proliferation IC_{50} values <100 nM in 91% of all cell lines tested (Laquerre et al., 2007). A few representative cell lines are shown in Table 14.11. The standard proliferation assay exposed the cells to the compound for 72 hours. A series of washout experiments were performed to determine the minimum exposure time necessary to commit the cells to death. Interestingly, the time varied by cell line, and p53 status seemed to be a key determinant of sensitivity (Degenhardt et al., 2007).

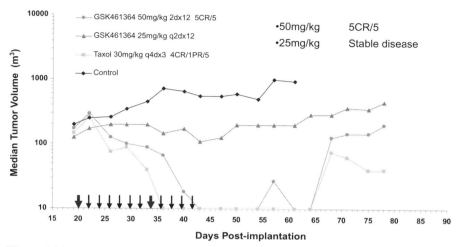

Figure 14.4. Response of Colo205 xenografts in mice to treatment with GSK461364.

GSK461364 has shown activity in human tumor xenograft experiments conducted in nude mice (Sutton et al., 2007). Dosing every other day in a Colo205 xenograft provided robust response (Figure 14.4). It was also demonstrated that when GSK461364 dosing was stopped, the tumors began to regrow. Reinitiation of dosing caused the tumors to shrink again (data not shown). Increasing the dose led to toxicity similar to other cytotoxics (neutropenia, GI degradation, weight loss); however, antitumor activity was demonstrated in many xenograft cell lines at nontoxic doses. We continue to learn more about the sensitivity of different tumor types to Plk1 inhibitors and the appropriate scheduling of doses to maximize antitumor activity.

14.4. SUMMARY

A thorough evaluation of the SAR around thiophene benzimidazoles led to the discovery of GSK461364, a potent, selective inhibitor of Plk1 and potential therapeutic for the treatment of cancer. GSK461364 is currently in Phase I clinical trials.

REFERENCES

Barr, F., Sillje, H., and Nigg, E. (**2004**). Polo-like kinases and the orchestration of cell division. *Nat Rev Mol Cell Biol.* 5, 429–440.

Bettencourt-Dias, M., Rodrigues-Martins, A., Carpenter, L., et al. (**2005**). SAK/PLK4 is required for centriole duplication and flagella development. *Curr Biol.* 15(24), 2199–2207.

Degenhardt, Y., Greshock, J., Laquerre, S., et al. (2007). Association of mutations in the TP53 gene and chromosome instability with sensitivity to the PLK1 inhibitor GSK461364. EORTC-AACR-NCI Meeting.

Erskine, S., Madden, L., Hassler, D., et al. (2007). Biochemical characterization of a novel, potent, and selective inhibitor of polo-like kinase-1 (Plk1). AACR National Meeting.

Goh, K., Wang, H., Yu, N., et al. (2004). PLK1 as a potential drug target in cancer therapy. *Drug Dev Res*. 62(4), 349–361.

Golsteyn, R., Schultz, S., Bartek, J., et al. (1994). Cell cycle analysis and chromosomal localization of human Plk1, a putative homologue of the mitotic kinases *Drosophila polo* and *Saccharomyces cerevisiae* Cdc5. *J Cell Sci*. 107(6), 1509–1517.

Holtrich, U., Wolf, G., Braeuninger, A., et al. (1994). Induction and down-regulation of PLK, a human serine/threonine kinase expressed in proliferating cells and tumors. *PNAS*. 91(5), 1736–1740.

Kuntz, K., Salovich, J., Mook, R., et al. (2007). Identification of GSK461364, a novel small molecule polo-like kinase 1 inhibitor for the treatment of cancer. AACR National Meeting.

Lansing, T., McConnell, R., Duckett, D., et al. (2007). In vitro biological activity of a novel small-molecule inhibitor of polo-like kinase 1. *Mol Cancer Ther*. 6(2), 450–459.

Laquerre, S., Sung, C., Gilmartin, A., et al. (2007). A potent and selective polo-like kinase 1 (Plk1) inhibitor (GSK461364) induces cell cycle arrest and growth inhibition of cancer cell. AACR National Meeting.

Lowery, D., Lim, D., and Yaffe, M. (2005). Structure and function of polo-like kinases. *Oncogene*. 24, 248–259.

Macurek, L., Lindqvist, A., Lim, D., et al. (2008). Polo-like kinase-1 is activated by Aurora A to promote checkpoint recovery. *Nature*. 455(7209), 119–123.

McInnes, C., Mezna, M., and Fischer, P. (2005). Progress in the discovery of polo-like kinase inhibitors. *Curr Topics Med Chem*. 5(2), 181–197.

Seeburg, D., Feliu-Mojer, M., Gaiottino, J., et al. (2008). Critical role of CDK5 and polo-like kinase 2 in homeostatic synaptic plasticity during elevated activity. *Neuron*. 58(4), 571–583.

Strebhardt, K., and Ullrich, A. (2006). Targeting polo-like kinase 1 for cancer therapy. *Nat Rev Cancer*. 6(4), 321–330.

Sutton, D., Diamond, M., Faucette, L., et al. (2007). Efficacy of GSK461364, a selective Plk1 inhibitor, in human tumor xenograft models. AACR National Meeting.

Takai, N., Hamanaka, R., Yoshimatsu, J., et al. (2005). Polo-like kinases (Plks) and cancer. *Oncogene*. 24, 287–291.

Walter, S., Cutler, R., Martinez, R., et al. (2003). Stk10, a new member of the polo-like kinase kinase family highly expressed in hematopoietic tissue. *J Biol Chem*. 278(20), 18221–18228.

Wood, K., Cornwell, W., and Jackson, J. (2001). Past and future of the mitotic spindle as an oncology target. *Curr Opin Pharmacol*. 1, 370–377.

Yang, Y., Bai, J., Shen, R., et al. (2008). Polo-like kinase 3 functions as a tumor suppressor and is a negative regulator of hypoxia-inducible factor-1.alpha. under hypoxic conditions. *Cancer Res*. 68(11), 4077–4085.

Yap, T., Molife, L., Blagden, S., et al. (2007). Targeting cell cycle kinases and kinesins in anticancer drug development. *Expert Opin Drug Discov*. 2(4), 539–560.

PART IV

RELATED SPECIAL TOPICS

15

PHARMACOGENOMICS OF DASATINIB (Sprycel™)

Fei Huang and Edwin A. Clark

15.1. INTRODUCTION

Utilizing the wealth of information gathered on cancer targets in the so-called genomics age, effective targeted therapies have been developed that benefit at least a subset of patients. Targeting the subset of patients who will benefit should be the developmental goal for such agents. Therefore new predictive molecular markers are needed to accurately predict a patient's response to therapies in development. Such markers would better assess a patient's sensitivity to a specific therapy, thus facilitating the individualization of therapy.

Dasatinib (Sprycel™) is a novel, oral, multitargeted kinase inhibitor that targets several important oncogenic pathways, including SRC family kinases (SFKs) and BCR-ABL; it demonstrates antitumor activity against a variety of tumor types including leukemia (Lombardo et al., 2004). Chronic myelogenous leukemia (CML) is a hematopoietic disorder that typically first appears as chronic phase and progresses usually via an accelerated phase to fatal blast crisis over 3–5 years (Sawyers, 1999). CML is caused by constitutively activated tyrosine kinase BCR-ABL, which has been identified as the key therapeutic target in CML. Imatinib, a selective inhibitor of BCR-ABL, represents current front-line therapy for CML with proven efficacy (O'Brien et al., 2003; Deininger et al., 2005). Although responses in chronic phase tend to be durable, relapse after an initial response is common in patients with more advanced disease (Sawyers et al., 2002; Talpaz et al., 2002). Development of BCR-ABL

Kinase Inhibitor Drugs. Edited by Rongshi Li and Jeffrey A. Stafford
Copyright © 2009 John Wiley & Sons, Inc.

kinase domain mutations is the major cause of imatinib resistance (Gorre et al., 2001; Shah and Sawyers, 2003). The significant medical need for new and more effective therapeutic interventions spurred the rapid development of second-generation tyrosine kinase inhibitors to overcome imatinib resistance. Dasatinib and nilotinib are new targeted drugs developed to treat imatinib-resistant CML (Weisberg et al., 2007). Preclinical and clinical investigations demonstrate that dasatinib effectively overcomes imatinib resistance (Hochhaus, 2007b; Jabbour et al., 2007; Olivieri and Manzione, 2007; Steinberg, 2007; Weisberg et al., 2007; Brave et al., 2008). Presently, dasatinib is approved for treatment of CML and Philadelphia chromosome-positive acute lympho-blastic leukemia (Ph+ ALL) with resistance or intolerance to prior therapy including imatinib. Due to its multitargeted activity, dasatinib also demonstrates in vitro and in vivo antitumor activity in multiple human solid tumor cell lines and xenograft models (Lombardo et al., 2004; Johnson et al., 2005; Lee et al., 2005; Nam et al., 2005; Song et al., 2006; Shor et al., 2007), suggesting opportunities for use outside CML. This chapter will review (1) how dasatinib is rationally designed to overcome the limitation of imatinib therapy that leads to resistance; (2) how biomarkers identified using preclinical models have been integrated into early clinical studies supporting the advancement of the drug into registrational studies in CML; (3) how preclinical cell line models were used to identify pharmocogenomic predictive biomarkers for dasatinib response in solid tumors; and (4) how a candidate dasatinib-responsive subpopulation was defined, generating a hypothesis that will be tested clinically. The strategy of using preclinical and clinical pharmacogenomic predictors in the development of a novel targeted agent provides a paradigm for future drug development.

15.2. DASATINIB, A MULTITARGETED KINASE INHIBITOR

15.2.1. Kinase Profile

Dasatinib is N-(2-chloro-6-methyl-phenyl)-2-(6-(4-(2-hydroxyethyl)-piperazin -1-yl)-2-methylpyrimidin-4-ylamino)-thiazole-5-carboxamide with chemical structure illustrated in Figure 15.1, and identified as a potent SRC/ABL kinase inhibitor with excellent antiproliferative activity against hematological and solid tumor cell lines (Lombardo et al., 2004). To test the kinase inhibition activity of dasatinib, in vitro kinase assays against a panel of glutathione-S -transferase fused kinases, including protein tyrosine kinase and serine/threo-nine kinase, were performed. Dasatinib is very potent, with an IC_{50} (the drug concentration required to achieve a 50% kinase inhibition as compared with untreated control) at subnanomolar to low nanomolar concentrations against SFK members (SRC = 0.55 nM, LCK = 1.1 nM, YES = 0.41 nM, FYN = 0.2 nM); BCR-ABL (<3 nM); c-KIT (13 nM); EPHA2 (17 nM); and PDGFß receptor (28 nM) (Lee et al., 2005). The activity spectrum of dasatinib against protein

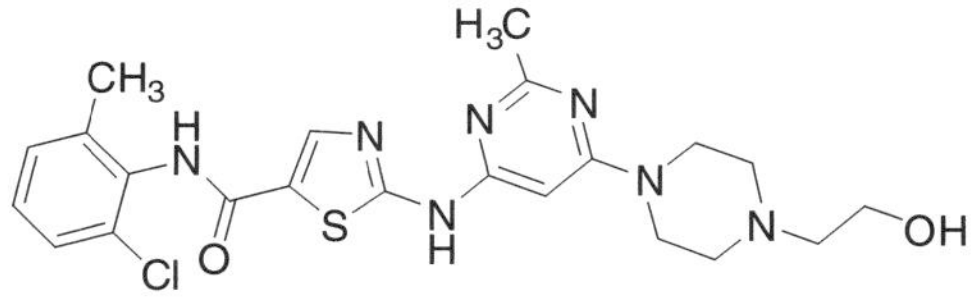

Figure 15.1. Chemical structure of dasatinib.

kinases could be classified into three groups based on potency: (1) high potency with single nanomolar inhibitory activity against kinases such as BCR-ABL and SFKs; (2) moderate potency with subnanomolar activity against c-KIT, PDGFβ, and EPHA2 receptor tyrosine kinases; and (3) low potency with 100- to 20,000-fold less potency than the first two categories against unrelated tyrosine kinases, for example, HER1/HER2 receptors, VEGF2 receptor, IGF-1 receptor, FGF receptor, FAK, MEK, MET, and serine–threonine kinases such as PKA, PKC, p38, GSK-3, and CaMKII. In addition, the activity of dasatinib was tested in two independent studies by different assay types. One assay was an in vitro competition binding assay against a panel of 317 protein kinases (Karaman et al., 2008); another was a high-throughput in vitro cellular proliferation assay on 35 activated tyrosine kinases (Melnick et al., 2006). The results from both studies revealed that dasatinib has additional activity against other members of EPH receptors, such as EPHA3, EPHA5, EPHA8, EPHB1, EPHB2, and EPHB4.

Dasatinib competes with ATP for the ATP-binding site in the kinase domain of selected kinases, inhibiting their autophosphorylation and phosphorylation of additional downstream targets, thus blocking oncogenic activity. In the in vitro cellular proliferation assay dasatinib is 325-fold more potent than imatinib against cells expressing wild-type BCR-ABL (Burgess et al., 2005; O'Hare et al., 2005) and is active against 14 out of 15 imatinib-resistant BCR-ABL mutants tested (Shah et al., 2004). In human CML K562 cells, dasatinib inhibits tyrosine phosphorylation of BCR-ABL and SFKs, including SRC, HCK, and LYN, and subsequently decreases the phosphorylation of downstream target Stat5, significantly resulting in inhibition of cellular proliferation and induction of apoptosis (Nam et al., 2007). In prostate cancer cell lines highly expressing SFK members SRC and LYN, it inhibits the cellular SRC and LYN autophosphorylation in a dose-dependent manner, blocks SFK/FAK/p130CAS signaling, and causes inhibition of cell adhesion, migration, and invasion (Nam et al., 2005). Dasatinib also potently inhibits autophosphorylation and kinase activity of wild-type, juxtamembrane domain mutant, and imatinib-resistant activation loop mutants of KIT isoforms; and it affects KIT-dependent activation of downstream pathways important for cell viability and survival (Schittenhelm et al., 2006). In summary, dasatinib targets multiple kinases that are important for tumor growth, apoptosis, and progression.

15.2.2. In Vitro and In Vivo Antitumor Activity

When tested in CML and Ph+ ALL cell lines K562, KU-812, MEG-01, and SUP-B15, dasatinib demonstrates very potent in vitro cell-killing activity with IC_{50} values ≤ 1 nM, which is 300–655-fold more potent than imatinib against these same cell lines (Lee et al., 2004). It blocks G1/S transition and inhibits cell growth in leukemic cells (Fabarius et al., 2006). In addition, dasatinib has markedly greater potency compared with imatinib against the majority of imatinib-resistant BCR-ABL mutants (Shah et al., 2004). Several preclinical imatinib-resistant cell models, which derived from SUP-B15, MEG-01, and K562 cell lines, have three- to sixfold increased resistance to imatinib with different resistant mechanisms. For example, the imatinib acquired-resistance SUP-B15/IM^R model has F359V mutation in BCR-ABL and MEG-01/IM^R has Q252H, respectively, whereas K562/IM^R develops resistance through a BCR-ABL independent mechanism (overexpression of FYN, a member of SFKs), which has been implicated in imatinib resistance (Donato et al., 2003). Dasatinib demonstrates equal activity against both parental and these imatinib-resistant models, and it is able to inhibit tyrosine phosphorylation of FYN at concentrations of 0.5–2.0 nM for K562/IM^R cells, whereas imatinib is unable to do so even at concentrations up to 900 nM. The lack of activity of imatinib against the FYN protein kinase could explain imatinib resistance of the K562/IM^R cells. Knockdown of FYN with shRNA slows leukemia cell growth, inhibits clonogenicity, and leads to increased sensitivity to imatinib, indicating that FYN mediates CML cell proliferation (Ban et al., 2008). These results demonstrate that dasatinib can overcome imatinib acquired resistance due to overexpression of SFKs. Dasatinib shows curative efficacy at a wide range of dose levels against imatinib-sensitive and -resistant CML mouse models in vivo. When administered orally once daily, dasatinib proves to be curative over a 40-fold dose range (2.5–100 mg/kg/day) in K562 xenograft mice. In contrast, imatinib fails to elicit cures even at its maximal tolerant dose of 450 mg/kg/day, although it does produce a highly significant growth delay (2.4 log cell kill). Against the imatinib-resistant K562/IM^R xenografts, dasatinib produces equally impressive activity, eliciting cures at doses as low as 5 mg/kg/day (Lee et al., 2004). It also significantly prolongs survival in BCR-ABL-driven CML mouse models and inhibits proliferation of BCR-ABL-positive bone marrow progenitor cells from patients with imatinib-sensitive and imatinib-resistant CML (Shah et al., 2004). In Ph+ ALL mice it induces complete remissions (Hu et al., 2006).

SFKs play a key role in many cellular signaling pathways that involve proliferation, differentiation, survival, motility, angiogenesis, adhesion, and migration (Thomas and Brugge, 1997; Bromann et al., 2004; Yeatman, 2004). Aberrant expression and activation of SFKs have been implicated in a number of human malignancies including lung, skin, colon, ovary, endometrium, head and neck, prostate, and breast (Thomas and Brugge, 1997; Irby and Yeatman, 2000; Summy and Gallick, 2003; Yeatman, 2004), so targeting SFKs by dasatinib may provide a valuable approach for treatment of these cancer types. Multiple studies in head and neck squamous cell carcinoma, lung, prostate, neuroblastoma, and sarcoma cell lines support the role of SRC inhibition with dasatinib to inhibit in vitro proliferation, reduce migration and invasion, and in some cases induce apoptosis (Johnson et al., 2005; Nam et al., 2005; Song et al., 2006; Shor et al., 2007; Timeus et al., 2008). Dasatinib is also able to bind and inhibit both wild-type and active mutant KIT, an oncoprotein involved in a number of cancers, including acute myelogenous leukemia, systemic mastocytosis, a subset of sinonasal natural killer/T-cell non-Hodgkin's lymphoma, seminoma/dysgerminoma, and imatinib-resistant gastrointestinal stromal tumor (GIST) (Olivieri and Manzione, 2007). Dasatinib is effective in inhibiting KIT D816V, an imatinib-resistant activating mutation that triggers neoplastic growth in most patients with systemic mastocytosis (Shah et al., 2006) and in patients with GIST (Evans et al., 2005). Dasatinib also demonstrates antiproliferative activity with varying degrees of potency in a wide spectrum of cancer cell lines including a large panel of breast (Finn et al., 2007; Huang et al., 2007), prostate (Wang et al., 2007), multiple myeloma (Deng et al., 2005), colon (Wainberg et al., 2008), and sarcomas (Kolb et al., 2008). In cellular proliferation assays, dasatinib at clinically achievable concentrations ($<1.0\,\mu M$) inhibits the proliferation of 11 of 23 (48%) lung, 9 of 31 (29%) colon, and 11 of 35 (31%) breast cancer cell lines. In vivo, in preclinical chemotherapy trials against a panel of 13 solid tumors grown in mice, clinically relevant doses of dasatinib significantly inhibit the growth of 6 of 13 (46%) xenografts; responsive tumor types include breast, prostate, colon, pancreatic, sarcoma, and small cell lung cancers (Lee et al., 2005). It also reduces primary pancreatic tumor growth and metastasis to liver and lymph node (Trevino et al., 2006). These results suggest that dasatinib may have therapeutic utilities in a broad spectrum of cancer types.

15.3. PHARMACOGENOMICS OF DASATINIB IN CML

CML is a disorder of hematopoietic stem cells that results in uncontrolled myeloproliferation. It is characterized by a genetic abnormality, the Philadelphia chromosome, resulting from a reciprocal translocation between chromosomes 9 and 22 to form a chimeric *Bcr-Abl* fusion gene, which occurs in >90% of patients (Nowell and Hungerford, 1960). The *Bcr-Abl* fusion gene codes for an oncoprotein, BCR-ABL, with constitutively activated tyrosine kinase activity. BCR-ABL is the underlying cause of CML and has been identified as the key therapeutic target. Currently, imatinib is the standard of care for the treatment of patients with CML. However, the development of resistance and intolerance to imatinib is of increasing clinical relevance, particularly in patients with advanced disease, where a substantial number of patients either are primarily resistant to treatment or develop resistance during the course of treatment (Sawyers et al., 2002; Talpaz et al., 2002; Druker et al., 2006). In the pivotal Phase III IRIS study, 31% of patients discontinued imatinib in ≤5 years, over half of these were due to intolerance or resistance to imatinib; in patients developing secondary resistance, 17% relapsed and 7% progressed to the accelerated phase or blast crisis at 5 years on imatinib treatment (Druker et al., 2006). Furthermore, patients with more advanced disease have a higher incidence of resistance with 60% in accelerated phase, and 90% in blast phase after 3 years (Hochhaus and La Rosee, 2004).

Multiple mechanisms define imatinib resistance, including BCR-ABL gene mutations (Gorre et al., 2001; Branford et al., 2002; Shah et al., 2002; Shah and Sawyers, 2003), overexpression or amplification of the BCR-ABL gene locus (Gorre et al., 2001), P-glycoprotein efflux pump overexpression (Illmer et al., 2004), and activation of BCR-ABL independent pathways, such as members of SFKs (Donato et al., 2003). Additionally, SFKs play an important role in the progression of CML and development of Ph+ ALL (Ban et al., 2008; Li, 2008), which may partially explain the aggressive nature of advanced CML and its relatively poor responsiveness to imatinib (Sawyers et al., 2002; Donato et al., 2003). The lack of therapeutic options for those patients who are refractory to imatinib treatment highlights the significant medical need for new and more effective therapeutic interventions that can target both wild-type and mutant BCR-ABL with greater potency and broader activity to overcome imatinib resistance. The extensive understanding of the mechanism of imatinib resistance has prompted the search for alternate BCR-ABL inhibitors. In particular, the use of agents that inhibit both BCR-ABL dependent and independent mechanisms of imatinib resistance would be a favorable approach to overcome imatinib resistance and delay transition to advanced phase disease. The use of combinations of BCR-ABL and SRC inhibitors to address these problems has been assessed preclinically, which provides the rationale to develop dual SRC/ABL inhibitors (Warmuth et al., 2003b; Tipping et al., 2004).

Structural biology studies have facilitated the design of new drugs to circumvent resistance, and several second-generation tyrosine kinase inhibitors, such as dasatinib and nilotinib, have been developed specifically for this purpose (Weisberg et al., 2007). Dasatinib was rationally designed with a structure distinct from imatinib (Tokarski et al., 2006), as one way to address the limitations of imatinib therapy that lead to resistance. It combines nanomolar inhibition of BCR-ABL kinase activity with similar potency against members of the SFKs, and shows 325-fold greater activity against wild-type BCR-ABL than imatinib in vitro (Burgess et al., 2005; O'Hare et al., 2005). Crystal structure analysis of the ABL kinase domain in complex with dasatinib showed dasatinib is capable of recognizing multiple conformations of the enzyme and binding to both the inactive and active forms of BCR-ABL, whereas imatinib binds only to the inactive form (Nagar et al., 2002; Tokarski et al., 2006; Lee et al., 2008). BCR-ABL mutations often induce a structural predisposition toward the active conformation of the protein, resulting in a shift in the equilibrium of BCR-ABL from inactive to active, which imatinib is unable to bind (Nagar et al., 2002; Lee et al., 2008). The lack of binding of imatinib to the active confirmation of BCR-ABL is a clear disadvantage in the long-term treatment of disease, where mutations are a common phenomenon. With continued imatinib treatment, resistant mutants are selected and eventually outgrow the sensitive leukemic cells. Since dasatinib has broad activity against all but one BCR-ABL mutation, including all mutations in the P-loop, it was hypothesized that dasatinib would be an effective treatment of CML and Ph+ ALL.

Another BCR-ABL independent mechanism of imatinib resistance is over-expression of the efflux protein multidrug resistance protein-1 (MDR1) in CML (Illmer et al., 2004). It is likely to reduce the intracellular concentrations of imatinib to a suboptimal level because imatinib is a substrate of MDR1 (Thomas et al., 2004). Unlike imatinib, dasatinib is not a substrate of the MDR1 protein and its activity is unaffected by overexpression of MDR1. This might be another advantage of dasatinib over imatinib to prevent both primary and acquired drug resistance.

With the following properties associated with it, dasatinib will offer an option to overcoming imatinib resistance in CML and Ph+ ALL, delaying progression to advanced phase disease: (1) dasatinib has less stringent confor-mational requirements to allow binding to both the inactive and active forms of BCR-ABL kinase domain, therefore inhibiting wild-type as well as mutated BCR-ABL kinase; (2) dasatinib is not a substrate of multidrug P-glycoprotein efflux pumps; and (3) dasatinib targets multiple oncogenic pathways including SFKs, PDGFRβ receptor, c-KIT, and ephrin family kinases. With this, dasat-inib has been taken into preclinical testing and clinical validation to demon-strate its efficacy in imatinib-resistant CML.

15.3.1. Preclinical Studies to Demonstrate Dasatinib Is Active Against BCR-ABL Mutations

Resistance to imatinib is commonly associated with BCR-ABL kinase domain mutations, resulting in amino acid substitutions (Gorre et al., 2001). Indeed, in CML patients who developed resistance to imatinib, 30–90% exhibit imatinib-resistant BCR-ABL mutations (Hughes et al., 2006). The therapeutic limita-tions of imatinib lead to in vitro testing of dasatinib against imatinib-resistant mutations. When tested in a panel of Ba/F3 cell lines expressing either wild-type or distinct imatinib-resistant BCR-ABL mutants, dasatinib was 325-fold more potent than imatinib against wild-type BCR-ABL and active in all imatinib-resistant BCR-ABL mutations tested except the T315I mutant (Burgess et al., 2005; O'Hare et al., 2005; Shah et al., 2004). The IC_{50} concen-trations range from 1 to 10 nM for the majority of mutants, whereas T315I requires much higher concentration of dasatinib (see Table 15.1). For example, compared with the wild-type BCR-ABL, the F317L and E255V mutants required 9- and 14-fold higher concentrations of dasatinib, respectively, whereas the Y253H mutant is as sensitive to dasatinib as wild-type BCR-ABL. Additionally, the IC_{90} values for all BCR-ABL mutants to dastinib are below 50 nM (O'Hare et al., 2005); if invoking inhibition at or above the IC_{90} value is an indicator of clinical benefit, dasatinib would be predicted to be an effective single-agent therapeutic for CML cells expressing wild-type BCR-ABL and all mutants tested except T315I at a trough level of 50 nM (O'Hare et al., 2005).

TABLE 15.1. Comparison of In Vitro Sensitivity Between Imatinib, Nilotinib, and Dasatinib on Different BCR-ABL Mutations, and the Correlation Between the Baseline BCR-ABL Mutation and Clinical Response to Dasatinib at 8 months' Follow-up in Phase II Studies

Baseline Mutation	Cellular Proliferation[a]						Clinical Response to Dasatinib at 8 moths' Follow-up[c]		
	Imatinib		Nilotinib		Dasatinib				
	IC$_{50}$ (nM)	Fold Change[b]	IC$_{50}$ (nM)	Fold Change[b]	IC$_{50}$ (nM)	Fold Change[b]	Total N (%)	MaHR[d] N (%)	MCyR[e] N (%)
No mutations							261 (51)	193 (74)	130 (50)
Any mutation							253 (49)	172 (70)	105 (42)
P-loop (amino acids 248–256)							91	77 (85)	43 (47)
A-loop (amino acids 379–398)							43	30 (70)	19 (44)
WT Bcr-Abl	260	1	13	1	0.8	1			
M244V	2,000	8	38	3	1.3	2	28	22 (79)	16 (57)
G250E	1,350	5	48	4	1.8	2	41	27 (66)	15 (37)
Q252H	1,325	5	70	5	3.4	4	3	2 (67)	1 (33)
Y253F	3,475	13	125	10	1.4	2	2	1 (50)	1 (50)
Y253H	>6,400	>25	450	35	1.3	2	22	16 (73)	10 (45)

E255K	5,200	20	200	15	5.6	7	18	6 (33)	5 (28)
E255V	>6,400	>25	430	33	11	14	5	5 (100)	2 (40)
T315I	>6,400	>25	>2,000	>154	>200	>250	25	1 (4)	1 (4)
F317L	1,050	4	50	4	7.4	9	8	8 (100)	1 (13)
M351T	880	3	15	1.2	1.1	1.4	12	9 (75)	3 (25)
F359V	1,825	7	175	13	2.2	3	13	11 (85)	4 (31)
V379I	1,630	6	51	4	0.8	1	6	3 (50)	3 (50)
H396R	1,750	7	41	3	1.3	2	19	13 (68)	7 (37)

[a] Cellular proliferation data was taken with permission from O'Hare et al. (2005) in *Cancer Research*.

[b] Fold change refers to the fold difference in the IC_{50}, relative to wild type, which is set to 1.

[c] Data are summarized from Guilhot et al. (2007), Cortes et al. (2007), Ottmann et al. (2007), Kantarjian et al. (2007), and Hochhaus et al. (2007a).

[d] MaHR indicates major hematologic response and includes both complete hematologic response (CHR) and no evidence of leukemia (NEL). CHR criteria: white blood cell (WBC) count no more than institutional ULN; absolute neutrophil count (ANC) $\geq 1 \times 10^9$/L (1000/mm^3); platelet count $\geq 100 \times 10^9$/L (100,000/mm^3); no blasts or promyelocytes in peripheral blood; bone marrow blasts $\leq 5\%$; less than 5% myelocytes plus metamyelocytes in peripheral blood; basophils in peripheral blood < 2% and basophils in the bone marrow < 2%; no extramedullary involvement (including no hepatomegaly or spleno-megaly). NEL criteria: WBC count no more than institutional ULN; no blasts or promyelocytes in peripheral blood; bone marrow blasts $\leq 5\%$; less than 5% myelocytes plus metamyelocytes in peripheral blood; no extramedullary involvement (including no hepatomegaly or splenomegaly); basophils in peripheral blood < 2% and at least one of the following: 20×10^9/L (20,000/mm^3) $\leq$ platelets < 100×10^9/L (100,000/mm^3) or 0.5×10^9/L (500/mm^3) $\leq$ ANC < 1.0×10^9/L (1000/mm^3).

[e] MCyR indicates major cytogenetic response and is the sum of complete cytogenetic response (CCyR) and partial cytogenetic response (PCyR). Cytogenetic response is evaluated by bone marrow aspirates/biopsies and calculated from the percentage of Ph+ cells in metaphase in the bone marrow sample and defined as CCyR (0%), PCyR (1–35%).

As dasatinib use broadens, it will be useful to predict the profile of mutations that confer drug resistance. To identify specific resistance mutations in BCR-ABL which could emerge under therapy with imatinib, dasatinib, or nilotinib, a second generation of BCR-ABL inhibitor that is more potent than imatinib (Golemovic et al., 2005; Weisberg et al., 2006), an in vitro mutagenesis screening using cell-based assays was conducted in the presence of graded concentrations of either drug to generate resistance mutation profiles for each drug (Bradeen et al., 2006). As summarized in Table 15.2, different spectrums of recovered mutations were observed, twenty different mutations identified with imatinib, ten with nilotinib, and nine with dasatinib, respectively. From the in vitro mutagenesis study, the two highest mutation incidences, Y253H and T315I, were found for imatinib and nilotinib. Y253H, accounting for 45% and 37% of total observed mutations for imatinib and nilotinib, was not detected for dasatinib even at the highest drug concentration, while T315I mutation confers resistance to all three drugs. The predominant mutations arising in the presence of dasatinib were T315I (78%) and F317I/L/C/V (total 17%). Overall, F317 is the most frequently involved residue besides T315, and four different mutations have been identified (F317I/L/C/V), implicating F317 as a potential vulnerable site for dasatinib resistance. Crystal structure analysis of the ABL kinase domain in complex with dasatinib has revealed that the compound binds an active conformation of ABL, with F317 as a contact residue directly interacting with the pyrimidine and thiazole rings of dasatinib (Tokarski et al., 2006). Additional mutants detected at 10–50 nM dasatinib include V299L, which is also a contact point, and Q252H in the P-loop. T315I emerges as the sole mutation at drug concentrations of at least 100 nM. These observations correspond well with reported IC_{50} values from cell proliferation assays (Burgess et al., 2005; O'Hare et al., 2005). Taken together, the findings indicate that dasatinb should be efficacious in most cases in which BCR-ABL point mutants cause imatinib resistance and suggest that dasatinib may be superior to imatinib in treated imatinib-resistant patients and in preventing the development of resistance.

These preclinical findings predict that dasatinib should be effective for patients with CML and Ph+ ALL resistant to imatinib who harbor either wild-type or mutated BCR-ABL. However, these results suggested that patients with T315I mutation might not benefit from dasatinib and mutations at residue T315 may account for dasatinib clinical resistance. As T315I mutation accounts for only approximately 10–15% of patients who developed imatinib-resistant mutations (Hughes et al., 2006), a substantial fraction of imatinib-resistant CML patients, including unmutated and mutated at other sites of BCR-ABL, could benefit from dasatinib. These hypotheses have now been tested and validated in CML and Ph+ ALL clinical studies of dasatinb.

15.3.2. Clinical Validation of In Vitro Results

With promising preclinical results, a Phase I trial with dasatinib began in November 2003 with the primary objective to define drug tolerability and

TABLE 15.2. Spectrum and Frequency of BCR-ABL Kinase Domain Mutations Recovered in the Presence of Imatinib, Nilotinib, or Dasatinib in the In Vitro Mutagenesis Screening

Mutation	Imatinib (2,000–16,000 nM)		Nilotinib (10–5,000 nM)		Dasatinib (5–500 nM)	
	Mutation Recovered	Percentage in Recovered Mutations	Mutation Recovered	Percentage in Recovered Mutations	Mutation Recovered	Percentage in Recovered Mutations
M244V	Yes	0.27	No	0	No	0
L248R	Yes	0.54	No	0	No	0
L248V	Yes	0.81	Yes	0.58	Yes	1.66
G250E	Yes	1.08	Yes	2.89	No	0
Q252H	Yes	1.34	No	0	Yes	0.55
Y253H	Yes	45.16	Yes	36.99	No	0
E255K	Yes	5.91	Yes	2.89	Yes	1.1
E255V	Yes	0.27	Yes	0.58	No	0
D276G	Yes	0.54	No	0	No	0
E292V	No	0	Yes	0.58	No	0
V299L	No	0	No	0	Yes	1.66
F311I	Yes	1.08	No	0	No	0
F311V	Yes	0.81	No	0	No	0
T315I	Yes	37.37	Yes	50.87	Yes	77.9
F317C	No	0	No	0	Yes	3.87
F317I	No	0	No	0	Yes	6.63
F317L	Yes	0.54	No	0	Yes	5.52
F317V	No	0	No	0	Yes	1.1
M351T	Yes	0.27	No	0	No	0
E355G	Yes	0.27	No	0	No	0
F359C	Yes	1.61	Yes	3.47	No	0
F359V	Yes	0.81	No	0	No	0
V379I	Yes	0.54	No	0	No	0
L384M	Yes	0.27	Yes	0.58	No	0
L387F	No	0	Yes	0.58	No	0
H396R	Yes	0.54	No	0	No	0

[a]Data summarized from Bradeen et al. (2006).

safety. Secondary objectives were to determine the pharmacokinetic proper-
ties and antileukemic activity of dasatinib, and to examine potential correlation of clinical response to the BCR-ABL genotype. Phase II studies began in
December 2004 in chronic phase CML (CP-CML), accelerated-phase CML
(AP-CML), myeloid blast crisis CML (MBC), lymphoid blast crisis CML
(LBC), or Ph+ ALL to determine clinical response and durability. Two Phase
III studies began in July 2005 to test dasatinib at different doses and schedules
in all stages of CML for patients who had resistance or intolerance to
imatinib.

Clinical Efficacy. The Phase I dose-escalation study tested dasatinib in a total
of 84 patients with 40 CP-CML and 44 AP-CML, MBC, and LBC/Ph+ ALL.
The rates of major hematologic response (MaHR, see Table 15.1 footnote for
definition) were 92%, 82%, 61%, and 70%, respectively, and the rates of
major cytogenetic response (MCyR, see Table 15.1 footnote for definition)
were 45%, 27%, 35%, and 80% for CP-CML, AP-CML, MBC, and LBC/Ph+
ALL, respectively (Talpaz et al., 2006). Data from long-term follow-up (≥27
months) of the Phase I study (Cortes et al., 2008) confirmed that dasatinib is
associated with high rates of hematologic and cytogenetic responses in
CP-CML patients who failed imatinib treatment; and the responses were
durable and translated into favorable progression-free survival (PFS) and
overall survival (OS). At 36 months, PFS and OS were 64% and 82%, respectively; patients who achieved a MCyR at any time versus those who did not
had improved rates of PFS (87% vs. 37%) and OS (95% vs. 66%). The dasatinib Phase II study in CP-CML with a median follow-up of 15.2 months
showed that 91% of patients maintained or achieved complete hematologic
response (CHR) (Hochhaus, 2007b; Hochhaus et al., 2008a). Responses were
rapid and durable, and 15 month PFS was 90% while OS was 96%. MCyR and
complete cytogenetic response (CCyR) were maintained or achieved in 59%
and 49% of patients, respectively. The 2 year data further demonstrated continuing efficacy of dasatinib with even higher MCyR (62%) and CCyR (53%)
rates; the responses were longlasting with 88% of patients in MCyR and 90%
in CCyR maintaining their response at 2 years (Cervantes et al., 2008; Mauro
et al., 2008). In Phase II studies with a minimum of 8 months' follow-up, dasatinib induced MaHR and MCyR in a significant number of CML patients with
advanced disease. In patients with AP-CML ($n = 107$), MBC ($n = 74$), and
LBC ($n = 42$), 64%, 34%, and 31% achieved MaHR, respectively; and 33%,
31%, and 50% of patients achieved MCyR, respectively, and a significant
proportion of these MCyRs were CCyRs (Cortes et al., 2007; Guilhot et al.,
2007). The 24 month data from blast phase CML further confirmed efficacy of
dasatinib; in patients with limited therapeutic options, dasatinib resulted in OS
rates of 38% and 26% in MBC and LBC, respectively (Saglio et al., 2008a).
The interim results of a Phase II study of dasatinib in Ph+ ALL with a
minimum follow-up of 8 months demonstrated that dasatinib resulted in a
MaHR and CCyR in 42% and 58% of patients, respectively (Ottmann et al.,

2007). The responses were achieved rapidly and were durable with a positive impact on survival with 2 year follow-up (Porkka et al., 2008).

To compare the response of 140 mg dasatinib with high-dose (800 mg) imatinib in patients with CP-CML, a randomized Phase II study was conducted. With a median follow-up of 15 months, CHR was observed in 93% and 82% of patients receiving dasatinib and high-dose imatinib, respectively (Kantarjian et al., 2007). In recent reports (Rousselot et al., 2008a,b) with a minimum 2 years' follow-up, the rates for MCyR were 53% versus 33% ($p = 0.017$), for CCyR they were 44% versus 18% ($p = 0.0025$) for patients receiving dasatinib and high-dose imatinib, respectively. The progression-free survival at 2 years also favored dasatinib (86% vs. 65%, $p = 0.0012$).

In a Phase III study to compare dasatinib 50 or 70 mg twice daily (bid), or 100 or 140 mg once daily (qd) in a total of 662 CP-CML patients, response rates were similar across all dosing groups (CHR: 88–93%; MCyR: 58–64%; CCyR: 46–50%) with a median follow-up of 11.5 months (Hochhaus et al., 2007b). In another study to compare 140 mg once daily or 70 mg twice daily in advanced phase CML or Ph+ ALL patients, 609 patients were treated, and response rates (MaHR and MCyR) were similar between the two dose schedules for AP-CML, MBC, LBC, and Ph+ ALL subgroups with a median follow-up of 6.4 months (Dombret et al., 2007).

Dasatinib as a highly effective second-line drug was one of the most rapidly developed drugs, taking just 25 months from first in human to the filing of the New Drug Application and 31 months to registration approval in the United States. Based on positive data in Phase I and Phase II trials, dasatinib received accelerated approval by the Food and Drug Administration (FDA) in June 2006, and the European Medicines Agency in November 2006, for the treatment of adults in all phases CML with resistance or intolerance to imatinib. Full approval was also granted for the treatment of adults with Ph+ ALL with resistance or intolerance to prior therapy. The Phase III dose optimization study (Hochhaus et al., 2007b) demonstrated that dasatinib 100 mg once daily is highly effective in patients with chronic phase CML resistant or intolerant to imaitinib, with less frequent key side effects. Based on these results, the approved dose of dasatinib for the treatment of CP-CML imatinib-resistant or -intolerant patients was changed from 70 mg twice daily to 100 mg once daily.

BCR-ABL Mutations Versus Clinical Response. The analysis of BCR-ABL mutation as biomarkers was implemented in the Phase I study and the results demonstrated that dasatinib has clinical activity in patients with a variety of BCR-ABL mutations except T315I at baseline (Talpaz et al., 2006). This result mirrors the preclinical findings (Shah et al., 2004; O'Hare et al., 2005). Furthermore, as summarized in Table 15.1, mutations were identified in 253 (49%) of 514 patients who had baseline mutational analysis data on the BCR-ABL kinase domain available when the results were reported from five Phase II trials (Cortes et al., 2007; Guilhot et al., 2007; Hochhaus et al., 2007a;

Kantarjian et al., 2007; Ottmann et al., 2007). Among these, G250E, M244V, T315I, Y253H, H396R, E255K, F359V, and M351T were the most common baseline mutations detected across all five studies, which may reflect the most frequent resistant mutations developed during imatinib treatment. Sixty-three patients were observed to have two mutations and 15 patients to have more than two mutations. As shown in Table 15.1, of the baseline mutations observed, approximately 36% and 17% were located within the P-loop (amino acids 248–256) and A-loop (amino acids 379–398) of the kinase domain, respectively; 60% of mutations were associated with moderate to very high resistance to imatinib (M244V, G250E, Q252H, Y253F, Y253H, E255K, E255V, T315I, F359V, V379I, and H396R), which was defined by more than a fivefold increase in IC_{50} compared with unmutated BCR-ABL in the in vitro cellular proliferation (O'Hare et al., 2005). The correlation of the BCR-ABL genotype with a clinical response to dasatinib demonstrated that the presence of BCR-ABL mutations conferring imatinib resistance did not preclude a response to dasatinib. Overall, both hematologic and cytogenetic responses to dasatinib were observed broadly across the mutation spectrum (Table 15.1). Specifically, patients with imatinib-resistant BCR-ABL mutations had achieved MaHR and MCyR with the rates not significantly different from either the unmutated patient population or the whole population for all disease stages. In addition, comparable response rates to dasatinib were observed in patients with mutations in the P-loop or activation-loop compared with mutations located elsewhere (Cortes et al., 2007; Guilhot et al., 2007; Hochhaus et al., 2007a; Kantarjian et al., 2007; Ottmann et al., 2007; Cervantes et al., 2008; Mauro et al., 2008; Porkka et al., 2008). This is a significant finding given that a previous study reported mutations in the P-loop may contribute to increased oncogenicity of the kinase and is associated with a very poor survival among patients treated with imatinib; the 1 year survival rate of patients with P-loop mutations was 15% versus 80% with non-P-loop mutations (Branford et al., 2003). More importantly, notable response rates were observed in patients having baseline mutations associated with moderate to very high resistance to imatinib except T315I (Table 15.1). For example, in the Phase II CP-CML study with a median follow-up of 15.2 months, 89.6% and 57.1% of patients with these highly imatinib-resistant mutations achieved CHR and MCyR, respectively, very close to the rates of unmutated patients (90.8% and 59.7% for CHR and MCyR, respectively) (Hochhaus et al., 2008a). Recent analyses (Hochhaus et al., 2008b,c) of a Phase III CP-CML study to compare the efficacy of different dasatinib dosing regimens administered with regard to commonly occurring individual baseline BCR-ABL mutations were reported, and results from 581 of 662 treated patients, who had baseline mutation evaluation performed and 1 year cytogenetic response data, demonstrated that similar MCyRs and CCyRs were observed across the four dosing groups in patients with different BCR-ABL mutations with the exception of T315I. For dasatinib 100 mg once daily, the MCyRs were 59% and 63%, and the CCyRs were 43% and 50% for the patients with baseline BCR-ABL mutations (except T315I) and patients with mutations in the P-loop, respectively, which were similar to those of other dosing schedules tested. These results confirmed dasatinib is highly effective in CP-CML patients with different baseline BCR-ABL mutations including those occurring in the P-loop.

Dasatinib also demonstrated favorable MCyR (58–69%) in CP-CML patients with BCR-ABL mutations such as Y253H, E255V/K, and F359C/V (Hochhaus et al., 2008c; Mauro et al., 2008), these mutations are less sensitive to nilotinib (Table 15.1) as defined by in vitro cellular $IC_{50} > 150\,nM$ (O'Hare et al., 2005). In contrast, nilotinib achieved MCyR only in 19% of patients with these mutations (Saglio et al., 2008b). These mutations account for 14–27% of the BCR-ABL mutated population that are resistant to imatinib in these study cohorts (Hochhaus et al., 2008c; Mauro et al., 2008; Saglio et al., 2008b). To conclude, dasatinib has broad efficacy in patients with a variety of mutations in the BCR-ABL kinase domain, including those associated with high levels of resistance to imatinib and nilotinib.

In the Phase I trial of dasatinib, three patients with T315I at baseline did not respond to dasatinib, and the presence or the emergence of the T315I mutation was identified in several patients at the time of relapse (Talpaz et al., 2006). The same results were observed in all Phase II studies (Cortes et al., 2007; Guilhot et al., 2007; Hochhaus et al., 2007a; Kantarjian et al., 2007; Ottmann et al., 2007; Hochhaus et al., 2008a); dasatinib had no activity in patients with the T315I mutation with one exception, a CP-CML patient who achieved a CHR and MCyR (Kantarjian et al., 2007). In the Phase III study in CP-CML, only 1 of 15 patients with baseline T315I mutation achieved a MCyR (Hochhaus et al., 2008c). A study by Müller et al. (2007) evaluated the emergence of new mutations in 22 imatinib-resistant CP-CML patients who had not achieved a molecular response to dasatinib after a median follow-up of 20 months. New emerged mutations on dasatinib were observed in several patients [F317L ($n = 7$), T315I ($n = 3$), and V299L ($n = 2$)]. Khorashad et al. (2008b) characterized the in vivo kinetics of kinase domain mutation evolving during dasatinib treatment in 12 patients with different baseline mutations and found they all responded to dasatinib. During the follow-up (range 6+ to 25+ months on dasatinib), four of them lost their mutations (E453V, F359V, and two with H396R) and remained undetectable. Three retained their mutations (L248V, G250R, and M244V) and another three lost their original mutations (M244V, M351T, and H396R) but developed a new mutation, F317L. Ten of 12 patients were still responsive to dasatinb at the time of the reported analysis; however, two patients developed a T315I mutation in addition to the original mutation (F311I and Y253H) and had disease progression. These data support the observations from in vitro mutagenesis studies with dasatinib (Table 15.2), suggesting that contact site mutants, notably T315I and F317L, may develop on dasatinib (Burgess et al., 2005; Bradeen et al., 2006). Interestingly, F317L was also reported in patients from Phase II studies with acquired resistance to dasatinib (Soverini et al., 2006). Whether developing the F317L is a more common phenomenon for acquired resistance to dasatinib remains to be seen as more data become available. Clearly, with T315I emerging as a "gatekeeper" mutation conferring resistance to imatinib, nilotinib, and dasatinib, an inhibitor of T315I will ultimately be required to effectively treat CML patients with T315I mutation.

In summary, preclinical studies of dasatinib in CML supported its selection as an outstanding clinical candidate to meet a significant unmet medical need—imatinib-resistant CML. The integration of biomarker (BCR-ABL mutations) testing in the Phase I study provided a molecular understanding of dasatinib in CML, supporting an accelerated clinical development. The studies discussed demonstrate that dasatinib is the most appropriate agent for patients with CML who have developed resistance to imatinib. Its efficacy in the imatinib-resistant nonmutated CML patient population has promoted the investigational trials of dasatinib in first-line setting, head-to-head with imatinib in newly diagnosed chronic phase Ph+ CML to compare CCyR within 12 months and duration of the response. Preliminary data suggests that dasatinib compares favorably with imatinib in first-line use (Hochhaus, 2007a).

15.4. PHARMACOGENOMICS OF DASATINIB IN BREAST CANCER

The SRC tyrosine kinase was the first protooncogene described and functions at the hub of a vast array of signal transduction cascades that influence cellular proliferation, differentiation, motility, and survival. Elevated levels and activation of SRC have been found in a variety of human solid cancers and correlate with disease progression (Thomas and Brugge, 1997; Irby and Yeatman, 2000; Summy and Gallick, 2003; Yeatman, 2004), so targeting SRC by dasatinib to reduce the activity may provide a valuable approach for the treatment of these cancer types. Accumulative data generated in preclinical models (Johnson et al., 2005; Lee et al., 2005; Nam et al., 2005; Song et al., 2006; Shor et al., 2007) demonstrated that dasatinib has potent antitumor activity in both in vitro cell lines and in vivo xenografts in a broad spectrum of cancer types, supporting SRC as a potential target for designing therapeutics (Susva et al., 2000; Warmuth et al., 2003a). For this reason, dasatinib is undergoing evaluation in a number of solid tumors.

Effective targeted therapies have been developed that benefit at least a subset of patients with defined molecular phenotypes. For example, trastuzumab is effective in breast cancer patients with HER2 amplification (Slamon et al., 2001). The responsiveness of non-small-cell lung cancer to EGFR inhibitors, gefitinib, or erlotinib is associated with EGFR mutations (Lynch et al., 2004; Pao et al., 2004). These results highlight the importance of identifying the fraction of cancer patients who will benefit from a given targeted therapy: to guide the use of targeted therapeutic agents based on a patient's molecular characteristics; and to provide an opportunity to better match the most effective drug with the right subset of patients. The importance and benefit of patient selection is best illustrated by the example of trastuzumab. The overall response rate to trastuzumab in breast cancer patients is about 10% without patient selection, while with selection of HER2 amplification the overall response rate increases to 35–50% (Vogel et al., 2002). The example demonstrates the need in clinical development to identify biomarkers that will guide patient selection and enable monitoring of drug efficacy at the molecular level. Identification and utilization of robust biomarkers in trials for innovative medicines could speed up clinical development, facilitate the individualization of therapy, and result in fast approval of developmental drug.

Since biomarkers correlated with the sensitivity to SFK inhibitors were not known before dasatinib began development, there was a need to search for biomarkers capable of predicting response to dasatinib. To this end, efforts have been made to characterize the subtypes of breast tumors more responsive to dasatinib; and to globally search for molecular markers predictive of response to dasatinib in these subtypes of breast cancer (Finn et al., 2007; Huang et al., 2007). These studies could provide valuable information for potential patient selection to support the clinical development of dasatinib in breast cancer.

15.4.1. Use of Preclinical Models to Identify Dasatinib Efficacy Predictive Biomarkers

Gene expression profiling studies have demonstrated the advantages of genomic "signatures" or marker sets generated by microarray analysis in predicting chemotherapeutic response (Iwao-Koizumi et al., 2005; Rouzier et al., 2005; Dressman et al., 2006; Hess et al., 2006). Huang et al. (2007) conducted preclinical pharmacogenomic studies in a panel of breast cancer cell lines to identify a molecular signature significantly correlated with in vitro sensitivity to dasatinib. Specifically, the sensitivity of dasatinib was tested in a panel of 23 breast cancer cell lines using an in vitro proliferation assay with the sensitivity expressed as an IC_{50} (the drug concentration required to inhibit cell proliferation to 50% compared to untreated control cells). The IC_{50} values ranged from 5.5 nM to >9.5 µM among these cell lines with a 3-log difference, suggesting that, if these cell lines are representative of breast cancer patients, the drug might be effective in only a subset of patients. Based on the IC_{50} value, each cell line was then classified as either sensitive or resistant to dasatinib using the sensitive/resistant demarcation of 0.6 µM. In parallel, the baseline gene expression profiles for these 23 cell lines were generated using Affymetrix high-density oligonucleotide array human HG-U133 set chips (containing >44,000 probe sets). Three statistical methods (signal-to-noise statistic with permutation test; Pearson correlation between the IC_{50} values and the gene expression level; and Welch t-test) were used to look for the intrinsic gene expression pattern that significantly correlated with dasatinib sensitive/resistant classification and to identify a 161 gene signature ("dasatinib sensitivity gene signature") differentially expressed between sensitive and resistant cell line groups as illustrated in Figure 15.2A. Among the 161 gene signature, 83 genes were highly expressed in the cell lines sensitive to dasatinib and 78 genes were highly expressed in the resistant cell lines. Many of these genes are linked

(A)   **(B)**

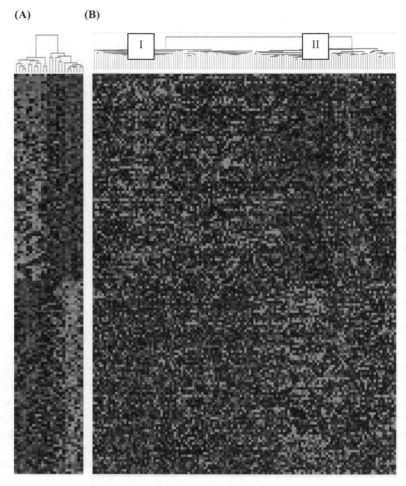

Figure 15.2. Hierarchical clustering analysis depicting the expression patterns of "dasatinib sensitivity gene signature." This figure is adopted from Huang et al. (2007). Each column represents a cell line or tumor and each row represents a gene. The matrix represents normalized expression patterns for each gene. Red indicates relatively high expression and green indicates relatively low expression. (**A**) The relative expression levels of 161 genes ("dasatinib sensitivity gene signature") that are highly correlated with dasatinib sensitivity/resistance classification in 23 breast cell lines. The sensitive cell lines are labeled in blue and resistant cell lines are labeled in red. (**B**) The expression patterns of "dasatinib sensitivity gene signature" in 134 breast tumors. Cluster I is the potential dasatinib nonresponder population labeled in red and cluster II is the potential dasatinib responder population labeled in blue. (See color insert.)

to signaling pathways of SFKs, including genes involved in cell cycle, cell growth and proliferation, apoptosis, adhesion, and migration. Interestingly, several direct targets of dasatinib (LYN, EphA2, and EphB2) as well as downstream targets of SFKs (CAV1 and CAV2) are highly expressed in the sensitive cell lines compared to the resistant ones.

The important questions to answer are: What is the utility of the "dasatinib sensitivity gene signature" and could it be used as a predictor to make dasatinib response prediction on other testing samples? To further assess this, the 161 gene signature was used to build a predictor based on their expression pattern in the 23 breast cell lines. This predictor was then utilized to predict response to dasatinib in an additional dataset of 12 breast cancer cell lines by a weighted-voting algorithm (Golub et al., 1999; Staunton et al., 2001). The 161 gene model correctly predicted three out of four sensitive and all eight resistant breast cancer cell lines, resulting in a sensitivity of 75% and a specificity of 100%. A prediction accuracy of 92% (11/12) was achieved ($p = 0.0182$, Fisher exact test). The positive predictive value (PPV) and negative predictive value (NPV) were 100% and 89%, respectively. While technologies now exist to examine thousands of genes simultaneously, the identification of a more limited number of markers that predict response to dasatinib might be more useful and feasible in clinical studies. Based on both statistical significance and biological relevance to the targeted pathway, six genes (EPHA2, CAV1, CAV2, ANXA1, PTRF, and IGFBP2) were selected to build a model for further assessment of its predictive ability. All six genes are either targets of dasatinib or substrates for SFKs, and/or expression level is modulated by dasatinib, suggesting they are part of signaling pathways downstream of SFKs. The predictive power of the six gene predictor was tested again on the 12 breast cancer cell lines. The same prediction result (Table 15.3) was obtained as using the 161 gene predictor. The results validated the utility of the six gene predictor in the same tissue type.

Since the value of a predictor that could be utilized across indications is greater than one that works in a single indication, the predictive accuracy of the six gene predictor was further evaluated in test datasets of 23 lung and 16 prostate cancer cell lines. As shown in Table 15.3, the prediction accuracy of

TABLE 15.3. Dasatinib Response Prediction on Additional Datasets of Testing Cell Lines Using the Six Gene Predictors Developed on 23 Breast Cell Lines

Dataset	Breast Cancer Cell Lines ($n = 12$)	Lung Cancer Cell Lines ($n = 23$)	Prostate Cancer Cell Lines ($n = 16$)
Sensitivity	75%	91%	82%
Specificity	100%	75%	80%
PPV	100%	77%	90%
NPV	89%	90%	67%
Overall accuracy	92% (11/12)	83% (19/23)	81% (13/16)

the six gene predictor was very similar for both lung and prostate datasets, 83% (19/23) and 81% (13/16), respectively. Furthermore, the ability of the six gene predictor was assessed for predicting the in vivo response to dasatinib in seven tumor xenograft models that were generated either from cancer cell lines (breast: MCF-7; prostate: PC3 and MDAPCa-2b; and colon: WiDr) or from pancreatic tumors (Pat-25, Pat-26, and Pat-27). Xenografts Pat 26, Pat27, PC3, and WiDr were predicted to be sensitive, while Pat 25, MCF-7, and MDAPCa-2b were predicted to be resistant to dasatinib; the predicted result matched perfectly with in vivo antitumor activity of dasatinib in these xenografts of different tumor types.

Taking a similar approach to that described by Huang et al. (2007), Finn et al. (2007) used a different microarray platform (Agilent) and a panel of 39 human breast cancer cell lines to identify a set of three biologically relevant genes (CAV1, MSN, and YAP1) to be highly expressed in dasatinib-sensitive breast cell lines. These three genes were able to discriminate "responsive" cell lines on the 39 breast cell line panel with an 88% sensitivity and 85% specificity, respectively. Interestingly, both CAV1 and MSN were identified in the study by Huang et al. (2007), and YAP1 was also observed to be expressed at higher levels in sensitive cell lines in their study but just missed the stringent statistical cutoff.

Whether the predictive biomarkers identified in these two preclinical studies can be utilized in the clinic to predict dasatinib response in cancer patients still remains to be evaluated. Other studies have shown that in vitro developed genomic signatures of chemotherapy sensitivity can predict clinical response with reasonable accuracy in individuals treated with these agents. For example, Potti et al. (2006) reported using NCI-60 cell lines as models coupling drug response data with microarray gene expression data to develop the in vitro signature of docetaxel sensitivity, and then further assess and validate the docetaxel response prediction model in an independent set of lung and ovarian cancer cell lines with the prediction accuracy exceeding 80%. The in vitro docetaxel sensitivity predictor was further tested retrospectively in the breast neoadjuvant setting, where it correctly predicted docetaxel response in 22 of 24 clinical samples for an overall accuracy of 91.6%. Similar accuracy was obtained when extending this result by predicting the response to docetaxel as salvage therapy for patients with ovarian cancer that was refractory to primary therapy. They applied this approach to identify expression signatures for various cytotoxic chemotherapeutic drugs. Another study by Hsu et al. (2007) showed that in vitro developed gene signatures of cisplatin sensitivity can be utilized to predict clinical response in patients treated with cisplatin. Baselga et al. (2009) also identified genes, such as estrogen receptor (ER), associated with in vitro sensitivity/resistance to the microtubule inhibitor ixabepilone using breast cell lines, and further validated retrospectively in a neoadjuvant study that ER expression level was inversely correlated with pathological response to ixabepilone. The results from those examples shed light on validity and robustness of in vitro developed drug-sensitivity signature in predicting clinical drug response.

15.4.2. "Dasatinib Sensitivity Gene Signature" and Predicted Response to Dasatinib in Tumor Samples

It seems that the predictive biomarkers identified in breast cell lines worked well to predict dasatinib response in preclinical models both in vitro and in vivo. Whether the predictive biomarkers have utility to select cancer patients likely to respond to dasatinib in the clinic needs to be tested in clinical studies. To explore whether the "dasatinib sensitivity gene signature" correlated with the in vitro response to dasatinib in breast cell lines also exists in primary breast tumors, an expression dataset of 134 primary breast cancer surgical specimens was examined. Hierarchical clustering analysis segregated the breast tumors into two distinct groups as illustrated in Figure 15.2B, with one group (cluster II) of tumors having similar expression pattern as the sensitive cell lines and the other group (cluster I) expressing the gene signature observed in the dasatinib-resistant cell lines. Similar patterns were also observed for lung tumors and ovarian tumors. It is reasonable to hypothesize that tumors in cluster II having a similar expression pattern as the dasatinib sensitive cell lines are more likely to respond to dasatinib.

To estimate the percentage of patients with different types of cancer that might be responsive to dasatinib, gene expression databases for 318 breast tumors, 93 lung, and 239 ovarian tumors were interrogated. The rate of patients predicted to be responsive to dasatinib by the six gene predictor identified in breast cancer cell lines was estimated to be 30–40% depending on the tumor type (Huang et al., 2007). Again, whether this would represent the actual percentage of patients benefiting from dasatinib treatment is still to be answered.

15.4.3. Clinical Characteristics of a Potential Dasatinib Responsive Breast Cancer Subpopulation

There are different molecular phenotypes observed among the breast tumors based on gene expression profiling (Perou et al., 2000; Sorlie et al., 2001; Sotiriou et al., 2003). In the study by Finn et al. (2007), the 39 breast cell lines were molecular profiled and classified into three subtypes: "luminal" type, expressing specific cytokeratins (CK8 and CK18); "basal" type based on the expression of cytokeratins CK5 and CK17; and "post-EMT" type, which had undergone an epithelial-to-mesenchymal transition based on their expression of vimentin and the loss of cytokeratin expression. When $1 \mu M$ dasatinib was tested on these cell lines, 8 of them were highly sensitive (>60% growth inhibition), 10 of them were moderately sensitive (40–59% growth inhibition), and 21 were resistant to dasatinib. A highly significant correlation between breast cancer subtypes and the sensitivity classification to dasatinib was observed ($x^2 = 9.66$ and $p = 0.008$) with basal-type and post-EMT breast cancer cell lines being most sensitive to growth inhibition by dasatinib. The cell lines sensitive to dasatinib tend to have negative expression of ER and unamplified Her2. As has been observed previously, the basal subtype of breast cancers are generally "triple-negative" (i.e., ER negative, progesterone receptor (PR) negative, and HER2 negative), with a clinical disease that is more invasive, has a higher mitotic index, and a worse clinical outcome (Thomas et al., 1999; Laakso et al., 2006).

The observation that dasatinib preferentially inhibits the growth of triple-negative breast cancer cell lines has also been made independently and simultaneously (Huang et al., 2007). As shown in Figure 15.2B, breast tumors can be clustered into two main clusters based on the expression pattern of the "dasatinib sensitivity gene signature" identified from breast cancer cell lines. Cluster II has an expression pattern similar to the dasatinib-sensitive cell lines and may represent a potential dasatinib-responsive subpopulation. One interesting question is: What clinical characteristics define this potential dasatinib-responsive subpopulation in breast cancer patients? When the expression levels of ER, PR, and HER2 were assessed for cluster I (dasatinib nonresponder) and cluster II (dasatinib responder), there were significant differences in the distribution of tumors expressing ER, PR, or HER2 between the two clusters: in cluster II, a higher percentage of tumors have low expression levels of ER, PR, or HER2 (Table 15.4). Furthermore, a higher percentage of tumors with high expression levels of CK5 and CK17 were observed in the dasatinib responders compared to nonresponders, suggesting dasatinib-responding tumors may include the "basal type" of breast cancer as defined

TABLE 15.4. Distribution of "High" (H) and "Low" (L) Expresser of ER, PR, HER2, CK5, and CK17 Between Dasatinib Potential Responder and Nonresponder Clusters of Breast Tumors Based on the 161 Gene Expression Pattern Analyzed by Hierarchical Clustering[a]

Gene	Expression Level[b]	Dasatinib Nonresponder (Cluster I, 71) N (%)	Dasatinib Responder (Cluster II, 63) N (%)	p Value in x^2 Test
HER2	H	45 (63.4)	22 (34.9%)	0.00095
	L	26 (36.6%)	41 (65.1%)	
ER	H	52 (73.2%)	15 (23.8%)	1.1E-08
	L	19 (26.8%)	48 (76.2%)	
PR	H	46 (64.8%)	21 (33.3%)	0.00026
	L	25 (35.2%)	42 (66.7%)	
CK17	H	28 (39.4%)	39 (61.9%)	0.00943
	L	43 (60.6%)	24 (38.1%)	
CK5	H	25 (35.2%)	42 (66.7%)	0.00028
	L	46 (64.8)	21 (33.3%)	

[a]See Figure 15.2B.
[b]The median expression level of a gene across the 134 tumors was used to define "high" (H) or "low" (L) expression. A tumor is designated as "L" if its expression is below the median level and designated as "H" if its expression is above the median.

by CK5/CK17 expression (van de Rijn et al., 2002; Laakso et al., 2006). Similar results were observed when the six gene predictor was used to predict the dasatinib-responsive subpopulation in the 134 breast cancer patients: the predicted dasatinib-responsive subgroup tends to have more tumors with lower expression of ER, PR, or HER2 gene and more tumors with higher expression of CK5/CK17. This patient population is one that currently does not benefit from conventional targeted therapies such as endocrine therapy or trastuzumab, leaving only chemotherapy in the therapeutic armamentarium. Because these patients express a dasatinib sensitivity gene signature, this drug may represent a valuable treatment option for this difficult-to-treat population of breast cancer patients.

15.4.4. Relationship Between SRC Pathway Deregulation and the Sensitivity to SRC Inhibitors

Although SRC expression is not correlated with the sensitivity of breast cancer cell lines to dasatinib, the activation status of the SRC pathway may be. In a study by Bild et al. (2006), gene expression signatures that reflect the activation status of several oncogenic pathways, including SRC pathway, were developed. These gene expression signatures can link pathway deregulation with sensitivity to therapeutics that target components of the pathway. For example, expression of the SRC oncogenic pathway gene signature can predict the sensitivity of human cancer cell lines to a SRC inhibitor, SU6656. This provides an opportunity to make use of the oncogenic pathway signatures to guide the use of targeted therapeutics. When using the SRC pathway gene signature to perform clustering analysis on the panel of breast caner cell lines, Huang et al. (2007) observed a pattern of cell lines very similar to the one shown in Figure 15.2A with dasatinib-sensitive cell lines separated from resistant ones, indicating that a SRC pathway gene signature can predict response to dasatinib in the cell lines even though these two gene signatures don't overlap. This observation further confirms the finding that cancer cell lines with an activated oncogenic pathway are more sensitive to therapeutic agents that target the components of that pathway. The results demonstrate that different analytical approaches may identify different sets of predictive biomarkers to agents targeting a specific oncogene. These different sets of biomarkers lead to the identification of the very similar subset of cell lines and could ultimately select patients who will benefit from such agents. As recently discussed by Fan et al. (2006), although different gene sets are being used for prognostication in patients with breast cancer, they each track a common set of biologic characteristics and result in similar predictions of outcome. The observation that the "dasatinib sensitivity gene signature" (Huang et al., 2007) and the SRC pathway gene signature (Bild et al., 2006) identified a similar set of breast cell lines as either sensitive or resistant to dasatinib supports the observation by Fan et al. (2006).

15.5. PHARMACOGENOMICS OF DASATINIB IN PROSTATE CANCER

SFKs and EphA2 play important roles in prostatic tumorigenesis (Walker-Daniels et al., 1999; Nam et al., 2005). Dasatinib inhibits activity of SFK members SRC and LYN and subsequently blocks the downstream signaling cascade, resulting in inhibition of cell adhesion, migration, and invasion in prostate cancer cell lines (Nam et al., 2005). To support the development of dasatinib in prostate cancer, Wang et al. (2007) employed prostate cancer cell lines as preclinical models to identify molecular biomarkers whose expression was correlated with the sensitivity to dasatinib and modulated by dasatinib treatment.

15.5.1. Efficacy Predictive Biomarkers Identification

Wang et al. (2007) tested 16 prostate cancer cell lines with dasatinib and found 11 cell lines were sensitive to dasatinib with IC_{50} values lower than 200 nM and another 5 cell lines were resistant with IC_{50} values greater than or equal to 2 μM. Thus 174 candidate predictive genes with baseline expression levels correlated with sensitivity to dasatinib were identified from these cell lines. Most strikingly, two important prostatic cell markers, prostate specific antigen (PSA) and androgen receptor (AR), were found to be overexpressed in the resistant cell lines, while CK5 was highly expressed in a majority of the sensitive cell lines. Since CK5 is a basal cell marker for the prostatic cell lineage, these data suggest that cells exhibiting the basal phenotype are sensitive to dasatinib, whereas the cells expressing lower levels of CK5 and high levels of PSA and AR are resistant to dasatinib. The expression pattern of PSA and AR, two luminal cell markers, complementarily reinforces the above observation.

In addition, EphA2, one of the targets of dasatinib, was found significantly correlated with dasatinib sensitivity in both prostate and breast cancer cell lines with higher expression seen in sensitive cell lines. It appears to be a strong candidate biomarker for dasatinib in prostate cancer. Furthermore, urokinase-type plasminogen activator (uPA), a gene with higher basal level expression in dasatinib-sensitive cell lines (Figure 15.3A) and reduced by dasatinib treatment (Figure 15.3B), was taken for further testing. When eight cell lines were treated with dasatinib, the magnitude of uPA reduction by dasatinib correlated nicely with the sensitivity of cells to dasatinib ($r = 0.72$), with the highest reduction seen in the most sensitive cell line (Wang et al., 2007). Both uPA mRNA level (Figure 15.3B) and amount of protein secretion into the growth medium (Figure 15.3C) were reduced upon dasatinib treatment in a dose-dependent fashion in PC3 prostate cancer cell line, suggesting uPA is a potential pharmacodynamic biomarker for the biological effect of dasatinib. This kind of marker is desirable in drug development for two reasons. First, markers linked to the mechanisms of action for the drug would enhance the understanding of what biological effects are achieved at what dose level. Second, demonstration that

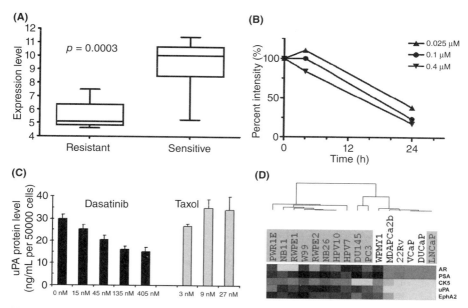

Figure 15.3. (**A**) Differential baseline expression of uPA gene between 11 sensitive and 5 resistant prostate cancer cell lines to dasatinib as detected by Affymetrix GeneChip. Y-axis is the RMA normalized expression value in $\log_2$ scale. The p-value is calculated from a t-test. (**B**) Dose-dependent downregulation of uPA mRNA expression in PC3 cells by dasatinib treatment compared to untreated control as measured by Affymetrix GeneChip. (**C**) Dasatinib inhibits secretion of uPA protein from PC3 cells in a dose-dependent manner as detected by ELISA assay. (**D**) Expression pattern of a five-gene set (AR, PSA, CK5, uPA, and EphA2) in prostate cell lines. Hierarchical clustering analysis of 16 cell lines using the five gene set with expression level highly correlated with dasatinib sensitivity/resistance classification. The sensitive cell lines are highlighted. This figure, courtesy of Dr. Xi-De Wang, is adapted from Wang et al. (2007). (See color insert.)

a drug inhibits its relevant molecular target at a tolerant dose is important in early stage of drug development, as this increases the probability of success in later Phase II and III clinical trials. In particular, while dasatinib is potent in inhibiting cell adhesion, migration, and invasion, it appears in preclinical models to be cytostatic rather than cytotoxic. Therefore it is not expected to have a high rate of clinical tumor response as monotherapy. uPA has been demonstrated to play an important role in prostatic tumorigenesis in numerous studies. For example, it is highly expressed in high-grade prostate tumors and metastases (Cozzi et al., 2006), and when a tumor progresses to androgen independence, the level of uPA expression is enhanced (Rocchi et al., 2004). In addition, RNA interference-induced knockdown of uPA inhibits invasion, survival, and in vivo tumorigenicity of prostate cancer cells (Pulukuri et al., 2005). In the clinic, elevated uPA plasma level or uPA-uPA receptor densities are correlated with prostate cancer invasion, metastasis, and poorer survival in prostate cancer (Miyake et al., 1999; Shariat et al., 2007). These warrant clinical testing of uPA as a potential pharmacodynamic biomarker for the biological effect of dasatinib.

In summary, five genes (AR, PSA, CK5, uPA, and EphA2) were identified as dasatinib efficacy predictive biomarkers for prostate cancer as illustrated in Figure 15.3D. Five dasatinib-resistant cell lines all expressed high levels of AR and PSA and low levels of CK5, uPA, and EphA2. In contrast, sensitive cell lines (with the exception of LNCaP) expressed low levels of AR and PSA, and high levels of uPA, EphA2, and/or CK5.

15.5.2. Defining a Dasatinib-Responsive Prostate Cancer Subpopulation

The dynamic range in the expression of the five candidate predictive biomarkers and the approximate patient population exhibiting dasatinib-responsive gene expression patterns were examined using a previously published prostate tumor dataset consisting of 52 tumor samples (Singh et al., 2002). Nearly 44% (23/52) of the prostate tumors showed the "dasatinib-responsive" expression patterns (i.e., low AR and PSA and high uPA, EphA2, and/or CK5). In the remaining approximately 56% of tumors, expression of AR and PSA was concordantly relatively high and the expression of uPA and EphA2 was relatively low. There were certain degrees of coexpression as well as mutually exclusive expression of AR and CK5 in this dataset, reminiscent of the expression patterns of these two genes in basal, intermediate, and luminal cells of normal prostatic epithelium (Wang et al., 2007). These markers are currently under early phase clinical evaluation using methods such as immunohistochemistry, ELISA, or RT-PCR to test the associations with dasatinib efficacy. If validated, they could facilitate patient stratification in trials of dasatinib.

15.6. OTHER FACTORS MAY AFFECT DASATINIB SENSITIVITY

Cross-talk and cooperation between SRC and EGFR/ErbB2 are necessary for transformation by EGFR. SRC directly modulates EGFR function through phosphorylation of tyrosine residues on EGFR that allows for coupling to downstream signaling events (Bromann et al., 2004; Ishizawar and Parsons, 2004). Based on the importance of EGFR signaling in lung cancer, the known cooperation between EGFR and SRC proteins, and evidence of elevated SRC activity in human lung cancers, EGFR may be one factor important in the sensitivity of lung cancer to dasatinib. Indeed, Song et al. (2006) evaluated the effectiveness of dasatinib in lung cancer cell lines and showed that cell fate (death versus growth arrest) in lung cancer cells exposed to dasatinib is dependent on EGFR status. Specifically, dasatinib reduces cell viability through the induction of apoptosis by downregulation of activated Akt and Stat3 survival proteins in cells with EGFR mutation that are dependent on EGFR for survival, while inducing a G1 cell cycle arrest with associated changes in cyclin D and p27 proteins, inhibition of activated FAK, and prevention of tumor cell invasion in cell lines with WT or EGFR mutations that are not sensitive to EGFR inhibition. These results show that dasatinib could be an effective therapy for patients with lung cancers through disruption of cell growth, survival, and tumor invasion; and suggest that EGFR status is important in deciding cell fate in response to dasatinib, so a priori determination of lung cancers dependent on EGFR for growth and/or survival may identify patient subsets who derive the maximum benefit from dasatinib.

Deng et al. (2005) demonstrated that myeloma cells are likely to be sensitive to dasatinib if they had higher baseline expression of genes responsible for proliferation and anti-apoptosis, such as MAF, MAFF, NFYC, PML, and YY1. Dasatinib sensitivity is also predicted by the presence of other genes for cell surface receptors (e.g., EphB4 and CXCR4) and proteosome subunits PSMC3, PSMD12, and PSME2, as well as the apoptotic regulators CIAP1 and IKKe.

Wainberg et al. (2008) recently reported a three gene set (PTK-7, PLK-2, and PLK-3) that was able to distinguish dasatinib-sensitive and -resistant colon cell lines. All three genes had relatively higher expression levels in the dasatinib-sensitive cell lines as compared to the dasatinib-insensitive cell lines. Interestingly, PLK-2 and PLK-3 are part of the Polo-like kinase family and have recently been identified as potential targets for cancer therapy, which suggest a rationale for combining dasatinib with PLK targeted agents for more effective therapies.

Among the candidate predictive biomarker genes for dasatinib sensitivity identified from breast and/or prostate cell lines, several are components of signaling pathways important for cell survival and proliferation, such as the EGF-EGFR, transforming growth factor receptor, fibroblast growth factor receptor, and Met (Huang et al., 2007; Wang et al., 2007). As an intracellular tyrosine kinase, SRC can act as a signal transducer downstream of these receptor kinases (Thomas and Brugge, 1997; Ishizawar and Parsons, 2004; Yeatman, 2004). Alternatively, SRC kinase may function independently in one or more pathways. Although the mechanisms of either cooperation or cross-talk of these pathways with the SRC-mediated pathway in breast and prostate cancer is not clear, they may still represent candidate target pathways for combination therapies to achieve optimal efficacy and may provide insights for future clinical development strategies for dasatinib or other SFK-targeting agents.

15.7. PERSPECTIVE ON PHARMACOGENOMICS OF DASATINIB

Analyzing the dynamics of BCR-ABL mutated clones in CML patients who experienced hematologic or cytogenetic relapse on imatinib revealed that mutations are detectable several months prior to relapse in CML patients of all phases, suggesting that the occurrence of mutations during imatinib therapy may be predictive of relapse (Ernst et al., 2008). A recent study analyzed the outcome of 319 patients with CP-CML who were treated with imatinib and routinely screened for mutations (Khorashad et al., 2008a). The results showed the 5 year cumulative incidence of mutations was 6.6% for early CP and 17% for later CP patients; and identification of a mutation was highly predictive for loss of CCyR and for progression to advanced phase. Therefore routine mutation screening of patients who appear to be responding to imatinib may identify those at high risk of disease progression. Currently, there is no accepted consensus on when patients should be screened for analysis of BCR-ABL kinase domain mutations. Expert recommendations suggest that mutations should be identified as early as possible (Hughes et al., 2006; Shah et al., 2006). From a pharmacogenomic viewpoint, systematically monitoring the BCR-ABL mutations will be helpful in the setting of clinical resistance to imatinib. Early identification of patients who are likely to relapse on imatinib by genetic testing (e.g., mutation analysis) could prompt the earlier use of an alternative drug, such as dasatinib, capable of combating the particular mutation identified, and may help to improve prognosis by initiating earlier responses to treatment and preventing the progression to advanced phase. In addition, identifying patients having a T315I mutation, which is resistant to the tyrosine kinase inhibitors imatinib, nilotinib, and dasatinib, may allow the patient to be referred for earlier allogeneic stem cell transplantation or offered investigational therapies with drugs that can inhibit T315I-bearing BCR-ABL.

The fact that dasatinib is effective in patients with imatinib-resistant disease without BCR-ABL mutations suggests that dasatinib may also overcome other possible mechanisms of imatinib resistance, including SFK dysregulation. Notably, 42% of patients who had not achieved a prior CyR of any level on prior imatinib treatment attained a MCyR with dasatinib (Hochhaus et al., 2008a). Therefore early detection of SFK activation in patients on imatinib treatment may also shed light on when patients should be switched to dasatinib to optimize clinical benefit.

"Triple-negative" breast cancer is one of the difficult-to-treat patient populations that currently does not benefit from conventional targeted therapies such as endocrine therapy or trastuzumab. The preclinical in vitro activity of dasatinib in "basal" type or "triple-negative" breast cancer provided a hypothesis that is now under testing in clinical studies. In addition, the "dasatinib sensitivity gene signature" (Huang et al., 2007), predictive markers (Finn et al., 2007; Wang et al., 2007), and SRC pathway signature (Bild et al., 2006) identified from in vitro cell lines will require validation in a clinical setting. Evaluation of predefined candidate predictive biomarkers in Phase II trials may have advantage over de novo response predictive biomarker discovery using gene expression profiling due to the confounding effect of coordinated expression of thousands of genes that are associated with clinical response in a relatively small number of patients as elucidated in a recent paper (Pusztai et al. 2007). A pharmacogenomic clinical trial is underway to simultaneously examine the "dasatinib sensitivity gene signature" (Huang et al., 2007), SRC pathway gene signature (Bild et al., 2006), and a signature consisting of targets for dasatinib in a single, parallel, multiarm study in breast cancer patients using the tandem two-step Phase II design as outlined by Pusztai et al., (2007). In a preclinical study in breast cancer cell lines, both the "dasatinib sensitivity gene signature" and the SRC pathway gene signature identified a similar subset of cell lines to be sensitive to dasatinib (Huang et al., 2007); it would be interesting to see whether this is the case clinically. While pharmacogenomic studies of dasatinib in solid tumor are still in their infancy, several hypotheses generated from preclinical studies will be tested clinically with the hope to target the right patients with this novel targeted agent.

REFERENCES

Ban, K., Gao, Y., Amin, H. M., et al. (**2008**). BCR-ABL1 mediates up-regulation of Fyn in chronic myelogenous leukemia. *Blood*. 111(5), 2904–2908.

Baselga, J., Zambetti, M., Llombart-Cussac, A., et al. (**2009**). Phase II genomics study of ixabepilone as neoadjuvant treatment for breast cancer. *J Clin Oncol*. 27(4), 526–534.

Bild, A. H., Yao, G., Chang, J. T., et al. (**2006**). Oncogenic pathway signatures in human cancers as a guide to targeted therapies. *Nature*. 439(7074), 353–357.

Bradeen, H. A., Eide, C. A., O'Hare, T., et al. (**2006**). Comparison of imatinib mesylate, dasatinib (BMS-354825), and nilotinib (AMN107) in an *N*-ethyl-*N*-nitrosourea (ENU)-based mutagenesis screen: high efficacy of drug combinations. *Blood*. 108(7), 2332–2338.

Branford, S., Rudzki, Z., Walsh, S., et al. (**2002**). High frequency of point mutations clustered within the adenosine triphosphate-binding region of BCR/ABL in patients with chronic myeloid leukemia or Ph-positive acute lymphoblastic leukemia who develop imatinib (STI571) resistance. *Blood*. 99(9), 3472–3475.

Branford, S., Rudzki, Z., Walsh, S., et al. (**2003**). Detection of BCR-ABL mutations in patients with CML treated with imatinib is virtually always accompanied by clinical resistance, and mutations in the ATP phosphate-binding loop (P-loop) are associated with a poor prognosis. *Blood*. 102(1), 276–283.

Brave, M., Goodman, V., Kaminskas, E., et al. (**2008**). Sprycel for chronic myeloid leukemia and Philadelphia chromosome-positive acute lymphoblastic leukemia resistant to or intolerant of imatinib mesylate. *Clin Cancer Res*. 14(2), 352–359.

Bromann, P., Korkaya, H., and Courtneidge, S. (**2004**). The interplay between Src family kinases and receptor tyrosine kinases. *Oncogene*. 23, 7957–7968.

Burgess, M. R., Skaggs, B. J., Shah, N. P., et al. (**2005**). Comparative analysis of two clinically active BCR-ABL kinase inhibitors reveals the role of conformation-specific binding in resistance. *Proc Natl Acad Sci USA*. 102(9), 3395–3400.

Cervantes, F., Baccarani, M., Lipton, J., et al. (**2008**). Dasatinib long-term efficacy in patients with chronic myeloid leukemia in chronic phase (CML-CP) with resistance or intolerance to imatinib: a two-year update of the START-C study. *Haematologica*. 92(Suppl 1), 372, Abst 0934.

Cortes, J., Rousselot, P., Kim, D. W., et al. (**2007**). Dasatinib induces complete hematologic and cytogenetic responses in patients with imatinib-resistant or -intolerant chronic myeloid leukemia in blast crisis. *Blood*. 109(8), 3207–3213.

Cortes, J., Sawyers, C. L., Kantarjian, H., et al. (**2008**). Dasatinib is associated with durable treatment responses in chronic phase chronic myeloid leukemia: long-term follow-up from the Phase I trial (CA180002). *Haematologica*. 92(Suppl 1), 58, Abst 0119.

Cozzi, P. J., Wang, J., Delprado, W., et al. (**2006**). Evaluation of urokinase plasminogen activator and its receptor in different grades of human prostate cancer. *Hum Pathol*. 37(11), 1442–1451.

Deininger, M., Buchdunger, E., and Druker, B. (**2005**). The development of imatinib as a therapeutic agent for chronic myeloid leukemia. *Blood*. 105, 2640–2653.

Deng, Q., Mitsiades, N., Negri, J., et al. (**2005**). Dasatinib (BMS-354825): a multi-targeted kinase inhibitor with activity against multiple myeloma. *Blood*. 106(11), 1654, Abst 1571.

Dombret, H., Ottmann, O., Goh, Y., et al. (**2007**). Dasatinib 140 mg qd vs 70 mg b.i.d. in advanced-phase CML or Ph(+) ALL resistant or intolerant to imatinib: results from a randomized, Phase-III trial (CA180035). *Haematologica*. 92(Suppl 1), 319, Abst 0859.

Donato, N. J., Wu, J. Y., Stapley, J., et al. (**2003**). BCR-ABL independence and LYN kinase overexpression in chronic myelogenous leukemia cells selected for resistance to STI571. *Blood*. 101(2), 690–698.

Dressman, H. K., Hans, C., Bild, A., et al. (**2006**). Gene expression profiles of multiple breast cancer phenotypes and response to neoadjuvant chemotherapy. *Clin Cancer Res*. 12(3 Pt 1), 819–826.

Druker, B. J., Guilhot, F., O'Brien, S. G., et al. (**2006**). Five-year follow-up of patients receiving imatinib for chronic myeloid leukemia. *N Engl J Med*. 355(23), 2408–2417.

Ernst, T., Erben, P., Muller, M. C., et al. (**2008**). Dynamics of BCR-ABL mutated clones prior to hematologic or cytogenetic resistance to imatinib. *Haematologica*. 93(2), 186–192.

Evans, T., Morgan, J., and Van den Abbeele, A. (**2005**). Phase I dose-escalation study of the SRC and multi-kinase inhibitor BMS-354825 in patients (pts) with GIST and other solid tumors. *J Clin Oncol*. 23(June 1 Suppl), 3034.

Fabarius, A., Giehl, M., Kraemer, A., et al. (**2006**). Centrosome aberrations, disturbed mitotic spindle formation and G1 arrest in normal and leukemic cells treated with the SRC/ABL inhibitor dasatinib. *Blood*. 108, 614a–615a, Abst 2167.

Fan, C., Oh, D. S., Wessels, L., et al. (**2006**). Concordance among gene-expression-based predictors for breast cancer. *N Engl J Med*. 355(6), 560–569.

Finn, R. S., Dering, J., Ginther, C., et al. (**2007**). Dasatinib, an orally active small molecule inhibitor of both the src and abl kinases, selectively inhibits growth of basal-type/"triple-negative" breast cancer cell lines growing in vitro. *Breast Cancer Res Treat*. 105(3), 319–326.

Golemovic, M., Verstovsek, S., Giles, F., et al. (**2005**). AMN107, a novel aminopyrimidine inhibitor of Bcr-Abl, has in vitro activity against imatinib-resistant chronic myeloid leukemia. *Clin Cancer Res*. 11(13), 4941–4947.

Golub, T. R., Slonim, D. K., Tamayo, P., et al. (**1999**). Molecular classification of cancer: class discovery and class prediction by gene expression monitoring. *Science*. 286(5439), 531–537.

Gorre, M. E., Mohammed, M., Ellwood, K., et al. (**2001**). Clinical resistance to STI-571 cancer therapy caused by BCR-ABL gene mutation or amplification. *Science.* 293(5531), 876–880.

Guilhot, F., Apperley, J., Kim, D. W., et al. (**2007**). Dasatinib induces significant hematologic and cytogenetic responses in patients with imatinib-resistant or -intolerant chronic myeloid leukemia in accelerated phase. *Blood.* 109(10), 4143–4150.

Hess, K. R., Anderson, K., Symmans, W. F., et al. (**2006**). Pharmacogenomic predictor of sensitivity to preoperative chemotherapy with paclitaxel and fluorouracil, doxorubicin, and cyclophosphamide in breast cancer. *J Clin Oncol.* 24(26), 4236–4244.

Hochhaus, A. (**2007a**). Management of Bcr-Abl-positive leukemias with dasatinib. *Expert Rev Anticancer Ther.* 7(11), 1529–1536.

Hochhaus, A. (**2007b**). Dasatinib for the treatment of Philadelphia chromosome-positive chronic myelogenous leukaemia after imatinib failure. *Expert Opin Pharmacother.* 8(18), 3257–3264.

Hochhaus, A., and La Rosee, P. (**2004**). Imatinib therapy in chronic myelogenous leukemia: strategies to avoid and overcome resistance. *Leukemia.* 18(8), 1321–1331.

Hochhaus, A., Kantarjian, H. M., Baccarani, M., et al. (**2007a**). Dasatinib induces notable hematologic and cytogenetic responses in chronic-phase chronic myeloid leukemia after failure of imatinib therapy. *Blood.* 109(6), 2303–2309.

Hochhaus, A., Kim, D. W., Rousselot, P., et al. (**2007b**). Dasatinib dose and schedule optimization in chronic-phase CML resistant or intolerant to imatinib: results from a randomized Phase-III trial (CA180034). *Haematologica.* 92(Suppl 1), 128–129, Abst 0359.

Hochhaus, A., Baccarani, M., Deininger, M., et al. (**2008a**). Dasatinib induces durable cytogenetic responses in patients with chronic myelogenous leukemia in chronic phase with resistance or intolerance to imatinib. *Leukemia.* 22(6), 1200–1206.

Hochhaus, A., Mueller, M., Cortes, J., et al. (**2008b**). Dasatinib efficacy after imatinib failure by dosing schedule and baseline BCR-ABL mutation status in patients with chronic phase CML. *Haematologica.* 92(Suppl 1), 371–372, Abst 0933.

Hochhaus, A., Mueller, M., Cortes, J., et al. (**2008c**). Dasatinib efficacy by dosing schedule across individual baseline BCR-ABL mutations in chronic phase chronic myelogenous leukemia (CML-CP) after imatinib failure. *J Clin Oncol.* 26(May 20 Suppl), Abst 7014.

Hsu, D. S., Balakumaran, B. S., Acharya, C. R., et al. (**2007**). Pharmacogenomic strategies provide a rational approach to the treatment of cisplatin-resistant patients with advanced cancer. *J Clin Oncol.* 25(28), 4350–4357.

Hu, Y., Swerdlow, S., Duffy, T. M., et al. (**2006**). Targeting multiple kinase pathways in leukemic progenitors and stem cells is essential for improved treatment of Ph+ leukemia in mice. *Proc Natl Acad Sci USA.* 103(45), 16870–16875.

Huang, F., Reeves, K., Han, X., et al. (**2007**). Identification of candidate molecular markers predicting sensitivity in solid tumors to dasatinib: rationale for patient selection. *Cancer Res.* 67(5), 2226–2238.

Hughes, T., Deininger, M., Hochhaus, A., et al. (**2006**). Monitoring CML patients responding to treatment with tyrosine kinase inhibitors: review and recommendations for harmonizing current methodology for detecting BCR-ABL transcripts and kinase domain mutations and for expressing results. *Blood.* 108(1), 28–37.

Illmer, T., Schaich, M., Platzbecker, U., et al. (2004). P-glycoprotein-mediated drug efflux is a resistance mechanism of chronic myelogenous leukemia cells to treatment with imatinib mesylate. *Leukemia*. 18(3), 401–408.

Irby, R. B., and Yeatman, T. J. (2000). Role of Src expression and activation in human cancer. *Oncogene*. 19(49), 5636–5642.

Ishizawar, R., and Parsons, S. J. (2004). c-Src and cooperating partners in human cancer. *Cancer Cell*. 6(3), 209–214.

Iwao-Koizumi, K., Matoba, R., Ueno, N., et al. (2005). Prediction of docetaxel response in human breast cancer by gene expression profiling. *J Clin Oncol*. 23(3), 422–431.

Jabbour, E., Cortes, J., and Kantarjian, H. (2007). Dasatinib for the treatment of Philadelphia chromosome-positive leukaemias. *Expert Opin Invest Drugs*. 16(5), 679–687.

Johnson, F. M., Saigal, B., Talpaz, M., et al. (2005). Dasatinib (BMS-354825) tyrosine kinase inhibitor suppresses invasion and induces cell cycle arrest and apoptosis of head and neck squamous cell carcinoma and non-small cell lung cancer cells. *Clin Cancer Res*. 11(19 Pt 1), 6924–6932.

Kantarjian, H., Pasquini, R., Hamerschlak, N., et al. (2007). Dasatinib or high-dose imatinib for chronic-phase chronic myeloid leukemia after failure of first-line imatinib: a randomized Phase 2 trial. *Blood*. 109(12), 5143–5150.

Karaman, M. W., Herrgard, S., Treiber, D. K., et al. (2008). A quantitative analysis of kinase inhibitor selectivity. *Nat Biotechnol*. 26(1), 127–132.

Khorashad, J. S., de Lavallade, H., Apperley, J. F., et al. (2008a). Finding of kinase domain mutations in patients with chronic phase chronic myeloid leukemia responding to imatinib may identify those at high risk of disease progression. *J Clin Oncol*. 26(29), 4806–4813.

Khorashad, J. S., Milojkovic, D., Mehta, P., et al. (2008b). In vivo kinetics of kinase domain mutations in CML patients treated with dasatinib after failing imatinib. *Blood*. 111(4), 2378–2381.

Kolb, E. A., Gorlick, R., Houghton, P. J., et al. (2008). Initial testing of dasatinib by the pediatric preclinical testing program. *Pediatr Blood Cancer*. 50(6), 1198–1206.

Laakso, M., Tanner, M., Nilsson, J., et al. (2006). Basoluminal carcinoma: a new biologically and prognostically distinct entity between basal and luminal breast cancer. *Clin Cancer Res*. 12(14 Pt 1), 4185–4191.

Lee, F. Y., Lombardo, L., Borzilleri, R., et al. (2004). BMS-354825—a potent dual SRC/ABL kinase inhibitor possessing curative efficacy against imatinib sensitive and resistant human CML models in vivo. *Cancer Res*. 46, 921, Abst 3987.

Lee, F., Lombardo, L., Camuso, A., et al. (2005). BMS-354825 potently inhibits multiple selected oncogenic tyrosine kinases and possesses broad-spectrum antitumor activities in vitro and in vivo. *Cancer Res*. 46, 159, Abst 675.

Lee, F., Fandi, A., and Voi, M. (2008). Overcoming kinase resistance in chronic myeloid leukemia. *Int J Biochem Cell Biol*. 40(3), 334–343.

Li, S. (2008). Src-family kinases in the development and therapy of Philadelphia chromosome-positive chronic myeloid leukemia and acute lymphoblastic leukemia. *Leuk Lymphoma*. 49(1), 19–26.

Lombardo, L. J., Lee, F. Y., Chen, P., et al. (2004). Discovery of *N*-(2-chloro-6-methyl-phenyl)-2-(6-(4-(2-hydroxyethyl)-piperazin-1-yl)-2-methylpyrimidin-4-ylamino) thiazole-5-carboxamide (BMS-354825), a dual Src/Abl kinase inhibitor with potent antitumor activity in preclinical assays. *J Med Chem.* 47(27), 6658–6661.

Lynch, T. J., Bell, D. W., Sordella, R., et al. (**2004**). Activating mutations in the epidermal growth factor receptor underlying responsiveness of non-small-cell lung cancer to gefitinib. *N Engl J Med.* 350(21), 2129–2139.

Mauro, M. J., Baccarani, M., Cervantes, F., et al. (**2008**). Dasatinib 2-year efficacy in patients with chronic-phase chronic myelogenous leukemia (CML-CP) with resistance or intolerance to imatinib (START-C). *J Clin Oncol.* 26(May 20 Suppl), Abst 7009.

Melnick, J. S., Janes, J., Kim, S., et al. (**2006**). An efficient rapid system for profiling the cellular activities of molecular libraries. *Proc Natl Acad Sci USA.* 103(9), 3153–3158.

Miyake, H., Hara, I., Yamanaka, K., et al. (**1999**). Elevation of urokinase-type plasminogen activator and its receptor densities as new predictors of disease progression and prognosis in men with prostate cancer. *Int J Oncol.* 14(3), 535–541.

Müller, M., Erben, P., Ernst, T., et al. (**2007**). Molecular response according to type of preexisting BCR-ABL mutations after second line dasatinib therapy in chronic phase CML patients. *Blood.* 110(11), 748, Abst 319.

Nagar, B., Bornmann, W. G., Pellicena, P., et al. (**2002**). Crystal structures of the kinase domain of c-Abl in complex with the small molecule inhibitors PD173955 and imatinib (STI-571). *Cancer Res.* 62(15), 4236–4243.

Nam, S., Kim, D., Cheng, J. Q., et al. (**2005**). Action of the Src family kinase inhibitor, dasatinib (BMS-354825), on human prostate cancer cells. *Cancer Res.* 65(20), 9185–9189.

Nam, S., Williams, A., Vultur, A., et al. (**2007**). Dasatinib (BMS-354825) inhibits Stat5 signaling associated with apoptosis in chronic myelogenous leukemia cells. *Mol Cancer Ther.* 6(4), 1400–1405.

Nowell, P., and Hungerford, D. (**1960**). A minute chromosome in human chronic granulocytic leukemia. *Science.* 132, 1497.

O'Brien, S. G., Guilhot, F., Larson, R. A., et al. (**2003**). Imatinib compared with interferon and low-dose cytarabine for newly diagnosed chronic-phase chronic myeloid leukemia. *N Engl J Med.* 348(11), 994–1004.

O'Hare, T., Walters, D. K., Stoffregen, E. P., et al. (**2005**). In vitro activity of Bcr-Abl inhibitors AMN107 and BMS-354825 against clinically relevant imatinib-resistant Abl kinase domain mutants. *Cancer Res.* 65(11), 4500–4505.

Olivieri, A., and Manzione, L. (**2007**). Dasatinib: a new step in molecular target therapy. *Ann Oncol.* 18(Suppl 6), vi42–46.

Ottmann, O., Dombret, H., Martinelli, G., et al. (**2007**). Dasatinib induces rapid hematologic and cytogenetic responses in adult patients with Philadelphia chromosome positive acute lymphoblastic leukemia with resistance or intolerance to imatinib: interim results of a Phase 2 study. *Blood.* 110(7), 2309–2315.

Pao, W., Miller, V., Zakowski, M., et al. (**2004**). EGF receptor gene mutations are common in lung cancers from "never smokers" and are associated with sensitivity of tumors to gefitinib and erlotinib. *Proc Natl Acad Sci USA.* 101(36), 13306–13311.

Perou, C. M., Sorlie, T., Eisen, M. B., et al. (**2000**). Molecular portraits of human breast tumours. *Nature.* 406(6797), 747–752.

Porkka, K., Martinelli, G., Ottman, O. G., et al. (**2008**). Dasatinib efficacy in patients with imatinib-resistant/-intolerant Philadelphia chromosome-positive acute lymphoblastic leukemia: 24-month data from START-L. *Haematologica*. 92(Suppl 1), 12, Abst 0001.

Potti, A., Dressman, H. K., Bild, A., et al. (**2006**). Genomic signatures to guide the use of chemotherapeutics. *Nat Med*. 12(11), 1294–1300.

Pulukuri, S. M., Gondi, C. S., Lakka, S. S., et al. (**2005**). RNA interference-directed knockdown of urokinase plasminogen activator and urokinase plasminogen activator receptor inhibits prostate cancer cell invasion, survival, and tumorigenicity in vivo. *J Biol Chem*. 280(43), 36529–36540.

Pusztai, L., Anderson, K., Kenneth, R., et al. (**2007**). Pharmacogenomic predictor discovery in Phase II clinical trials for breast cancer. *Clin Cancer Res*. 13(20), 6080–6086.

Rocchi, P., Muracciole, X., Fina, F., et al. (**2004**). Molecular analysis integrating different pathways associated with androgen-independent progression in LuCaP 23.1 xenograft. *Oncogene*. 23(56), 9111–9119.

Rousselot, P., Corm, S., Paquette, R., et al. (**2008a**). Dasatinib compared with high-dose imatinib in patients with chronic myelogenous leukemia in chronic phase (CML-CP) after failure of standard-dose imatinib—a two-year update of the START-R study. *Haematologica*. 92(Suppl 1), 48, Abst. 0122.

Rousselot, P., Facon, T., Paquette, R., et al. (**2008b**). Dasatinib or high-dose imatinib for patients with chronic myelogenous leukemia chronic-phase (CML-CP) resistant to standard-dose imatinib: 2-year follow-up data from START-R. *J Clin Oncol*. 26(May 20 Suppl), Abst 7012.

Rouzier, R., Perou, C. M., Symmans, W. F., et al. (**2005**). Breast cancer molecular subtypes respond differently to preoperative chemotherapy. *Clin Cancer Res*. 11(16), 5678–5685.

Saglio, G., Dombret, H., Rea, D., et al. (**2008a**). Dasatinib efficacy in patients with imatinib-resistant/-intolerant chronic myeloid leukemia (CML) in blast phase: 24-month data from the START program. *Haematologica*. 92(Suppl 1), 360, Abst 0880.

Saglio, G., Radich, J., Kim, D., et al. (**2008b**). Response to nilotinib in chronic myelogenous leukemia patients in chronic phase (CML-CP) according to BCR-ABL mutations at baseline. *J Clin Oncol*. 26(May 20 Suppl), Abst 7060.

Sawyers, C. L. (**1999**). Chronic myeloid leukemia. *N Engl J Med*. 340(17), 1330–1340.

Sawyers, C. L., Hochhaus, A., Feldman, E., et al. (**2002**). Imatinib induces hematologic and cytogenetic responses in patients with chronic myelogenous leukemia in myeloid blast crisis: results of a Phase II study. *Blood*. 99(10), 3530–3539.

Schittenhelm, M. M., Shiraga, S., Schroeder, A., et al. (**2006**). Dasatinib (BMS-354825), a dual SRC/ABL kinase inhibitor, inhibits the kinase activity of wild-type, juxtamembrane, and activation loop mutant KIT isoforms associated with human malignancies. *Cancer Res*. 66(1), 473–481.

Shah, N. P., and Sawyers, C. L. (**2003**). Mechanisms of resistance to STI571 in Philadelphia chromosome-associated leukemias. *Oncogene*. 22(47), 7389–7395.

Shah, N. P., Nicoll, J. M., Nagar, B., et al. (**2002**). Multiple BCR-ABL kinase domain mutations confer polyclonal resistance to the tyrosine kinase inhibitor imatinib (STI571) in chronic phase and blast crisis chronic myeloid leukemia. *Cancer Cell*. 2(2), 117–125.

Shah, N. P., Tran, C., Lee, F. Y., et al. (**2004**). Overriding imatinib resistance with a novel ABL kinase inhibitor. *Science*. 305(5682), 399–401.

Shah, N. P., Lee, F. Y., Luo, R., et al. (**2006**). Dasatinib (BMS-354825) inhibits KITD816V, an imatinib-resistant activating mutation that triggers neoplastic growth in most patients with systemic mastocytosis. *Blood*. 108(1), 286–291.

Shariat, S. F., Roehrborn, C. G., McConnell, J. D., et al. (**2007**). Association of the circulating levels of the urokinase system of plasminogen activation with the presence of prostate cancer and invasion, progression, and metastasis. *J Clin Oncol*. 25(4), 349–355.

Shor, A. C., Keschman, E. A., Lee, F. Y., et al. (**2007**). Dasatinib inhibits migration and invasion in diverse human sarcoma cell lines and induces apoptosis in bone sarcoma cells dependent on SRC kinase for survival. *Cancer Res*. 67(6), 2800–2808.

Singh, D., Febbo, P. G., Ross, K., et al. (**2002**). Gene expression correlates of clinical prostate cancer behavior. *Cancer Cell*. 1(2), 203–209.

Slamon, D. J., Leyland-Jones, B., Shak, S., et al. (**2001**). Use of chemotherapy plus a monoclonal antibody against HER2 for metastatic breast cancer that overexpresses HER2. *N Engl J Med*. 344(11), 783–792.

Song, L., Morris, M., Bagui, T., et al. (**2006**). Dasatinib (BMS-354825) selectively induces apoptosis in lung cancer cells dependent on epidermal growth factor receptor signaling for survival. *Cancer Res*. 66(11), 5542–5548.

Sorlie, T., Perou, C. M., Tibshirani, R., et al. (**2001**). Gene expression patterns of breast carcinomas distinguish tumor subclasses with clinical implications. *Proc Natl Acad Sci USA*. 98(19), 10869–10874.

Sotiriou, C., Neo, S. Y., McShane, L. M., et al. (**2003**). Breast cancer classification and prognosis based on gene expression profiles from a population-based study. *Proc Natl Acad Sci USA*. 100(18), 10393–10398.

Soverini, S., Martinelli, G., Colarossi, S., et al. (**2006**). Presence or the emergence of a F317L BCR-ABL mutation may be associated with resistance to dasatinib in Philadelphia chromosome-positive leukemia. *J Clin Oncol*. 24(33), e51–52.

Staunton, J. E., Slonim, D. K., Coller, H. A., et al. (**2001**). Chemosensitivity prediction by transcriptional profiling. *Proc Natl Acad Sci USA*. 98(19), 10787–10792.

Steinberg, M. (**2007**). Dasatinib: a tyrosine kinase inhibitor for the treatment of chronic myelogenous leukemia and Philadelphia chromosome-positive acute lymphoblastic leukemia. *Clin Ther*. 29(11), 2289–2308.

Summy, J. M., and Gallick, G. E. (**2003**). Src family kinases in tumor progression and metastasis. *Cancer Metastasis Rev*. 22(4), 337–358.

Susva, M., Missbach, M., and Green, J. (**2000**). Src inhibitors: drugs for the treatment of osteoporosis, cancer or both? *Trends Pharmacol Sci*. 21, 489–495.

Talpaz, M., Silver, R. T., Druker, B. J., et al. (**2002**). Imatinib induces durable hematologic and cytogenetic responses in patients with accelerated phase chronic myeloid leukemia: results of a Phase 2 study. *Blood*. 99(6), 1928–1937.

Talpaz, M., Shah, N. P., Kantarjian, H., et al. (**2006**). Dasatinib in imatinib-resistant Philadelphia chromosome-positive leukemias. *N Engl J Med*. 354(24), 2531–2541.

Thomas, S. M., and Brugge, J. S. (**1997**). Cellular functions regulated by Src family kinases. *Annu Rev Cell Dev Biol*. 13, 513–609.

Thomas, P. A., Kirschmann, D. A., Cerhan, J. R., et al. (**1999**). Association between keratin and vimentin expression, malignant phenotype, and survival in postmenopausal breast cancer patients. *Clin Cancer Res.* 5(10), 2698–2703.

Thomas, J., Wang, L., Clark, R. E., et al. (**2004**). Active transport of imatinib into and out of cells: implications for drug resistance. *Blood.* 104(12), 3739–3745.

Timeus, F., Crescenzio, N., Fandi, A., et al. (**2008**). In vitro antiproliferative and antimigratory activity of dasatinib in neuroblastoma and Ewing sarcoma cell lines. *Oncol Rep.* 19(2), 353–359.

Tipping, A. J., Baluch, S., Barnes, D. J., et al. (**2004**). Efficacy of dual-specific Bcr-Abl and Src-family kinase inhibitors in cells sensitive and resistant to imatinib mesylate. *Leukemia.* 18(8), 1352–1356.

Tokarski, J. S., Newitt, J. A., Chang, C. Y., et al. (**2006**). The structure of dasatinib (BMS-354825) bound to activated ABL kinase domain elucidates its inhibitory activity against imatinib-resistant ABL mutants. *Cancer Res.* 66(11), 5790–5797.

Trevino, J. G., Summy, J. M., Lesslie, D. P., et al. (**2006**). Inhibition of SRC expression and activity inhibits tumor progression and metastasis of human pancreatic adenocarcinoma cells in an orthotopic nude mouse model. *Am J Pathol.* 168(3), 962–972.

van de Rijn, M., Perou, C. M., Tibshirani, R., et al. (**2002**). Expression of cytokeratins 17 and 5 identifies a group of breast carcinomas with poor clinical outcome. *Am J Pathol.* 161(6), 1991–1996.

Vogel, C. L., Cobleigh, M. A., Tripathy, D., et al. (**2002**). Efficacy and safety of trastuzumab as a single agent in first-line treatment of HER2-overexpressing metastatic breast cancer. *J Clin Oncol.* 20(3), 719–726.

Wainberg, Z., Dering, J., Ginther, C., et al. (**2008**). Identification of predictive markers of response in colorectal cancer following treatment with dasatinib, an orally active tyrosine kinase inhibitor of ABL and SRC. *J Clin Oncol.* 26(May 20 Suppl), Abst 14688.

Walker-Daniels, J., Coffman, K., Azimi, M., et al. (**1999**). Overexpression of the EphA2 tyrosine kinase in prostate cancer. *Prostate.* 41(4), 275–280.

Wang, X. D., Reeves, K., Luo, F. R., et al. (**2007**). Identification of candidate predictive and surrogate molecular markers for dasatinib in prostate cancer: rationale for patient selection and efficacy monitoring. *Genome Biol.* 8(11), R255.

Warmuth, M., Damoiseaux, R., Liu, Y., et al. (**2003a**). SRC family kinases: potential targets for the treatment of human cancer and leukemia. *Curr Pharm Des.* 9(25), 2043–2059.

Warmuth, M., Simon, N., Mitina, O., et al. (**2003b**). Dual-specific Src and Abl kinase inhibitors, PP1 and CGP76030, inhibit growth and survival of cells expressing imatinib mesylate-resistant Bcr-Abl kinases. *Blood.* 101(2), 664–672.

Weisberg, E., Manley, P., Mestan, J., et al. (**2006**). AMN107 (nilotinib): a novel and selective inhibitor of BCR-ABL. *Br J Cancer.* 94(12), 1765–1769.

Weisberg, E., Manley, P. W., Cowan-Jacob, S. W., et al. (**2007**). Second generation inhibitors of BCR-ABL for the treatment of imatinib-resistant chronic myeloid leukaemia. *Nat Rev Cancer.* 7(5), 345–356.

Yeatman, T. J. (**2004**). A renaissance for SRC. *Nat Rev Cancer.* 4(6), 470–480.

16

PRACTICAL USE OF COMPUTATIONAL CHEMISTRY IN KINASE DRUG DISCOVERY

JAMES M. VEAL

16.1. INTRODUCTION

Intense investigation of protein kinases as therapeutic targets has occurred over the past decade. The approval of Gleevec in 2001 for the treatment of leukemia validated kinases, more specifically their ATP-binding sites, as legitimate drug discovery targets. They now comprise a substantial fraction of the pharmaceutical discovery portfolio, particularly in the areas of cancer and inflammation. In coordination with the general increase in kinase discovery research has been an expansion in the application of computational chemistry, cheminformatics, and bioinformatics techniques to kinase drug discovery. Kinases as a target class are arguably the most favorable set of proteins for use of computational techniques. Although each is distinct, they nonetheless share broad overlapping features that allow learnings from past target efforts to be applied prospectively. The determinants of ligand binding to the ATP site are spatially concentrated, allowing for effective use of docking techniques, and the availability of hydrophobic pockets to target improves the probabilities of effective inhibitor design and modification. Selectivity considerations and, more recently, resistance have always been important in kinase drug discovery and modeling techniques have utility in evaluating and understanding these issues. Perhaps most importantly, protein kinases have proved highly amenable to crystallography and the wealth of X-ray data available has allowed for legitimate structure-aided drug discovery techniques to be employed.

The goal of this chapter is to provide a survey of how computational techniques may be applied as part of a project team effort toward drug discovery. It incorporates specific examples from the literature as well as some personal experiences and viewpoints. It is beyond the scope of the chapter to be in any way comprehensive. In researching the chapter, PubMed searches were done for kinase inhibitors followed by secondary searches using keywords such as "modeling," "docking," "computational," "structure-based," and "structure–activity." For late 2003 to the present or roughly the past 5 years, the number of references was in excess of 400! Instead, the hope is that the examples will illustrate how computational techniques can be effectively incorporated into the drug discovery paradigm. Particular objectives are to focus on how techniques can be used in a pragmatic time-bound manner and can be effectively integrated with the skills of other team members such as medicinal chemists and screening biologists.

16.2. OVERVIEW OF THE PROTEIN KINASE BINDING SITE AND CONFORMATIONAL VARIABILITY

16.2.1. Binding Site

The characteristics of the protein kinase ATP-binding site and its vicinity have recently been described in detail elsewhere (Liao, 2007; Liao and Andrews, 2007). Nonetheless, for the sake of completeness, a concise summary incorporating personal observations is provided here as well. As indicated, X-ray crystallography has been essential in understanding the range of possible conformations available for inhibitors to target (Marsden and Knapp, 2008). The insulin receptor bound to a nonhydrolyzable ATP analog (Figures 16.1 and 16.2) provides a starting reference point from which to understand binding modes (Hubbard, 1997). The protein is observed to be in a catalytically active conformation capable of phosphorylating a target peptide. The adenine moiety forms two hydrogen bonds, via N1 and exocyclic amine N6, to backbone peptide atoms that compose the "hinge" region of the protein. Over time, a jargon has developed around protein kinase structures and the hinge naming derives from the fact that it is a flexible linker region connecting the primary N and C terminal domains of the kinase. ATP and analogs reside in a binding cleft formed by these two domains with the adenine also being sandwiched by a series of hydrophobic residues both above and below the aromatic plane. The tetrahydrofuran portion of the ribose sugar also makes additional hydrophobic interactions, more so with the N-terminal domain region, and may engage in hydrogen bonding as well with a series of more polar residues that sit at the front of the binding site at the solvent interface.

It is worthwhile to note that the residues that form the adenine and ribose portions of the ATP-binding site are not conserved in sequence although some do show high homology. Instead, conserved residues occur in the

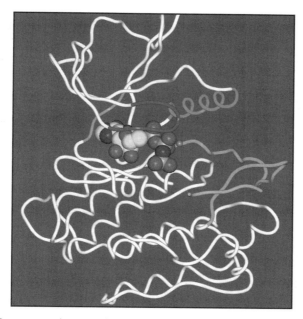

Figure 16.1. Representative protein kinase structure (Hubbard, 1997; pdb code 1IR3). ATP (nonhydrolyzable analog in this structure) binds into a cleft formed between the primary N (top) and C (bottom) terminal domains and engages in hydrogen bonding with the flexible hinge region (orange) that links the two domains. Key regulatory regions are the glycine-rich loop colored in magenta and draping over the phosphate-binding site; the activation loop colored in cyan; and the C-helix colored in green. A subset of kinase inhibitors target variations in conformation of these regulatory regions. Peptide inhibitor is shown is light green. (See color insert.)

phosphate-binding region (Figure 16.2), where they are responsible for both the correct phosphate group orientation and chemistry functions required for catalysis. A central question for protein kinases has always been the issue of attaining appropriate selectivity (Thaimattam et al., 2007), although increasingly what that means is less well defined. Regardless, strategies for modulating selectivity are apparent from analysis of ligand X-ray structures. A useful example to consider is that of the 4-anilinoquinazoline Tarceva bound to EGFR (Figure 16.2) (Stamos et al., 2002). Comparison to the insulin receptor structure shows that the ligand occupies substantial additional space relative to that occupied by ATP. In particular, the aniline moiety projects back into a hydrophobic region, past the so-called gatekeeper residue. This area is frequently targeted in kinase inhibitor design, shows sequence variability, and, although hydrophobic as indicated, also offers additional potential hydrogen-bonding opportunities. The gatekeeper residue derives its name because its steric size in part determines the availability of this back binding region. As can be seen, it is a methionine in IR versus a threonine in EGFR and the steric

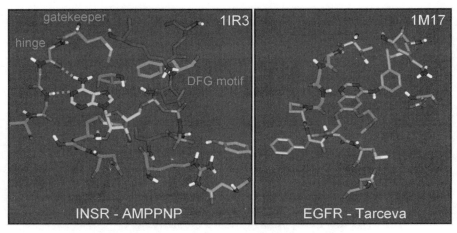

Figure 16.2. (*Left*) Close-up view of the insulin receptor ATP-binding site as determined by X-ray (Hubbard, 1997; pdb code 1IR3). Backbone atoms of the hinge region (orange) engage in hydrogen bonds with adenine N1 and exocylic amine N6 while the adenine ring system lies sandwiched between hydrophobic residues. Conserved catalytic residues are shown in magenta. The phenylalanine of the DFG motif is highlighted in cyan and the conformation is DFG in. On bottom left a portion of an inhibitor peptide (light green) is shown with tyrosine hydroxyl group proximal to gamma phosphate of AMPPNP analog. (*Right*) EGFR–Tarceva active sight as determined by X-ray (Stamos et al., 2002; pdb code 1M17). The anilino group projects into a back hydrophobic pocket made accessible by a small gatekeeper residue (Thr790). The catechol ether moiety of Tarceva also projects into a hydrophobic space, and then to solvent, at the front of the binding site. Both of these regions are unoccupied by ATP. (See color insert.)

bulk of the methionine side chain, if in an extended conformation, diminishes the ability to target this area. Even more pronounced examples are the CDKs and FLT3, which possess a phenylalanine at this position. The gatekeeper residue's importance to inhibitor binding is seen in the clinical manifestations of resistance to kinase inhibitors. T790M is a mutation (selected allele) that occurs in 50% of patients who initially respond to Tarceva and then relapse (Pao et al., 2005; Balak et al., 2006). Similarly, the T315I mutation in BCR-ABL confers resistance to Gleevec (Gorre et al., 2001).

In addition to the back hydrophobic pocket, there is also a second hydrophobic region that occurs in front of the binding site as shown in Figure 16.2, off the ATP C2 and N3 positions. Almost all kinases have a strongly hydrophobic residue (Ile, Val, Leu, Met, Phe, etc.) that forms the top of this site (the residue is not shown in the figure to keep from obscuring the ligand). The catechol ether moiety of Tarceva utilizes this binding area. This front region also shows a series of variable polar residues, proximal to the ribose hydroxyl's in ATP-bound structures, and additional affinity and selectivity may be gained by appropriate interactions. Another point is that the front of the site, where the ends of the ether linkages of Tarceva project, is solvent exposed. Structurally related quinazoline analogs (e.g., Iressa, Zactima, Tykerb) as well as a wide range of other ligand classes incorporate an amine basic functionality in this vicinity for solubility and modulation of physicochemical properties. An exception to the above statements is the AGC family kinase members (PKA, AKT, etc.), which largely close off the front hydrophobic region through insertion of a phenylalanine residue from the end of the protein C-terminal domain.

16.2.2. Conformational Variability

Because of their central role in cellular signaling pathways, it is not surprising that protein kinases are extensively regulated. From a structural viewpoint, at least three distinct mechanisms are available to provide appropriate regulatory control, and targeting the resulting conformational states has been a central strategy in the design and optimization of kinase inhibitors (Bogoyevitch and Fairlie, 2007). The first mechanism is modulation of the conformation of the glycine-rich loop region of the N-terminal domain (Figure 16.1). Phosphorylation (e.g., CDK2 by Wee1) and interactions of Hsp90 with cochaperone CDC37 are examples of endogenous regulation (Den Haese et al., 1995; Terasawa et al., 2006). Owing to its inherent conformation plasticity, the glycine-rich loop has been observed to mold to various ligand inhibitors with a recent example being a pyrazolopyridazine analog targeting ERK2 (Kinoshita et al., 2006).

Perhaps the most important mode of regulation is via the "activation loop" (T-loop) that spans from a consensus DFG motif at the back of the ATP-binding site to residues just upstream of a second, albeit lesser conserved, APE motif. This loop undergoes a wide range of conformational motions spanning from the "DFG-in" conformation seen for insulin receptor to a "DFG-out" orientation in which the phenylalanine may dock into the ATP-binding region and autoinhibit the kinase. The activation loop is a primary site of regulatory phosphorylation and is central to the trans-activating autophosphorylation mechanisms that occur when receptor tyrosine kinases bind their peptide ligands and homo- or heterodimerize. The DFG-out conformation is targeted by a range of inhibitors including Gleevec and BIRB 796 (Figure 16.3) (Schindler et al., 2000; Pargellis et al., 2002). A common feature for these inhibitors is a diaryl amide, urea, or related isostere; one aromatic group binds into the region vacated by the phenylalanine and the amide/urea functionalities form multiple hydrogen bonds involving the conserved glutamate from the kinase C-helix (Figure 16.1) and backbone NH of the aspartic acid of the DFG triad. Portions of the binding regions occupied by these ligands are now well removed spatially from the area occupied by ATP. Different kinases seem to exhibit a range of propensities for adopting the DFG-out conformation, and it is important to view the range of conformations available to the activation loop as an equilibrium-based phenomenon in which the conformational energy to adopt any one orientation will be an essential consideration as to its likelihood of occurring and being targeted by an inhibitor.

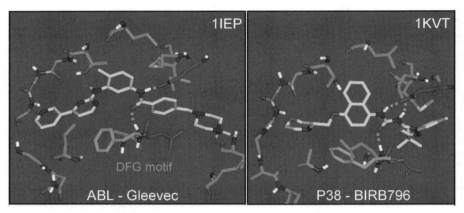

Figure 16.3. (*Left*) ABL–Gleevec structure as determined by X-ray crystallography (Schindler et al., 2000; pdb code 1IEP). The structure exemplifies the DFG-out kinase motif in which the phenylalanine is relocated from its position in a catalytically active kinase to, in this case, a position roughly adjacent to where the ATP ribose would be. The phenyl amide moiety occupies the region where the phenylalanine normally resides and makes hydrogen bonds to both the backbone NH of the DFG aspartate and carboxyl group of the catalytic glutamate from the C-helix. The piperazine group reaches solvent on the backside of the protein. (*Right*) P38–BIRB796 structure as a second example of the DFG-out binding motif (Pargellis et al., 2002; pdb code 1KVT). A *tert*-butyl-pyrazole-urea functionality provides pharmacophore elements analogous to the phenyl-amide group of Gleevec. Because of the strong interactions with the allosteric binding region, the ligand has a diminished need for strong interactions in the adenine-binding region, which is occupied by the morpholino group. (See color insert.)

A third mechanism of regulatory control involves modulation of the C-helix, which contains a conserved glutamic acid residue responsible in part for maintaining appropriate phosphate orientation prior to catalysis. Endogenous regulation (e.g., of Src kinase or CDK2) involves this helix being in an inactive form in the absence of appropriate factors such as cyclins. Recently, examples have emerged of inhibitors that likewise target an inactive C-helix formation. Notably, the dual EGFR/Her2 inhibitor Tykerb targets, at least for EGFR, a displaced C-helix conformation (Wood et al., 2004). Another class of allosteric ligands, which inhibit MEK kinase, exert this effect in part by again binding to a conformation in which the C-helix is inappropriately aligned for catalysis (Ohren et al., 2004). As with the activation loop, C-helix conformational changes represent an equilibrium process and as such they may or may not be readily targeted for a particular kinase.

16.2.3. Summary on Binding Site and Conformational Flexibility

Two general points emerge from the brief description just given. First, there are multiple regions of the protein kinase in the vicinity of the ATP-binding site that may be targeted for improved affinity once a core scaffold of interest is identified. Additionally, the conformational variability of certain regions of the kinase structure, owing largely to regulatory mechanisms, provides an additional strategy for gaining both potency and selectivity beyond just target-ing specific amino acids. A conceptual point is that there is sometimes a frus-tration among researchers that the high concentration of ATP in the cell (low millimolar, mM) makes the hurdles of achieving cellular activity and in vivo efficacy more difficult due to simple competitive effects. Binding affinities (K_d) of 100 nM or better are often required in order to begin to see low micromolar (μM) or better cellular activities. The nature of the enzymatic assay, for example, IC_{50} only determination (vs. a true K_d) at low ATP concentrations, may further confuse the situation. However, it is argued here that the presence of a high intracellular ATP concentration ultimately is really a boon for the kinase drug discovery effort. Concomitant with the high ATP concentration is that the K_m for ATP is low (typically 20–100 μM) for protein kinases, meaning that there is no strong natural pressure to have an optimized binding site for ATP for a given kinase. Thus there is high variability and "looseness" to the ATP-binding site in protein kinases and these properties can be properly exploited for the design of good inhibitors.

16.3. APPLICATION OF COMPUTATIONAL TECHNIQUES WITHIN THE DRUG DISCOVERY PROCESS

16.3.1. Overview

The goal of this main section is to provide recent examples of how different computational techniques have been utilized within the scope of the standard drug discovery process (Figure 16.4). For the discussion here, the process today

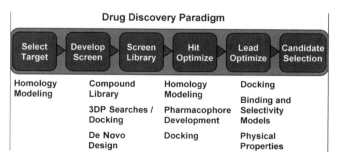

Figure 16.4. Overview of the typical process for a drug discovery program. The types of computational techniques that are most likely to be applied at different steps in the process are indicated. As described in the text, computational methods are particularly useful in developing libraries or novel templates for screening, and at the hit and lead optimization steps.

generally begins with identification of a target of interest via emerging literature or internal biological data. There are strong personal feelings as to whether
this is the best strategy (or should be the only strategy), and these are a subject
of a different discussion, but the "target-based approach" seems to have
become a widely engrained methodology in the era of the human genome
effort. In order to prosecute a target, a screen is then set up; the screen may
vary from an enzymatic assay designed to assess a limited or focused set of
compounds to a high-throughput screen (HTS) intended for an entire compound collection. Both types may actually be run with the focused screen
typically providing early data and the HTS, which generally takes longer to
set up, providing subsequent data. If successful, the screen will provide a series
of compounds of interest or hits that show affinity for the target of interest
and provide the initial input into medicinal chemistry efforts. Chemical analysis and exploration of these hits yields molecules that now possess more
impressive qualities and can be termed leads. The hit versus lead distinction
is arbitrary, and a lead definition can range from something having cellular
activity to in vivo activity (pharmacokinetic or efficacy). Practically, multiple
hits, each with limited medicinal chemistry evaluation, triage to one or two
leads that are subjected to extended medicinal chemistry exploration. If all
hurdles are met, one of the leads successfully advances to candidate status and
enters development. What follows is how computational techniques may be
applied within each of the above domains of the discovery process.

16.3.2. Target Selection

The view here is that, overall, computational techniques have relatively
limited impact at the target selection stage for protein kinases. The chief technique that may be employed is binding site evaluation via either analysis of
X-ray data or homology modeling, if such data are unavailable. As a general
note, homology modeling, as defined here, is a term meant to include the
underlying bioinformatics components of sequence alignment and so on in
addition to the computational chemistry component of protein model building. Homology modeling and binding site assessment generally can allow for
informed evaluation of the likely tractability of a target for small molecule
inhibitor design. Since the central ATP-binding site of protein kinases is well
established as a target for small molecules, this utility is not relevant. A possible use is to assess whether a kinase should be pursued as a target based on
its homology to related kinases that could clearly be viewed as off-targets.
Again, it is thought that this effort is generally not productive; a desirable
biological target will be pursued regardless of selectivity issues and usually
these issues can at least to some degree be overcome. A case in point is the
effort to discover selective small molecule kinase inhibitors for the cancer
target IGF-1R despite its high homology to insulin receptor; such efforts
appear to have succeeded to a reasonable degree (García-Echeverría et al.,
2004; Ji et al., 2007). Homology models and underlying sequence alignments
are useful at this stage of discovery in flagging up what likely may be

off-targets to be concerned about and this effort may in turn allow early development of relevant counterscreens.

16.3.3. Focused Compound Collections, Library Design, and Novel Scaffolds for Screening

The design and selection of compound sets for screening has proved to be an area of high value for the application of computational chemistry and cheminformatics techniques. There are multiple reasons for finding particular utility here. First, the adenine moiety of ATP provides a defined scaffold from which to derive a range of core templates, which can then be incorporated into two-dimensional (2D) descriptor-based searches. This comment can actually be a bit more formalized to state that the protein kinase ATP-binding pocket provides a well-defined pharmacophore target in terms of a hydrophobic cleft, designed for an aromatic ring system, and an adjacent acceptor–donor–acceptor hydrogen-bonding motif afforded by the hinge region. The majority of kinase inhibitors, including many that target the DFG-out motif, contain an aromatic adenine isostere and utilize some element of hydrogen bonding to the hinge region. This motif leads to a list of templates as exemplified in Figure 16.5 as being suitable substructures around which to base library design and acquisition efforts. Additionally, the kinase-binding site beyond the hinge

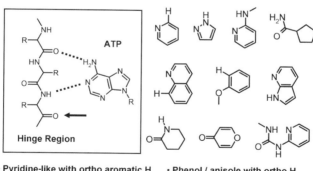

- Pyridine-like with ortho aromatic H
- Pyrazole-like with free NH
- 2-amino-pyridine-like
- Primary amide attached to ring
- Quinazoline-like (aromatic H at C8)

- Phenol / anisole with ortho H
- Azaindole
- Cyclic secondary amide
- Flavone-like
- Urea at 2-position of pyridine

Figure 16.5. Representative substructures that can be used in developing screening libraries. The structures all have precedent as adenine mimetics for protein kinases. They offer the potential to satisfactorily replace the two hydrogen bonds formed by ATP to the backbone groups of the kinase hinge region. Sufficiently polar aromatic hydrogens may act as isosteres for the exocyclic N6 amino group of ATP. Note also that combining or substituting the various mimetics allows for targeting an additional backbone carbonyl group in the hinge region that is well positioned for hydrogen bonding.

region, as indicated in the binding site overview, is relatively well defined owing to the extensive X-ray crystallography efforts directed at kinases. Given that, for screening, the goal is generally to identify hit templates in the 100 nM to 5 μM range, this information can be generalized and incorporated into docking or pharmacophore studies, including ones that are more three-dimensional (3D) in their nature. There is always a trade-off between the time, resources, and quality of results when comparing 2D descriptor searches versus 3D based full docking. Appropriate consideration of the goals and timelines is essential in evaluating which techniques are appropriate for the given situation.

Two side points are worth mentioning here as well. First, a somewhat unusual feature of the interactions between inhibitor and hinge region is that it frequently involves aromatic hydrogens from the ligand interacting at short distance (<2.5 Å) with a backbone carbonyl oxygen from the hinge region. The definition of this interaction is not formally a hydrogen bond, but the aromatic hydrogens are, nonetheless, also typically more "acidic" in nature as they are usually bonded to carbons that are in turn ortho, or otherwise polarized, by aromatic nitrogens. These interactions have recently been surveyed in some detail (Pierce et al., 2002; Tóth et al., 2007). A second note is that the emergence of DFG-out and inactive C-helix targeted ligands has diminished the absolute importance of having an adenine mimetic as part of the scaffold. Still, DFG-out ligands at least have their own defined pharmacophore as well, the aryl-amide and urea-type motifs, which may in turn be incorporated into design principles. Moreover, an attractive selectivity strategy (molecular weight considerations withstanding) is to attempt to span the full adenine and DFG-out binding regions with an inhibitor. If good hydrogen bonds that are remote in distance can be achieved, the prospects for selectivity are enhanced as even subtle conformational changes between two kinases will likely lead to a detuning and reduced value of such hydrogen bonds for the off-target.

16.3.3.1. *Focused Screening.*

Kinases are particularly good targets for focused screening for the reasons outline previously. Corporate and academic focused screening sets are now common and are designed, augmented, and/or maintained via computational methods (Prien, 2005; Brenk et al., 2008). These methods typically cull and cluster proven inhibitors as well as incorporate new templates from internal synthetic efforts and external compound acquisition. A well-designed compound set that is on the order of 10–50K compounds should produce hits and can usually be screened rapidly, much more so than an HTS, which involves significant setup efforts and longer times to screen, analyze, and follow-up. However, these arguments are in no way meant to disparage HTS as a valuable mechanism for kinase hit discovery. Hit rates should be substantially lower, but an HTS may produce more unusual or novel templates that perturb the kinase protein in unexpected ways and thus provide valuable new chemical matter. This matter can then be iteratively incorporated into new focused library designs. Thus focused screening and HTS are viewed as fully complementary and their combined and integrated use provides the highest probability for success. Virtual screening, in which a database is searched and evaluated, leading to a specific screening set for a specific target is now also routinely employed as a method to identify hits or starting compounds of interest for a given kinase. The methodology used may involve direct docking of compounds into a kinase X-ray or model structure or the development of a 3D pharmacophore model that is then used to search a database.

There are numerous representative examples from the literature since 2005 where computational methods have been used to provide a focused compound set for screening with subsequent identification of hits. Virtual screen docking was combined with a novel chromatography and mass spectrometry based screening technique to identify inhibitors of EphB2 (Toledo-Sherman et al., 2005). In silico docking using a receptor grid strategy produced a pyrazolo-pyrimidine as an EGFR inhibitor (Cavasotto et al., 2006). Chk1 inhibitors were identified by docking compounds to the ATP-binding site followed by selected screening of top scoring compounds (Foloppe et al., 2006). High-throughput docking led to CDK inhibitors, which were subsequently optimized into isoform selective binders (Thomas and McInnes, 2006) in one study and optimized for selectivity over GSK-3 in another effort (Richardson et al., 2007). High-throughput docking also was used to discover additional inhibitors for CDK2 as well as Plk1 and CK2 (Golub et al., 2008; Taylor et al., 2008). A 3D pharmacophore model was used to screen a corporate database and identified previously unreported scaffolds that targeted the DFG-out binding conformation of p38 (Angell et al., 2008b). Similarly, CDK2 and GSK-3 inhibitors were found via 3D pharmacophore models followed by virtual screening (Kim et al., 2007; Kim et al., 2008; Taha et al., 2008). Development of pharmacophore models for Src based on known inhibitors, followed by commercial database searches, yielded 1,3,4-thiadiazoles and pyrazolydine-3,5-diones as new inhibitors (Manetti et al., 2006). A detailed homology model for RSK1 was used to find inhibitors from the NCI repository (Nguyen et al., 2006). Receptor models were also utilized to identify compounds for synthesis that would bind to KGFR, yielding cell active analogs (Hackett et al., 2007). Aurora kinases have been cancer targets of much interest and fragment-based virtual screening followed by synthesis led to a pyrrolopyrimidine inhibitor (Warner et al., 2006), whereas a virtual screen of a 60K compound collection produced a 6,7-dihydro-4H-pyrazolo-[1,5-a] pyrrolo[3,4-d]pyrimidine-5,8-dione novel scaffold (Coumar et al., 2008). Pyrazolo[1,5-a][1,3,5]triazines were identified as a CK2 binding scaffold via computational screening methodologies and subsequently optimized to potent inhibitors (Nie et al., 2007). Recently, energy-based docking strategies yielded EphB4 inhibitors (Kolb et al., 2008a,b), and high-throughput docking to Pim-1 kinase successfully provided multiple hits on which to initiate optimization efforts (Pierce et al., 2008).

16.3.3.2. Novel Scaffold Identification. An increasing role for computational chemistry in the realm of kinase drug discovery is to assist in the design of novel scaffolds. The intellectual property environment for kinases is highly competitive, increasingly crowded, and now a central issue in discovery efforts. One method for addressing this challenge is to design and synthesize novel templates, including so-called scaffold morphing or hopping, and as such de novo design has arguably been used more in the kinase target space than in any other protein systems class. As with computational screening methods, there have been multiple publications in the last three years that demonstrate practical application. Scaffold morphing from a purine scaffold led to novel triazolo[1,5-*a*]pyrimidines targeting CDK2 (Richardson et al., 2006); similarly, migration of a thiazole core template to a pyrimidine based on matching electrostatic characteristics yielded new inhibitors, one of which ultimately progressed to clinical trials (Chu et al., 2006). New granulatimide analogs and macrocyclic pyridyl ureas, the latter using a *cis*-amide bond as an adenine isostere, have been designed as Chk1 inhibitors (Conchon et al., 2007; Tao et al., 2007). A macrocylic design strategy based on X-ray data was also used to identify a novel constrained pyrazolo[1,5-*a*] [1,3,5]triazine inhibitor of CK2. For GSK-3, modeled alterations to a VEGFR2 furo[2,3-*d*]pyrimidine scaffold converted it to a GSK-3 inhibitor (Miyazaki et al., 2008) and de novo design yielded a 7-hydroxy-benzimidazole scaffold (Shin et al., 2007). Multiple p38 targeted novel scaffolds have been derived from assessment of BIRB 796 binding followed by chemical modification (Goldberg et al., 2007; Cogan et al., 2008; Montalban et al., 2008).

New scaffold design has also recently been directed at receptor tyrosine kinases. For ALK, one strategy that was successfully employed to identify novel pyridone inhibitors was to develop models that could identify known inhibitors and then apply that model to virtual libraries to prioritize them for syntheses (Li et al., 2006). Overlapping of distinct compounds into an X-ray structure allowed combining them to yield a modified oxindole FGF1R inhibitor (Kammasud et al., 2007). VEGF receptors have been the focus of much investigation with a range of new scaffolds, derived using structure and modeling components, being reported (Tripathy et al., 2006; Uno et al., 2008; Abou El Ella et al., 2008; Peifer et al., 2008). Finally, structure-guided modeling aided in the elaboration of a novel pyrimido-diazepine core scaffold that produced potent inhibitors of VEGFR2, Flt3, and c-Kit (Gracias et al., 2008).

16.3.4. Hit Optimization

After the screening process is complete, there will typically be a range of hits, hopefully with some diversity in structure that will provide initial input into medicinal chemistry efforts. The goal of the computational chemist at this point is to develop plausible models that can provide insight into binding modes, offer strategies for optimization, and suggest routes to pursue to improve selectivity if that is an issue. The goal is not to provide the designed candidate molecule; actually that should never be the goal, rather it should be to facilitate the discovery process that leads a project team to a candidate molecule.

A central initial objective, if not done already as part of the screening process, is to develop reasonable protein models in which to dock ligands. The degree of effort needed is largely dependent on the X-ray data available. The possibilities range from the need to develop full homology models for the kinase of interest, to developing a DFG-out model when a DFG-in X-ray is available (or vice versa), to developing a series of models that take into account possible side chain rotamers of key residues (e.g., gatekeeper or catalytic lysine). There is a range of software available that offer the potential to build homology models in an automated fashion. That is fine and they may facilitate the process, but the homology model is a case where the computational chemist should put in detailed and often manual effort to develop as accurate as possible models. This effort requires thorough review of the available protein structures. Typically, the model will be based off one primary structure; however, significant components may best derive from alternative structures and evaluation of local homology is thus as important as global homology. The same rules apply to evaluation of side chain rotamer populations. The rationale for expending significant effort toward the development of models is that it is by and large a one-time effort for a given project; the week or two of effort to derive good models will be well served over the course of a two year medicinal chemistry discovery program.

Following development of the models as necessary, binding modes for compounds are then developed. The goal should be to establish all viable models and, if there are multiple plausible binding modes, strategies for distinguishing them. Because kinase pharmacophores are often rich in aromatic nitrogens and amine groups, there are often multiple legitimate binding models, and it is much preferred to present the variations until there is confidence about the correct model. An example of the potential pitfalls is a 3-amino-pyrazole series, which showed alternative binding modes to CDK2 depending on substituent patterns (Sato et al., 2006). Similarly, a pyrazolylpyrrole showed significantly different binding modes to ERK and JNK3 (Aronov et al., 2007), and the phenomenon of a kinase-dependent binding mode was also recently reported for the binding of an anilino-bipyridine to JNK1 and JNK3 (Swahn et al., 2006).

A particularly valuable objective, if it can be achieved, is to understand how different hit molecules overlap one another, as often that may provide rapid strategies for combining features into a single molecule with enhanced novelty and/or potency. The framework of a binding site is especially helpful as it is common to derive overlaps using protein structural information that would not necessarily be the most intuitive or computationally preferred in the absence of structural guidance. Table 16.1 provides a representative sampling of the recent use of hit optimization techniques to prospectively aid kinase programs. The designation of hit optimization versus lead optimization, as already noted, is somewhat arbitrary but the aim here was to identify efforts

**TABLE 16.1. Summary of Representative Recent Literature References Where
Computational Chemistry Techniques Were Applied to the Hit Optimization Process**

Kinase	Core Scaffold	Reference	Comment
Aurora-A	Indazole-benzimidazole	Poulsen et al. (2008)	Improved potency from substitutions
B-RAF	Diaryl-imidazole	Wolin et al. (2008)	Incorporation of urea to target both ATP and allosteric binding sites
EphB4	Dianilino-pyrimidine	Bardelle et al. (2008)	Optimization from merging based on overlap of pyrimidine and quinazoline hits
CaMKIId	Pyrimidine	Mavunkel et al. (2008)	Improved potency from substitutions
MK2	Indole	Xiong et al. (2008)	Improved potency from substitutions
Abl	Pyrazolo[3,4-d] pyrimidines	Manetti et al. (2008)	Improved potency from substitutions
CDK1/GSK3	9-Oxo-thiazolo[5,4-f] quinazoline	Loge et al. (2008)	Binding model to identify target positions for substitution
Chk1	Biphenyl pyrazole	Teng et al. (2007)	Modifications to maintain enzyme binding but improve cell activity
Abl	Benzotriazine	Cao et al. (2007)	Targeting C-helix glutamic acid
Chk1	Pyrazoloquinolinone	Brnardic et al. (2007)	Improved potency and solubility from substitutions
CDK5	Quinolin-2(1H)-one	Zhong et al. (2007)	Improved potency using active site homology model
VEGFR2/TIE2	Benzimidazole	Hasegawa et al. (2007)	Modeling to understand and guide SAR
Lck	Pyrimidine	Bamborough et al. (2007)	Binding models to guide indazole isostere design for improved PK
EGFR/Her2	Pyrrolotriazine	Mastalerz et al. (2007)	Modeling to understand and guide SAR

TABLE 16.1. *Continued*

Kinase	Core Scaffold	Reference	Comment
ROCK II	Indazole	Iwakubo et al. (2007)	Further optimization of designed scaffold
p38	Benzimidazolone	Hammach et al. (2006)	Energy calculation-based modifications to improve potency
CDKs	Quinoxalin-2-one macrocycle	Kawanishi et al. (2006)	Improved potency from substitutions
VEGFR2	1,4-Dihydroindeno[1, 2-*c*]pyrazole	Dinges et al. (2006)	Modeling to understand and guide SAR
IKKβ	Thienopyridine	Morwick et al. (2006)	Pharmacophore model to aid transition to more tractable scaffold
TrkA	Isothiazole	Lippa et al. (2006)	Improved potency from substitutions
FAK	7*H*-Pyrrolo[2,3-*d*] pyrimidine	Choi et al. (2006)	Improved potency from substitutions
EGFR	Anilino-quinazoline	Ballard et al. (2006)	Guided design of compounds targeting ribose pocket
PKB	Iosoquinoline-5-sulfonamide	Collins et al. (2006)	Identification of potent substituents via screening virtual libraries
CDK2/CDK4	Pyrazolopyrimidinone	Rossi et al. (2005)	Improved potency from substitutions; selectivity SAR
CDKs	Imidazo[1,2-*a*]pyridine	Hamdouchi et al. (2005)	Improved selectivity from substitutions
VEGFR2	Aryl-oxazole	Harris et al. (2005)	Improved selectivity from substitutions
CDK1	Alsterpaullone	Kunick et al. (2005)	Improved potency from substitutions
PKB	Azepines	Breitenlechner et al. (2005)	Improved selectivity from substitutions, relative to PKA

that involved more hit series overlap and early optimization prior to the point of in vivo efficacy and other later stage type studies.

16.3.5. Lead Optimization

At the point lead optimization is initiated, there are typically one to two front running series that demonstrate structure–activity relationships that are presumably positive and tractable. From the computational chemistry perspective, there are hopefully well-defined binding models or sets of models that can be used to assist in optimization. Optimization should not be assumed to be synonymous with increased potency but may also reflect improving physicochemical properties (e.g., solubility or lowered molecular weight) while maintaining potency. Selectivity issues may also be an ongoing consideration that can be improved through an understanding of binding modes. Identifying strategies for introducing conformational restraint, to improve potency or other properties, is also an area where models are valuable.

High-throughput docking, or more specifically restrained docking, is a particularly useful computational technique to apply to the process of lead optimization. The scenario that occurs frequently in the lead optimization process is as follows. There is a lead molecule whose binding mode is reasonably well established. Medicinal chemists have identified a series of synthetic schemes that allow optimization at distinct positions on the molecule. The chemistries involved are sufficiently robust and involve starting materials that are widely available, say, amines or carboxylic acids or aromatic bromides. The objective for the computational chemist should be to first help in prioritizing which substitution positions are likely to be most beneficial and then, in cases where reagents are widely available, to prioritize a set of analogs for synthesis. Reagents such as carboxylic acids and amines number in the thousands of commercially available analogs, and even robust parallel syntheses procedures require reduced numbers of such analogs. Docking procedures thus require several steps. First, in silico synthesis of analogs of interest from the lead template and reagent class is carried out. Second, the product molecules are docked in a flexible but restrained mode, for example, based on established hydrogen bonds to the hinge region of the core scaffold. Conformational searching of the substituent region and possibly the entire molecule should then be pursued followed by minimization of preferred conformers. Scoring of different possible analogs is a subject of much literature incorporated in the referenced examples below. However, the personal view is that docking or scoring energies should be used as a filter to winnow down possible analogs of interest to a number on the order of 20% of the original possibilities and from that point both binding energies and visual inspection, often in conjunction with medicinal chemists, should be used to guide selection of the final set of analogs to pursue synthetically.

Recent examples of the use of computational techniques in lead optimization span a range of kinase targets and include reports on molecules now undergoing clinical development. Pan receptor tyrosine kinase profile inhibitors are an area of active investigation; docking of thienopyrimidine and indazole core scaffolds helped guide optimization of urea moieties targeting the adjacent allosteric pocket of RTKs, leading to a clinical candidate (Dai et al., 2005, 2007). Discovery of a Src and VEGFR2 dual inhibitor clinical candidate incorporated design strategies for making interactions with the conserved C-helix glutamate (Palanki et al., 2008). For VEGFR2 specifically, modeling aided successful transition from a benzimidazole template to an optimized benzoxazole that showed in vivo activity (Potashman et al., 2007). Computational overlaps of quinazoline and pyrimidine scaffolds and subsequent docking studies also facilitated discovery of a VEGFR2 clinical candidate (Harris et al., 2008) as did modeling efforts to identify optimal locations for modifications to improve solubility and PK aspects of a pyrrolo[2,1-*f*][1,2,4]triazine (Bhide et al., 2006). Achieving selectivity for LCK tyrosine kinase over VEGFR2 for a pyrimido[1,2-*a*]benzimidazol-5(6*H*)-one template was accomplished through structural analysis of binding modes followed by targeting the gatekeeper threonine of LCK (Martin et al., 2008). IGF-1R computational models were used in discovery and optimization of orally active imidazo[1,5-*a*]pyrazines that utilize a quinoline to target the back binding region (Mulvihill et al., 2008). For serine–threonine kinases, computational techniques have also been recently applied in lead optimization. For example, docking studies identified substitution at the 8-position of a cyano quinoline template as a way to successfully establish selectivity for Tpl2 kinase versus EGFR (Green et al., 2007). Use of polar surface area calculations led to improvement in cellular potency of an indolylquinolinone scaffold targeting Chk1 (Huang et al., 2006). CoMFA models were used to help prioritize synthesis efforts targeting the MEK allosteric inhibitor site (Spicer et al., 2007), and binding models aided in optimization of biphenyl amides as allosteric inhibitors of p38 (Angell et al., 2008a).

16.4. TWO APPLICATION EXAMPLES

Two brief examples are provided from personal experience. One involves general design of a small focused screening library from commercial vendors. The library was intended for purine-binding proteins of which protein kinases are a major subset. The second effort involves lead optimization efforts toward CDK2 involving an oxindole scaffold.

16.4.1. Focused Library Development

The objective was to select and acquire from commercial vendors a quality set of 5–10K compounds with a biased likelihood for targeting the purine-binding proteome. The core methodology was to first select a comprehensive set of compounds that were sufficiently like a "modified" adenosine (adenosine plus a phenyl group to provide additional hydrophobicity). From that set, a maximally diverse and representative subset was then chosen. The methodology is outlined in Figure 16.6.

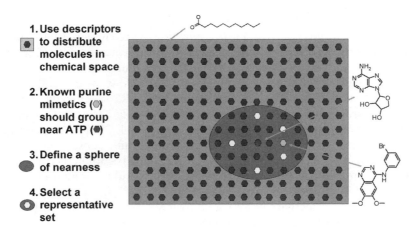

1. Use descriptors to distribute molecules in chemical space

2. Known purine mimetics (○) should group near ATP (●)

3. Define a sphere of nearness

4. Select a representative set

Figure 16.6. General schematic outlining strategy for development of a focused screening library. Descriptors are developed to allow distribution of compounds (blue hexagons) into a dimensional chemical space. If descriptor design is done successfully, known adenosine mimetics such as quinazolines will map close in space to adenosine, whereas non-mimics, for example, a fatty acid, will map far away. A cutoff defines a selection region which is then sampled representatively to provide a compound set for screening.

The first step was to obtain, in SDF format, vendor lists of compounds for purchase. A set of vendors can be obtained through the ACD directory lists, and SDF files for ~2.4 million compounds were compiled from 19 vendors. A central component of the entire compound selection process is the idea that two molecules can be related in terms of "similarity" or "diversity." It is important to realize that these types of classifications are totally relative to the comparisons used. Typically, these descriptor measurements are derived from a dissection of molecular topology (bonds, connectivities, rings, etc.) and features such as hydrogen-bonding groups, hydrophobic moieties, or other functional groups. In-house algorithms were developed to analyze each molecule and determine these characteristics from the provided atom and bond information such that at the end of the process, a detailed characterization was available for each molecule. Included in the characterization was an analysis for adenine mimetics (Figure 16.5).

Molecular profile information was initially utilized as a way to filter molecules that had chemically reactive groups or other undesirable features related to general properties (e.g., molecular weight and rotatable bonds) and functional group counts. A set of 85 filters were used, leading to elimination of more than 50% of some vendor collections from the selection process. The calculated topologies and descriptors were then used to identify compounds that had sufficient similarity to the modified adenosine template. Fingerprints (arrays containing counts of each property) were weighted such that a group of ~30 known kinase inhibitors, inserted into the compound set as controls,

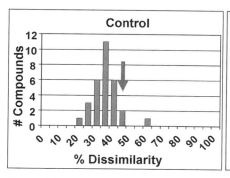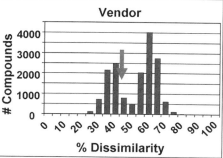

Figure 16.7. Profiling of compounds using descriptors. Optimized weighted descriptors are used to calculate a Sorensen coefficient measuring the likeness of a compound to an adenosine analog (0% dissimilariy would be an identical match). A cutoff value of ~45% captures >90% of a control group of known kinase inhibitors. Using this cutoff then allows selection of a set of compounds for purchase from a vendor (following clustering, representative selection, and visual inspection). The biphasic nature of the profiles derives from the inclusion of adenine isosteres as part of the compound profiling.

were preferentially selected from the set when Sorensen or Tanimoto coefficient calculations were performed. A cutoff criteria (Figure 16.7) that identified >90% of the kinase inhibitors returned a subset of approximately 150K molecules of interest.

Fingerprints were then used to pick as representative (i.e., dissimilar) a set of molecules as possible from this subset of molecules that had survived the selection process so far. A first molecule was arbitrarily picked and then the process was to proceed iteratively through the collection, evaluating at each step, all unselected molecules against all those already selected. A penultimate target set of 15K molecules was identified. The final, and perhaps most important, step was to use visual inspection to reduce the compound set down to approximately 8000 molecules. This step concluded the selection process and compounds were then purchased. The library was actually developed as a 5000 member initial screening set followed by a second round of 3000 compounds. Screening results versus 10 kinases are summarized in Figure 16.8; the screen yielded multiple hits of less than 5 μM and less than 1 μM versus all kinases tested. Also shown as part of Figure 16.8 are two examples of a novel 2,8-disubstituted naphthyridine scaffold identified as part of the screen. The scaffold was subsequently successfully expanded via medicinal chemistry efforts (Hanson et al., 2006).

16.4.2. Lead Optimization of a CDK2 Inhibitor

As part of a CDK2 inhibitor discovery program a 1*H*-indole-2,3-dione-3-phenylhydrazone scaffold was identified as an attractive lead series to pursue

Kinase	IC$_{50}$ <5µM	IC$_{50}$ <1µM	Kinase	IC$_{50}$ <5µM	IC$_{50}$ <1µM
ALK	37	6	EphB1	37	9
AXL	37	3	Her2	55	13
EGFR	46	8	PDK1	62	15
EphA2	64	15	SKY	24	4
EphA4	45	10	Tie2	50	14

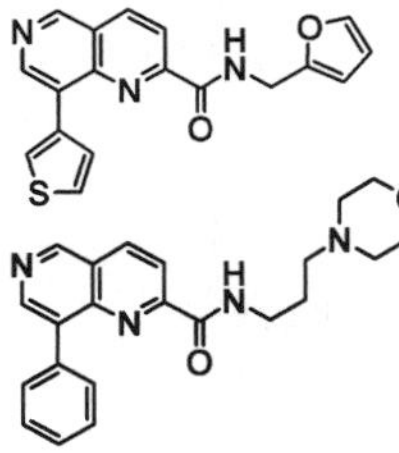

Figure 16.8. Summary screening results of 8000 member acquired library. Library was designed for purine-binding proteins generally but was profiled against 10 protein kinases and hits identified as summarized. Compounds at right are an example of a novel template identified from the screening process (2,8-disubstituted naphthyridines).

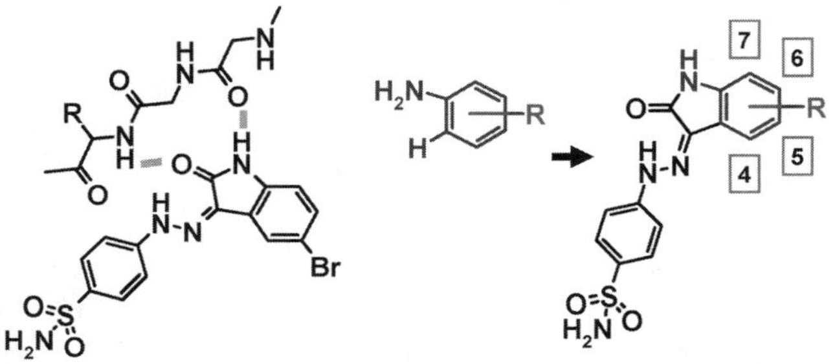

Figure 16.9. Oxindole CDK2 inhibitor. (*Left*) Schematic of initial lead oxindole structure showing hydrogen-bonding interactions with hinge region. (*Right*) Schematic showing incorporation of substituted aniline starting reagent into oxindole final product. Oxindole numbering is shown.

for further optimization (Bramson et al., 2001). In particular, a *para*-sulfonamide on the pendant phenyl ring, coupled with a 5-position bromo substitution on the oxindole moiety, was a 60 nM starting point (Figure 16.9). X-ray data were also available for this compound bound to CDK2 (but in absence of cyclin A). The objective was to replace the bromo group, while retaining its increase in potency relative to the unsubstituted oxindole, by exploring positions 4–7 of the oxindole. These substitutions derived from aniline precursors containing a free 2-H (Figure 16.9). The objective of the computational chemistry effort was to identify a subset of anilines for synthesis to facilitate rapid optimization of the template.

Anilines from commercial sources were compiled and filtered based on molecular weight and chemical reactivity criteria leading to a set of 410 anilines for evaluation in docking studies. SMILES string based virtual chemistry, using in-house developed algorithms, was employed to transform the anilines to corresponding benzene-sulfonamide derivatives. Note that for meta-substituted anilines, both 4- and 6-substituted oxindoles were possible synthetic products, and both were evaluated. Conformational searching (without protein) was

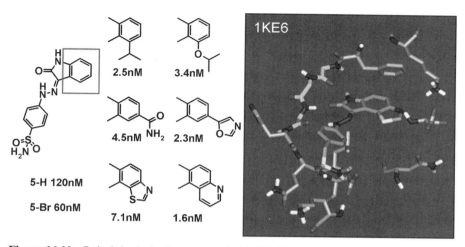

Figure 16.10. Oxindole derivatives potently inhibit CDK2. (*Left*) Hydrophobic substitutions at 4-position or hydrogen bond acceptors at 5-position substantially improved potency, relative to unsubstituted oxindole and 5-Br lead. Fused analogs also showed high potency. (*Right*) X-ray of a fused thiazole derivatve bound to CDK2 (Bramson et al., 2001; pdb code 1KE6).

done via a high-temperature molecular dynamics (MD) based script. One hundred conformations were generated by a repeated cycle consisting of: MD 2000 °C/0.5 ps; MD 100 °C/0.2 ps; minimization 200 steps. Additional rejection criteria were to discard conformations with energy of 7.5 kcal/mol above the lowest energy structure and identical conformations as defined by a sum root mean square (rms) deviation of less that 0.25 Å for heavy atoms. Partial atomic charges were established for each molecule via semiempirical PM3 minimization of low-energy conformer followed by a Hartree–Fock 3-21G* single-point calculation to set up for CHELPG charge determination.

Ligand docking was done to a protein conformation derived from an in-house X-ray complex of CDK2, cyclin A, and flavopiridol using the X-ray data from the 5-Br analog to position the oxindole scaffold initially. Energy minimization was performed with GB/SA solvation; proximal protein atoms were allowed free minimization but those beyond 8 Å from the ligand starting atomic coordinates were subjected to positional restraints. Solvation energy differences, ligand–protein interaction energies, and ligand only conformation energy differences were used to compute a binding energy score, which in turn was used to rank order possible substitutions. This ranking, coupled with visual inspection of the compounds docked into the CDK2 binding site, led to selection of a set of 40 anilines of which ~25 were ultimately incorporated into syntheses. Multiple analogs were identified with single-digit nanomolar potency and were primarily modeled to provide either additional favorable hydrophobic interactions with Val18 or hydrogen bonding to Lys33 via 4- and 5-position substitutions, respectively (Figure 16.10). 4,5-Fused thiazole and quinoline analogs were particularly promising, providing the potential for both types of interactions. 6-Position analogs and especially 7-position analogs showed steric crowding due to the Phe80 gatekeeper residue. Ultimately, a clinical candidate was identified from this series.

16.5. SUMMARY

The purpose of this chapter has been to demonstrate how computational chemistry and cheminformatics techniques may be incorporated into the kinase drug discovery process to aid in the discovery of inhibitors and ultimately new medicines. Strategies and examples have been provided that span from new template generation to lead optimization. A central underlying theme has been how to use computational methodologies in a practical and *prospective* manner. To be clear, there is certainly value in post-rationalizations of binding modes and retrospective analyses of which scoring function best reproduced the data that were generated, but these efforts are, nonetheless, outside the direct process of drug discovery. There is now a substantial body of examples where computational techniques have provided significant contributions toward the development of screening libraries and discovery of new scaffolds, promising hits, and optimized leads that have ultimately become drug candidates. The wealth of protein structural data, coupled with ever-improving computational power, has made the past decade a particularly exciting one for computational chemistry-based research applied to kinases. Hopefully, kinase inhibitors will continue to progress through the clinic to become new medicines, and in doing so will promote continuing discovery efforts directed at kinases. Computational methodologies are well suited to play an integral role in those efforts.

REFERENCES

Abou El Ella, D. A., Ghorab, M. M., Noaman, E., et al. (**2008**). Molecular modeling study and synthesis of novel pyrrolo[2,3-*d*]pyrimidines and pyrrolotriazolopyrimidines of expected antitumor and radioprotective activities. *Bioorg Med Chem.* 16(5), 2391–2402.

Angell, R. M., Angell, T. D., Bamborough, P., et al. (**2008a**). Biphenyl amide p38 kinase inhibitors 2: optimisation and SAR. *Bioorg Med Chem Lett.* 18(1), 324–328.

Angell, R. M., Bamborough, P., Cleasby, A., et al. (**2008b**). Biphenyl amide p38 kinase inhibitors 1: Discovery and binding mode. *Bioorg Med Chem Lett.* 18(1), 318–323.

Aronov, A. M., Baker, C., Bemis, G. W., et al. (**2007**). Flipped out: structure-guided design of selective pyrazolylpyrrole ERK inhibitors. *J Med Chem.* 50(6), 1280–1287.

Balak, M. N., Gong, Y., Riely, G. J., et al. (**2006**). Novel D761Y and common secondary T790M mutations in epidermal growth factor receptor-mutant lung adenocarcinomas with acquired resistance to kinase inhibitors. *Clin Cancer Res.* 12(21), 6494–6501.

Ballard, P., Bradbury, R. H., Harris, C. S., et al. (**2006**). Inhibitors of epidermal growth factor receptor tyrosine kinase: novel C-5 substituted anilinoquinazolines designed to target the ribose pocket. *Bioorg Med Chem Lett.* 16(6), 1633–1637.

Bamborough, P., Angell, R. M., Bhamra, I., et al. (**2007**). N-4-Pyrimidinyl-1H-indazol-4-amine inhibitors of Lck: indazoles as phenol isosteres with improved pharmacokinetics. *Bioorg Med Chem Lett.* 17(15), 4363–4368.

Bardelle, C., Cross, D., Davenport, S., et al. (**2008**). Inhibitors of the tyrosine kinase EphB4. Part 1: Structure-based design and optimization of a series of 2,4-bis-anilinopyrimidines. *Bioorg Med Chem Lett.* 18(9), 2776–2780.

Bhide, R. S., Cai, Z. W., Zhang, Y. Z., et al. (**2006**). Discovery and preclinical studies of (R)-1-(4-(4-fluoro-2-methyl-1H-indol-5-yloxy)-5-methylpyrrolo[2,1-f][1,2,4]triazin-6-yloxy)propan-2-ol (BMS-540215), an in vivo active potent VEGFR-2 inhibitor. *J Med Chem.* 49(7), 2143–2146.

Bogoyevitch, M. A., and Fairlie, D. P. (**2007**). A new paradigm for protein kinase inhibition: blocking phosphorylation without directly targeting ATP binding. *Drug Discov Today.* 12(15–16), 622–633.

Bramson, H. N., Corona, S., Davis, S. T., et al. (**2001**). Oxindole-based inhibitors of cyclin-dependent kinase 2 (CDK2): design, synthesis, enzymatic activities, and X-ray crystallographic analysis. *J Med Chem.* 44(25), 4339–4358.

Breitenlechner, C. B., Friebe, W. G., Brunet, E., et al. (**2005**). Design and crystal structures of protein kinase B-selective inhibitors in complex with protein kinase A and mutants. *J Med Chem.* 48(1), 163–170.

Brenk, R., Schipani, A., James, D., et al. (**2008**). Lessons learnt from assembling screening libraries for drug discovery for neglected diseases. *ChemMedChem.* 3(3), 435–444.

Brnardic, E. J., Garbaccio, R. M., Fraley, M. E., et al. (**2007**). Optimization of a pyrazoloquinolinone class of Chk1 kinase inhibitors. *Bioorg Med Chem Lett.* 17(21), 5989–5994.

Cao, J., Fine, R., Gritzen, C., et al. (**2007**). The design and preliminary structure–activity relationship studies of benzotriazines as potent inhibitors of Abl and Abl-T315I enzymes. *Bioorg Med Chem Lett.* 17(21), 5812–5818.

Cavasotto, C. N., Ortiz, M. A., Abagyan, R. A., et al. (**2006**). In silico identification of novel EGFR inhibitors with antiproliferative activity against cancer cells. *Bioorg Med Chem Lett.* 16(7), 1969–1974.

Choi, H. S., Wang, Z., Richmond, W., et al. (**2006**). Design and synthesis of 7H-pyrrolo[2,3-d]pyrimidines as focal adhesion kinase inhibitors. Part 2. *Bioorg Med Chem Lett.* 16(10), 2689–2692.

Chu, X. J., DePinto, W., Bartkovitz, D., et al. (**2006**). Discovery of [4-amino-2-(1-methanesulfonylpiperidin-4-ylamino)pyrimidin-5-yl](2,3-difluoro-6-methoxyphenyl)methanone (R547), a potent and selective cyclin-dependent kinase inhibitor with significant in vivo antitumor activity. *J Med Chem.* 49(22), 6549–6560.

Cogan, D. A., Aungst, R., Breinlinger, E. C., et al. (**2008**). Structure-based design and subsequent optimization of 2-tolyl-(1,2,3-triazol-1-yl-4-carboxamide) inhibitors of p38 MAP kinase. *Bioorg Med Chem Lett.* 18(11), 3251–3255.

Collins, I., Caldwell, J., Fonseca, T., et al. (**2006**). Structure-based design of isoquinoline-5-sulfonamide inhibitors of protein kinase B. *Bioorg Med Chem.* 14(4), 1255–1273.

Conchon, E., Anizon, F., Aboab, B., et al. (**2007**). Synthesis and biological activities of new checkpoint kinase 1 inhibitors structurally related to granulatimide. *J Med Chem.* 50(19), 4669–4680.

Coumar, M. S., Wu, J. S., Leou, J. S., et al. (**2008**). Aurora kinase A inhibitors: identification, SAR exploration and molecular modeling of 6,7-dihydro-4*H*-pyrazolo-[1,5-*a*]pyrrolo[3,4-*d*]pyrimidine-5,8-dione scaffold. *Bioorg Med Chem Lett.* 18(5), 1623–1627.

Dai, Y., Guo, Y., Frey, R. R., et al. (**2005**). Thienopyrimidine ureas as novel and potent multitargeted receptor tyrosine kinase inhibitors. *J Med Chem.* 48(19), 6066–6083.

Dai, Y., Hartandi, K., Ji, Z., et al. (**2007**). Discovery of *N*-(4-(3-amino-1*H*-indazol-4-yl) phenyl)-*N'*-(2-fluoro-5-methylphenyl)urea (ABT-869), a 3-aminoindazole-based orally active multitargeted receptor tyrosine kinase inhibitor. *J Med Chem.* 50(7), 1584–1597.

Den Haese, G. J., Walworth, N., Carr, A. M., et al. (**1995**). The Wee1 protein kinase regulates T14 phosphorylation of fission yeast Cdc2. *Mol Biol Cell.* 6(4), 371–385.

Dinges, J., Ashworth, K. L., Akritopoulou-Zanze, I., et al. (**2006**). 1,4-Dihydroindeno[1,2-*c*]pyrazoles as novel multitargeted receptor tyrosine kinase inhibitors. *Bioorg Med Chem Lett.* 16(16), 4266–4271.

Foloppe, N., Fisher, L. M., Howes, R., et al. (**2006**). Identification of chemically diverse Chk1 inhibitors by receptor-based virtual screening. *Bioorg Med Chem.* 14(14), 4792–4802.

García-Echeverría, C., Pearson, M. A., Marti, A., et al. (**2004**). In vivo antitumor activity of NVP-AEW541—a novel, potent, and selective inhibitor of the IGF-IR kinase. *Cancer Cell.* 5(3), 231–239.

Goldberg, D. R., Hao, M. H., Qian, K. C., et al. (**2007**). Discovery and optimization of p38 inhibitors via computer-assisted drug design. *J Med Chem.* 50(17), 4016–4026.

Golub, A. G., Yakovenko, O. Y., Prykhod'ko, A. O., et al. (**2008**). Evaluation of 4,5,6,7-tetrahalogeno-1*H*-isoindole-1,3(2*H*)-diones as inhibitors of human protein kinase CK2. *Biochim Biophys Acta.* 1784(1), 143–149.

Gorre, M. E., Mohammed, M., Ellwood, K., et al. (**2001**). Clinical resistance to STI-571 cancer therapy caused by BCR-ABL gene mutation or amplification. *Science.* 293(5531), 876–880.

Gracias, V., Ji, Z., Akritopoulou-Zanze, I., et al. (**2008**). Scaffold oriented synthesis. Part 2: Design, synthesis and biological evaluation of pyrimido-diazepines as receptor tyrosine kinase inhibitors. *Bioorg Med Chem Lett.* 18(8), 2691–2695.

Green, N., Hu, Y., Janz, K., et al. (**2007**). Inhibitors of tumor progression loci-2 (Tpl2) kinase and tumor necrosis factor alpha (TNF-alpha) production: selectivity and in vivo antiinflammatory activity of novel 8-substituted-4-anilino-6-aminoquinoline-3-carbonitriles. *J Med Chem.* 50(19), 4728–4745.

Hackett, J., Xiao, Z., Zang, X. P., et al. (**2007**). Development of keratinocyte growth factor receptor tyrosine kinase inhibitors for the treatment of cancer. *Anticancer Res.* 27(6B), 3801–3806.

Hamdouchi, C., Zhong, B., Mendoza, J., et al. (**2005**). Structure-based design of a new class of highly selective aminoimidazo[1,2-*a*]pyridine-based inhibitors of cyclin dependent kinases. *Bioorg Med Chem Lett.* 15(7), 1943–1947.

Hammach, A., Barbosa, A., Gaenzler, F. C., et al. (**2006**). Discovery and design of benzimidazolone based inhibitors of p38 MAP kinase. *Bioorg Med Chem Lett.* 16(24), 6316–6320.

Hanson, G. J., Ware, R. W., Barta, T. E., et al. (**2006**). 2,8-Disubstituted naphthyridine derivatives. PCT International Application WO2006/017672.

Harris, P. A., Cheung, M., Hunter, R. N., et al. (**2005**). Discovery and evaluation of 2-anilino-5-aryloxazoles as a novel class of VEGFR2 kinase inhibitors. *J Med Chem.* 48(5), 1610–1619.

Harris, P. A., Boloor, A., Cheung, M., et al. (**2008**). Discovery of 5-[[4-[(2,3-dimethyl-2H-indazol-6-yl)methylamino]-2-pyrimidinyl]amino]-2-methyl-benzenesulfonamide (Pazopanib), a novel and potent vascular endothelial growth factor receptor inhibitor. *J Med Chem.* 51(15), 4632–4640.

Hasegawa, M., Nishigaki, N., Washio, Y., et al. (**2007**). Discovery of novel benzimidazoles as potent inhibitors of TIE-2 and VEGFR-2 tyrosine kinase receptors. *J Med Chem.* 50(18), 4453–4470.

Huang, S., Garbaccio, R. M., Fraley, M. E., et al. (**2006**). Development of 6-substituted indolylquinolinones as potent Chek1 kinase inhibitors. *Bioorg Med Chem Lett.* 16(22), 5907–5912.

Hubbard, S. R. (**1997**). Crystal structure of the activated insulin receptor tyrosine kinase in complex with peptide substrate and ATP analog. *EMBO J.* 16(18), 5572–5581.

Iwakubo, M., Takami, A., Okada, Y., et al. (**2007**). Design and synthesis of Rho kinase inhibitors (II). *Bioorg Med Chem.* 15(1), 350–364.

Ji, Q. S., Mulvihill, M. J., Rosenfeld-Franklin, M., et al. (**2007**). A novel, potent, and selective insulin-like growth factor-I receptor kinase inhibitor blocks insulin-like growth factor-I receptor signaling in vitro and inhibits insulin-like growth factor-I receptor dependent tumor growth in vivo. *Mol Cancer Ther.* (8), 2158–2167.

Kammasud, N., Boonyarat, C., Tsunoda, S., et al. (**2007**). Novel inhibitor for fibroblast growth factor receptor tyrosine kinase. *Bioorg Med Chem Lett.* 17(17), 4812–4818.

Kawanishi, N., Sugimoto, T., Shibata, J., et al. (**2006**). Structure-based drug design of a highly potent CDK1,2,4,6 inhibitor with novel macrocyclic quinoxalin-2-one structure. *Bioorg Med Chem Lett.* 16(19), 5122–5126.

Kim, M. K., Min, J., Choi, B. Y., et al. (**2007**). Discovery of cyclin-dependent kinase inhibitor, CR229, using structure based drug screening. *J Microbiol Biotechnol.* 17(10), 1712–1716.

Kim, H. J., Choo, H., Cho, Y. S., et al. (**2008**). Novel GSK-3beta inhibitors from sequential virtual screening. *Bioorg Med Chem.* 16(2), 636–643.

Kinoshita, T., Warizaya, M., Ohori, M., et al. (**2006**). Crystal structure of human ERK2 complexed with a pyrazolo[3,4-c]pyridazine derivative. *Bioorg Med Chem Lett.* 16(1), 55–58.

Kolb, P., Huang, D., Dey, F., et al. (**2008a**). Discovery of kinase inhibitors by high-throughput docking and scoring based on a transferable linear interaction energy model. *J Med Chem.* 51(5), 1179–1188.

Kolb, P., Kipouros, C. B., Huang, D., et al. (**2008b**). Structure-based tailoring of compound libraries for high-throughput screening: discovery of novel EphB4 kinase inhibitors. *Proteins.* 73(1), 11–18.

Kunick, C., Zeng, Z., Gussio, R., et al. (**2005**). Structure-aided optimization of kinase inhibitors derived from alsterpaullone. *Chembiochem.* 6(3), 541–549.

Li, R., Xue, L., Zhu, T., et al. (**2006**). Design and synthesis of 5-aryl-pyridone-carboxamides as inhibitors of anaplastic lymphoma kinase. *J Med Chem.* 49(3), 1006–1015.

Liao, J. J. (**2007**). Molecular recognition of protein kinase binding pockets for design of potent and selective kinase inhibitors. *J Med Chem.* 50(3), 409–424.

Liao, J. J., and Andrews, R. C. (**2007**). Targeting protein multiple conformations: a structure-based strategy for kinase drug design. *Curr Top Med Chem.* 7(14), 1394–1407.

Lippa, B., Morris, J., Corbett, M., et al. (**2006**). Discovery of novel isothiazole inhibitors of the TrkA kinase: structure–activity relationship, computer modeling, optimization, and identification of highly potent antagonists. *Bioorg Med Chem Lett.* 16(13), 3444–3448.

Loge, C., Testard, A., Thiery, V., et al. (**2008**). Novel 9-oxo-thiazolo[5,4-*f*]quinazoline-2-carbonitrile derivatives as dual cyclin-dependent kinase 1 (CDK1)/glycogen synthase kinase-3 (GSK-3) inhibitors: synthesis, biological evaluation and molecular modeling studies. *Eur J Med Chem.* 43(7), 1469–1477.

Manetti, F., Locatelli, G. A., Maga, G., et al. (**2006**). A combination of docking/dynamics simulations and pharmacophoric modeling to discover new dual c-Src/Abl kinase inhibitors. *J Med Chem.* 49(11), 3278–3286.

Manetti, F., Brullo, C., Magnani, M., et al. (**2008**). Structure-based optimization of pyrazolo[3,4-*d*]pyrimidines as Abl inhibitors and antiproliferative agents toward human leukemia cell lines. *J Med Chem.* 51(5), 1252–1259.

Marsden, B. D., and Knapp, S. (**2008**). Doing more than just the structure–structural genomics in kinase drug discovery. *Curr Opin Chem Biol.* 12(1), 40–45.

Martin, M. W., Newcomb, J., Nunes, J. J., et al. (**2008**). Structure-based design of novel 2-amino-6-phenyl-pyrimido[5′,4′:5,6]pyrimido[1,2-*a*]benzimidazol-5(6*H*)-ones as potent and orally active inhibitors of lymphocyte specific kinase (Lck): synthesis, SAR, and in vivo anti-inflammatory activity. *J Med Chem.* 51(6), 1637–1648.

Mastalerz, H., Chang, M., Chen, P., et al. (**2007**). New C-5 substituted pyrrolotriazine dual inhibitors of EGFR and HER2 protein tyrosine kinases. *Bioorg Med Chem Lett.* 17(7), 2036–2042.

Mavunkel, B., Xu, Y. J., Goyal, B., et al. (**2008**). Pyrimidine-based inhibitors of CaMKIIdelta. *Bioorg Med Chem Lett.* 18(7), 2404–2408.

Miyazaki, Y., Maeda, Y., Sato, H., et al. (**2008**). Rational design of 4-amino-5,6-diaryl-furo[2,3-*d*]pyrimidines as potent glycogen synthase kinase-3 inhibitors. *Bioorg Med Chem Lett.* 18(6), 1967–1971.

Montalban, A. G., Boman, E., Chang, C. D., et al. (**2008**). The design and synthesis of novel alpha-ketoamide-based p38 MAP kinase inhibitors. *Bioorg Med Chem Lett.* 18(6), 1772–1777.

Morwick, T., Berry, A., Brickwood, J., et al. (**2006**). Evolution of the thienopyridine class of inhibitors of IkappaB kinase-beta: Part I: Hit-to-lead strategies. *J Med Chem.* 49(10), 2898–2908.

Mulvihill, M. J., Ji, Q. S., Coate, H. R., et al. (**2008**). Novel 2-phenylquinolin-7-yl-derived imidazo[1,5-*a*]pyrazines as potent insulin-like growth factor-I receptor (IGF-IR) inhibitors. *Bioorg Med Chem.* 16(3), 1359–1375.

Nguyen, T. L., Gussio, R., Smith, J. A., et al. (**2006**). Homology model of RSK2 N-terminal kinase domain, structure-based identification of novel RSK2 inhibitors, and preliminary common pharmacophore. *Bioorg Med Chem.* 14(17), 6097–6105.

Nie, Z., Perretta, C., Erickson, P., et al. (**2007**). Structure-based design, synthesis, and study of pyrazolo[1,5-*a*][1,3,5]triazine derivatives as potent inhibitors of protein kinase CK2. *Bioorg Med Chem Lett.* 17(15), 4191–4195.

Ohren, J. F., Chen, H., Pavlovsky, A., et al. (**2004**). Structures of human MAP kinase kinase 1 (MEK1) and MEK2 describe novel noncompetitive kinase inhibition. *Nat Struct Mol Biol.* 11(12), 1192–1197.

Palanki, M. S., Akiyama, H., Campochiaro, P., et al. (**2008**). Development of prodrug 4-chloro-3-(5-methyl-3-{[4-(2-pyrrolidin-1-ylethoxy)phenyl]amino}-1,2,4-benzotriazin-7-yl)phenyl benzoate (TG100801): a topically administered therapeutic candidate in clinical trials for the treatment of age-related macular degeneration. *J Med Chem.* 51(6), 1546–1559.

Pao, W., Miller, V. A., Politi, K. A., et al. (**2005**). Acquired resistance of lung adenocarcinomas to gefitinib or erlotinib is associated with a second mutation in the EGFR kinase domain. *PLoS Med.* 2(3), e73.

Pargellis, C., Tong, L., Churchill, L., et al. (**2002**). Inhibition of p38 MAP kinase by utilizing a novel allosteric binding site. *Nat Struct Biol.* 9(4), 268–272.

Peifer, C., Selig, R., Kinkel, K., et al. (**2008**). Design, synthesis, and biological evaluation of novel 3-aryl-4-(1*H*-indole-3yl)-1,5-dihydro-2*H*-pyrrole-2-ones as vascular endothelial growth factor receptor (VEGF-R) inhibitors. *J Med Chem.* 51(13), 3814–3824.

Pierce, A. C., Sandretto, K. L., and Bemis, G. W. (**2002**). Kinase inhibitors and the case for CH···O hydrogen bonds in protein–ligand binding. *Proteins.* 49(4), 567–576.

Pierce, A. C., Jacobs, M., and Stuver-Moody, C. (**2008**). Docking study yields four novel inhibitors of the protooncogene Pim-1 kinase. *J Med Chem.* 51(6), 1972–1975.

Potashman, M. H., Bready, J., Coxon, A., et al. (**2007**). Design, synthesis, and evaluation of orally active benzimidazoles and benzoxazoles as vascular endothelial growth factor-2 receptor tyrosine kinase inhibitors. *J Med Chem.* 50(18), 4351–4373.

Poulsen, A., William, A., Lee, A., et al. (**2008**). Structure-based design of Aurora A & B inhibitors. *J Comput Aided Mol Des.* 22(12), 897–906.

Prien, O. (**2005**). Target-family-oriented focused libraries for kinases—conceptual design aspects and commercial availability. *Chembiochem.* 6(3), 500–505.

Richardson, C. M., Williamson, D. S., Parratt, M. J., et al. (**2006**). Triazolo[1,5-*a*] pyrimidines as novel CDK2 inhibitors: protein structure-guided design and SAR. *Bioorg Med Chem Lett.* 16(5), 1353–1357.

Richardson, C. M., Nunns, C. L., Williamson, D. S., et al. (**2007**). Discovery of a potent CDK2 inhibitor with a novel binding mode, using virtual screening and initial, structure-guided lead scoping. *Bioorg Med Chem Lett.* 17(14), 3880–3885.

Rossi, K. A., Markwalder, J. A., Seitz, S. P., et al. (**2005**). Understanding and modulating cyclin-dependent kinase inhibitor specificity: molecular modeling and biochemical evaluation of pyrazolopyrimidinones as CDK2/cyclin A and CDK4/cyclin D1 inhibitors. *J Comput Aided Mol Des.* 19(2), 111–122.

Sato, H., Shewchuk, L. M., and Tang, J. (**2006**). Prediction of multiple binding modes of the CDK2 inhibitors, anilinopyrazoles, using the automated docking programs GOLD, FlexX, and LigandFit: an evaluation of performance. *J Chem Inf Model.* 46(6), 2552–2562.

Schindler, T., Bornmann, W., Pellicena, P., et al. (**2000**). Structural mechanism for STI-571 inhibition of abelson tyrosine kinase. *Science.* 289(5486), 1938–1942.

Shin, D., Lee, S. C., Heo, Y. S., et al. (**2007**). Design and synthesis of 7-hydroxy-1*H*-benzoimidazole derivatives as novel inhibitors of glycogen synthase kinase-3beta. *Bioorg Med Chem Lett.* 17(20), 5686–5689.

Spicer, J. A., Rewcastle, G. W., Kaufman, M. D., et al. (**2007**). 4-Anilino-5-carboxamido-2-pyridone derivatives as noncompetitive inhibitors of mitogen-activated protein kinase kinase. *J Med Chem.* 50(21), 5090–5102.

Stamos, J., Sliwkowski, M. X., and Eigenbrot, C. (**2002**). Structure of the EGF receptor kinase domain alone and in complex with a 4-anilinoquinazoline inhibitor. *J Biol Chem.* 277(48), 46265–46272.

Swahn, B. M., Xue, Y., Arzel, E., et al. (**2006**). Design and synthesis of 2'-anilino-4,4'-bipyridines as selective inhibitors of c-Jun N-terminal kinase-3. *Bioorg Med Chem Lett.* 16(5), 1397–1401.

Taha, M. O., Bustanji, Y., Al-Ghussein, M. A., et al. (**2008**). Pharmacophore modeling, quantitative structure–activity relationship analysis, and in silico screening reveal potent glycogen synthase kinase-3beta inhibitory activities for cimetidine, hydroxychloroquine, and gemifloxacin. *J Med Chem.* 51(7), 2062–2077.

Tao, Z. F., Wang, L., Stewart, K. D., et al. (**2007**). Structure-based design, synthesis, and biological evaluation of potent and selective macrocyclic checkpoint kinase 1 inhibitors. *J Med Chem.* 50(7), 1514–1527.

Taylor, P., Blackburn, E., Sheng, Y. G., et al. (**2008**). Ligand discovery and virtual screening using the program LIDAEUS. *Br J Pharmacol.* 153(Suppl 1), S55–67.

Teng, M., Zhu, J., Johnson, M. D., et al. (**2007**). Structure-based design and synthesis of (5-arylamino-2*H*-pyrazol-3-yl)-biphenyl-2',4'-diols as novel and potent human CHK1 inhibitors. *J Med Chem.* 50(22), 5253–5256.

Terasawa, K., Yoshimatsu, K., Iemura, S., et al. (**2006**). Cdc37 interacts with the glycine-rich loop of Hsp90 client kinases. *Mol Cell Biol.* 26(9), 3378–3389.

Thaimattam, R., Banerjee, R., Miglani, R., et al. (**2007**). Protein kinase inhibitors: structural insights into selectivity. *Curr Pharm Des.* 13(27), 2751–2765.

Thomas, M. P., and McInnes, C. (**2006**). Structure-based discovery and optimization of potential cancer therapeutics targeting the cell cycle. *IDrugs.* 9(4), 273–278.

Toledo-Sherman, L., Deretey, E., Slon-Usakiewicz, J. J., et al. (**2005**). Frontal affinity chromatography with MS detection of EphB2 tyrosine kinase receptor. 2. Identification of small-molecule inhibitors via coupling with virtual screening. *J Med Chem.* 48(9), 3221–3230.

Tóth, G., Bowers, S. G., Truong, A. P., et al. (**2007**). The role and significance of unconventional hydrogen bonds in small molecule recognition by biological receptors of pharmaceutical relevance. *Curr Pharm Des.* 13(34), 3476–3493.

Tripathy, R., Reiboldt, A., Messina, P. A., et al. (**2006**). Structure-guided identification of novel VEGFR-2 kinase inhibitors via solution phase parallel synthesis. *Bioorg Med Chem Lett.* 16(8), 2158–2162.

Uno, M., Ban, H. S., Nabeyama, W., et al. (**2008**). De novo design and synthesis of *N*-benzylanilines as new candidates for VEGFR tyrosine kinase inhibitors. *Org Biomol Chem.* 6(6), 979–981.

Warner, S. L., Bashyam, S., Vankayalapati, H., et al. (**2006**). Identification of a lead small-molecule inhibitor of the Aurora kinases using a structure-assisted, fragment-based approach. *Mol Cancer Ther.* 5(7), 1764–1773.

Wolin, R. L., Bembenek, S. D., Wei, J., et al. (**2008**). Dual binding site inhibitors of B-RAF kinase. *Bioorg Med Chem Lett.* 18(9), 2825–2829.

Wood, E. R., Truesdale, A. T., McDonald, O. B., et al. (**2004**). A unique structure for epidermal growth factor receptor bound to GW572016 (Lapatinib): relationships among protein conformation, inhibitor off-rate, and receptor activity in tumor cells. *Cancer Res.* 64(18), 6652–6659.

Xiong, Z., Gao, D. A., Cogan, D. A., et al. (**2008**). Synthesis and SAR studies of indole-based MK2 inhibitors. *Bioorg Med Chem Lett.* 18(6), 1994–1999.

Zhong, W., Liu, H., Kaller, M. R., et al. (**2007**). Design and synthesis of quinolin-2(1*H*)-one derivatives as potent CDK5 inhibitors. *Bioorg Med Chem Lett.* 17(19), 5384–5389.

17

APPROACHES TO KINASE HOMOLOGY MODELING: SUCCESSES AND CONSIDERATIONS FOR THE STRUCTURAL KINOME

VICTORIA A. FEHER AND J. DAVID LAWSON

17.1. INTRODUCTION

This chapter focuses on the characteristics of protein kinases that avail themselves to homology modeling (also known as comparative protein modeling) as part of a structure-based drug design/discovery (SBDD) process. We explore the extent of the kinome accessible to SBDD via homology modeling. We also demonstrate the advantages conferred by modeling members of this protein superfamily that contains conserved elements and conserved dynamics and has an ever-growing body of chemogenomic data. In addition, successes of and caveats for kinase homology modeling are discussed.

The kinome is recognized as highly druggable through the confluence of two recent advances in drug discovery: the sequencing of the human genome and the assurgency of SBDD as a tool for rapid lead discovery and optimization. In 2002 a comprehensive inventory of human kinases was distilled from human genome data (Manning et al., 2002). This set of kinases, now known collectively as the human kinome, contains 519 putative members (Source: Manning's www.kinase.com as of June 2008). Additional analysis indicates that at least 164 kinases are associated with oncologic diseases and 80 additional kinases are associated with other major diseases such as diabetes and inflammation, making the kinome an extremely rich source of potential drug

Kinase Inhibitor Drugs. Edited by Rongshi Li and Jeffrey A. Stafford
Copyright © 2009 John Wiley & Sons, Inc.

targets (Manning et al., 2002). Concurrent with the elucidation of the kinome, SBDD has gained acceptance as a standard methodology in pharmaceutical discovery, as evidenced by a growing number of drugs discovered and optimized via these methods (Cohen, 2002; Noble et al., 2004; Vieth et al., 2005).

In addition to the above scientific advances, kinases have several characteristics that make them popular SBDD targets. The kinase catalytic domain (which catalyzes phosphorylation of the target protein) can often be excised from the full-length protein and still maintain a soluble, natively folded, bilobed structure of ~270 amino acids. This makes the catalytic domain amenable to structure determination via X-ray crystallography (Breitenlechner et al., 2003) (also see Chapter 19 of this volume). In addition, the catalytic domain contains a nucleotide binding pocket of an appropriate size and shape to accommodate small molecules that, when bound, inhibit phosphorylation and thus signal transduction downstream of the kinase. It is through this signal transduction that kinases participate in disease-related intracellular processes.

Because of the relative ease in obtaining kinase crystal structures and the importance of kinases to pathological processes, it is not surprising that there are an abundance of published kinase catalytic domain structures. As of June 2008, we have tallied at least 133 unique members of the kinome (Figure 17.1) that have a representative catalytic domain structure in the Protein Data Base (PDB) (Berman et al., 2000). Highlighted in green on Figure 17.2 are those kinases with structures currently deposited in the PDB. By this count, ~25% of

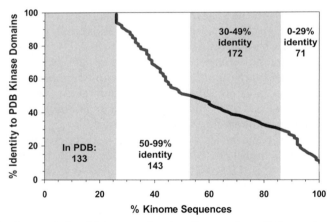

Figure 17.1. A cumulative histogram showing the number of kinase domains in the human kinome (*x*-axis) with better than a given sequence identity (*y*-axis) to any kinase in the PDB. Kinome catalytic domains were compared to sequences from the PDB using BLAST (Altschul et al., 1997). The closest PDB neighbor of each kinome member was hand annotated to confirm whether or not it was, in fact, the identified kinase. Once the completed set of PDB available kinase domains were annotated, pairwise identities to the remainder of the kinome were generated in ClustalW (Larkin et al., 2007). The highest identity for each kinome sequence is represented in the plot.

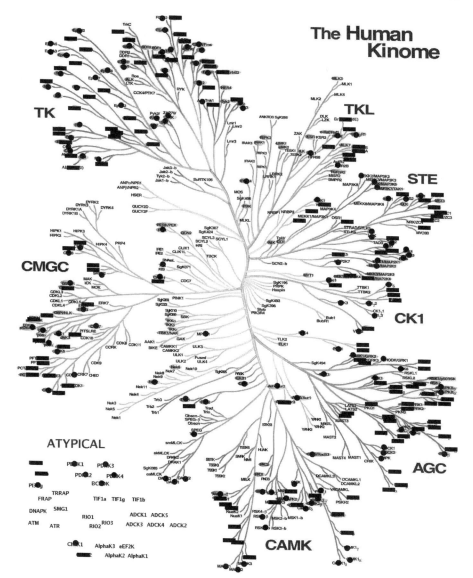

Figure 17.2. The Human Kinome dendogram illustrating >500 protein kinases, organized by their sequence identity and families. Kinases with at least one structure deposited in PDB as of June 2008 are noted with circles and those with at least 50% identity to a kinase with a deposited crystal structure are noted by rectangles. "The Human Kinome" dendogram is reproduced with the kind permission of Cell Signaling Technology, Inc. We have added several kinases from the Atypical family, including the PI3Ks.

the kinome is directly accessible for structure-based drug design methodologies. Homology modeling, however, allows us to extend the SBDD "druggable" portion of the kinome beyond the 25% based on crystal structures alone.

Interestingly, the close catalytic domain homology that makes kinases amenable to homology modeling reduces the likelihood that a given kinase catalytic domain structure will be determined by one of the structural genomics initiatives. These major contributors of high-resolution three-dimensional (3D) structures over the past decade include the Protein Structure Initiative (PSI) of the United States; the Riken Structural Genomics/Proteomics Initiative (RSGI) of Japan; the Structural Genomics Consortium (SGC) of Canada, the United Kingdom, and Sweden; and the now-defunct Structural Proteomics in Europe (SPINE). SGC's targets are picked by their funding sponsors (which include several pharmaceutical companies) and focus on medically relevant proteins. Thus SBC has contributed over 40 kinase structures—including over 30 novel structures—to the PDB in the last five years (Fedorov et al., 2007; Marsden and Knapp, 2008). Conversely, while RSGI, SPINE, and the four large-scale centers of the PSI have deposited a combined 5229 structures into the PDB as of June 2008, only eleven of those were protein kinase catalytic domain structures (of which seven were novel). This is largely due to these initiatives focusing on enlarging the breadth of our structural knowledge rather than selecting targets due to their interesting biological or commercial application. In general, proteins with greater than 25% identity to protein structures already in the public domain are not targeted. As seen in Figure 17.1, only ~9% of the kinome falls below this cutoff. Thus it is unlikely that RGSI and PSI will be providing a significant number of structures relevant to kinase inhibitor design in the near future.

Regardless of their source, the number of publicly available kinase structures will continue to accrue. Nevertheless—because drug discovery projects are often started before a target structure is available; because a particular kinase may not be amenable to crystallization; and because even when a structure does exists, the conformation does not support the modeling of a chemotype of interest—we foresee that homology modeling will have continued utility in driving kinase drug discovery projects.

Homology modeling covers a broad range of purposes in biochemistry, from exploring the putative fold or function of a protein to the refinement of an active site for virtual screening or drug design purposes. The resolution of the structure required for these different purposes varies dramatically and dictates (1) the methodology used for determining the homology model and (2) the sequence identity requirements of the protein template(s) used for modeling. SBDD exacts the most stringent requirements for resolution because details of the ligand–protein interactions significantly impact the ability to distinguish between ligand binding modes, binding energies for strong versus weak ligands, and selectivity of a ligand for one kinase over another. So although low resolution homology models have been determined for protein pairs with as little as 30% sequence identity, it has been suggested the more stringent demands of for SBDD require a sequence identity of at least 50% (Madhusudhan et al., 2005). Given the current number of known structures and their distribution within the kinome phylogeny, this cutoff yields ~55% of kinome catalytic domains as currently accessible for drug discovery via SBDD (Figures 17.1 and 17.2). We would like to suggest, however, that due to the characteristics of the kinase superfamily, a much larger percentage is likely accessible to homology modeling. To illustrate how these characteristics alter the homology modeling process, we first describe kinase homology modeling using traditional methods.

17.2. EXAMPLES OF KINASE HOMOLOGY MODELING UTILIZING TRADITIONAL MODELING METHODS

A flowchart of a standard homology modeling protocol illustrates that the first steps are template selection and sequence alignment (Figure 17.3). The large number of kinase crystal structures and the coverage of structures across kinome subfamilies usually allows for straightforward selection of multiple templates with >50% sequence identity to the target. Searching for the template structure(s) with the closest sequence identity to the target of interest can be performed using structural databases such as those at ExPASy or PDB (Berman et al., 2000; UniProt Consortium, 2008) or in any homology modeling

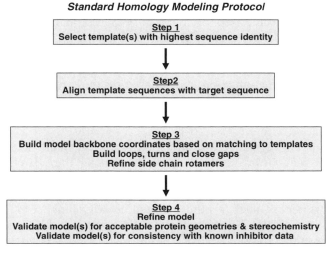

Figure 17.3. Flowchart outlining general steps for homology modeling. The reader is referred to reviews by Madhusudhan et al. (2005) and Xiang (2006) for detailed methods, software, and protocol options.

software package with a built-in structural database (e.g., Modeller, Composer, ICM-Homology, MOE—Sali and Blundell, 1993; Sutcliffe et al., 1987; Molsoft L.L.C., www.molsoft.com; Chemical Computing Group, www.chemcomp.com). There are a large number of literature examples of kinase homology modeling performed in this way, not all to be recounted here. Rather, the readers are referred to a recent review containing examples and references (Rockey and Elcock, 2006). However, we discuss several examples in order to demonstrate that the methods outlined in Figure 17.3 produce homology models useful for SBDD.

One such example is a homology model constructed for Fyn kinase, a nonreceptor tyrosine kinase involved in T-cell signal transduction (Jelić et al., 2007). The authors report that this model is in "excellent agreement" with the general catalytic domain fold and staurosporine binding orientation when compared to a published Fyn crystal structure (PDB code: 2DQ7; Kinoshita et al., 2006) that was released while the paper by Jelić et al. (2007) was in press. To construct the model, the authors followed the general steps outlined in Figure 17.3. First, they selected four template structures with sequence identities ranging over 62–77% with respect to the Fyn catalytic domain. Second, the templates and target sequences were aligned and compared in order to identify regions of conserved and nonconserved structural elements using the sequence alignment program MultAlig (Corpet, 1988). The third step was accomplished using the Composer homology modeling suite in SYBYL (Sutcliffe et al., 1987; Tripos Inc., www.tripos.com). Composer first builds structurally conserved regions (SCRs) where target residues are imposed on the coordinates for the most closely related template structure. This methodology is common to several modeling packages and generally functions to build the SCRs first, leaving gaps for variable regions—typically comprised of loops, turns, and small insertions—to be modeled later (Sutcliffe et al., 1987; Sali and Blundell, 1993). The program then searches a library containing all known protein structures in order to find the best match for the variable regions between the SCRs, subsequently fitting the backbone atom coordinates based on these matches. Note that it is not unusual for variable regions to be modeled using nonkinase protein structures. This process provides the backbone coordinates of the initial model(s).

Model building continues with the addition of the amino acid side chains to the backbone coordinates. In the present example, the side chain torsions were defined by a rotamer library within the Composer program. Side chain refinement can also be achieved through side chain libraries of low-energy side chain rotamers, such as those found in MOE or SCWRL/MolIDE (Canutescu et al., 2003). Not all modelers rely solely on such libraries; others have used examples of homologous kinase structures for guidance on the side chain torsion angles (Takami et al., 2004). This latter approach relies less on automated methods from standard modeling packages and more on the structure building prowess of the modeler.

The final step is refinement and validation of the model(s). Refinement commonly refers to a geometry optimization process that acts to relieve molecular strain from side chain atom clashes, corrects bond lengths and angles, and generally moves the structure toward a local energy minimum. This was achieved with the AMBER force field for the Jelić et al. (2007) Fyn model, but a number of suitable methods have been documented (see "Other Advances in Model Refinement" in Xiang, 2006; Nayeem et al., 2006). Model validation requires first confirming that the model's backbone and side chain Cα–Cβ (χ_1) torsion angles fall within acceptable ranges (as can be visualized in a Ramachandran plot). This is typically performed with programs such as PROCHECK (Laskowski et al., 1996) or WHAT IF (Vriend, 1990). We would like to encourage researchers who find out-of-range torsions to check their template structure. More often than not, they will find that this is the source of the torsion outliers. Secondly, the model should be validated as being consistent with available empirical data for the target, such as binding data for known inhibitors or mutagenesis data. The Jelić et al. (2007) Fyn model was successfully validated for SBDD by docking known ligands for the nucleotide binding site, AMP, and staurosporine (and ultimately by comparison to a Fyn crystal structure).

Some researchers, using variations on the above method, have published results that kinase catalytic domain templates with <50% overall sequence identity to the target can be utilized for homology modeling and still produce models that are useful for SBDD. For example, a Plk1 model was built using PKA as a template which, in 2005, had the closest overall sequence identity at 31%. To get around the identity limitation, three kinase templates (PKA, CDK2, and Erk2) were aligned to give segments of ~50 residues where the identity to Plk1 was 44–48%. The resulting model was useful for docking known inhibitors and noting features unique to the Plk1 kinase pocket (McInnes et al., 2005). Similarly, Takami and co-workers developed a very successful homology model for Rho kinase based on PKA (37% overall sequence identity). The resulting Rho kinase model was used to identify four hinge binding scaffolds: pyridine, indazole, isoquinoline, and phthalimide. This was followed by identifying a set of linkers that could bridge interactions to small molecule fragments having shape complementarity to a part of the binding pocket they termed the "D pocket" (Takami et al., 2004). Subsequent medicinal chemistry efforts combined with iterative rounds of modeling for these chemical series led to published accounts of low nanomolar compounds for two of these scaffolds (Iwakubo et al., 2007a,b).

Examples such as these are evidence that the published homology modeling guideline for a 50% sequence identity cutoff between template and target sequences (Madhusudhan et al., 2005) can, for many targets in the kinase superfamily, be reduced to ~30% and still provide models suitable for SBDD. There are two explanations as to why one can effectively model more distantly related homologs when modeling kinases but cannot with other proteins: fold conservation of the catalytic domain and sequence conservation within the ATP binding pocket.

Both the tertiary fold of the kinase domain and the secondary structure elements therein are well conserved across the kinome—with the exception of the atypical kinases (Manning et al., 2002). Hanks and Quinn (1991) note that about 90% of the kinase catalytic domains fall within the range of 247–290 amino acids in length and any that exceed this have a large insertion of ~20 residues. Our analysis of the kinome sequences maintained at www.kinase.com (which contains approximately fivefold more sequences than the Hanks–Quinn analysis a decade ago) indicate that, for non-atypical kinases, the catalytic domain averages 272 residues with 85% of the sequences between 245 and 300 residues in length. In a comparison of the backbone RMSDs for all 104 solved kinase domain structures in 2006, the median deviation was ~1.2 Å and ranged to a maximum of ~2.5 Å (Rockey and Elcock, 2006), suggesting that using any kinase template would produce backbone coordinates with a generally accurate fold. This obviates the need for mixing and matching multiple templates to generate the model unless there are special regions such as the ATP pocket or activation loop that require more precise modeling or special modifications. Indeed, one finds, when the literature is surveyed for examples of kinase homology models, that most are constructed using a single template. Five to ten years ago this was most likely because fewer kinase domain crystal structures were available. More recently, the reliance on a single template is related to the recognition that the kinase catalytic domain fold and secondary structure elements are well conserved.

In addition to the overall fold conservation among kinase catalytic domains, there is also a high degree of sequence similarity within the ATP binding pocket with ten highly conserved or invariant residues in the pocket. One set of conserved residues, known variously as the Walker A motif, the P-loop, and the glycine-rich loop (i.e., Gly50-X-Gly-X-X-Gly-X-Val57), is associated with ATP binding (sequence numbering based on PKA; Taylor, 1989). A second set, known as the DFG motif (i.e., Asp184-Phe-Gly186), anchors the N terminus of the activation loop (A-loop) and is thus associated with regulation of the enzymatic function. The third set are those residues required for catalyzing the transfer of the γ-phosphate from ATP to the target protein, namely, Lys72, Glu91, and Asp184. Several additional catalytic domain residues are also highly conserved: Asp166, Asn171, Gly186, Glu208, Asp220, Gly225, and Arg280 (Hanks and Hunter, 1995). These invariant and conserved residues serve to assist in the alignment process (step 2 in Figure 17.3), a critical step in determining the accuracy of the model.

This modeling simplification can extend even to side chain refinement. Rockey and Elcock (2006) show that although the number of side chain clashes can be high in raw models—upwards of 20—they are usually found in the less conserved C-terminal lobe of the catalytic domain and not near the nucleotide binding site. Implementing protocols that relieve the clashes through "repacking" methods, especially those that alter backbone coordinates, introduces different clashes in other parts of the model, sometimes in the nucleotide pocket and detrimental to subsequent SBDD efforts. Although

Rockey and Elcock are not advocating sloppy model building, they point out there is a danger in overrefining models in regions unnecessary for drug design.

Investing time in the details of the nucleotide binding pocket, however, is worthwhile. For example, special care must be taken for the correct modeling of torsions in the hinge region. Insertions of one to two amino acids in the target sequence relative to the template can have dramatic effects in successful modeling of hinge–ligand H-bonding because of the precise directionality required for H-bonding partners. Rockey and Elcock (2006) found that by simply eliminating the insertion and retaining the hinge backbone torsions from the template gave the best results when attempting to reproduce staurosporine docking. Any further refinement of the insertion diminishes the success rate of the docking. Note, however, that these are cases where the template structure had the molecule they were docking (i.e., staurosporine) bound and does not address the ability to dock other known chemotypes into the model. As always, validation of the model by docking known inhibitors will provide an understanding of the utility of the model. The model may yield consistent results with the known inhibition data for one chemical series (and thus will be useful for SBDD within that series) but not for a series with a different chemotype.

As discussed previously, the close homology between members of the kinase superfamily extends the utility of homology modeling tools to provide better accuracy and subsequent SBDD results than one would expect when homology modeling in the rest of the proteome. However, as we describe next, the utility of homology modeling can be extended even further when the target and templates are in the same subfamily.

17.3. ADVANTAGES OF SUBFAMILY HOMOLOGY

The kinome dendrogram (Figure 17.2) illustrates that kinases can be further classified into families and subfamilies. Often subfamily members will share sequence identities greater than 70% for the kinase domain and have as few as one to five conservative residue substitutions within the ATP binding pocket (Hanks et al., 1988). In the absence of a three-dimensional structure for the target kinase, using a subfamily member for homology modeling or chimera development has proven to be highly successful for SBDD. Not only is sequence alignment relatively straightforward, thus enhancing model accuracy, but the subfamily members can also be used as experimental surrogates during the design process. In addition, most drug discovery programs will run enzymatic assays against subfamily members in order to determine the selectivity of a chemical series. These assays can be used to (1) validate the homology model with SAR data, that is, a good model should be able to explain selectivity differences between the target and template; and (2) identify inhibitors that one may want to co-crystallize with the subfamily member in order to confirm inhibitor binding modes or better understand selectivity profiles. A series of papers published over the past eight years describing CDK4 drug discovery projects illustrate both successes and caveats with these approaches.

McInnes et al. (2004) used standard protocols for developing their CDK4 model based on two template homologs: CDK2 co-crystallized with purvalanol (47% sequence identity), and CDK6 co-crystallized with p19INK4d (72% sequence identity). Using a commercially available homology modeling package, SCRs were built using the CDK2 backbone coordinates as a template. Nonconserved loop regions were modeled using coordinates from either CDK2 or CDK6 or were modeled de novo. The raw model coordinates were refined with energy minimization and molecular dynamics (MD). Final validation for this model came from the consistency found between predicted binding energies (from inhibitors docked into CDK2 and the CDK4 model) and experimental inhibition data. The authors found two sequence differences between CDK4 and CDK2 at the edge of the ATP binding pocket that appear to influence specificity: Q131E and K89T (the first residue of each pair is from CDK2 and the second is the analogous residue in CDK4; numbering is from CDK2) (Figure 17.4). The Q131E substitution is sterically conservative but introduces an acidic group and negative charge while the K89T substitution removes both steric bulk and an amino cation. Combined, these substitutions result in a larger and substantially more electronegative binding surface. This understanding allowed the modeling and successful optimization of novel CDK4

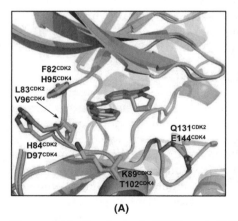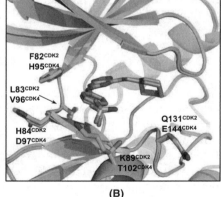

(A)   (B)

Figure 17.4. Overlays of CDK2 and CDK2/CDK4 chimeras. For both panels, the ligand and residues that impact residue specificity are shown in stick representations. (**A**) The crystal structures from Ikuta et al. (2001) of CDK2 (PDB code: 1GII, blue) and a CDK2/CDK4 chimera (PDB code: 1GIJ, green). Residues His84 and Gln131, which can impact specificity but aren't mutated, are colored orange. (**B**) The crystal structures from Pratt et al. (2006) of two different CDK2/CDK4 chimeras (PDB codes: 2IW9, blue and 2IW8, green). Residue Gln131, which can impact specificity but isn't mutated in either of the chimeras, is colored orange. (See color insert.)

analogs based on a previously reported CDK2 inhibitor series, 2-anilino-4-(thiazol-5-yl) pyrimidines (Wang et al., 2004). Guided by this model, the authors added positively charged substituents to the aniline and generated an interaction with the Glu144 carboxylate side chain. As one would predict, this resulted in compounds with up to a 30-fold increase in potency versus CDK4 while only increasing CDK2 potency twofold.

An alternate method to homology modeling within a subfamily is to experimentally generate a chimeric protein construct, making several mutations within the binding pocket in order to mimic the pocket of the target protein. Ideally, this can be achieved without altering the favorable crystallization properties of the template protein. While this is not technically in silico homology modeling, this method is driven by correct in silico sequence alignment and structural comparisons. This was the approach used by Honma, Ikuta, and colleagues (Honma et al., 2001a,b; Ikuta et al., 2001). The authors generated a chimeric protein for X-ray crystallographic structure determination and subsequently analyzed the inhibitor specificity between CDK2 and CDK4 (PDB codes: 1GII, 1GIJ). The chimera, based on CDK2, replaced three residues with corresponding residues from the aligned sequence of CDK4: F82H, L83V, and K89T (Figure 17.4A). The chimera was subsequently crystallized with an inhibitor that is approximately equipotent for both enzymes. Note that the steric change when Lys89 is substituted with Thr in the chimera guided the authors to design an analogous compound with a bulkier moiety in that region, resulting in a ~2 nM CDK4 inhibitor with 190-fold selectivity over CDK2 (Honma et al., 2001b). Pratt and co-workers (2006) followed a similar approach, making combinations of F82H, L83V, H84D, and K89T mutants to find which ones most impacted the selectivity of two different inhibitor chemotypes: disubstituted purine, NU6102, and bisanilinopyrimidine, AZ2 (Figure 17.4B). The authors used these results to generate two CDK2/CDK4 chimeras in order to aid the interpretation of their SAR data. One chimera was based on CDK2 with three CDK4 binding site substitutions: F82H, L83V, and H84D. The second chimera was based on CDK2 with a single binding site substitution, K89T.

It is interesting to note that while the CDK2/CDK4 chimera developed by Ikuta et al. (2001) was successful in developing a more selective CDK4 inhibitor in their study, the choice of mutations has been limiting in other studies. As described earlier, McInnes et al. (2004) chose to create an in silico CDK4 homology model rather than use the chimera. Specifically, the Q131E substitution is missing in the chimera but is a key interaction point with their compounds. Similarly, Tsou et al. (2008) mutated the Ikuta et al. (2001) chimera in silico to make it even more similar to CDK4. Tsou and colleagues found that hinge substitution H84D was needed to explain their series' specificity between CDK2 and CDK4 and that the Q131E substitution was likely also relevant though not directly interpretable from their model. We note, however, that the Pratt et al. (2006) chimera would have been adequate for this study. These results underline a key caveat for making chimeras either in silico or as physical proteins for crystallograpy: namely, the key residue(s) important in defining selectivity for one chemical series may differ from the key residue(s) responsible for kinase selectivity in another series. Davies and colleagues, however, demonstrate that if a structural biology team is diligent in designing all of the relevant selectivity residues into their chimera (PDB codes 2JDV, etc.), the resulting structure can be used to confirm binding modes for multiple chemical series, help understand selectivity profiles between the two parent kinases (in this case, PKA and PKB), and help drive the overall SBDD process (Davies et al., 2007; Caldwell et al., 2008).

17.4. ACCOMMODATING ACTIVE VERSUS INACTIVE KINASE CONFORMATIONS

The above examples focus on homology modeling of the catalytic domain's active conformation. It has been discussed in the literature that there are regions of flexibility around the nucleotide binding pocket (i.e., the glycine-rich P-loop, the A-loop, and hinge opening) that give rise to small variations in the pocket size and shape while in its active conformation (Johnson et al., 2001; Lu et al., 2005). Co-crystal structures for inhibitors such as imatinib, sorafenib, and lapatinib have shown that there are also some large conformational differences in the kinases within inactivated forms. Jacobs et al. (2008) have clustered the inactive kinase conformations into two major groups (Figure 17.5). One conformation is named "DFG-out" in reference to the

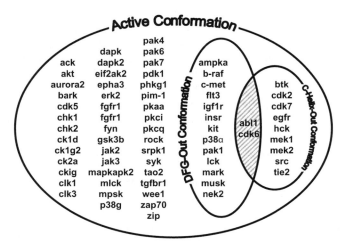

Figure 17.5. Venn diagram showing conformational classifications for public domain kinase crystal structures; adapted from Jacobs et al. (2008). Presumably, all kinases can access the active conformation (large oval) and many kinases have only been observed in this conformation. By contrast, only those kinases listed in the smaller ovals have been observed in the DFG-out of C-helix-out conformations. Furthermore, only two kinases (listed in the overlap section) have been observed in both DFG-out and C-helix-out conformations. Please see the original reference for classification criteria.

greater than 10 Å position change for the phenylalanine located in the N-terminal region of the activation loop anchor relative to the active conformation. The second conformation is termed "C-helix out" referring to the position of the C-helix relative to the N-terminal lobe of the catalytic domain. This conformation opens an additional binding pocket and ablates the canonical salt bridge between Lys72 and C-helix residue Glu91. Next, we discuss what implications these various conformations have on homology modeling and subsequent SBDD.

One example of the successful generation of a DFG-out conformation homology model comes from a study that investigated the structural factors driving the selectivity of PDGFRβ and Flt3 for inhibitor drug imatinib (STI-571) (Böhmer et al., 2003). STI-571 is known to bind Bcr-Abl, PDGFRβ, and Kit kinases with similar affinities (IC_{50} ~100–300 nM) but does not bind a closely related tyrosine kinase, Flt3. Böhmer et al. (2003) assert that the gatekeeper residue is the key determinant in the selectivity differences observed: Abl, Kit, and PDGFRβ have a threonine at the gatekeeper position, whereas Flt3 has a phenylalanine that is too bulky to permit STI-571 binding. To illustrate that there are not other differences present in the extended binding pocket, homology models for PDGFRβ and for a Flt3 F691T mutant were constructed. Because the closest homolog structures at the time were only in the DFG-in conformation (VEGFR2 and FGFR1) or were in a DFG-out conformation that occluded the active site (IRK), these were used to model SCRs in the portions of the protein distal to the active site. Abl, which has only 38% and 40% identity to the two targets, was used to model the active site and activation loop based on two experimental observations: inhibition by STI-571 is approximately equipotent for Abl and PDGFRβ and is similarly reduced in the phosphorylated (i.e., activated) enzymes. Thus the remaining backbone coordinates, the inhibitor pose, and the crystallographic waters were derived entirely from the STI-571/Abl crystal structure (PDB code: 1IEP; Nagar et al., 2002) and the resulting model was energy minimized. The homology models converged quickly despite seven residue differences in the extended binding pocket between Abl and the PDGFRβ or Flt3 F691T models. Böhmer et al. (2003) point out that this is consistent with the lack of additional clashes between the inhibitor and the binding pocket, which thereby support the hypothesis that the sole selectivity determinant is the gatekeeper residue. The Flt3 F691T mutant protein has an $IC_{50} \approx 200$ nM by STI-571, a value similar to that of PDGFRβ and Abl, further validating the modeling results.

Subsequent to the Böhmer et al. (2003) publication, new crystal structures with STI-571 bound have been solved for Kit, Lck, Syk, and Src (Atwell et al., 2004; Mol et al., 2004; Seeliger et al., 2007; Jacobs et al., 2008). The Kit, Lck, and Src structures show a remarkable conservation of the backbone conformation in the DFG-out ATP binding pocket relative to Abl. And in the case of Lck and Src, even the side chains are nearly superposable. Other than the activation loop, the region with the highest RMSD is the glycine-rich loop, which folds over the ATP binding cleft in the Abl/STI-571 co-crystal structure but is more extended over the activation loop in the three other structures.

Interestingly, the Syk/STI-571 structure shows STI-571 binding in a completely different binding mode, one that does not require a DFG-out conformation. This demonstrates that binding modes are not always transferable between kinases—something to keep in mind when picking a template structure and, perhaps more importantly, when validating a model.

A more recent example of PDGFRβ homology modeling (Mori et al., 2008) was not as complex as the Böhmer et al. (2003) model building. It utilized the structure of a single close homolog Flt3 (~50% sequence identity) in the DFG-out conformation [something not available to Böhmer et al. (2003)]. The DFG-out conformation was important in this case as the quinoxalin-2-one inhibitors of interest prevent autophosphorylation in both Flt3 and PDGFRβ, consistent with adoption of a DFG-out conformation in both cases. The authors chose Flt3 as a template because, in addition to the close homology and appropriate conformational dynamics, the quinoxalin-2-one ligands demonstrate similar inhibition profiles in both Flt3 and PDGFRβ. The resulting homology model performed well in being able to explain the SAR data.

These results suggest that even when the closest homolog doesn't have the desired conformation (i.e., DFG-in, DFG-out, or C-helix out) one can still expect to have success in modeling the backbone conformations for the ATP nucleotide binding region, the anchor of the activation loop and the extended "back pocket." This is supported by Figure 17.6C, which shows that for a total of 25 crystal structures of Abl in DFG-in, DFG-out, and C-helix out conformations, all of the pairwise comparisons have a less than ~2.5 Å RMSD for their active site Cα atoms. In other words, even with significant changes in the active site, most residues will maintain similar positions in the overall fold. The hard part is figuring out what is the desired conformation (i.e., what is moving—or not moving) and what template to pick in order to best model that conformation. Thus it would likely be worthwhile to develop a customized loop database based solely on existing kinase structures rather than the entire PDB. Such a

---

Figure 17.6. A comparison of active site sequence identity and active site Cα RMSD for three sets of kinase crystal structures. (*Note*: We've defined the active site as residues within 6 Å of the bound ligand.) For each set, the active sites were aligned as a group and subsequently analyzed in a pairwise fashion within the set (note that multiple protein–ligand complexes in the asymmetric unit were split out and also compared). (**A**) The analysis for the structures of 34 protein kinase catalytic domains with the pan-kinase inhibitor staurosporine bound in the active site. The isolated overlaid staurosporine ligands are shown in the inset. All of the outlier data points in the upper left quadrant of the plot are from the 1E8Z structure of PI3K, an Atypical kinase. The staurosporine molecule from this structure can also be seen in the inset to be shifted relative to the remainder of the ligands. (**B**) The analysis of 45 protein kinase catalytic domains with the ATP analog AMPPNP bound in the active site. The isolated overlaid AMPPNP ligands are shown in the inset. (**C**) Plots of the frequency of the pairwise RMSDs for 25 active sites of ABL co-complexed with various ligands in the active site. Both DFG-in and DFG-out protein conformations were used.

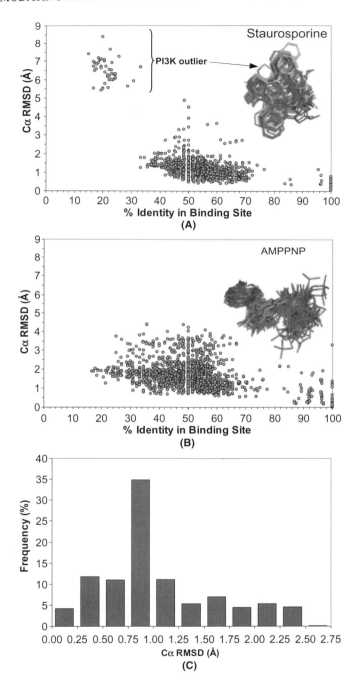

database could contain known glycine-rich P-loop and A-loop coordinates to limit the conformational space searched and facilitate homology model refinement of these regions.

17.5. A CHEMOGENOMIC APPROACH TO KINASE HOMOLOGY MODELING

The extensive selectivity data and the deposition of multiple liganded crystal structures for many kinases provide the modeler many choices for template selection beyond a simple sequence identity query. As was pointed out earlier, selecting the template based on a similar SAR relative to the target (rather than by sequence identity) may result in a higher quality model for the binding pocket—a desirable outcome when pursuing a SBDD program. Several examples illustrate the successes found via what some have termed "SAR homology modeling" or "SARAH" (Frye, 1999).

Tuccinardi and colleagues (2007) used compounds known to inhibit their target kinase, RET, to screen available crystal structures for chemically similar bound inhibitors. This study led them to select two kinase templates: FGFR1 and Lck. FGFR1 was selected because, of the available template structures, it had the closest overall sequence identity to RET (55%). In addition, a FGFR1 structure was available with indolinone inhibitor inhibitor SU5402 bound—one of a class of inhibitors that binds multiple tyrosine kinases including RET. Lck was also selected despite its lower sequence identity (38% identity to RET), because a structure was available with PP2 bound—a potent RET inhibitor whose binding induces a more open conformation of the glycine-rich loop. Both models were built using standard protocols and validated by docking 12 known inhibitors. The second model, based on the Lck/PP2 structure, was validated with literature data and is consistent with mutational analysis causing resistance to three RET inhibitors, PP1, PP2, and ZD6474 (Carlomagno et al., 2004). Virtual screening of the model led to the testing of a focused library and identification of ten compounds with 10–71% RET inhibition at 10 µM (Tuccinardi et al., 2007). Subsequent to their homology modeling studies, the crystal structures for RET were determined with PP1 and ZD6474 bound. Tuccinardi et al. (2007) compared the structures to their homology models and found a high degree of accuracy. They concluded that their decision to choose the RET template based on SAR instead of sequence identity alone resulted in a model more comparable to the crystal structure. The RMSD for the 30 nucleotide binding site residues within 7 Å of the ligand in the model and the crystal structure is 0.7 Å for backbone heavy atoms and 1.2 Å for all heavy atoms; the ligand positions are also close with RMSDs for PP1 and ZD6474 at 1.2 Å and 2.1 Å, respectively.

Selectivity data can also substitute for sequence identity in target selection. Pan and colleagues (2007) found a purine analog that yielded 8.2 nM inhibition of the putative rheumatoid arthritis target, BTK. Rather than solely utilizing the BTK crystal structure, solved in the unphosphorylated apo form, they submitted this inhibitor to Ambit Biosciences (San Diego, CA), a company that provides binding assay screens for more than 400 kinases (Fabian et al., 2005). The compound was found to inhibit several Tec and Src subfamily members. This was in agreement with another study that reported the compound inhibits Lck—a Tec subfamily member—at 4.6 nM (Arnold et al., 2000). Based on these data, the authors chose to generate the homology model using a combination of the apo BTK crystal structure and a Lck structure with a similar inhibitor bound. The resulting homology model revealed a Cys residue in the active site that was found only in ten other kinases out of an alignment of 491 kinases from across the kinome. This led to the Cys residue becoming a target for the design of an irreversible inhibitor. The final series of inhibitors resulting from this SBDD program demonstrated >500-fold selectivity for BTK over Lyn or Syk in anti-IgM stimulated Ramos cells and demonstrated dose-dependent in vivo efficacy in mouse rheumatoid arthritis models (Pan et al., 2007).

To better understand how the bound ligand impacts active site conformation in kinase catalytic domains, we analyzed several sets of public domain kinase catalytic domain structures (Figure 17.6) and found that the amount of structural variation for kinases bound with a single chemotype varies depending on the properties of the chemotype. For 34 structures coliganded with pan-kinase inhibitor staurosporine (Omura et al., 1977), most of the pairwise backbone RMSD comparisons of active site (i.e., within 6 Å of the ligand) residues are within 2.5 Å. Likewise, the backbone RMSD for most of the pairs of the 45 kinase catalytic domains liganded with ATP analog AMPPNP (Yount et al., 1971) fall in the same 2.5 Å range. However, due to the flexibility of the imidodiphosphate tail (Figure 17.6B—inset), the P-loop and A-loop segments of the kinases are not uniformly ligated and demonstrate considerable flexibility that is reflected in the hysteresis of RMSD measurements. Note that for neither the AMPPNP nor the staurosporine-bound structural alignments are examples found with RMSDs under 1.0 Å when sequence similarity dips into the "twilight zone," that is, protein sequences with less than 30% identity (Doolittle, 1986). An extreme example is the 1E8Z structure of an atypical kinase family member, PI3K, bound to staurosporine (Walker et al., 2000). Due to the lack of a good structural alignment to the other complexes, the RMSDs for 1E8Z to all other kinases in the set are relatively high. The poor structural alignment can actually be seen in the inset of Figure 17.6A, showing the ligands from the overlaid structures. While choosing a template based on chemotype alone will often lead to an adequate model, as can be seen in Figures 17.6A and 17.6B, it is not always the case. Furthermore, is not likely to be accurate in twilight zone cases.

For the sake of comparison, we also performed an overlay of 25 structures of liganded Abl catalytic domains. Not surprisingly, almost all of the backbone RMSDs were relatively low (<2.5 Å). However, when one considers that DFG-in, DFG-out, and C-helix out conformations were included in the analysis, this is a little surprising. Closer analysis demonstrates that with the exception of the A-loop, P-loop, and C-helix, the structures are in fact very close. Also, the

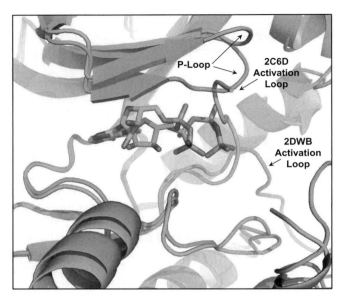

Figure 17.7. Two different crystal structures of Aurora-A bound to AMPPNP. The structure of the T287D construct (PDB code: 2C6D; Heron et al., 2006) is shown in blue. The wild-type construct is shown in green (PDB code: 2DWB). There is a significant amount of structural divergence between the two structures—mainly in the regions of the activation loop and P-loop. This is likely arising due to a combination of the T287D mutation and crystallization conditions. Note that for the sake of clarity, only one of the two conformations of the 2C6D AMPPNP molecule is shown. Also, the γ-phosphate of the 2CSD AMPPNP is disordered. (See color insert.)

number of residues moving a significant distance is less than those that are essentially static. This skews the RMSD measurement toward a smaller number. It also suggests that with careful loop modeling, inactive conformations can be modeled successfully on an active template and vice versa.

These results are consistent with observations previously published (Taylor et al., 2005) noting that it is not the general fold nor the high conservation of residues around the kinase catalytic site that creates chemical diversity for an individual kinase's function, but rather the surface residues that create its selectivity and differences in protein–protein interactions. So perhaps it isn't surprising that the backbone deviations are small.

Of interest in Figure 17.6B is the outlier on the 100% abscissa representing a comparison between Aurora-A/AMPPNP structures 2C6D and 2DWB. The former is of activation mutant T287D (Heron et al., 2006) while the latter is a wild-type construct. The >3 Å RMSD arises from different conformations of the activation loop and the P-loop (Figure 17.7). Interestingly, even though the 2C6D structure contains an activation mutation, it is in an inactive conformation. Heron et al. (2006) speculate that this may be due to the low pH (3.8) of the crystallization buffer protonating Asp287, which thus loses its electronegative character and ability to salt bridge to Arg255 and isn't able to stabilize the activated conformation. Even more interesting is that while the "activated" mutant doesn't adopt the activated conformation, the wild-type mutant does. This can clearly be seen by overlaying (data not shown) the 2DWB structure with the structure of active PKA (1ATP) (Zheng et al., 1993). This is a good example of how, in addition to ligand chemotype and sequence identity, the researcher also must consider other factors when evaluating template structures such as construct mutations, phosphorylation states, other proteins in the complex (which can often influence the active site conformation), and even the buffer used for crystallization, making sure that they are appropriate for the desired target conformation/activation state.

The bottom line is that when picking a template, a closely related kinase is better than a distant relative—however, even better is a close relative with a ligand bound that is similar in chemotype to the series that you wish to study. When homology modeling for a SBDD project, if you have to choose between either a close neighbor or a close chemotype, the close chemotype template should be chosen first (as long as it is better than 30% homology). If the resulting model does not adequately explain your SAR, try again using the close neighbor or a chimera between the two templates.

17.6. CONSIDERATIONS FOR "TWILIGHT ZONE" KINASE HOMOLOGS

The atypical kinase family (lower left portion of Figure 17.2), as well as kinases with catalytic domains that have less than 30% sequence identity to any other kinase, provides a challenge for homology modeling. These models are far less accurate, largely because of difficulties in properly aligning sequences (Ginalski, 2006, and CASP references therein). Considerable research efforts have focused on trying to obtain better sequence alignments for these "twilight zone" sequences (Li et al., 2002; Orengo and Thornton, 2005; Dunbrack, 2006). One solution utilizes ortholog sequence alignment, that is, aligning multiple sequences from various species for the target protein and likewise aligning multiple sequences of the template sequence (Orengo and Thornton, 2005). This artifical increase in the conserved residue matches improves the template to target alignment step. It is our view that homology modeling of twilight zone kinases will become increasingly important due to the recent interest in the atypical family. Several members of this family are now recognized as attractive oncology and anti-inflammation drug targets (Smith, 2007; Gridelli et al., 2008; Mavrou et al., 2008).

A recent example of pushing the limits of homology modeling into the twilight zone comes from Tobak (2007), who took advantage of the kinase superfamily's familiar traits and a multispecies alignment method to develop a homology model of mTOR kinase, also known as FRAP kinase. Tobak used

PI3Kγ, a structure with 22% sequence identity to the target, as the model template. The initial alignment performed used human mTOR and eight orthologs from across seven different species. This identified Asp2357 (from the DFG motif) and Arg2339 as conserved across the homologs aligned. Subsequent alignment of the mTOR and PI3Kγ sequences demonstrated that 13 of the 22 ATP binding site residues were identical, including Arg2339 and Asp2357, and an additional three were similar. This boded well for being able to recreate the binding site based on the template despite the low overall sequence identity. The mTOR versus PI3Kγ alignment also revealed the presence of three gaps and three insertions in the mTOR sequence. All but one of these gaps and insertions were one to four residues in length. The remaining insertion was 37 residues long (2247–2283). No homologous sequence for this insertion could be found in PDB; thus it was decided to model the loop de novo. Using the mTOR versus PI3Kγ alignment as a starting point, multiple models were generated in three different homology modeling programs (Sali and Blundell, 1993; Bates and Sternberg, 1999; Martí-Renom et al., 2000; Bates et al., 2001; Petrey et al., 2003). Evaluation and selection of the final model was based on several factors: structural conservation (relative to the template) of binding site residues, especially Arg2339 and Asp2357; agreement with secondary structure predictions, especially within the 2247–2283 insertion; and structural stability during MD simulations. In addition to the above considerations, Tobak (2007) also used chemogenomic information to evaluate the models. Wortmannin and LY294002, compounds known to inhibit both mTOR and PI3Kγ, were docked into the models and only those with interactions consistent with strong binding were considered. Although it may be some time before the accuracy of the mTOR model can be assessed with a known crystal structure, several compounds identified through docking with this model have been validated as inhibitors of mTOR by in vitro assay testing.

Another approach to modeling kinases in the twilight zone can be through "brain transplant" methods, that is, simple mutation of one or a few key residues in the ATP binding pocket. This is similar to the generation of chimeras for crystallography, as discussed earlier, except that it is done only in silico. This is likely to be most successful if the resulting model can then be refined using a ligand with known SAR for validation purposes. However, some subtleties may be missed, as is illustrated in the positional shift in staurosporine binding to PI3K relative to other kinases seen in Figure 17.6A.

17.7. SUMMARY

While the general approach to homology modeling is (1) template selection, (2) template–target sequence alignment, (3) model building, and (4) evaluation of the models (Figure 17.3), each paper reviewed in this chapter

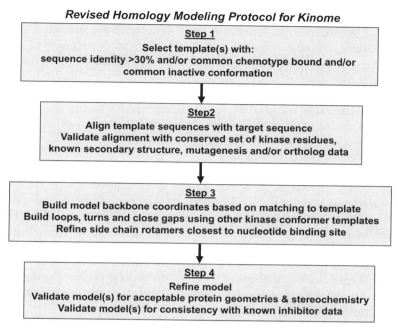

Revised Homology Modeling Protocol for Kinome

Step 1

Select template(s) with:
sequence identity >30% and/or common chemotype bound and/or
common inactive conformation

Step2

Align template sequences with target sequence
Validate alignment with conserved set of kinase residues,
known secondary structure, mutagenesis and/or ortholog data

Step 3

Build model backbone coordinates based on matching to template
Build loops, turns and close gaps using other kinase conformer templates
Refine side chain rotamers closest to nucleotide binding site

Step 4

Refine model
Validate model(s) for acceptable protein geometries & stereochemistry
Validate model(s) for consistency with known inhibitor data

Figure 17.8. A flowchart for homology modeling steps revised to incorporate additional data and characteristics associated with the kinase superfamily.

uses the template information in different ways. Hence, for best results, there is no "one-size-fits-all" approach. Rather, the researcher must approach kinase homology modeling on a case-by-case basis. For a protein superfamily rich in structural information, sequence, and chemogenomic information, there are always multiple ways to generate a model and some methods will yield better results than others. Therefore we propose a homology modeling flowchart that makes use of these superfamily advantages in Figure 17.8.

In the literature, there are examples ranging from the simple—for example, using an ortholog template or standard BLAST search for template selection followed by model building and evaluation within protein modeling packages (Vangrevelinghe et al., 2003; Sandberg et al., 2005; Verma et al., 2005)—to the intermediate, for example, constructing a basic model and further modifying it based on structural details found in other templates (Takami et al., 2004)—to the complex, for example, extracting ligands for manual docking and subsequent pocket opening modifications via MD and energy minimization cycles (Tuccinardi et al., 2007). Despite the variety of protocols described, there are some clear trends observed in successful homology modeling for the kinome.

When selecting the template, consideration of the chemical series or the compound library to be screened will more likely lead to a binding site model amenable to SBDD than a model based on close sequence identity alone. This phenomenon arises from the regions of deformability within the nucleotide binding site. The glycine-rich P-loop and A-loop can have a multitude of positions, opening or closing the size and shape of the binding pocket based on an induced fit. This tertiary plasticity superposed on the ability of the binding pocket side chains to adopt multiple torsions and the ability of the two lobes to open relative to each other makes prediction of the pocket shape difficult in the absence of the bound ligand.

For this reason, some researchers choose to use a large binding pocket conformation as a starting template, selecting a staurosporine-bound or apo form of the kinase for modeling. This method is suggested for virtual screening exercises due to the larger binding site being able to accommodate a wider diversity of chemotypes—a desirable trait when trying to find hits in general compound collections. One thing, however, is clear: use of the ATP or ADP bound form for a model can lead to failure in virtual screening or lead optimization because of the very closed nature of the ATP pocket in this form—a conformation that is important for efficient catalysis but not as useful for inhibitor design (Diller and Li, 2003).

Other researchers choose a kinase template with a chemotype as similar as possible to their compound series of interest. The chemogenomic information within common SARs can be leveraged in multiple ways to provide a model that will best allow for optimization of a specific series. SAR homology can assist in aligning those nucleotide binding site details most important for a chemical series, which can be especially helpful when the template and target are not closely related. This was demonstrated in the example of mTOR modeling discussed earlier where ortholog conservation and SAR homology were used to drive both initial sequence alignment and final model validation (Tobak, 2007). Using a template with close SAR homology also helps optimize the structural details of the binding site for use in studying a specific series as was shown by Rockey and Elcock (2006), who performed an elegant study cross-docking staurosporine into homology models based on staurosporine-bound templates. It is not, however, without pitfalls as the Rockey–Elcock study also revealed relatively worse results with PIM1, a kinase with an insertion in the hinge.

Our analysis of AMPPNP and staurosporine structures discussed earlier also demonstrates that SAR-based template selection is an excellent approach with the caveat that the template should be checked carefully to be sure it is actually in the expected and desired conformation. The propensity for some kinases to adopt dramatically different conformations of the activation loop (DFG-in vs. DFG-out vs. C-helix out—Figure 17.5) requires some knowledge on the part of the modeler as to what form he/she is most interested in targeting with inhibitors. The good news is that there are multiple example templates for each conformation from which to start—though not necessarily closely related to your kinase of interest so a multitemplate model may be necessary to assist with reducing side chain clashes. When investigating a kinase with few or no known inhibitors, one of the biggest challenges is predicting whether or not it can adopt these special conformations. In this way, template(s) selection for homology modeling a given target mirrors selection of the appropriate crystal structure for docking when multiple crystal structures are available for a single protein. Homology modeling only differs in that one selects from different orthologous or paralogous kinases.

The accessibility of commercial kinase profiling assays from vendors such as Millipore, Novascreen, Invitrogen, and Ambit Biosciences provides a distinct advantage to those modelers looking to utilize SAR homologies for kinase comparative modeling. These companies have enzymatic assays developed for upwards of half the known kinome. An inhibitor for the target kinase could be submitted to a panel of these assays to "fish" for other kinases with similar inhibition profiles, as was shown in the BTK modeling example. Perhaps it would be useful to devise a "structurally enabled" kinase panel to more easily identify SAR homologs that can be used for modeling or co-crystallization efforts. This combined with ~25% of the kinome being "structurally enabled" greatly promotes kinase SBDD.

Not addressed in this chapter is the potential to build kinase homology models for allosteric inhibitor pockets such as those reported for MEK, CHK, and the myristoyl pocket of Bcr-Abl (Ohren et al., 2004; Adrián et al., 2006; Converso, 2008). At the time of this writing, we are unaware of published examples of homology models based on these sites. It is certainly straightforward to build a kinase homology model using the published co-crystal structures for MEK1 or MEK2 bound to their allosteric inhibitors as a template. It remains to be experimentally verified, however, whether or not other kinases adopt pockets similar to those reported, thus questioning the validity of such models in the first place. In the case of MEK1 and MEK2, kinase selectivity screenings by Ohren and colleagues suggest that PD184352-like inhibitors are highly specific to these kinases alone and cannot induce similar binding pockets in other kinases. Unfortunately, because allosteric sites appear to be ligand-induced conformations and depend on the plasticity of kinase conformations, they are difficult to predict a priori. However, as new allosteric inhibitors are discovered, a rational approach to developing related kinase homology models would be to combine experimental kinase selectivity panel data with chemogenomic homology modeling.

Overall, if we hold to Madhusudhan's guideline of 50% sequence identity between target and template being necessary for a quality model, over half of the kinome either has a structure in PDB or is amenable to SBDD via homology modeling (Figure 17.1). If we leverage the special characteristics of the kinome such as conserved fold, conserved structural elements, conformational homology, and SAR homology during the homology modeling process, even the most distantly related kinase in the kinome should not be dismissed as a possible target for homology modeling.

REFERENCES

Adrián, F. J., Ding, Q., Sim, T., et al. (**2006**). Allosteric inhibitors of Bcr-Abl-dependent cell proliferation. *Nat Chem Biol.* 2(2), 95–102.

Altschul, S. F., Madden, T. L., Schäffer, A. A., et al. (**1997**). Gapped BLAST and PSI-BLAST: a new generation of protein database search programs. *Nucleic Acids Res.* 25(17), 3389–3402.

Arnold, L. D., Calderwood, D. J., Dixon, R. W., et al. (**2000**). Pyrrolo[2,3-*d*]pyrimidines containing an extended 5-substituent as potent and selective inhibitors of lck I. *Bioorg Med Chem Lett.* 10(19), 2167–2170.

Atwell, S., Adams, J. M., Badger, J., et al. (**2004**). A novel mode of Gleevec binding is revealed by the structure of spleen tyrosine kinase. *J Biol Chem.* 279(53), 55827–55832.

Bates, P. A., and Sternberg, M. J. (**1999**). Model building by comparison at CASP3: using expert knowledge and computer automation. *Proteins Suppl.* 3, 47–54.

Bates, P. A., Kelley, L. A., MacCallum, R. M., et al. (**2001**). Enhancement of protein modeling by human intervention in applying the automatic programs 3D-JIGSAW and 3D-PSSM. *Proteins Suppl.* 5, 39–46.

Berman, H. M., Westbrook, J., Feng, Z., et al. (**2000**). The Protein Data Bank. *Nucleic Acids Res.* 28(1), 235–242.

Böhmer, F. D., Karagyozov, L., Uecker, A., et al. (**2003**). A single amino acid exchange inverts susceptibility of related receptor tyrosine kinases for the ATP site inhibitor STI-571. *J Biol Chem.* 278(7), 5148–5155.

Breitenlechner, C., Gassel, M., Hidaka, H., et al. (**2003**). Protein kinase A in complex with Rho-kinase inhibitors Y-27632, Fasudil, and H-1152P: structural basis of selectivity. *Structure* 11(12), 1595–1607.

Caldwell, J. J., Davies, T. G., Donald, A., et al. (**2008**). Identification of 4-(4-aminopiperidin-1-yl)-7*H*-pyrrolo[2,3-*d*]pyrimidines as selective inhibitors of protein kinase B through fragment elaboration. *J Med Chem.* 51(7), 2147–2157.

Canutescu, A. A., Shelenkov, A. A., and Dunbrack, R. L. (**2003**). A graph-theory algorithm for rapid protein side-chain prediction. *Protein Sci.* 12(9), 2001–2014.

Carlomagno, F., Guida, T., Anaganti, S., et al. (**2004**). Disease associated mutations at valine 804 in the RET receptor tyrosine kinase confer resistance to selective kinase inhibitors. *Oncogene.* 23(36), 6056–6063.

Chemical Computing Group, MOE molecular modeling package. Available at http://www.chemcomp.com.

Cohen, P. (**2002**). Protein kinases—the major drug targets of the twenty-first century? *Nat Rev Drug Discov.* 1(4), 309–315.

Converso, A. (**2008**). Development of thioquinazolinones, allosteric Chk1 kinase inhibitors. 236th ACS National Meeting, Philadelphia, PA.

Corpet, F. (**1988**). Multiple sequence alignment with hierarchical clustering. *Nucleic Acids Res.* 16(22), 10881–10890.

Davies, T. G., Verdonk, M. L., Graham, B., et al. (**2007**). A structural comparison of inhibitor binding to PKB, PKA and PKA-PKB chimera. *J Mol Biol.* 367(3), 882–894.

Diller, D. J., and Li, R. (**2003**). Kinases, homology models, and high throughput docking. *J Med Chem*. 46(22), 4638–4647.

Doolittle, R. (**1986**). *Of Urfs and Orfs: A Primer on How to Analyze Derived Amino Acid Sequences*. Sausalito, CA: University Science Books.

Dunbrack, R. L. (**2006**). Sequence comparison and protein structure prediction. *Curr Opin Structural Biol*. 16(3), 374–384.

Fabian, M. A., Biggs, W. H., Treiber, D. K., et al. (**2005**). A small molecule–kinase interaction map for clinical kinase inhibitors. *Nat Biotechnol*. 23(3), 329–336.

Fedorov, O., Sundström, M., Marsden, B., et al. (**2007**). Insights for the development of specific kinase inhibitors by targeted structural genomics. *Drug Discov. Today*. 12(9–10), 365–372.

Frye, S. V. (**1999**). Structure–activity relationship homology (SARAH): a conceptual framework for drug discovery in the genomic era. *Chem Biol*. 6(1), R3–7.

Ginalski, K. (**2006**). Comparative modeling for protein structure prediction. *Curr Opin Structural Biol*. 16(2), 172–177.

Gridelli, C., Maione, P., and Rossi, A. (**2008**). The potential role of mTOR inhibitors in non-small cell lung cancer. *Oncologist*. 13(2), 139–147.

Hanks, S. K., and Hunter, T. (**1995**). Protein kinases 6. The eukaryotic protein kinase superfamily: kinase (catalytic) domain structure and classification. *FASEB J*. 9(8), 576–596.

Hanks, S. K., and Quinn, A. M. (**1991**). Protein kinase catalytic domain sequence database: identification of conserved features of primary structure and classification of family members. In: B. M. Sefton and T. Hunter (eds.), *Methods in Enzymology*, Vol. 200, pp. 38–62. Hoboken, NJ: Wiley.

Hanks, S. K., Quinn, A. M., and Hunter, T. (**1988**). The protein kinase family: conserved features and deduced phylogeny of the catalytic domains. *Science*. 241(4861), 42–52.

Heron, N. M., Anderson, M., Blowers, D. P., et al. (**2006**). SAR and inhibitor complex structure determination of a novel class of potent and specific Aurora kinase inhibitors. *Bioorg Med Chem Lett*. 16(5), 1320–1323.

Honma, T., Hayashi, K., et al. (**2001a**). Structure-based generation of a new class of potent Cdk4 inhibitors: new de novo design strategy and library design. *J Med Chem*. 44(26), 4615–4627.

Honma, T., Yoshizumi, T., et al. (**2001b**). A novel approach for the development of selective Cdk4 inhibitors: library design based on locations of Cdk4 specific amino acid residues. *J Med Chem*. 44(26), 4628–4640.

Ikuta, M., Kamata, K., Fukasawa, K., et al. (**2001**). Crystallographic approach to identification of cyclin-dependent kinase 4 (CDK4)-specific inhibitors by using CDK4 mimic CDK2 protein. *J Biol Chem*. 276(29), 27548–27554.

Iwakubo, M., Takami, A., Okada, Y., et al. (**2007a**). Design and synthesis of Rho kinase inhibitors (II). *Bioorg Med Chem*. 15(1), 350–364.

Iwakubo, M., Takami, A., Okada, Y., et al. (**2007b**). Design and synthesis of rho kinase inhibitors (III). *Bioorg Med Chem*. 15(2), 1022–1033.

Jacobs, M. D., Caron, P. R., and Hare, B. J. (**2008**). Classifying protein kinase structures guides use of ligand-selectivity profiles to predict inactive conformations: structure of lck/imatinib complex. *Proteins*. 70(4), 1451–1460.

Jelić, D., Mildner, B., Kostrun, S., et al. (**2007**). Homology modeling of human Fyn kinase structure: discovery of rosmarinic acid as a new Fyn kinase inhibitor and in silico study of its possible binding modes. *J Med Chem.* 50(6), 1090–1100.

Johnson, D. A., Akamine, P., Radzio-Andzelm, E., et al. (**2001**). Dynamics of cAMP-dependent protein kinase. *Chem Rev.* 101(8), 2243–2270.

Kinoshita, T., Matsubara, M., Ishiguro, H., et al. (**2006**). Structure of human Fyn kinase domain complexed with staurosporine. *Biochem Biophys Res Commun.* 346(3), 840–844.

Larkin, M. A., Blackshields, G., Brown, N. P., et al. (**2007**). Clustal W and Clustal X version 2.0. *Bioinformatics (Oxford, England)*, 23(21), 2947–2948.

Laskowski, R. A., Rullmannn, J. A., MacArthur, M. W., et al. (**1996**). AQUA and PROCHECK-NMR: programs for checking the quality of protein structures solved by NMR. *J Biomol NMR.* 8(4), 477–486.

Li, W., Jaroszewski, L., and Godzik, A. (**2002**). Sequence clustering strategies improve remote homology recognitions while reducing search times. *Protein Eng.* 15(8), 643–649.

Lu, B., Wong, C. F., and McCammon, J. A. (**2005**). Release of ADP from the catalytic subunit of protein kinase A: a molecular dynamics simulation study. *Protein Sci.* 14(1), 159–168.

Madhusudhan, M. S., Marti-Renom, M. A., Eswar, N., et al. (**2005**). Comparative protein structure modeling. *In*: J. M. Walker (ed.), *The Proteomics Protocols Handbook*. Totowa, NJ: Humana Press, p. 1016.

Manning, G., Whyte, D. B., Martinez, R., et al. (**2002**). The protein kinase complement of the human genome. *Science.* 298(5600), 1912–1934.

Marsden, B. D., and Knapp, S. (**2008**). Doing more than just the structure–structural genomics in kinase drug discovery. *Curr Opin Chem Biol.* 12(1), 40–45.

Martí-Renom, M. A., Stuart, A. C., Fiser, A., et al. (**2000**). Comparative protein structure modeling of genes and genomes. *Annu Rev Biophys Biomol Structure.* 29, 291–325.

Mavrou, A., Tsangaris, G. T., Roma, E., et al. (**2008**). The ATM gene and ataxia telangiectasia. *Anticancer Res.* 28(1B), 401–405.

McInnes, C., Wang, S., Anderson, S., et al. (**2004**). Structural determinants of CDK4 inhibition and design of selective ATP competitive inhibitors. *Chem Biol.* 11(4), 525–534.

McInnes, C., Mezna, M., and Fischer, P. M. (**2005**). Progress in the discovery of polo-like kinase inhibitors. *Curr Top Med Chem.* 5(2), 181–197.

Mol, C. D., Dougan, D. R., Schneider, T. R., et al. (**2004**). Structural basis for the autoinhibition and STI-571 inhibition of c-Kit tyrosine kinase. *J Biol Chem.* 279(30), 31655–31663.

Molsoft L. L. C., ICM-Homology Module. Available at http://www.molsoft.com/.

Mori, Y., Hirokawa, T., Aoki, K., et al. (**2008**). Structure-activity relationships of quinoxalin-2-one derivatives as platelet-derived growth factor beta receptor (PDGFRβ) inhibitors, derived from molecular modeling. *Chem Pharm Bull.* 56, 682–687.

Nagar, B., Bornmann, W. G., Pellicena, P., et al. (**2002**). Crystal structures of the kinase domain of c-Abl in complex with the small molecule inhibitors PD173955 and imatinib (STI-571). *Cancer Res.* 62(15), 4236–4243.

Nayeem, A., Sitkoff, D., and Krystek, S. (**2006**). A comparative study of available software for high-accuracy homology modeling: from sequence alignments to structural models. *Protein Sci.* 15(4), 808–824.

Noble, M. E. M., Endicott, J. A., and Johnson, L. N. (**2004**). Protein kinase inhibitors: insights into drug design from structure. *Science.* 303(5665), 1800–1805.

Ohren, J. F., Chen, H., Pavlovsky, A., et al. (**2004**). Structures of human MAP kinase kinase 1 (MEK1) and MEK2 describe novel noncompetitive kinase inhibition. *Nat Structural Mol Biol.* 11(12), 1192–1197.

Omura, S., Iwai, Y., Hirano, A., et al. (**1977**). A new alkaloid AM-2282 of *Streptomyces* origin. Taxonomy, fermentation, isolation and preliminary characterization. *J Antibiotics.* 30(4), 275–282.

Orengo, C. A., and Thornton, J. M. (**2005**). Protein families and their evolution—a structural perspective. *Annu Rev Biochem.* 74, 867–900.

Pan, Z., Scheerens, H., Li, S., et al. (**2007**). Discovery of selective irreversible inhibitors for Bruton's tyrosine kinase. *ChemMedChem.* 2(1), 58–61.

Petrey, D., Xiang, Z., Tang, C. L., et al. (**2003**). Using multiple structure alignments, fast model building, and energetic analysis in fold recognition and homology modeling. *Proteins.* 53(Suppl 6), 430–435.

Pratt, D. J., Bentley, J., Jewsbury, P., et al. (**2006**). Dissecting the determinants of cyclin-dependent kinase 2 and cyclin-dependent kinase 4 inhibitor selectivity. *J Med Chem.* 49(18), 5470–5477.

Rockey, W. M., and Elcock, A. H. (**2006**). Structure selection for protein kinase docking and virtual screening: homology models or crystal structures? *Curr Protein Peptide Sci.* 7(5), 437–457.

Sali, A., and Blundell, T. L. (**1993**). Comparative protein modelling by satisfaction of spatial restraints. *J Mol Biol.* 234(3), 779–815.

Sandberg, E. M., Ma, X., He, K., et al. (**2005**). Identification of 1,2,3,4,5,6-hexabromo-cyclohexane as a small molecule inhibitor of jak2 tyrosine kinase autophosphorylation [correction of autophophorylation]. *J Med Chem.* 48(7), 2526–2533.

Seeliger, M. A., Nagar, B., Frank, F., et al. (**2007**). c-Src binds to the cancer drug imatinib with an inactive Abl/c-Kit conformation and a distributed thermodynamic penalty. *Structure.* 15(3), 299–311.

Smith, S. M. (**2007**). Clinical development of mTOR inhibitors: a focus on lymphoma. *Rev Recent Clin Trials.* 2(2), 103–110.

Sutcliffe, M. J., Haneef, I., Carney, D., et al. (**1987**). Knowledge based modelling of homologous proteins, Part I: Three-dimensional frameworks derived from the simultaneous superposition of multiple structures. *Protein Eng.* 1(5), 377–384.

Takami, A., Iwakubo, M., Okada, Y., et al. (**2004**). Design and synthesis of Rho kinase inhibitors (I). *Bioorg Med Chem.* 12(9), 2115–2137.

Taylor, S. S. (**1989**). cAMP-dependent protein kinase. Model for an enzyme family. *J Biol Chem.* 264(15), 8443–8446.

Taylor, S. S., Kim, C., Vigil, D., et al. (**2005**). Dynamics of signaling by PKA. *Biochim Biophys Acta.* 1754(1–2), 25–37.

Tobak, A. T. (**2007**). Construction of the 3D structure of the mTOR kinase-domain and discovery of novel mTOR inhibitors. PhD thesis, Rutgers University.

Tripos, Inc., SYBYL molecular modeling package. Available at http://www.tripos.com.

Tsou, H., Otteng, M., Tran, T., et al. (**2008**). 4-(Phenylaminomethylene)isoquinoline-1,3(2H,4H)-diones as potent and selective inhibitors of the cyclin-dependent kinase 4 (CDK4). *J Med Chem.* 51(12), 3507–3525.

Tuccinardi, T., Manetti, F., Schenone, S., et al. (**2007**). Construction and validation of a RET TK catalytic domain by homology modeling. *J Chem Inf Modeling.* 47(2), 644–655.

UniProt Consortium (**2008**). The universal protein resource (UniProt). *Nucleic Acids Res.* 36(Database issue), D190–195.

Vangrevelinghe, E., Zimmermann, K., Schoepfer, J., et al. (**2003**). Discovery of a potent and selective protein kinase CK2 inhibitor by high-throughput docking. *J Med Chem.* 46(13), 2656–2662.

Verma, S., Nagarathnam, D., Shao, J., et al. (**2005**). Substituted aminobenzimidazole pyrimidines as cyclin-dependent kinase inhibitors. *Bioorg Med Chem Lett.* 15(8), 1973–1977.

Vieth, M., Sutherland, J. J., Robertson, D. H., et al. (**2005**). Kinomics: characterizing the therapeutically validated kinase space. *Drug Discov. Today.* 10(12), 839–846.

Vriend, G. (**1990**). WHAT IF: a molecular modeling and drug design program. *J Mol Graphics.* 8(1), 52–56, 29.

Walker, E. H., Pacold, M. E., Perisic, O., et al. (**2000**). Structural determinants of phosphoinositide 3-kinase inhibition by wortmannin, LY294002, quercetin, myricetin, and staurosporine. *Mol Cell.* 6(4), 909–919.

Wang, S., Meades, C., Wood, G., et al. (**2004**). 2-Anilino-4-(thiazol-5-yl)pyrimidine CDK inhibitors: synthesis, SAR analysis, X-ray crystallography, and biological activity. *J Med Chem.* 47(7), 1662–1675.

Xiang, Z. (**2006**). Advances in homology protein structure modeling. *Curr Protein Peptide Sci.* 7(3), 217–227.

Yount, R. G., Babcock, D., Ballantyne, W., et al. (**1971**). Adenylyl imidodiphosphate, an adenosine triphosphate analog containing a P–N–P linkage. *Biochemistry.* 10(13), 2484–2489.

Zheng, J., Trafny, E. A., Knighton, D. R., et al. (**1993**). 2.2 Å refined crystal structure of the catalytic subunit of cAMP-dependent protein kinase complexed with MnATP and a peptide inhibitor. *Acta Crystallogr D. Biol.* 49(Pt 3), 362–365.

18

FRAGMENT-BASED DRUG DISCOVERY OF KINASE INHIBITORS

Daniel A. Erlanson

18.1. INTRODUCTION

Fragment-based drug discovery has emerged in the past decade as a powerful complement to other methods of finding lead compounds. The basic concept stems from the recognition that far more possible small molecules exist than could ever be assembled and tested. A widely quoted estimate is that there are roughly 10^{63} possible drug-like molecules with molecular weights less than about 500 Da (Bohacek et al., 1996) while the worldwide screening collection is estimated to be only 100 million molecules (Hann and Oprea, 2004). However, just as there are many fewer two-letter words than four-letter words, there are fewer possible molecules with molecular weights less than 250 Da than 500 Da. Indeed, one analysis puts the number of molecules with molecular weights less than or equal to 160 Da at "only" between 14 and 44 million (Fink et al., 2005). In principle, lead discovery could be accelerated over traditional screening (Figure 18.1A) if it were possible to screen these small "fragments," and then either expand the resulting hits (Figure 18.1B) or link them together (Figure 18.1C).

Although reducing this concept to practice poses serious challenges, the potential benefits of fragment-based approaches are sufficient to generate widespread interest. In addition to covering more chemical space, fragment-based drug discovery could be very efficient. The hit rate should be higher for smaller, simpler fragments since the more complex the molecule, the greater

Kinase Inhibitor Drugs. Edited by Rongshi Li and Jeffrey A. Stafford
Copyright © 2009 John Wiley & Sons, Inc.

a) Traditional HTS

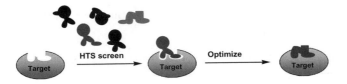

b) Fragment-based drug discovery, growing fragments

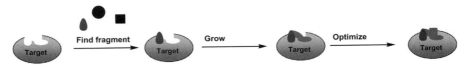

c) Fragment-based drug discovery, linking fragments

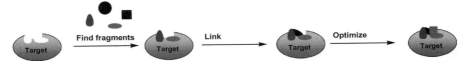

Figure 18.1. Different methods of drug discovery. (**A**) Traditional high-throughput screening (HTS) relies on large libraries of relatively large molecules. Hits may bind suboptimally (lower left), and near hits may be missed due to interfering substituents (upper right). (**B**) Fragment-based drug discovery screens fewer, smaller fragments. Once identified, a fragment can be grown to improve its potency, or (**C**) linked with another fragment. Note that in all three cases some degree of optimization is likely needed.

chance of substituents that block interactions with a protein target; such substituents will be more common than those that can productively engage with the target. This was elegantly demonstrated computationally by Hann et al. (2001) but can also be appreciated in Figure 18.1A, where one member of the HTS library has all of the correct binding elements, but also contains a blocking element that prevents it from binding to the target.

Just as fragments are less likely to have blocking elements than are larger molecules, they are also less likely to have extraneous chemical moieties that may not productively engage the target, but only increase the size of the molecule. This is captured in the concept of "ligand efficiency," which is defined as the free energy of binding divided by the number of heavy atoms (Kuntz et al., 1999; Hopkins et al., 2004; Abad-Zapatero and Metz, 2005; Reynolds et al., 2008). A molecule with high ligand efficiency will be smaller than an equipotent molecule with a lower ligand efficiency and is thus more likely to conform to the "Rule-of-5" criteria that correlate with oral bioavailability (Lipinski et al., 1997).

In this chapter I review the application of fragment-based drug discovery to the discovery of kinase inhibitors, highlighting areas where fragment-based methods were particularly useful as well as areas that could still be improved.

18.2. HISTORICAL DEVELOPMENT

Given the potential advantages, it is perhaps surprising that fragment-based approaches to drug discovery only recently became widespread. In fact, the theoretical underpinnings of the approach were proposed in the early 1980s by William Jencks, who described the energetic advantages of finding and linking two fragments, each of which has low affinity for a target (Jencks, 1981). However, practical limitations prevented much experimental follow-up: small fragments, with their smaller surface areas, generally bind a target with lower affinity than larger molecules, and detecting low-affinity binders can be challenging. The simplest method for discovering small-molecule binders is a biochemical assay that detects inhibition. Such assays are readily amenable to high-throughput formats and miniaturization, but, unfortunately, they are also susceptible to a wide variety of artifacts. Although some of these artifacts arise when impure or reactive molecules are screened (Rishton, 2003), many small molecules can also form aggregates that cause inhibition in a biochemical assay without binding stoichiometrically to the protein (McGovern et al., 2002; McGovern et al., 2003; Ryan et al., 2003). This effect can be particularly pronounced at the high concentrations needed to discover low-affinity inhibitors and, relevant to this book, can even occur with legitimate kinase inhibitors (McGovern and Shoichet, 2003). Worse, this phenomenon was not appreciated until the early 21st century, so for many years low-affinity molecules were justifiably regarded with suspicion and disdain in the pharmaceutical industry.

Widespread interest in fragment-based drug discovery is traced back to 1996, with the publication of a paper in *Science* by Abbott researchers describing the use of NMR spectroscopy to identify two fragments that each bound weakly to FK506 binding protein (FKBP); structural information revealed how to productively link them (Shuker et al., 1996). This was followed a year later by a paper that used the approach to discover nonpeptidic inhibitors of stromelysin, revealing that fragment-based drug discovery was not only practical but could also be used to discover novel leads against challenging targets (Hajduk et al., 1997). Within the next few years, numerous researchers developed strategies for fragment-based drug discovery, using a variety of techniques including NMR, X-ray crystallography, mass spectrometry, computational approaches, dynamic combinatorial chemistry, surface plasmon resonance, and even functional screening. A full consideration of these techniques is beyond the scope of this chapter. However, at least one book and numerous reviews cover various aspects of fragment-based drug discovery (Jahnke and Erlanson, 2006; Erlanson et al., 2004a; Rees et al.,

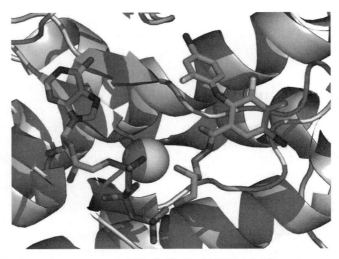

Figure 18.2. Crystal structure of ATP (*left*), PD318088 (*right*), and a magnesium ion (sphere) bound to MEK1. In total, there are 58 nonhydrogen atoms making up these three ligands (not counting water molecules), with a total molecular weight of more than 1000 Da. Although the high molecular weight is due in part to the halogens and phosphorus atoms, the number of heavy atoms is roughly the molecular weight of *two* good-sized drugs. Figure made using PyMOL (DeLano, PyMOL graphics system).

2004; Erlanson, 2006; Hajduk and Greer, 2007; Congreve et al., 2008). In addition, an earlier review covering fragment-based drug discovery as applied to kinases has also been published (Gill, 2004).

18.2.1. Kinases and Fragment-Based Drug Discovery

As a class, protein kinases are well suited for fragment-based drug discovery. Their active sites have evolved to bind both ATP as well as a peptide or protein substrate, thus providing numerous subpockets capable of binding fragments. Liao (2007) has provided a thorough analysis of the structural features of kinases, but the following example illustrates the point.

The kinases MEK1 and MEK2 are actively pursued anticancer targets (Wang et al., 2007). Researchers at Pfizer have discovered a class of inhibitors that bind in an adaptive pocket of both MEK1 and MEK2; these compounds are exquisitely selective for MEK and, surprisingly, bind in the presence of ATP and a magnesium ion (Ohren et al., 2004). Figure 18.2 shows a structure of one of these compounds (PD318088), ATP, and a magnesium ion bound to MEK1. As seen in the figure, the volume of available space for binding makes kinases ideal for drug discovery in general, and especially for fragment-based drug discovery.

Although the binding mode (in the adaptive pocket with no extension into the purine binding site) observed for the MEK inhibitors is unusual, many kinase inhibitors extend from the purine-binding site into the adaptive pocket.

Indeed, imatinib (Hunter, 2007), the first kinase inhibitor clinically approved in the United States, binds in just such an extended fashion (Schindler et al., 2000; Nagar et al., 2002). Such inhibitors lend themselves particularly well to fragment-based drug discovery: the purine-binding element and adaptive-site binder can be discovered as independent fragments. Moreover, because the adaptive pocket is less conserved than the ATP-binding pocket, there is theoretically greater potential for developing selective kinase inhibitors by making use of this pocket. However, it is possible to achieve highly specific kinase inhibitors that do not bind in the adaptive binding site (Karaman et al., 2008), and, as illustrated later, fragment-based drug discovery is also useful for discovering these types of inhibitors.

18.2.2. Precedents: Inhibitors from Fragment-like Hits

A few well-known examples of kinase inhibitors that did not formally arise from fragment-based drug discovery are particularly illustrative of how the approach could be used.

Raf-1. One of the first kinase inhibitors to reach the market was sorafenib, an inhibitor of Raf-1, VEGFR, and several other kinases. The molecule was discovered at Onyx Pharmaceuticals and received FDA approval for treatment of advanced renal cell carcinoma in late 2005 (Kane et al., 2006). The discovery process started with a classic high-throughput screen (HTS) of 200,000 compounds, resulting in the identification of the 17 μM hit shown in Figure 18.3A, which was subsequently optimized through medicinal chemistry (Lowinger et al., 2002). The starting compound is a fairly weak hit from an HTS campaign, where most compounds that are pursued by medicinal chemists tend to be single-digit micromolar or even nanomolar. That said, it is not quite as weak as a typical fragment hit; these tend to be high micromolar or even millimolar in their affinities. However, there are a number of examples of fragment screens that have yielded hits of comparable potency (Erlanson, 2006). Regarding the chemical properties of the hit, it has a molecular weight of 332 Da, with 23 heavy (nonhydrogen) atoms. This is on the large size for fragments, which generally have molecular weights of less than 300 Da, or about 20 heavy atoms (Erlanson, 2006). Indeed, this could perhaps be more properly considered a "lead-like" than "fragment-like" molecule, albeit a somewhat lipophilic one (Teague et al., 1999). Nonetheless, one could imagine a slightly smaller starting molecule, with a slightly weaker affinity, being identified from a fragment screen and leading to the final compound. Indeed, the analog without the methyl ester substituent still shows measurable activity and is less ambiguously fragment-like (with a molecular weight of 288 Da and 20 heavy atoms) (Lowinger et al., 2002).

p38. A similar case can be made for the p38 inhibitor BIRB 796, which was also derived from a biaryl urea discovered through HTS at Boehringer Ingelheim (Figure 18.3B) (Pargellis et al., 2002). In this case, crystallography

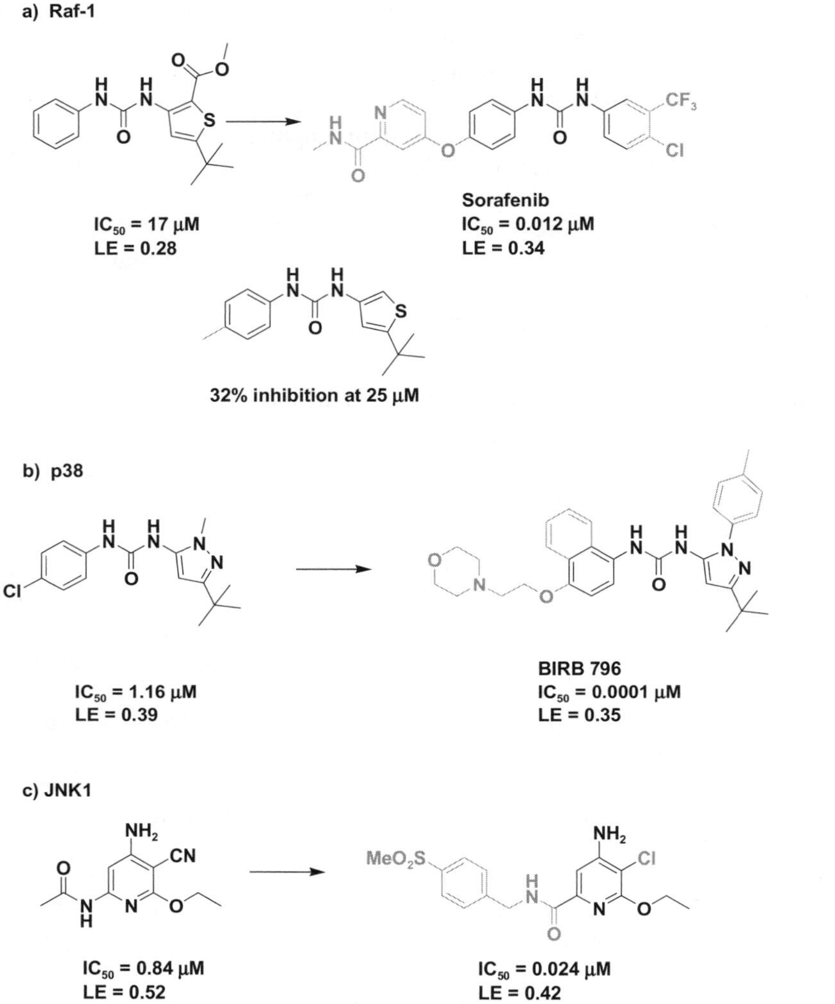

Figure 18.3. Examples of molecules that could have been discovered through fragment-based methods, but were actually identified using more traditional methods. LE = ligand efficiency.

revealed that the HTS hit was binding in the adaptive binding pocket of the kinase, with no extension into the purine-binding pocket. In fact, the compound binds to a "DFG-out" form of the protein, which is incompatible with ATP binding. Structure-based design led to subsequent improvements in potency by building into the purine-binding site, ultimately leading to the picomolar inhibitor BIRB 796, which subsequently entered clinical trials for Crohn's disease (Schreiber et al., 2006).

As in the case of sorafenib, the final clinical candidate incorporates portions of the initial fragment. In fact, in this case, both sides of the biaryl urea contain recognizable elements of the initial fragment. Although the initial hit is slightly larger than many of the fragments that will be discussed later (with a molecular weight of 307 Da and 21 heavy atoms), it is still distinctly fragment-like. Its distinguishing characteristic is really the fact that it has a sufficiently high potency that it could be detected in an HTS format.

JNK1. The two previous examples highlight fragment-like hits that bind in the adaptive pocket and were subsequently grown into the purine-binding site. However, fragment-like hits have also been identified that bind in the purine-binding site itself. An example is the c-Jun NH_2 terminal kinase 1 (JNK1) hit shown in Figure 18.3C, which was identified in a high-throughput screen at Abbott Laboratories (Zhao et al., 2006). Unlike the two earlier examples, this is unambiguously a fragment, with only 16 heavy atoms and a molecular weight of 220 Da. However, it is a very potent fragment, with an affinity of better than 1 μM. Subsequent medicinal chemistry led to a 24 nM inhibitor that is orally bioavailable, has good pharmacokinetic properties, and is selective for JNK1 and JNK2 over a panel of 76 other kinases. What distinguishes this from most examples of fragment-based drug discovery is the fact that the starting hit, although small, was also very potent, and therefore could be detected in a conventional screening assay. The high potency and ligand efficiency of the initial hit also meant that less than two orders of magnitude improvement in binding energy was sufficient to achieve low nanomolar inhibitors.

18.3. FRAGMENT-BASED DRUG DISCOVERY OF KINASE INHIBITORS

A key difference between HTS and fragment-based approaches is that the starting points are usually smaller and less potent. However, as shown next, it is possible to achieve highly potent compounds even starting from much weaker initial binders.

B-Raf. The previous section described how a high-throughput screen resulted in a fragment-like hit that was subsequently optimized to the approved anticancer drug sorafenib, which inhibits Raf as well as other kinases. However, Raf has also been the target of fragment-based screening, or "scaffold-based drug design," as Plexxikon refers to its methodology (Card et al., 2005). In this case, researchers screened a library of 20,000 compounds ranging in size from 150 to 350 Da in a functional assay against a panel of kinases at the relatively high concentration of 200 μM. Of these, 238 inhibited Pim-1, p38, and the kinase CSK at least 30%. These were subsequently characterized in more than 100 co-crystal structures. The compound 7-azaindole (Figure 18.4) bound in the adenine-binding site of Pim-1, although multiple binding modes were

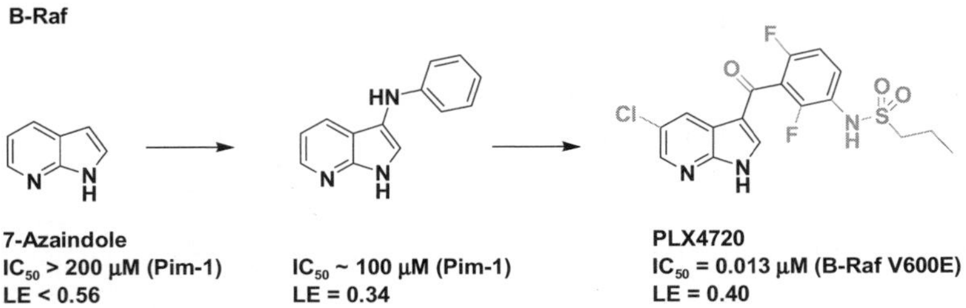

Figure 18.4. Discovery of a B-Raf kinase inhibitor using fragment-based methods.

observed in crystallographically distinct monomers. Subsequent chemistry resulted in the 3-aminophenyl-substituted azaindole (Figure 18.4), which was found by crystallography to have a single binding mode. This led to the synthesis of a series of libraries, screening against multiple kinases, and medicinal chemistry, culminating in the compound PLX4720, which is selective for the oncogenic B-raf mutant V600E (with an IC_{50} of 13 nM) over wild-type B-Raf ($IC_{50} = 160$ nM) (Tsai et al., 2008). The compound is also selective for the B-raf mutant relative to a panel of 70 other kinases, including Pim-1.

Crystallographic characterization of PLX4720 with B-Raf revealed, interestingly, two distinct conformations of protein: the predominant binding mode appeared to be an active DFG-in form of the protein, although a lower occupancy inactive DFG-out binding mode was also observed. In both cases, the azaindole forms two hydrogen bonds to the hinge region of the protein. The compound is active in cells and causes tumor regressions in xenograft mouse models, and a compound believed to be related to PLX4720 has entered clinical trials for melanoma.

This example illustrates several features of fragment-based drug discovery. First, unlike in the case of sorafenib, this program started unambiguously from a fragment; 7-azaindole has a molecular weight of only 118 Da, with 9 non-hydrogen atoms. Thus a weak fragment can be advanced to a potent molecule. Second, although fragment screening was applied against one set of kinases, inhibitors could be identified against a different kinase not included in the original screening set. This is similar to other, more conventional kinase inhibitor programs, where it is common to screen existing compounds against new kinases to look for hits. Finally, although the initial fragment was quite promiscuous, the molecule derived from it was highly selective. Although the advantages of promiscuous versus selective fragments are debated, this example demonstrates that a promiscuous starting point does not prevent subsequent selectivity.

A potential criticism is that, as most readers of this book are aware, 7-azaindole is a privileged (or highly established) kinase-binding element. Indeed, this fragment makes another appearance in the context of AKT (see later and Figure 18.6). However, it should be noted that although most kinase researchers today are well aware of 7-azaindole as a hinge-binding element,

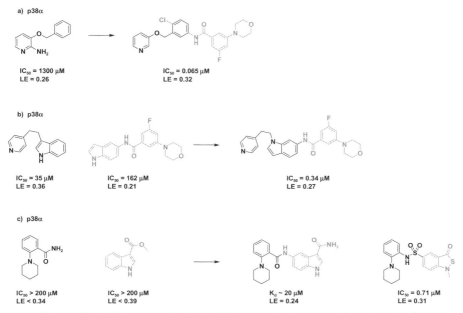

Figure 18.5. Discovery of p38α inhibitors using fragment-based methods.

this was not the case several years ago, when the research described in these papers occurred. Moreover, even if a fragment is common, it may still be worth pursuing, although with an eye toward rapidly establishing novelty.

p38. Unlike Plexxikon, which relies heavily on functional screening of medium-sized libraries, researchers at Astex have developed a screening technology based largely on crystallography with smaller fragment collections, containing as few as a few hundred compounds. One of their early reports described the discovery of a series of inhibitors of the kinase p38α, an attractive target for a variety of inflammatory diseases (Cook et al., 2007). In one case, a simple aminopyridine compound discovered in a crystallographic screen was found to have a very weak affinity for p38α (1.3 mM, Figure 18.5A). However, by applying knowledge from previous medicinal chemistry programs to this target, the researchers were able to rapidly improve the potency to 65 nM (Gill et al., 2005a). This molecule was characterized crystallographically and found to bind in the DFG-out conformation.

A similar strategy was applied to a different chemical starting point (Figure 18.5B). In this case, an indole-substituted pyridine was found to bind competitively to the hinge region of p38 (Gill et al., 2005b). The indole moiety of this fragment was combined with the phenyl morpholino fragment previously identified to generate a new fragment that bound with only high micromolar potency, but which could be crystallographically characterized as binding to the protein in the DFG-out conformation. Merging this molecule with the aminopyridyl moiety initially identified led to the high-nanomolar compound shown. Crystallography revealed that this molecule binds in the same mode as the component fragments.

Another fragment-based approach to p38 inhibitors was reported by researchers at the Burnham Institute (Chen et al., 2007). In this case, the authors used an innovative NMR (nuclear magnetic resonance) strategy called ILOE (interligand nuclear Overhauser effect), which allows the detection of two ligands that bind to a protein in close proximity (Becattini et al., 2006). By screening an inactive form of p38α against a mixture of 96 compounds, the researchers found two fragments that bind in close proximity to one another, even though the affinities of both fragments were worse than 200 µM. However, linking the two fragments together produced a molecule with an affinity of roughly 20 µM for the inactive form of the protein. A second molecule was discovered by computationally searching a commercial library for compounds with similar features to the two fragments; when tested, this molecule inhibited the kinase in the high nanomolar range, with good selectivity against other p38 isoforms (Figure 18.5c).

Akt/PKB. An elegant example of a fragment-growing approach has been reported by researchers at Astex Therapeutics and the Institute of Cancer Research in a series of papers. The target they chose is Akt (or protein kinase B, PKB), a hotly pursued oncology target (Cheng et al., 2005). An initial virtual screen of about 300,000 commercially available fragments yielded a number of promising hits that were confirmed by biochemical screening and high-throughput crystallography using a closely related protein, PKA, that had been mutagenized to increase its similarity to Akt (Gassel et al., 2003). One of the fragments identified as binding in the purine-binding site was 7-azaindole, a privileged kinase pharmacophore (see the earlier discussion of Raf). Although this fragment did not show activity in the biochemical assay, crystallography and knowledge of other inhibitors (particularly the importance of a basic amine) provided ideas for rapid optimization, leading to a low-micromolar compound shown in Figure 18.6A. Further structure-based drug design yielded the low-nanomolar inhibitor shown, which also displayed growth inhibition and target modulation in multiple cellular assays (Donald et al., 2007).

A second series of compounds also traces its origin to the 7-azaindole fragment (Caldwell et al., 2008). In an effort to modulate the lipophilicity of the molecules, researchers swapped the original phenyl group off the hinge-binding fragment for piperidine (Figure 18.6B). Subsequent medicinal chemistry led to a low-nanomolar Akt inhibitor with an impressive 30-fold selectivity versus the closely related PKA. This compound also demonstrated reasonable potency in a cellular assay and encouraging pharmaceutical properties in mice, including a high volume of distribution and low CYP inhibition.

The researchers also found a second fragment through crystallography-based screening; this substituted pyrazole also binds to the hinge region of

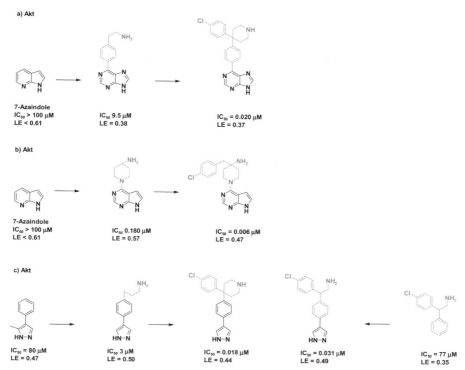

Figure 18.6. Discovery of Akt inhibitors using fragment-based methods.

the protein, forming two hydrogen bonds and, unlike the azaindole fragment, shows measurable activity in a biochemical assay (Figure 18.6C). As before, structure-based optimization led to low-nanomolar inhibitors (Saxty et al., 2007). One nice feature of this study was the ability to dissect the energetic contributions of each fragment of the molecule to overall binding affinity, with the conclusion that the majority of the binding energy resides in the pyrazole (hinge-binding) fragment. Nonetheless, the authors were able to remove the pyrazole moiety and retain micromolar binding affinity as well as demonstrate that the resulting fragment binds in roughly the same manner as the final compound (Figure 18.6C, furthest right). This could be considered an example of fragment-merging or fragment-linking, albeit in retrospect, as the exercise was done after the final molecule had been discovered. Moreover, the free energy of binding of the final molecule is greater than the sum of the free energies of binding of the two fragments, demonstrating at least some of the entropic advantages that would be expected (Murray and Verdonk, 2002).

Collectively, these three examples on a single target demonstrate the ability of fragment-based drug discovery to rapidly yield multiple series of drug leads. Akt has proven to be a very challenging target throughout the pharmaceutical industry, with many programs ultimately abandoned. Although it remains too early to say whether Astex's efforts will yield a drug, the company has chosen a preclinical development candidate, AT13148 (Congreve et al., 2008).

PDK1. Immediately upstream of Akt in the PI3-kinase signaling pathway lies PDK1, an intriguing but less actively pursued cancer target (Mora et al., 2004). Researchers at Vernalis have described an example of fragment growing and merging to identify inhibitors against this target, starting from a library of some 1400 fragments tested in a staurosporine displacement assay (Hubbard et al., 2007). Over 80 active fragments were identified, of which more than 40 also showed binding in two additional orthogonal assays, and a number of crystal structures were solved. One of these fragments was the substituted imidazole shown in Figure 18.7 (top left). Structure-based design led to a low-micromolar inhibitor.

Another attractive fragment identified was the substituted pyrazole shown in Figure 18.7, with mid-micromolar potency. A second, benzimidazole-containing fragment was designed and synthesized based on a series of known kinase inhibitors and was found to bind to PDK1 with low-micromolar potency. By combining elements of these two fragments with elements of the previous series, the researchers were able to produce a compound with mid-nanomolar potency.

This example provides an interesting case of fragment-inspired medicinal chemistry, in which low-affinity fragments discovered de novo were merged with more potent known fragments to identify a new molecule. Although the final molecule could conceivably have been arrived at using traditional

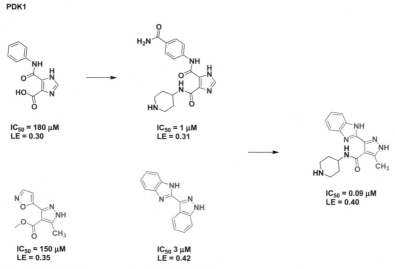

Figure 18.7. Discovery of a PDK1 inhibitor using fragment-based methods.

medicinal chemistry, the use of fragment-derived information may have accelerated the process.

CDK2. Cyclin-dependent kinase 2 (CDK2) is the target of multiple anticancer drugs in the clinic (Fischer, 2004). An unusual, dynamic combinatorial approach to fragment-based lead discovery was described by researchers at Astex several years ago (Congreve et al., 2003). Dynamic combinatorial chemistry involves the reversible formation of bonds between individual molecules, usually with some selection pressure to favor molecules that have a desired property such as binding to a receptor (Ramstrom and Lehn, 2002; Rowan et al., 2002). The Astex researchers realized that a previously reported inhibitor of CDK2 containing a hydrazone moiety could form from two fragments in aqueous conditions (Bramson et al., 2001). They found that, by soaking component fragments into crystals of CDK2, they could identify the high-affinity hydrazone product shown in Figure 18.8A (top right) using X-ray crystallography, even from a mixture containing up to 30 different hydrazones. Although it is not clear whether the ligands first form in solution and then diffuse into the CDK2 crystals, or whether CDK2 actually catalyzes the formation of the hydrazone bond, either provides proof of concept for applying dynamic combinatorial chemistry to fragment-based drug discovery.

A more traditional (if such a word can be used in such a young field) use of fragment-based drug discovery to identify CDK2 inhibitors has recently been disclosed by Astex (Wyatt et al., 2008). In this case, a library of 500 fragments was screened in pools of four against the protein using high-throughput crystallography, resulting in about 30 structures. Several were pursued to

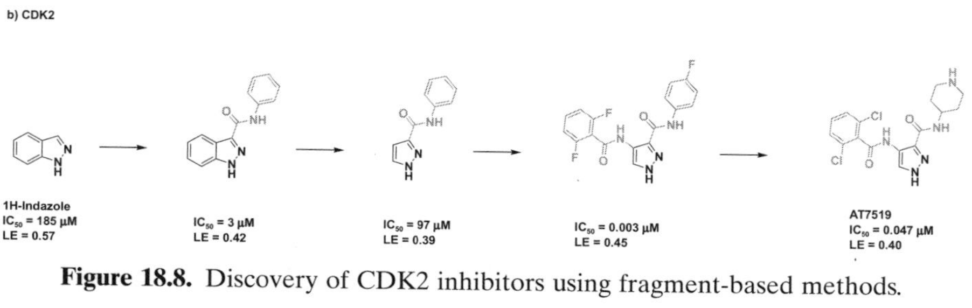

Figure 18.8. Discovery of CDK2 inhibitors using fragment-based methods.

micromolar or nanomolar inhibitors, with the most productive series starting with the indazole shown in Figure 18.8B, which had an IC_{50} of 185 µM. The addition of a phenyl linked through an amide bond increased potency, and crystallography revealed that the amide bond was making a third hydrogen bond in the hinge region in addition to the two to the indazole moiety. Paring back the indazole to a pyrazole reduced potency, but building a second amide off the pyrazole led to a 3 nM inhibitor. Finally, replacing one of the aromatic rings with a piperidine moiety improved the solubility without reducing potency too much, yielding AT7519 (Figure 18.8B). The compound shows a good tumor-to-plasma ratio, caused tumors to regress in mouse xenograft models, and, as of early 2008, was in Phase II clinical testing for cancer treatment (Wyatt et al., 2008).

Aurora. The Aurora kinases are key mitotic regulators and, as such, have been actively pursued as anticancer targets by numerous researchers using a variety of methods, including fragment-based approaches (Keen and Taylor, 2004). Researchers at the University of Arizona took a computational fragment approach (Warner et al., 2006). Using the crystal structure of Aurora-A, they applied the program LUDI to screen fragments that could bind to the protein (Bohm, 1992). This procedure identified a number of fragments, all of which had previously been reported as kinase inhibitors, though not necessarily against Aurora. The tricyclic molecule shown in Figure 18.9A was synthesized and found to inhibit the enzyme with low-micromolar potency. Interestingly, the sulfonamide shown in Figure 18.9A, which LUDI had docked in the phosphate-binding region, also showed measurable inhibition. Modeling suggested a strategy for linking the two fragments, yielding an ATP-competitive inhibitor with an IC_{50} of 94 nM.

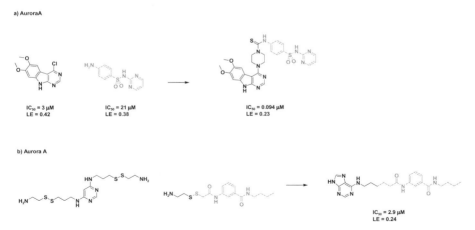

Figure 18.9. Discovery of Aurora-A inhibitors using fragment-based methods.

Another series of Aurora inhibitors was discovered by researchers at Sunesis, using a different fragment-linking approach (Cancilla et al., 2008). Sunesis originally developed a fragment-discovery technology called Tethering®, which uses a transient disulfide bond to identify fragments that bind to a protein in the vicinity of a natural or an introduced cysteine residue (Erlanson et al., 2000, 2004b). A second-generation version of the technology, Tethering with extenders, solved the linking dilemma by first covalently attaching a small-molecule "extender" to a cysteine on the protein and then using this to identify a second fragment through a transient disulfide bond (Erlanson et al., 2003). In the case of Aurora-A, the researchers used a variant of this approach, Tethering with dynamic extenders, in which the extender contains two disulfide moieties; the protein forms a disulfide bond with both the extender as well as with any fragment that binds in the vicinity. The researchers discovered one fragment that, when combined with the diaminopyrimidine-binding element of the extender, gave a 17 µM inhibitor. Optimization improved the potency to 2.9 µM, and crystallography confirmed that the molecule binds with the purine moiety in the purine-binding pocket and the newly identified fragment in the adaptive region, in a DFG-out conformation (Figure 18.9B) (Cancilla et al., 2008).

Other Examples. The kinase inhibitors described previously were chosen because they were either reported recently or exemplify specific methods of fragment-based drug discovery particularly clearly. Several older examples are worth mentioning. One of the first instances of fragment-based discovery applied to kinases was from researchers at the University of California, Berkeley, who used an iterative screening-linking procedure called combinatorial target-guided ligand assembly to discovery nanomolar inhibitors of the kinase c-Src (Maly et al., 2000). Researchers at Roche also used a fragment-based approach (this one relying heavily on crystallography) against the Src protein to discover nanomolar inhibitors that bind to the SH2 domain rather than the kinase domain (Lesuisse et al., 2002; Lange et al., 2003).

Another early report of fragment-based drug discovery, this one using an NMR-based screening technique called SHAPES (Fejzo et al., 1999), produced high-nanomolar inhibitors against the kinase JNK3; subsequent optimization guided by X-ray crystallography took the potency to less than 10 nM (Fejzo et al., 2003). An early fragment-based drug discovery company, Triad Therapeutics, used NMR to discover low-nanomolar p38α inhibitors (Sem, 2006). More recently, researchers at SGX Pharmaceuticals have reported the use of crystallography-driven fragment approaches to discover highly selective inhibitors of the oncology target c-Met, although chemical structures have not been disclosed (Burley, 2008). One of these compounds, SGX523, entered the clinic in 2008, although trials were suspended because of unexpected toxicity. Finally, an excellent recent review compiles a number of additional kinase targets that have been pursued using fragment-based drug discovery, including

CHK1, CK2, FMS/KIT, JNK2, KDR, REDK, SYK, and other examples of Akt and Aurora (Hajduk and Greer, 2007).

18.4. RELATED APPROACHES

In addition to fragment-based discovery of small-molecule kinase inhibitors, a number of researchers have explored the conceptually similar approach of linking peptides to small molecules in order to develop potent, specific inhibitors. Some of the earliest work along these lines, predating most small-molecule fragment-based drug discovery, consisted of using the "bisubstrate approach," in which an ATP mimetic was conjugated to a substrate-peptide (Ricouart et al., 1991). In one of the first examples, researchers at the Institut Pasteur in France linked an isoquinoline-5-sulfonamide moiety to a Ser-$(Arg)_6$ oligopeptide via a flexible linker to yield a 4 nM inhibitor of cyclic AMP-dependent protein kinase (PKA) (Ricouart et al., 1991). More recently, a variant of 3'-deoxyadenosine was conjugated to hexa-(D-arginine) through an alkyl linker to produce somewhat selective, low-nanomolar inhibitors of cAMP-dependent protein kinase (Enkvist et al., 2007). Similar approaches have involved conjugating small molecules to proteins, large or small, to develop selective kinase inhibitors (Shen and Cole, 2003; Schneider et al., 2005).

An interesting fragment-inspired approach using phage display was reported in 2007 by researchers from the University of Arizona (Erlanson, 2007; Meyer et al., 2007). A small molecule that binds kinases (staurosporine) was conjugated to the protein Jun, and a library of small cyclic oliogopeptides with six variable amino acids was built at the N terminus of its dimer partner, Fos, which was displayed on phage. Next, the modified Jun was mixed with the Fos library and screened against a target kinase. The idea is that when Fos and Jun dimerize, those dimers in which *both* the small molecule and the variable oligopeptide bind to a target protein will bind preferentially. The libraries were screened against cAMP-dependent protein kinase, or protein kinase A (PKA). One cyclic oligopeptide thus identified had modest affinity on its own, but when conjugated to staurosporine via a long, flexible linker the resulting molecule had a potency of 2.6 nM, more than 90-fold better than staurosporine and more than five orders of magnitude more potent than the cyclic peptide. The conjugate also displayed some selectivity against other kinases.

Finally, researchers at the Burnham Institute have reported a clever NMR-based method for finding novel kinase inhibitors (Vazquez et al., 2008). They start with an ATP-directed fragment to which they conjugate a paramagnetic probe; this serves as a reporter element for compounds that bind in the vicinity of the probe. In a proof-of-concept study targeted against the JNK kinases, the researchers demonstrated that they could use this technique to detect the binding of a peptide taken from a scaffolding protein that binds to a docking site outside the kinase active site. By linking a tripeptide portion of this scaffolding protein to the small-molecule probe through a glycine–glycine

linker, the researchers were able to produce an inhibitor with nanomolar activity against both JNK1 and JNK2.

18.5. COMPARISON OF FRAGMENT-DERIVED MOLECULES TO OTHER INHIBITORS

Because the large active sites of kinases are particularly capable of accommodating rather sizable "small" molecules, many kinase inhibitors are in fact quite large, and often lipophilic. In fact, a recent review comparing the properties of 45 orally bioavailable anticancer protein kinase inhibitors in clinical development to those of marketed oral drugs found that the kinase inhibitors are, on average, larger (by an average of 119 Da), more lipophilic (by an average of 1.7 log units in $C\log P$), and more complex (roughly two more rotatable bonds) (Gill et al., 2007). The average molecular weight of the 45 compounds is 457 Da, with an average $C\log P$ of 4.1.

Will fragment-based drug discovery improve these properties? Of the 14 examples provided here, the average molecular weight of the final compound is 394 Da, with an average $C\log P$ of 2.99. These values are still higher than most orally bioavailable drugs, though not as high as many of the kinase inhibitors in clinical development. Of course, the comparison is not entirely fair, as only one of the examples (AT7519) is actually in the clinic, and many others are clearly only research tools or proof-of-concept molecules. Still, the trends bode favorably for fragment-based drug discovery.

18.6. OUTLOOK

At the beginning of this chapter, fragment-based ligand discovery was proposed to have several strengths, including high coverage of chemical space, accelerated discovery of starting points, and more ligand-efficient leads. While it is difficult to measure some of these metrics (e.g., most publications don't disclose how much time and how many researchers it took to achieve a milestone) and data are still limited, the preliminary analysis suggests that fragment-derived molecules may be more ligand-efficient than leads derived from more traditional methods.

Operationally, fragment-based drug discovery has the significant advantage that it requires a much smaller library of molecules than a typical HTS; the largest fragment libraries are only 20,000 members or so, and typically much less. The reduction in up-front costs and ongoing compound handling and curation efforts allows smaller biotech companies and even academic laboratories to rapidly discover active molecules. That said, the reduced costs of these smaller fragment libraries are at least partially offset by the specialized infrastructure necessary to screen them: often dedicated NMR, crystallography, or mass spectrometry facilities. Working with fragments requires a shift

in approach, particularly in the early stages where affinity may be low. In these situations, ligand efficiency can be very useful for choosing and advancing the most promising hits. Strategies vary a great deal according to technique, protein, and starting components; indeed, an entire book has been devoted to the practice of fragment-based drug discovery (Jahnke and Erlanson, 2006).

Could the fragment-derived kinase inhibitors described here have been discovered using more traditional techniques, such as HTS, structure-based design, and "patent-busting"? In some cases the answer is almost certainly yes. As the dozen-plus single drug-focused chapters in this book illustrate, there are many effective ways to discover kinase inhibitors. However, it is clear that fragment-based drug discovery works: there are at least five kinase inhibitors in clinical trials that started from fragments, although the structures and details of most of these have not been reported (Congreve et al., 2008). How these compounds fare in the clinic, and how many compounds follow them, remains to be seen.

Of the two main strategies for fragment-based drug discovery outlined in Figure 18.1, growing and linking, there are slightly more successful examples of the former. A clear example of growth is Astex's CDK2 inhibitor AT7519 (Figure 18.3), which was iteratively built from an initial indazole fragment. In contrast, the two Aurora-A inhibitors discussed (Figure 18.7) were each built from two separate fragments that were linked together. The different approaches here could reflect differences in kinase architectures, with CDK2 requiring smaller, more compact molecules, while Aurora-A can tolerate larger, more extended molecules. But it is important not to focus too much on these distinctions, as sometimes the difference between the methods can be more semantic than real: How does one categorize the PDK1 example (Figure 18.7), in which multiple fragments were merged?

It is easy to slip into "technique fundamentalism," in which overly broad claims are made about specific varieties of fragment-based drug discovery or even about the superiority of the overall strategy to other methods of drug discovery. In reality, of course, every technology has its strengths and weaknesses. This chapter has discussed published examples of fragment-based drug discovery applied to kinases and has attempted to demonstrate where the technique has provided value, as well as what challenges remain. However, drug discovery is such a difficult problem that resourceful researchers will use every technique at their disposal. The beginning of this chapter described how HTS provided two fragment-like starting points that eventually entered the clinic and, in the case of sorafenib, ultimately became a drug. Fragment-based drug discovery seeks to explicitly search for such starting points, and provides both a justification and a conceptual framework for how to advance them.

DEDICATION

This chapter is dedicated to the researchers of Sunesis Pharmaceuticals, Inc., for expanding the limits of fragment-based drug discovery.

ACKNOWLEDGMENTS

I thank Monya L. Baker and Robert S. McDowell for helpful suggestions on the text.

REFERENCES

Abad-Zapatero, C., and Metz, G. (2005). Ligand efficiency indices as guideposts for drug discovery. *Drug Discov Today*. 10, 464–469.

Becattini, B., Culmsee, C., Leone, M., et al. (2006). Structure–activity relationships by interligand NOE-based design and synthesis of antiapoptotic compounds targeting Bid. *Proc Natl Acad Sci USA*. 103, 12602–12606.

Bohacek, R. S., McMartin, C., and Guida, W. C. (1996). The art and practice of structure-based drug design: a molecular modeling perspective. *Med Res Rev*. 16, 3–50.

Bohm, H. J. (1992). The computer program LUDI: a new method for the de novo design of enzyme inhibitors. *J Comput Aided Mol Des*. 6, 61–78.

Bramson, H. N., Corona, J., Davis, S. T., et al. (2001). Oxindole-based inhibitors of cyclin-dependent kinase 2 (CDK2): design, synthesis, enzymatic activities, and X-ray crystallographic analysis. *J Med Chem*. 44, 4339–4358.

Burley, S. K. (2008). Discovery and development of selective, orally bioavailable tyrosine kinase inhibitors for targeted treatment of human cancers. *In: CHI's Third Annual Drug Discovery Chemistry 2008: Tools, Targets & Therapies*, La Jolla, CA.

Caldwell, J. J., Davies, T. G., Donald, A., et al. (2008). Identification of 4-(4-aminopiperidin-1-yl)-7*H*-pyrrolo[2,3-*d*]pyrimidines as selective inhibitors of protein kinase B through fragment elaboration. *J Med Chem*. 51, 2147–2157.

Cancilla, M. T., He, M. M., Viswanathan, N., et al. (2008). Discovery of an Aurora kinase inhibitor through site-specific dynamic combinatorial chemistry. *Bioorg Med Chem Lett*. 18, 3978–3981.

Card, G. L., Blasdel, L., England, B. P., et al. (2005). A family of phosphodiesterase inhibitors discovered by cocrystallography and scaffold-based drug design. *Nat Biotechnol*. 23, 201–207.

Chen, J., Zhang, Z., Stebbins, J. L., et al. (2007). A fragment-based approach for the discovery of isoform-specific p38alpha inhibitors. *ACS Chem Biol*. 2, 329–336.

Cheng, J. Q., Lindsley, C. W., Cheng, G. Z., Yang, H., and Nicosia, S. V. (2005). The Akt/PKB pathway: molecular target for cancer drug discovery. *Oncogene*. 24, 7482–7492.

Congreve, M. S., Davis, D. J., Devine, L., et al. (2003). Detection of ligands from a dynamic combinatorial library by X-ray crystallography. *Angew Chem Int Ed Engl*. 42, 4479–4482.

Congreve, M., Chessari, G., Tisi, D., and Woodhead, A. J. (2008). Recent developments in fragment-based drug discovery. *J Med Chem*. 51, 3661–3680.

Cook, R., Wu, C. C., Kang, Y. J., and Han, J. (2007). The role of the p38 pathway in adaptive immunity. *Cell Mol Immunol*. 4, 253–259.

DeLano, W. L. PyMOL molecular graphics system on World Wide Web. http://pymol.sourceforge.net/.

Donald, A., McHardy, T., Rowlands, M. G., et al. (**2007**). Rapid evolution of 6-phenylpurine inhibitors of protein kinase B through structure-based design. *J Med Chem*. 50, 2289–2292.

Enkvist, E., Raidaru, G., Vaasa, A., Pehk, T., Lavogina, D., and Uri, A. (**2007**). Carbocyclic 3′-deoxyadenosine-based highly potent bisubstrate-analog inhibitor of basophilic protein kinases. *Bioorg Med Chem Lett*. 17, 5336–5339.

Erlanson, D. A. (**2006**). Fragment-based lead discovery: a chemical update. *Curr Opin Biotechnol*. 17, 643–652.

Erlanson, D. A. (**2007**). Fragment-based ligand discovery meets phage display. *ACS Chem Biol*. 2, 779–782.

Erlanson, D., Braisted, A., Raphael, D., et al. (**2000**). Site-directed ligand discovery. *Proc Natl Acad Sci USA*. 97, 9367–9372.

Erlanson, D. A., Lam, J. W., Wiesmann, C., et al. (**2003**). In situ assembly of enzyme inhibitors using extended tethering. *Nat Biotechnol*. 21, 308–314.

Erlanson, D. A., McDowell, R. S., and O'Brien, T. (**2004a**). Fragment-based drug discovery. *J Med Chem*. 47, 3463–3482.

Erlanson, D. A., Wells, J. A., and Braisted, A. C. (**2004b**). Tethering: fragment-based drug discovery. *Annu Rev Biophys Biomol Struct*. 33, 199–223.

Fejzo, J., Lepre, C. A., Peng, J. W., et al. (**1999**). The SHAPES strategy: an NMR-based approach for lead generation in drug discovery. *Chem Biol*. 6, 755–769.

Fejzo, J., Lepre, C., and Xie, X. (**2003**). Application of NMR screening in drug discovery. *Curr Top Med Chem*. 3, 81–97.

Fink, T., Bruggesser, H., and Reymond, J. L. (**2005**). Virtual exploration of the small-molecule chemical universe below 160 daltons. *Angew Chem Int Ed Engl*. 44, 1504–1508.

Fischer, P. M. (**2004**). The use of CDK inhibitors in oncology: a pharmaceutical perspective. *Cell Cycle*. 3, 742–746.

Gassel, M., Breitenlechner, C. B., Ruger, P., et al. (**2003**). Mutants of protein kinase A that mimic the ATP-binding site of protein kinase B (AKT). *J Mol Biol*. 329, 1021–1034.

Gill, A. (**2004**). New lead generation strategies for protein kinase inhibitors—fragment based screening approaches. *Mini Rev Med Chem*. 4, 301–311.

Gill, A., Cleasby, A., and Jhoti, H. (**2005a**). The discovery of novel protein kinase inhibitors by using fragment-based high-throughput X-ray crystallography. *Chembiochem*. 6, 506–512.

Gill, A. L., Frederickson, M., Cleasby, A., et al. (**2005b**). Identification of novel p38alpha MAP kinase inhibitors using fragment-based lead generation. *J Med Chem*. 48, 414–426.

Gill, A. L., Verdonk, M., Boyle, R. G., and Taylor, R. (**2007**). A comparison of physicochemical property profiles of marketed oral drugs and orally bioavailable anticancer protein kinase inhibitors in clinical development. *Curr Top Med Chem*. 7, 1408–1422.

Hajduk, P. J., and Greer, J. (**2007**). A decade of fragment-based drug design: strategic advances and lessons learned. *Nat Rev Drug Discov*. 6, 211–219.

Hajduk, P. J., Sheppard, G., Nettesheim, D. G., et al. (**1997**). Discovery of potent nonpeptide inhibitors of stromelysin using SAR by NMR. *J Am Chem Soc*. 119, 5818–5827.

Hann, M. M., and Oprea, T. I. (**2004**). Pursuing the leadlikeness concept in pharmaceutical research. *Curr Opin Chem Biol*. 8, 255–263.

Hann, M. M., Leach, A. R., and Harper, G. (**2001**). Molecular complexity and its impact on the probability of finding leads for drug discovery. *J Chem Inf Comput Sci*. 41, 856–864.

Hopkins, A. L., Groom, C. R., and Alex, A. (**2004**). Ligand efficiency: a useful metric for lead selection. *Drug Discov Today*. 9, 430–431.

Hubbard, R. E., Davis, B., Chen, I., and Drysdale, M. J. (**2007**). The SeeDs approach: integrating fragments into drug discovery. *Curr Top Med Chem*. 7, 1568–1581.

Hunter, T. (**2007**). Treatment for chronic myelogenous leukemia: the long road to imatinib. *J Clin Invest*. 117, 2036–2043.

Jahnke, W., and Erlanson, D. A. (eds.) (**2006**). *Fragment-Based Approaches in Drug Discovery*, Vol. 34. Weinheim, Germany: Wiley-VCH.

Jencks, W. P. (**1981**). On the attribution and additivity of binding energies. *Proc Natl Acad Sci USA*. 78, 4046–4050.

Kane, R. C., Farrell, A. T., Saber, H., et al. (**2006**). Sorafenib for the treatment of advanced renal cell carcinoma. *Clin Cancer Res*. 12, 7271–7278.

Karaman, M. W., Herrgard, S., Treiber, D. K., et al. (**2008**). A quantitative analysis of kinase inhibitor selectivity. *Nat Biotechnol*. 26, 127–132.

Keen, N., and Taylor, S. (**2004**). Aurora-kinase inhibitors as anticancer agents. *Nat Rev Cancer*. 4, 927–936.

Kuntz, I. D., Chen, K., Sharp, K. A., and Kollman, P. A. (**1999**). The maximal affinity of ligands. *Proc Natl Acad Sci USA*. 96, 9997–10002.

Lange, G., Lesuisse, D., Deprez, P., et al. (**2003**). Requirements for specific binding of low affinity inhibitor fragments to the SH2 domain of (pp60)Src are identical to those for high affinity binding of full length inhibitors. *J Med Chem*. 46, 5184–5195.

Lesuisse, D., Lange, G., Deprez, P., et al. (**2002**). SAR and X-ray. A new approach combining fragment-based screening and rational drug design: application to the discovery of nanomolar inhibitors of Src SH2. *J Med Chem*. 45, 2379–2387.

Liao, J. J. (**2007**). Molecular recognition of protein kinase binding pockets for design of potent and selective kinase inhibitors. *J Med Chem*. 50, 409–424.

Lipinski, C. A., Lombardo, F., Dominy, B. W., and Feeney, P. J. (**1997**). Experimental and computational approaches to estimate solubility and permeability in drug discovery and development settings. *Adv Drug Deliv Rev*. 23, 3–25.

Lowinger, T. B., Riedl, B., Dumas, J., and Smith, R. A. (**2002**). Design and discovery of small molecules targeting raf-1 kinase. *Curr Pharm Des*. 8, 2269–2278.

Maly, D. J., Choong, I. C., and Ellman, J. A. (**2000**). Combinatorial target-guided ligand assembly: identification of potent subtype-selective c-Src inhibitors. *Proc Natl Acad Sci USA*. 97, 2419–2424.

McGovern, S. L., and Shoichet, B. K. (**2003**). Kinase inhibitors: not just for kinases anymore. *J Med Chem*. 46, 1478–1483.

McGovern, S. L., Caselli, E., Grigorieff, N., and Shoichet, B. K. (**2002**). A common mechanism underlying promiscuous inhibitors from virtual and high-throughput screening. *J Med Chem*. 45, 1712–1722.

McGovern, S. L., Helfand, B. T., Feng, B., and Shoichet, B. K. (**2003**). A specific mechanism of nonspecific inhibition. *J Med Chem*. 46, 4265–4272.

Meyer, S. C., Shomin, C. D., Gaj, T., and Ghosh, I. (**2007**). Tethering small molecules to a phage display library: discovery of a selective bivalent inhibitor of protein kinase A. *J Am Chem Soc*. 129, 13812–13813.

Mora, A., Komander, D., van Aalten, D. M., and Alessi, D. R. (**2004**). PDK1, the master regulator of AGC kinase signal transduction. *Semin Cell Dev Biol*. 15, 161–170.

Murray, C. W., and Verdonk, M. L. (**2002**). The consequences of translational and rotational entropy lost by small molecules on binding to proteins. *J Comput Aided Mol Des*. 16, 741–753.

Nagar, B., Bornmann, W. G., Pellicena, P., et al. (**2002**). Crystal structures of the kinase domain of c-Abl in complex with the small molecule inhibitors PD173955 and imatinib (STI-571). *Cancer Res*. 62, 4236–4243.

Ohren, J. F., Chen, H., Pavlovsky, A., et al. (**2004**). Structures of human MAP kinase kinase 1 (MEK1) and MEK2 describe novel noncompetitive kinase inhibition. *Nat Struct Mol Biol*. 11, 1192–1197.

Pargellis, C., Tong, L., Churchill, L., et al. (**2002**). Inhibition of p38 MAP kinase by utilizing a novel allosteric binding site. *Nat Struct Biol*. 9, 268–272.

Ramstrom, O., and Lehn, J. M. (**2002**). Drug discovery by dynamic combinatorial libraries. *Nat Rev Drug Discov*. 1, 26–32.

Rees, D. C., Congreve, M., Murray, C. W., and Carr, R. (**2004**). Fragment-based lead discovery. *Nat Rev Drug Discov*. 3, 660–672.

Reynolds, C. H., Tounge, B. A., and Bembenek, S. D. (**2008**). Ligand binding efficiency: trends, physical basis, and implications. *J Med Chem*. 51, 2432–2438.

Ricouart, A., Gesquiere, J. C., Tartar, A., and Sergheraert, C. (**1991**). Design of potent protein kinase inhibitors using the bisubstrate approach. *J Med Chem*. 34, 73–78.

Rishton, G. M. (**2003**). Nonleadlikeness and leadlikeness in biochemical screening. *Drug Discov Today*. 8, 86–96.

Rowan, S. J., Cantrill, S. J., Cousins, G. R. L., Sanders, J. K. M., and Stoddart, J. F. (**2002**). Dynamic covalent chemistry. *Angew Chem Int Ed*. 41, 898–952.

Ryan, A. J., Gray, N. M., Lowe, P. N., and Chung, C. W. (**2003**). Effect of detergent on "promiscuous" inhibitors. *J Med Chem*. 46, 3448–3451.

Saxty, G., Woodhead, S. J., Berdini, V., et al. (**2007**). Identification of inhibitors of protein kinase B using fragment-based lead discovery. *J Med Chem*. 50, 2293–2296.

Schindler, T., Bornmann, W., Pellicena, P., Miller, W. T., Clarkson, B., and Kuriyan, J. (**2000**). Structural mechanism for STI-571 inhibition of Abelson tyrosine kinase. *Science*. 289, 1938–1942.

Schneider, T. L., Mathew, R. S., Rice, K. P., Tamaki, K., Wood, J. L., and Schepartz, A. (**2005**). Increasing the kinase specificity of k252a by protein surface recognition. *Org Lett*. 7, 1695–1698.

Schreiber, S., Feagan, B., D'Haens, G., et al. (**2006**). Oral p38 mitogen-activated protein kinase inhibition with BIRB 796 for active Crohn's disease: a randomized, double-blind, placebo-controlled trial. *Clin Gastroenterol Hepatol*. 4, 325–334.

Sem, D. S. (**2006**). NMR-guided fragment assembly. In: W. Jahnke and D. A. Erlanson (eds.). *Fragment-Based Approaches in Drug Discovery*, Vol. 34. Weinheim, Germany: Wiley-VCH, pp. 149–180.

Shen, K., and Cole, P. A. (**2003**). Conversion of a tyrosine kinase protein substrate to a high affinity ligand by ATP linkage. *J Am Chem Soc*. 125, 16172–16173.

Shuker, S. B., Hajduk, P. J., Meadows, R. P., and Fesik, S. W. (**1996**). Discovering high-affinity ligands for proteins: SAR by NMR. *Science*. 274, 1531–1534.

Teague, S. J., Davis, A. M., Leeson, P. D., and Oprea, T. (**1999**). The design of leadlike combinatorial libraries. *Angew Chem Int Ed Engl*. 38, 3743–3748.

Tsai, J., Lee, J. T., Wang, W., et al. (**2008**). Discovery of a selective inhibitor of oncogenic B-Raf kinase with potent antimelanoma activity. *Proc Natl Acad Sci USA*. 105, 3041–3046.

Vazquez, J., De, S. K., Chen, L. H., et al. (**2008**). Development of paramagnetic probes for molecular recognition studies in protein kinases. *J Med Chem*. 51, 3460–3465.

Wang, J. Y., Wilcoxen, K. M., Nomoto, K., and Wu, S. (**2007**). Recent advances of MEK inhibitors and their clinical progress. *Curr Top Med Chem*. 7, 1364–1378.

Warner, S. L., Bashyam, S., Vankayalapati, H., et al. (**2006**). Identification of a lead small-molecule inhibitor of the Aurora kinases using a structure-assisted, fragment-based approach. *Mol Cancer Ther*. 5, 1764–1773.

Wyatt, P. G., Woodhead, A. J., Berdini, V., et al. (**2008**). Identification of *N*-(4-piperidinyl)-4-(2,6-dichlorobenzoylamino)-1*H*-pyrazole-3-carboxamide (AT7519), a novel cyclin dependent kinase inhibitor using fragment-based X-ray crystallography and structure based drug design. *J Med Chem*. 51, 4986–4999.

Zhao, H., Serby, M. D., Xin, Z., et al. (**2006**). Discovery of potent, highly selective, and orally bioavailable pyridine carboxamide c-Jun NH(2)-terminal kinase inhibitors. *J Med Chem*. 49, 4455–4458.

19

PROTEIN KINASE STRUCTURAL BIOLOGY: METHODS AND STRATEGIES FOR TARGETED DRUG DISCOVERY

CLIFFORD D. MOL, KENGO OKADA, AND DAVID J. HOSFIELD

19.1. INTRODUCTION

Protein kinases are attractive targets for structure-based drug discovery (SBDD) projects. All protein kinases share the same global architecture, consisting of the conserved kinase two-domain fold, yet regulatory elements that exist at the amino or carboxyl termini can influence the molecular state of the enzyme and complicate the tractability of any particular protein kinase for structural analysis. Of the approximately 500 enzymes encoded in the human kinome, many have been implicated in the pathology of human diseases (Manning et al., 2002), but only a small fraction have thus far proved to be amenable to X-ray co-crystallography in support of directed chemistry efforts. As these protein kinases are a substantial and growing part of most major pharmaceutical companies' drug target portfolios (Cohen, 2002), there is increasing pressure on the structural biologist to provide the atomic-level description of any particular kinase with lead compounds or even smaller weak-binding fragments. Such fragment-based drug discovery (FBDD) can provide novel insights early in the design process, and X-ray crystallography is the best method to obtain this information, but not all protein kinase systems are readily amenable to SBDD or FBDD techniques. Often a surrogate kinase is employed based on the tractability of the crystal system and the similarity

Kinase Inhibitor Drugs. Edited by Rongshi Li and Jeffrey A. Stafford
Copyright © 2009 John Wiley & Sons, Inc.

of its inhibition profile to the target of interest. In this chapter we present an overview of the steps required to move a kinase from a target wish list to a stage where co-crystal structure information can readily be obtained to support chemistry efforts. We further discuss how kinase structural biology studies have defined three distinct structural states that are amenable to structure-based drug discovery and provide examples of kinases bound to drugs that target each particular state.

19.2. METHODS FOR KINASE STRUCTURAL BIOLOGY

19.2.1. Kinase Construct Design

Each individual protein kinase target selected for SBDD presents unique challenges for the expression and purification of soluble material that is suit-able for crystallization and structural studies. In the past 10 years, advances in modern molecular biology technologies have led to an explosion in the avail-ability of protein expression plasmids ideally tailored to support protein pro-duction in *Escherichia coli*, insect, yeast, and mammalian cells. For protein kinases, a major advance has been the development of baculovirus expression systems in insect cells as many kinases cannot be expressed in suitable amounts using bacteria. Constructs are typically designed by using molecular cloning techniques to transplant the kinase domain of the target of interest into the expression plasmid and than testing protein expression levels to guide con-struct optimization. Optimization procedures generally include generating multiple N- and C-terminal boundaries at the start and at the end of the pre-dicted kinase domain, changing the location and nature of affinity-purification and secretion tags, introducing proteolytic sites for tag removal, removal of internal insertion sequences, and introduction of site-specific amino acid modi-fications to enhance expression or mimic phosphorylation events (Lee et al., 2006). It is not uncommon to test dozens of expression constructs in an effort to find a single one that will support the high-level expression required to support structural biology work.

For many challenging kinase targets, the very act of overexpression leads to cell toxicity since the overexpressed kinase can phosphorylate and activate not only itself but also essential host cell proteins, thus disrupting normal cell function. For these difficult-to-express kinases, it is often imperative to include in the expression construct additional domains and/or control elements, which maintain the kinase in a stable and inactive conformation. Typically, an iterative optimization process is used to identify the correct combination of control elements, kinase domain boundaries, and affinity tags that will support high-level expression of the kinase of interest. In some cases, specific kinase inhibitors can be added to the expression media to improve production of soluble material (Strauss et al., 2007). Illustrative examples of the necessity of kinase control elements for successful expression include the expression of the lipid kinase PI3K family of enzymes and the

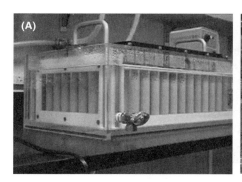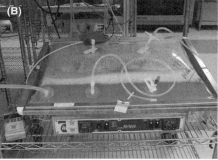

Figure 19.1. High-throughput expression of kinase constructs. (**A**) The fermenter for *E. coli* expression contains 96 tubes to allow for multiple constructs to be expressed simultaneously. Note the heating/cooling coil at left to adjust the expression temperature. (**B**) Wave bags and rocker for baculovirus expression. This experiment is expressing 10 liters of a single construct.

kinase domain of the cKIT proto-oncogene. For PI3Kα and PI3Kγ, successful expression requires constructs containing the kinase domain in combination with the regulatory RAS binding, C2, and helical domains (Huang et al., 2007). For cKIT, only constructs with the internal insertion sequence deleted and containing residues from the inactivating N-terminal juxtamembrane domain produced protein that could easily be expressed and purified for structural biology experiments (Mol et al., 2003, 2004a,b).

19.2.2. Kinase Microscale and Large-Scale Expression

Analysis of the protein expression level supported by each construct is routinely determined using microscale procedures that assess the total expression levels of the target as well as the percentage of material that is soluble and generally useful for SBDD. Standard electrophoretic procedures such as SDS-PAGE or Caliper Chip technologies (www.caliperls.com) are typically used in a semiautomated fashion to measure and catalog the expression levels. Promising constructs that demonstrate high levels of soluble protein expression (>5 mg/L) are scaled up for large-scale studies. For kinases that can be expressed in *E. coli*, large-scale expression is carried out in standard laboratory shake flasks or in fermenter systems that allow the bacteria to grow to very high cell densities, potentially increasing the yield of purified protein (Figure 19.1A). For baculovirus-expressed kinases, large-scale expression can also be performed using shake-flask methods, yet in recent years disposable wave bag technology (www.wavebiotech.net) has been adopted by a large number of organizations. These wave bags provide good scalability up to 20 liters or more, reduce the danger of contamination, and eliminate the labor associated with fermenter maintenance (Figure 19.1B).

19.2.3. Kinase Purification and Characterization

Kinases expressed from constructs that yield significant amounts of protein are purified by a battery of methods required to isolate the high-quality and conformationally homogeneous material needed for subsequent crystallization experiments. As with other proteins, nickel-chelate affinity purification is a typical first step used to isolate 6-His-tagged kinases from the majority of the cellular debris in which it was expressed. For well-behaved kinases, this first step can sometimes be sufficient to progress directly to crystallization experiments. Unfortunately, most protein kinases are not well behaved and additional purification methods such as ion-exchange chromatography, hydrophobic-interaction chromatography, and gel-filtration chromatography are required. These methods not only remove contaminating proteins that bind nonspecifically to the nickel resin, but they also ensure that aggregated material is removed and that the sample delivered for crystallographic experiments is conformationally pure.

Throughout the purification process, analytical methods such as size-exclusion chromatography, light scattering, and mass spectrometry are routinely used to assess sample molecular weight and purity, and also to determine levels and sites of post-translational modifications. These analytical results guide future experiments and provide key quality-control measures for ensuring reproducible crystallization. Mass spectrometry can be particularly useful for assessing the phosphorylation status of a kinase. Many kinases expressed in insect cells, as well as some kinases expressed in bacterial systems, are found to be multiply and heterogeneously phosphorylated and additional purification steps are needed to isolate the species of interest (Figure 19.2A). For programs targeting the active kinase conformation, purification of the singly or multiply phosphorylated species may be required. This approach was needed to crystallize the very first protein kinase to have its X-ray crystal structure determined, cyclic AMP-dependent protein kinase, also known as protein kinase A (PKA) (Knighton et al., 1991; Herberg et al., 1993; Davies et al., 2007). An alternative approach when targeting an active kinase is to design phosphomimetic mutants that mimic the active phosphorylated residues (Lei et al., 2005). This approach is more straightforward for the Ser/Thr kinases, where substitution with Asp and Glu residues can provide a reasonable structural analog for the phosphoserine and phosphothreonine residues, while Glu substitutions can provide some activation as an approximate analog for phosphotyrosine resides in the tyrosine kinases.

In some cases, such as the autoinhibited structures of cKit (Mol et al., 2004a) and Flt3 (Griffith et al., 2004), the completely unphosphorylated protein may be needed for crystallization experiments. If significant amounts of the unphosphorylated protein can be obtained from the cell pellet, then the desired kinase species can be purified away from the phosphorylated forms using ion-exchange chromatography. An alternative approach proven to be useful for the MEK1 (Smith et al., 2007) and ASK1 kinases (Bunkoczi et al., 2007) is to

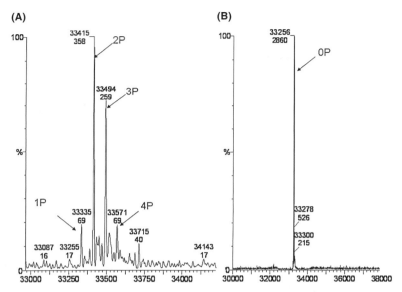

Figure 19.2. Mass spectrophotometric analysis of a kinase expressed as a multiply phosphorylated species: (**A**) initial partially purified protein showing a heterogeneous mixture of at least four separate phosphorylated species; (**B**) the same protein preparation after treatment with phosphatase to generate a single homogeneous nonphosphorylated sample.

treat the phosphorylated kinase preparation with a phosphatase to generate the unphosphorylated, and perhaps inactive, form of the kinase (Figure 19.2B).

19.2.4. High-Throughput Kinase Crystallization

Kinases that express at high levels and are well behaved can often be crystallized using standard methods that are employed for other proteins. These techniques include sitting-drop and hanging-drop vapor diffusion experiments (McPherson, 1999), which have now been automated at most pharmaceutical companies and structural genomics centers (Stevens, 2000). In the pharmaceutical and biotechnology industry, nanovolume crystallization technologies are employed in a high-throughput structural biology factory that can rapidly and reproducibly assess the crystallizability of a kinase sample using small amounts of purified material (Hosfield et al., 2003). For these experiments it is highly advantageous to image the crystal drops with automatic imagers on a regular basis to document which drops contain crystals, and also to allow the crystallographer to assess when a particular crystal has attained a size suitable for harvesting and X-ray diffraction analyses. A crystal growth time-course for the co-crystal of cKit bound to the inhibitor STI-571 is illustrated in Figure 19.3.

Kinase crystals grown from the nanodrop experiments are typically small, but when obtained from well-behaved material, they can diffract X-rays to

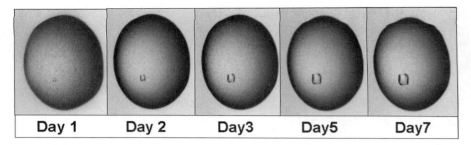

Figure 19.3. Time lapse of co-crystal growth for cKit:STI-571. A small crystal has already appeared by day 1 and reached full size by day 7. Note the small additional crystal in the upper right that appears on day 5.

high resolution. These crystals are often amenable to inhibitor soaking experiments, which enable fragment-based methods for kinase discovery. Generally, however, kinase crystallization remains a challenging undertaking since many kinases can only be expressed in low amounts and in many cases sample conformational heterogeneity hinders crystallization. In these difficult, yet common cases, nonstandard methods, which can include co-crystallization and co-concentration with inhibitors and/or substrate peptides, additive screening, and streak seeding, often improve the success of a given experiment. In many cases, a large number of kinase constructs need to be expressed and purified, and then each sample must be assessed by a skilled crystallographer who can determine the suitability of each sample for its propensity to yield reproducible crystals that can support a drug discovery program.

19.2.5. Kinase Structure Determination and Refinement

As protein kinases all belong to a common enzyme family sharing a similar bilobal protein fold, molecular replacement methods enjoy high rates of success for solving X-ray structures of new protein kinases. In these methods, standard sequence comparison tools are used to identify a previously determined kinase structure that can serve as a template to allow the crystallographer to "bootstrap" his/her way to a solution of the new kinase of interest. In some cases where the amino acid sequence homology is particularly low, it may be necessary to use a search model that contains only the more structurally conserved and mostly helical C-lobe of the kinase in order to obtain a solution. If the structure solution by molecular replacement proves intractable, then phases can be obtained by co-crystallizing with a ligand or compound containing an atom with a strong anomalous signal, such as an iodine, which was employed successfully to determine the structure of MEK1 bound with an allosteric compound (Ohren et al., 2004)). It may also be possible to express the kinase in a system that incorporates selenomethionine in place of the normal methionine residues, allowing the structure to be solved using multiwavelength anomalous dispersion (MAD) (reviewed in Ealick, 2000). For a construct that can be expressed in bacterial systems, this procedure is relatively straightforward, whereas recent advances using the baculovirus system might also be exploited to obtain selenomethionyl-incorporated protein (Cronin et al., 2007).

19.3. KINASE ARCHITECTURE

The overall structural architecture of any protein kinase reflects the fact that they all perform a common chemical reaction—the specific transfer of a phosphate group from ATP to a target protein Ser/Thr or Tyr residue. The conserved kinase two-domain fold consists of a smaller, amino-terminal N-lobe, comprised of mostly β-strands, connected via a single polypeptide chain termed the hinge to a larger, primarily α-helical, carboxy-terminal C-lobe (Figure 19.4). The active site is located at the cleft between these lobes and includes

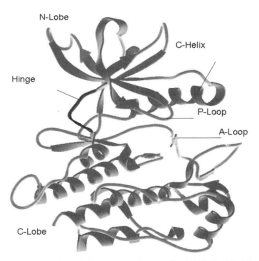

Figure 19.4. Kinase structural architecture. The typical bilobal fold of an active kinase is shown, with the smaller N-lobe (*top*) comprised of mostly β-sheet secondary structure, and the larger mostly α-helical C-lobe (*bottom*). The two lobes are connected via a single polypeptide chain termed the hinge, which provides key contacts to bound nucleotides and/or compounds. The phosphate-loop, or P-loop, is a glycine-rich stretch of sequence that packs closely with the nucleotide phosphate groups and typically contains a single, large hydrophobic residue that shields the active center from bulk solvent to facilitate the phosphoryl transfer reaction. The N-lobe also contains a conspicuous α-helix, termed the control or C-helix, whose exact positioning is critical for maintaining an active kinase. The C-lobe contains the activation-loop, or A-loop, which forms a platform for binding of the substrate polypeptide when it is in the extended conformation shown.

a hydrophobic pocket bounded by the hinge that binds the adenine portion of ATP. This pocket is commonly targeted as a subsite for the binding of drug compounds, and the hinge region contains a particular residue, termed the gatekeeper, whose chemical nature can affect the binding of drug compounds, and which is often mutated in kinases that have acquired resistance to specific drugs. The N-lobe has a single α-helix, termed the control- or C-helix, with a conserved glutamic acid residue that forms a salt bridge with the side chain of a buried lysine. This lysine positions the phosphates of bound ATP for the phosphoryl transfer reaction. The phosphates of the bound ATP are also contacted by the the phosphate-loop (P-loop), which is a short glycine-rich stretch of sequence that can pack closely against the nucleotide phosphates. The P-loop also typically contains a bulky phenylalanine or tyrosine residue that can shield the active site from solvent to facilitate the transphosphorylation reaction. The kinase catalytic loop, anchored by the N-terminal HRD motif, is located in the kinase C-lobe, and plays a key role in orienting an activation loop (A-loop) Asp and the substrate peptide hydroxyl during catalysis.

The A-loop and the DFG motif are two key structural components that control whether a kinase exists in an inactive or active state. Kinase activation is often triggered by the enzymatic phosphorylation of a particular residue(s) within the A-loop sequence, which leads to the A-loop assuming an extended conformation that forms a platform for substrate binding, and this conformation is stabilized by ionic interactions between positively charged residues and the newly phosphorylated A-loop residue as well as by an intramolecular β-sheet formed with the C-lobe (Dibb et al., 2004). The DFG motif, which lies near the beginning of the A-loop, is named after the single-letter amino acid codes for its three conserved Asp-Phe-Gly residues. With the A-loop in an active, extended state and ATP bound, the DFG motif is in the "Phe-in" conformation with the Asp residue coordinating the Mg^{2+} ion bridging the ATP phosphates and the phenylalanine positioned to allow binding of the ATP to the hinge region. If the kinase is in an inactive state and hence no ATP is bound, the A-loop is often folded back and the DFG motif is in the "Phe-out" conformation, where the phenylalanine residue blocks ATP from binding. Combined inhibition and structural biology work over the last 10 years has demonstrated that both kinase conformations can be exploited for designing potent inhibitors. In the following sections examples of inhibitors that target distinct kinase conformations are discussed.

19.4. KINASE INHIBITION BY TARGETING ACTIVE CONFORMATIONS

A straightforward strategy for producing a kinase inhibitor with a desired pharmacologic response in cell and animal models, and ultimately in clinical studies, is to produce an inhibitor targeted against the activated kinase responsible for the disease state. Many kinase inhibitor drug discovery programs have

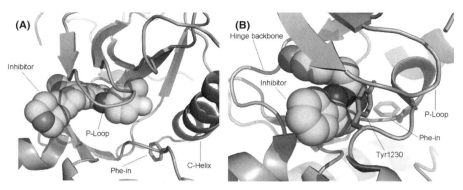

Figure 19.5. Inhibitor binding to active cMET kinase. (**A**) The inhibitor binds to the active kinase structure with an extended A-loop conformation and the Phe residue of the DFG motif in the Phe-In configuration. (**B**) Aromatic π-electron interactions between the inhibitor and the side chain of Tyr1230 are believed to provide specificity for active cMET.

developed drug compounds that target active conformations. All of these compounds bind in the nucleotide-binding site, forming specific hydrogen bonds to the hinge region and gaining selectivity through interactions with the gatekeeper residue, yet the kinase remains in the "Phe-in" configuration of the DFG motif (Figure 19.5). Constrained by the chemical necessity to perform the transphosphorylation reaction, the active-site structures of activated protein kinases in the "Phe-in" conformation are generally quite similar. It can be challenging to develop both highly potent and selective active kinase inhibitors compared to targeting the more structurally diverse conformations of inactive kinases. Some informative, recent crystal structures of protein kinases, however, have revealed that inhibitors that bind to the active conformation can be very selective against desirable targets, such as the receptor tyrosine kinases EGFR (Yun et al., 2007) and cMET (Albrecht et al., 2008). Low molecular weight (~300–350 daltons) cMET inhibitors with potencies in the single-digit nanomolar range have been developed that target the active kinase state. These compounds bind to the hinge in a bent-shaped manner (Figure 19.5A). One side of the inhibitor forms direct hydrogen bonds with the backbone atoms of hinge residues, whereas the other face of the inhibitor engages in π-electron stacking interactions with the aromatic side chain of a tyrosine residue. This aromatic stacking interaction is a specific feature observed only in cMET co-crystal structures and likely contributes to the high degree of selectivity against the other kinases (Figure 19.5B). These cMET inhibitors are currently undergoing human clinical trials for the treatment of various cancer indications. This strategy of exploiting distinctive features of active kinase conformations for the design of specific drug compounds is being actively pursued to develop the next generation of kinase inhibitors.

19.5. KINASE INHIBITION BY TARGETING INACTIVE CONFORMATIONS

The remarkable success of the targeted cancer drug STI-571 (Imatinib, Gleevec, or Glivec) and of sorafenib (BAY43-9006 or Nexavar) is due to the ability of the drug to bind to and stabilize an inactive kinase conformation. Unlike active kinase conformations, the "Phe-out" inactive conformation can be distinct for each kinase and can undergo a variety of induced fit interactions upon inhibitor binding. It is therefore preferable to be guided by co-crystal structures in order to develop these highly potent and selective inhibitors (Noble et al., 2004). The structure of STI-571 bound to ABL kinase provided the first molecular description of an inhibitor bound to a kinase conformation that is frequently referred to today as the inactive DFG-out conformation (Schindler et al., 2000). The structure illustrated that STI-571 adopts a fully extended conformation to make numerous contacts with the entire interlobal cleft of the kinase (Figure 19.6). Like inhibitors that target

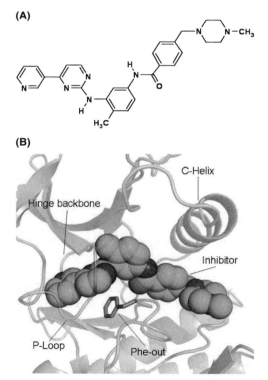

Figure 19.6. STI-571 and binding to inactive kinases: (**A**) chemical structure of STI-571 and (**B**) binding of STI-571 to cKit kinase. The compound assumes a bent shape and occupies both the nucleotide-binding site near the hinge, as well as the DFG-out pocket created when the Phe residue of the DFG motif is in an inactive conformation.

active kinase conformations, STI-571 forms key hinge-binding interactions via its pyridine and directly attached aminopyrimidine groups. Unlike active kinase inhibitors, however, the remainder of the inhibitor does not contact residues in the nucleotide-binding site, but instead, extends beyond the gate-keeper residue allowing the amide-linked diaryl group to form interactions with residues in a hydrophobic region termed the kinase back pocket. Of critical importance to STI-571 being able to access the ABL back pocket is the amide linker, which forms two key bridging hydrogen-bonding interactions that link together the C-helix Glu and the backbone NH of the catalytic Asp in the DFG motif. These interactions stabilize the extended binding mode of the compound and allow for, or induce, the kinase to change conformation to accommodate the entire inhibitor. Notably, the C-helix is displaced away from the ATP site and the A-loop adopts a folded-back conformation such that the Phe of the DFG motif occupies a position close to the ATP site, exposing a hydrophobic region in the back pocket targeted by hydrophobic inhibitor atoms. Remarkably, the structure adopted by ABL kinase when bound to Gleevec appears to represent a stable autoinhibitory conformation that many kinases adopt to remain in an "off-state" in the cell. Elegant structural studies of the full-length ABL kinase (Nagar et al., 2002, 2003), as well as the type III receptor tyrosine kinases cKIT (Mol et al., 2004a) and Flt3 (Griffith et al., 2004), demonstrated two distinct mechanisms for attaining and stabilizing the inactive state (Figure 19.7). In ABL kinase, binding of its internal SH2 and SH3 domains, with the aid of an N-terminal capping region, to the kinase domain stabilizes the kinase DFG-out conformation and maintains the enzyme in an off state (Nagar et al., 2006). In the cKIT and Flt3 structures, a short ~40 residue peptide encoded by juxtamembrane domain binds to the kinase domain and maintains the enzyme in a DFG-out conformation (Figure 19.7B).

The discovery of the DFG-out inactive kinase conformation has provided a significant opportunity for the development of new cancer drugs through the discovery of novel mechanisms used by kinases to maintain a DFG-out conformation in different cellular environments and tumor settings. Two excellent reviews on DFG-out kinase inhibitors (Mol et al., 2004b; Hosfield and Mol, 2008), which discuss how different compound classes exploit similar kinase structural features that are only present in the DFG-out conformation, are recommended to the reader seeking additional details.

19.6. KINASE INHIBITION BY TARGETING ALLOSTERIC SITES

The success of the DFG-out class of kinase inhibitors has spurred increasing interest and research into the discovery of novel drug compounds that are true allosteric inhibitors. By a strict definition, the class of compounds typified by STI-571 are not purely allosteric compounds as they do still bind to the nucleotide-binding site and merely exploit a pseudo-allosteric site that can be uncovered owing to the structural regulation of a particular kinase. Not

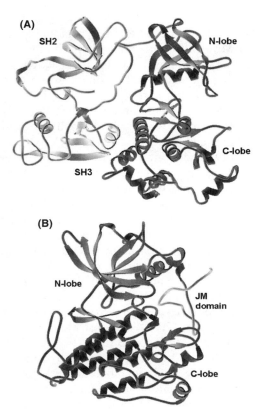

Figure 19.7. cABL and cKIT inactive kinases. (**A**) cABL kinase is maintained in the inactive state through the SH2 and SH2 domains that pack against and rigidify the kinase N- and C-lobes. (**B**) cKIT kinase is held in an inactive state by insertion of a small juxtamembrane (JM) domain into the cleft between the kinase N- and C-lobes.

all kinases undergo the DFG structural switch, and this fact contributes to the selectivity of this compound class. A true allosteric inhibitor is noncompetitive for both ATP and the substrate-binding site and would target a unique site. An example of such an allosteric compound is illustrated in the structures of unphosphorylated MEK1 and MEK2 kinases (Ohren et al., 2004), where the inhibitor binds to a distinct site in the N-lobe next to the ATP-binding site (Figure 19.8). Although the structure resembles that of other active kinases in the relationship of the N- and C-lobes to each other, significant structural changes have occurred to accommodate the allosteric inhibitor. The A-loop adopts an α-helical conformation and displaces the beginning of the C-helix from its active position. The C-helix, which contains a critical, conserved glutamate residue, shifts up and away from the active center resulting in a disruption of the catalytic Glu-Lys ion pair. Thus the binding of this

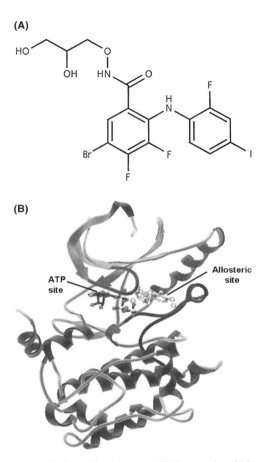

Figure 19.8. Allosteric inhibitor binding to MEK protein: (**A**) chemical structure of the allosteric MEK kinase inhibitor and (**B**) ribbon diagram of MEK co-crystal structure illustrating that the allosteric site is distinct from the nucleotide-binding site.

unique allosteric compound induces shifts in both the A-loop and C-helix that contribute to forming this novel, inactive kinase conformation, and it is doubtful that meaningful structure–activity relationships for this class of compounds could have been discerned lacking the crystal structure information. Whether similar allosteric-binding pockets that disrupt the C-helix can be discovered in other protein kinases, or if new sites for allosteric inhibitors can be elucidated, remains a challenging and exciting area for development of targeted drugs and structural biology results are poised to make seminal contributions in this area.

19.7. SUMMARY AND PERSPECTIVES

The field of kinase structural biology has moved forward markedly in the past decade. Advances in baculovirus- and even mammalian-cell expression systems have allowed for the production of increasing yields of soluble protein, while the intelligent use of purification tags can simplify and facilitate the rapid purification of recombinantly produced kinases. The advent of highly specific proteases to remove the purification tag, if desired, and the development and use of analytical techniques, such as mass spectrometry, to determine and monitor any post-translational modifications, particularly the phosphorylation state of the kinase, have all aided the structural biologist in obtaining homogeneous protein samples for crystallization experiments. Automated nanovolume crystallization robots and crystal drop imagers allow the crystallographer to search through a large number of conditions to find suitable crystals, while simultaneously minimizing the amount of protein needed—reducing both the material costs and human effort required to produce it.

The repertoire of protein kinases whose crystal structures have been determined has also grown substantially in the past decade. Although even the most optimistic and naïve structural biology program could not hope to determine the structures of all of the approximately 500 proteins in the human kinome, it is not unreasonable to expect that a significant number of important human drug targets will be amenable to SBDD techniques in the not too distant future. Since the completion of the Human Genome Project, substantial progress has already been made, and with each public disclosure of a heretofore intractable target succumbing to crystallographic analysis the determination of related kinase structures becomes more feasible.

REFERENCES

Albrecht, B. K., Harmange, J. C., Bauer, D., et al. (**2008**). Discovery and optimization of triazolopyridazines as potent and selective inhibitors of the c-Met kinase. *J Med Chem*. 51(10), 2879–2882.

Bunkoczi, G., Salah, E., Filippakopoulos, P., et al. (**2007**). Structural and functional characterization of human protein kinase ASK1. *Structure*. 15, 1215–1226.

Cohen, P. (**2002**). Protein kinases—the major drug targets of the twenty-first century? *Nat Rev Drug Discov*. 1, 309–315.

Cronin, C. N., Lim, K. B., and Rogers, J. (**2007**). Production of selenomethionyl-derivatized protein in baculovirus-infected cells. *Protein Sci*. 16, 2023–2029.

Davies, T. G., Verdonk, M. L., Graham, B., et al. (**2007**). A structural comparison of inhibitor binding to PKB, PKA and a PKA-PKB chimera. *J Mol Biol*. 367, 882–894.

Dibb, N. J., Dilworth, S. M., and Mol, C. D. (**2004**). Switching on kinases—the oncogenic activation of b-Raf and the PDGF receptor family. *Nat Rev Cancer*. 4, 718–727.

Ealick, S. E. (**2000**). Advances in multi-wavelength diffraction crystallography. *Curr Opin Chem Biol*. 4, 495–499.

Griffith, J., Black, J., Faerman, C., et al. (**2004**). The structural basis for autoinhibition of FLT3 by the juxtamembrane domain. *Mol Cell.* 13, 169–178.

Herberg, F. W., Bell, S. M., and Taylor, S. S. (**1993**). Expression of the catalytic subunit of cAMP-dependent protein kinase in *Escherichia coli*: multiple isozymes reflect different phosphorylation states. *Protein Eng.* 6, 771–777.

Hosfield, D. J., and Mol, C. D. (**2008**). Targeting inactive kinases: structure as a foundation for cancer drug discovery. *In: Cancer Drug Discovery and Development.* San Diego, CA: Academic Press, pp. 229–252.

Hosfield, D., Palan, J., Hilgers, M., et al. (**2003**). A fully integrated protein crystallization platform for small-molecule drug discovery. *J Struct Biol.* 142, 207–217.

Huang, C. H., Mandelker, D., Schmidt-Kittler, O., et al. (**2007**). The structure of a human p110alpha/p85alpha complex elucidates the effects of oncogenic PI3Kalpha mutations. *Science.* 318, 1744–1748.

Knighton, D. R., Zheng, J., Ten Eyck, L. F., et al. (**1991**). Crystal structure of the catalytic subunit of cyclic adenosine monophosphate-dependent protein kinase. *Science.* 253, 407–414.

Lee, S. J., Zhou, T., and Goldsmith, E. J. (**2006**). Crystallization of MAP kinases. *Methods.* 40(3), 224–233.

Lei, M., Robinson, M. A., and Harrison, S. C. (**2005**). The active conformation of the PAK1 kinase domain. *Structure.* 3(5), 769–778.

Manning, G., Whyte, D. B., Martinez, R., Hunter, T., and Sudarsanam, S. (**2002**). The protein kinase complement of the human genome. *Science.* 298, 1912–1932.

McPherson, A. (**1999**). *Crystallization of Biological Macromolecules.* Cold Spring Harbor, NY: Cold Spring Harbor Laboratory Press.

Mol, C. D., Lim, K. B., Sridhar, V., et al. (**2003**). Structure of a c-kit product complex reveals the basis for kinase transactivation. *J Biol Chem.* 278, 31461–31464.

Mol, C. D., Dougan, D. R., Schneider, T. R., et al. (**2004a**). Structural basis for the autoinhibition and STI-571 inhibition of c-Kit tyrosine kinase. *J Biol Chem.* 279, 31655.

Mol, C. D., Fabbro, D., and Hosfield, D. J. (**2004b**). Structural insights into the conformational selectivity of STI-571 and related kinase inhibitors. *Curr Opin Drug Discov Dev.* 7(5), 639–648.

Nagar, B., Bornmann, W. G., Pellicena, P., et al. (**2002**). Crystal structures of the kinase domain of c-Abl in complex with the small molecule inhibitors PD173955 and imatinib (STI-571). *Cancer Res.* 62(15), 4236–4243.

Nagar, B., Hantschel, O., Young, M. A., et al. (**2003**). Structural basis for the autoinhibiton of c-Abl tyrosine kinase. *Cell.* 112, 859–871.

Nagar, B., Hantschel, O., Seeliger, M., et al. (**2006**). Organization of the SH3-SH2 unit in active and inactive forms of the c-Abl tyrosine kinase. *Mol Cell.* 21(6), 787–798.

Noble, M. E., Endicott, J. A., and Johnson, L. N. (**2004**). Protein kinase inhibitors: insights into drug design from structure. *Science.* 303(5665), 1800–1805.

Ohren, J. F., Chen, H., Pavlovsky, A., et al. (**2004**). Structures of human MAP kinase kinase 1 (MEK1) and MEK2 describe novel non-competitive kinase inhibition. *Nat Struct Mol Biol.* 11, 1192–1197.

Schindler, T., Bornmann, W., Pellicena, P., Miller, W. T., Clarkson, B., and Kuriyan, J. (**2000**). Structural mechanism for STI-571 inhibition of abelson tyrosine kinase. *Science*. 289, 1938–1942.

Smith, C. K., Carr, D., Mayhood, T. W., Jin, W., Gray, K., and Windsor, W. T. (**2007**). Expression and purification of phosphorylated and non-phosphorylated human MEK1. *Protein Expression Purification*. 52, 446–456.

Stevens, R. C. (**2000**). High-throughput protein crystallization. *Curr Opin Struct Biol*. 10, 558–563.

Strauss, A., Fendricha, G., Horisbergera, M. A., et al. (**2007**). Improved expression of kinases in baculovirus-infected insect cells upon addition of specific kinase inhibitors to the culture helpful for structural studies. *Protein Expression Purification*. 56(2), 167–176.

Yun, C. H., Boggon, T. J., Li, Y., et al. (**2007**). Structures of lung cancer-derived EGFR mutants and inhibitor complexes: mechanism of activation and insights into differential inhibitor sensitivity. *Cancer Cell*. 11(3), 217–227.

INDEX

A431 xenograft, treatment with motesanib, 126
Abbott Laboratories, 467
ABL mutants, 271
ABT-869, 80–108
    cell-based antiproliferative activity, 96
    combination studies with chemotherapeutics in animal models, 103–4
    critical elements to the discovery process, 107–8
    discovery from 3-aminoindazole scaffold, 90
    efficacy in HT1080 tumor xenograft model, 101
    efficacy in leukemia models, 102
    human pharmacokinetic profile, 106
    inhibition of cell-based phosphorylation, 95–96
    kinase inhibition profile, 94–95
    PK-PD correlation studies, 104–5
    plasma protein binding, 95
    preclinical pharmacokinetic profiles, 98–99
    safety pharmacology, 91, 106
    solubility and formulation, 93–94
    structure-activity relationships, 93
    synthesis, 92
activation loop, 440
    in Aurora-A, 269
    conformation in EGFR structures, 52
    in MEK, 218
    in VEGFR2, 174
acute myelogenous leukemia. *See* AML
AG-013736. *See* axitinib
AG-028262, 19
alkaline phosphatases, cleavage of phosphate prodrug, 318
allosteric site, discovery and birth of MEK inhibitor program, 207
A-loop. *See* activation loop
American Association of Cancer Research, 64
amino acid ester prodrugs, use in brivanib discovery, 147
3-aminoindazole series, chemical synthesis, 91
3-aminopyrazole moiety, small-molecule hinge-binding motif, 286